HEALTH PROMOTION IN PRACTICE

Sherri Sheinfeld Gorin
Joan Arnold
Editors

Foreword by Lawrence W. Green

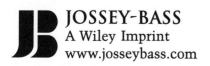

JOSSEY-BASS
A Wiley Imprint
www.josseybass.com

Published by Jossey-Bass
A Wiley Imprint
989 Market Street, San Francisco, CA 94103-1741   www.josseybass.com

Jossey-Bass books and products are available through most bookstores. To contact Jossey-Bass directly
call our Customer Care Department within the U.S. at 800-956-7739, outside the U.S. at 317-572-3986,
or fax 317-572-4002.

Jossey-Bass also publishes its books in a variety of electronic formats. Some content that appears in print
may not be available in electronic books.

Library of Congress Cataloging-in-Publication Data

Health promotion in practice / Sherri Sheinfeld Gorin, Joan Arnold, editors
   ; foreword by Lawrence W. Green. — 1st ed.
     p. ; cm.
   Includes bibliographical references and index.
   ISBN-13: 978-0-7879-7961-4 (alk. paper)
   ISBN-10: 0-7879-7961-9 (alk. paper)
   1. Health promotion.   2. Medicine, Preventive.   3. Physician and
patient.
   I. Gorin, Sherri Sheinfeld.   II. Arnold, Joan Hagan.
     [DNLM: 1. Health Promotion—methods.   2. Health Behavior.   3. Pre-
ventive Medicine—methods.   4. Public Health.   WA 525 H4363 2006]
   RA427.8H49752 2006
   613—dc22
2005036043

Printed in the United States of America
FIRST EDITION
PB Printing   10 9 8 7 6 5 4 3 2 1

CONTENTS

PART TWO: PRACTICE FRAMEWORKS FOR HEALTH PROMOTION

וכל המקיים נפש אחת מישראל מעלה עליו הכתוב כאילו קיים עולם מלא

He who saves a single life is as if he has saved the entire world.
—Babylonian Talmud, *Sanhedrin* 37a

מים רבים לא יוכלו לכבות את האהבה

Vast floods cannot quench love, no river can sweep it away.
—Song of Songs 8

For my beloved family.
—Sherri Sheinfeld Gorin

◆ ◆ ◆

But let there be no scales to weigh your unknown treasure;
And seek not the depths of your knowledge with staff or sounding line.
For self is a sea boundless and measureless.
—Kahlil Gibran, *The Prophet,* on Self-Knowledge

For Rick, Michael, and Matthew, knowing your love and support.
—Joan Arnold

TABLES, FIGURES, AND EXHIBITS

Tables

Figures

Exhibits

FOREWORD

Striking the right balance between theory, evidence-based guidelines, and the practical experience and wisdom of practitioners is the challenge of every generation of health workers, but that balance has become more challenging with the proliferation of theories, evidence, and varied circumstances of practice. Health promotion adds additional challenges, with its subject matter involving the complexities of human behavior, above and beyond the complexities of human biology.

Sherri Sheinfeld Gorin and Joan Arnold have waded courageously into these challenges and complexities with a creative approach designed to sort out and frame the various theories and problems of behavior and of practice. They wisely focused their health promotion matrix in the first edition on clinical practice, acknowledging the greater complexities presented by the social, cultural, and economic forces affecting health in the broader community. But they related clinical practice to that broader reality with their placement of clinical practice within an ecological framework of community influences.

With this second edition they have stretched their courage and have challenged their readers to stretch beyond the clinical to organizational wellness, with a stronger emphasis on health management, policy, and community disaster preparedness. This book links clinical practice with the social ecology of health behavior, emphasizing cultural competence and the broader contexts of economic and even global influences.

This book also reviews (in Chapter Two) theoretical and conceptual models of health, health behavior, and social behavior as they pertain to health. This emphasis on ecological models and approaches sets the stage for subsequent discussions of health promotion practice in relation to specific health issues and settings.

From the conceptual and context-setting frameworks in Part One, this book moves in Part Two into collaborative analyses of applications of the frameworks to the leading issues in health behavior change and health promotion in clinical practice. The authors of these chapters are leading professionals in their respective areas.

Finally, this book closes with a chapter titled "Future Directions for Health Promotion." This chapter invites students and health professionals to look forward and to create the future of their practice, not just react to it.

This book will help health professionals and students preparing for practice to find applications of theory in understanding the problems they face in practice, but even more important will be the solutions to problems in practice that will grow out of their greater understanding. Much has been made in the writings of scientists of the need for theory and evidence to guide practice, but this plea often sounds hollow to practitioners who perceive the theory and the scientific evidence to have come from outside the realities of everyday practice situations. The applications in this book should help to bridge that gap between theory and practice.

January 2006   Lawrence W. Green
                                                                                  University of California
                                                                                  at San Francisco

PREFACE AND ACKNOWLEDGMENTS

Health Promotion in Practice addresses health promotion for individuals, families, groups, and communities. As a practice-driven book it is designed to translate theories of health promotion into step-by-step clinical approaches for engaging with clients. The intended audience for this book includes practicing health care professionals and advanced students in a variety of health-related fields, including public health, nursing, health management and policy, medicine, and social work.

Health Promotion in Practice is the second edition of the *Health Promotion Handbook* (Sheinfeld Gorin and Arnold, 1998). In this new edition the Health Promotion Matrix (HPM) has been integrated into Chapter Two, "Models of Health Promotion," in order to better highlight the full range of models that apply to each of the specific practice frameworks. Further, the practice frameworks have been expanded to include violence prevention and disaster preparedness and a new view of organizational wellness. We have integrated contemporary themes such as cultural competence, resilience, genetic susceptibility, and survivorship. Replacing the uniform script at the end of each chapter with clinical interventions that are unique to the practice frameworks also strengthens the clinical relevance of this book.

The audience for this book is consequently expanded to include advanced students of health care such as upper-level undergraduates and graduate students. *Health Promotion in Practice,* because of its clinical focus, will also continue to serve as a valued resource for practitioners worldwide.

Organization

The four chapters in Part One, "Health, Health Promotion, and the Health Care Professional," describe the theoretical frameworks on which the work rests. Chapter One, "Images of Health," begins that description by presenting various constructions of health, such as health as a balanced state, health as goodness of fit, health as transcendence, and health as power. Such images represent the clustering of views on health and provide a framework to explain the dynamics of client change.

"Models of Health Promotion," Chapter Two, explores contemporary theoretical approaches to health promotion. It integrates the images of health with models of health promotion, from the macrolevel, such as the social ecology model, to the microlevel, including the health belief model. It highlights the moral underpinnings for these varied models of health promotion, as well as the cross-cutting constructs of empowerment and cultural competence. Approaches to the evaluation of health promotion programs founded on these contemporary models, and their consequent measures of change, are also discussed.

In Chapter Three, "Contexts for Health Promotion," the myriad political and economic forces influencing health promotion are detailed. With the expanding influence of international bodies like the World Health Organization, global legislation and policy mandates are changing the purview of national health promotion. States are playing a larger role in the maintenance of health for their citizens and in the protection of the most vulnerable. These initiatives are found in legislation, policy, and economic incentives, from the perspectives of governmental and private programs and insurers.

"Agents for Health Promotion," Chapter Four, describes who the current health care professionals are and the principles of practice that unify them across disciplines. Underlying these principles are the assumed values and skills of collaboration and cross-disciplinary partnering, cultural competence and proficiency, health communication and literacy, and using a strengths-based approach for changing systems for health promotion.

Part Two of this book, "Practice Frameworks for Health Promotion," is organized around clinical approaches specific to eleven healthy behaviors: eating well, physical activity, sexual health, oral health, smoking cessation, substance safety, injury prevention, violence prevention, disaster preparedness, organizational wellness, and enhancing development. The introduction to each chapter establishes the importance of the area and provides an evidence-based literature review. The chapter then moves on to suggest clinical interventions. Each chapter concludes with practice-related resources for engaging with clients in a dialogue about health promotion.

Chapter Five, "Eating Well," describes the role food plays in daily life, especially given the increased attention to obesity as a national health concern. Unlike behaviors such as smoking, eating is not something that clients can just stop doing. In changing eating behaviors, the health care professional must recognize that clients ingest food, not nutrients. Throughout the chapter, food is described as a promoter and sustainer of health. The health care professional assists clients in using nutritional appraisals, reorienting choices in food selection, and evaluating programs designed to encourage healthy eating.

Chapter Six, "Physical Activity," explores activity as a major contributor to risk reduction for multiple diseases, including non–insulin-dependent diabetes mellitus, and as central to weight control and the maintenance of bone mass. Using transtheoretical theory, techniques for assisting sedentary clients are described as well as mechanisms for engaging moderately or highly active clients. The Patient-Centered Assessment and Counseling for Exercise (PACE) program, an empirically tested program for systematic exercise development, is explored in depth.

Chapter Seven, "Sexual Health," looks at sexuality as a healthy dimension of being human. With an understanding of the diversity of sexual health needs across varied subgroups, the chapter examines how sexual health is defined and promoted. After assessing the evidence for the effectiveness of sexual health promotion, the chapter presents two interventions for clinical care settings: taking sexual histories and promoting individual safer sex.

In Chapter Eight, "Oral Health," the effects of common oral diseases and health conditions that place clients at risk of periodontal diseases, dental decay, and oral cancer are reviewed. An emphasis is placed on recognizing symptoms of these oral diseases through clinical assessment. Evidence-based preventive health activities are provided for health care professionals to use with their clients to prevent new disease and to reduce the severity of existing disease.

Chapter Nine, "Smoking Cessation," highlights the population subgroups that continue to smoke despite the enormous resources applied to both national and worldwide smoking cessation education and legislation. It addresses the causes of smoking, including emerging findings on genetic susceptibility. Further, the chapter explores key interventions for smoking cessation, particularly among the vulnerable oncology and psychiatric populations.

Chapter Ten, "Substance Safety," details the benefits of such safety promotion. It classifies drugs into several types: prescribed and over-the-counter drugs; banned street drugs, such as marijuana, cocaine, and heroin; alternative medicines, such as herbs and vitamins; and social drugs, such as nicotine, caffeine, and alcohol. Alcohol, the most widely used of the risky substances, is the focus of the remainder of the chapter. Differing rates and impacts of immoderate drinking in the various gender, age, and ethnic and racial groups may influence the strategies health care professionals adopt.

Chapter Eleven, "Injury Prevention," investigates injuries as a public health problem. It begins with the causes and magnitude of the problem, detailing the epidemiology of injuries. Axioms for injury prevention are then provided to guide efforts to control this problem. The chapter describes strategies for health promotion, education and behavioral change, legislation and law enforcement, use of engineering and technology, and use of combined behavioral and environmental approaches to injury prevention.

Resting on an epidemiologic base, Chapter Twelve, "Violence Prevention," details the significant advances that have been made in understanding violence as a public health issue. Using a taxonomy of types of violence and an ecological framework, violent behavior is thoughtfully examined. A framework for violence prevention and intervention is outlined as are strategies for program evaluation. The process of implementing and disseminating effective interventions is illustrated through discussion of the use of consensus documents and evidence-based guidelines and the involvement of those public health agencies that are leading the efforts to reduce violence.

Chapter Thirteen, "Disaster Preparedness," examines emerging concerns about threats to safety and security, now omnipresent in the United States. In the prologue, it explores the social ecological determinants of population health following disasters. It also discusses approaches to threat detection, vehicles for terrorism, and human responses to potential disasters. Detailing protocols for systemwide evacuations, triage, and treatment, this chapter explores a new area of public health that is now in the forefront of public health professionals' attention.

Chapter Fourteen, "Organizational Wellness," adopts a comprehensive definition that strategically integrates business, interpersonal, and individual needs to optimize overall human and organizational well-being. Applying a myriad of concepts derived from psychology and sociology to the understanding of the worksite as a venue for and an influence on health promotion, this chapter suggests a set of innovative approaches to enhance workplace wellness.

As Chapter Fifteen, "Enhancing Development," unfolds, development is explored as an ongoing and evolving process in individuals, families, groups, and communities. Viewed from a life course perspective, development is seen as complex, unique, and patterned. Resilience, spirituality, and grieving are discussed as significant forces in human systems as they develop. Throughout the chapter, loss and growth are viewed as intrinsically linked, at no time more than at the end of life.

Part Three of this book, "Economic Applications and Forecasting the Future of Health Promotion," explores some of the factors shaping the present and the future of the field.

Chapter Sixteen, "Economic Considerations in Health Promotion," recognizes the pivotal role economics plays in directing health promotion practice at present. Practical tools for analyzing the economic advantages of health promotion practices are offered. A detailed example of the process of implementing a health promotion program in a managed care organization anchors the chapter.

The final chapter, "Future Directions for Health Promotion," points to the larger influences on health promotion practice yet to come. It is likely that the opportunities will include addressing the needs of the growing elderly population, designing health promotion for a diverse populace, harnessing the forces of global change to promote health, measuring community change, and engaging in an ongoing ethical dialogue. The future of health promotion is predicated on actions taken by and for communities.

Acknowledgments

It is with deep appreciation that we thank the following individuals for their contributions to this book:

Andrew Pasternack at Jossey-Bass for proposing the idea of a second edition and for his support, guidance, and encouragement throughout the publication process. Seth Schwartz for his ongoing and informed support as we moved toward the completion of this book. Susan Geraghty for handling the production of the book and keeping us on deadline. Elspeth MacHattie for her meticulous copyediting that transformed this work.

Lawrence W. Green for his gracious foreword and his own storied contributions to the field of public health.

Stephen L. Sheinfeld, Sherri's beloved brother, for his knowledgeable guidance on the complexities of legal research and for his wise counsel.

Rebeca Franco for her expert and steadfast assistance when deadlines were pressing.

Rabbi Howard Hoffman for his considered review of the Hebrew text.

Linda Weinberg, librarian at Adelphi University, and Mark Haber, Jennifer Ransom, and Shannon Weidemann, librarians at The College of New Rochelle, for their helpful library research, and Christina Blay, circulation manager, Carolyn Reid, inter-library loan manager, and the entire staff of the Inter-Library Loan Department, The College of New Rochelle.

Linda Thomas at Elsevier for expediting the transfer of copyright.

The outstanding contributors, each of whom greatly shaped this text and to whom we are extraordinarily indebted. It was a privilege and a distinct pleasure for each of us to work with our esteemed colleagues who shared their time, expertise, and insights so willingly. The joy of writing this book rests on our relationships with them.

Finally, although this book is dedicated to our families, we wish to again express our appreciation and special affections for our spouses, Brian Gorin and Rick Arnold, and children, Aaron and Evan Gorin and Michael and Matthew Arnold, as well as our parents, Al and Trudy Sheinfeld and Marjorie and the late Robert Hagan. By sharing their immense love with us, they helped us to complete this work.

January 2006

Sherri Sheinfeld Gorin
New York, New York

Joan Arnold
New Rochelle, New York

THE CONTRIBUTORS

Sherri Sheinfeld Gorin, PhD
Associate Professor
Columbia University
Teachers College
and Senior Member, Herbert Irving Comprehensive Cancer Center
and
Director, New York Physicians against Cancer (NYPAC)
Columbia University
New York, NY

Joan Arnold, PhD, RN
Professor
The College of New Rochelle
School of Nursing
New Rochelle, NY

Kristen Lawton Barry, PhD
Research Associate Professor
Department of Psychiatry
University of Michigan
and

Associate Director
Department of Veterans Affairs National Serious Mental
Illness Treatment Research and Evaluation Center
Department of Veterans Affairs
Ann Arbor Health Care System
Ann Arbor, MI

Frederic C. Blow, PhD
Associate Professor and Research Associate Professor
Department of Psychiatry
University of Michigan
and
Director
Department of Veterans Affairs National Serious Mental
Illness Treatment Research and Evaluation Center
Department of Veterans Affairs
Ann Arbor Health Care System
Ann Arbor, MI

Laurel Janssen Breen, RN, MA, PhD Candidate
Assistant Professor
Nursing Department
St. Joseph's College
Patchogue/Brooklyn, NY

Karen J. Calfas, PhD
Professor and Director of Health Promotion
Student Health Services
San Diego State University
San Diego, CA

Wendy Dahar, MPH
Programmer Analyst
Population Care Management and Prevention
Kaiser Permanente
Brooklyn Heights, OH

Thomas Diamante, PhD
Consultant
DOAR Litigation Consulting
New York, NY

Sandro Galea, MD, DrPH
Associate Professor
Department of Epidemiology
University of Michigan School of Public Health
Ann Arbor, MI

Penelope Buschman Gemma, MS, RN, APRN BC, FAAN
Assistant Professor Clinical Nursing
School of Nursing
Columbia University
New York, NY

Andrea Carlson Gielen, ScD, ScM
Professor and Director
Center for Injury Research and Policy
Johns Hopkins Bloomberg School of Public Health
Baltimore, MD

Susanne K. Giorgio, RDH
Dental Hygienist in Private Practice
Elkins Park, PA

Joan I. Gluch, PhD, RDH
Director Community Health and Adjunct Associate Professor
School of Dental Medicine
University of Pennsylvania
Philadelphia, PA

Aaron P. Gorin, MHA
Analyst
The Frankel Group
New York, NY

Lawrence W. Green, PhD
Adjunct Professor
Department of Epidemiology and Biostatistics
School of Medicine and Comprehensive Cancer Center
University of California at San Francisco
San Francisco, CA

Craig Hadley, PhD
Robert Wood Johnson Health and Society Scholar
Center for Social Epidemiology and Population Health
University of Michigan
Ann Arbor, MI

Athena S. Hagler, MS, PhD Candidate
Joint Doctoral Program in Clinical Psychology
San Diego State University and the University of California at San Diego
San Diego, CA

Manuel London, PhD
Associate Provost
Faculty Director, Undergraduate College of Leadership and Service
Professor of Management and Director of the
Center for Human Resource Studies
State University of New York at Stony Brook
Stony Brook, NY

Lorraine E. Matthews, MS, RD, LDN
Food and Nutrition Consultant
Formerly Manager, Health Education & Community Programs
Division of Maternal, Child and Family Health
Philadelphia Department of Public Health
Philadelphia, PA

Stephen S. Morse, PhD
Associate Clinical Professor
Director
Center for Public Health Preparedness
National Center for Disaster Preparedness
Mailman School of Public Health
Columbia University
New York, NY

Samuel M. Natale, DPhil (Oxon.)
Professor
School of Business
Adelphi University
Garden City, NY
and

Senior Research Associate
Department of Educational Studies
University of Oxford
Oxford, England

Duncan Neuhauser, PhD
The Charles Elton Blanchard MD Professor of Health Management
Professor of Epidemiology and Biostatistics
Co-Director, Health Systems Management Center
Case Western Reserve University
Cleveland, OH

Lloyd B. Potter, PhD, MPH
Director
Center for the Study and Prevention of Injury, Violence,
and Suicide Education Development Center (EDC), Inc.
Newton, MA

Theo Sandfort, PhD
Associate Professor
HIV Center for Clinical and Behavioral Studies
New York State Psychiatric Institute and Columbia University
New York, NY

Robert A. Schnoll, PhD
Assistant Professor
Transdisciplinary Tobacco Use Research Center
Department of Psychiatry
University of Pennsylvania
Philadelphia, PA

David A. Sleet, PhD
Associate Director for Science
Division of Unintentional Injury Prevention
National Center for Injury Prevention and Control
Centers for Disease Control and Prevention (CDC)
Atlanta, GA

Barbara J. Steinberg, DDS
Clinical Professor of Surgery
College of Medicine
Drexel University
Philadelphia, PA

PART ONE

HEALTH, HEALTH PROMOTION, AND THE HEALTH CARE PROFESSIONAL

CHAPTER ONE

IMAGES OF HEALTH

Joan Arnold
Laurel Janssen Breen

What do you imagine when you think about health—your health? Do you view yourself as healthy? What health goals do you possess now for yourself and your family? Do factors in your community contribute to your personal health and your family's health? Is your community healthy? In your own unique way, how do you define health? These critical questions beckon examination by the client and the health care professional. Searching for their clarification provides opportunities for discovery about images of health and direction for professional health care interactions and interventions. Once conceptualized, an image of health provides direction for health promotion actions.

Health is baffling. Contemporary thinking about health emphasizes empowering nations, community groups, and individuals to realize their own health aims. In the face of widespread interest in defining health at the theoretical level, the development and the use of clinical practice frameworks to support interventions are increasing. These practice frameworks and theoretical models both reflect and affect clients' and health care professionals' *images of health*. This chapter describes ten categories of images of health, each reflecting a unique view (Exhibit 1.1).

Each image category may include aspects that are also found in other images, and some words may have different meanings in the contexts of different images. These images portray health as the antithesis of disease, a balanced state,

EXHIBIT 1.1. IMAGES OF HEALTH.

Antithesis of disease

Balanced state

Growth

Functionality

Goodness of fit

Wholeness

Well-being

Transcendence

Empowerment

Resource

growth, a functional capacity, goodness of fit, wholeness, well-being, transcendence, empowerment, and finally, a resource. Reflecting on these images of health reveals the complexities of health.

Imagining Health

Health is an elusive term because the state of being healthy can be viewed from a multitude of perspectives. Health may be considered a reference for disease, defined by determining forces, or a panacea. It may be thought of as autonomy and integrity projected by the human system. It may refer to the uniquely characteristic strengths of a person, a family, a group or population, a community, a nation, or the world. It may also mean a self-sustaining or self-replenishing capacity. Health may be thought unattainable, impossible to achieve because of limitations, oppression, and depleting forces. Curiously, health care professionals, regardless of discipline, know more about disease, pathology, and dysfunction than they do about health. Although health is valued and desired as a goal, the diagnostic precision found in dealing with conditions of illness, disease, and social problems is not evident in the study of health. Our clients look to us, as providers of health care, to assist them to achieve their desire to be and feel healthy. As clients strive to shape personal pictures of health, the health care professional bears witness to the coalescing of images of health into the client's own unique composite. This unique image may differ from the health care professional's image of health and expectations for client health. While the client and health care professional interact as partners, the health care professional recognizes these differences and enfolds them into the therapeutic process. Inherent in this challenge is the necessity to accept the client's right to self-determination and to commit to assisting the client in reducing barriers and achieving health goals. The images of health presented in this chapter reflect a clustering of views on health. These images are offered to stimulate a re-visioning of health. Health cannot remain an enigma; it stands on its own as a life process, to be imagined and realized within the unique capacity of everything human.

Health as the Antithesis of Disease

In the image of health as the antithesis of disease, health and disease are viewed as opposite states, with health as the absence of disease. Dubos (1965) referred to "the states of health and disease [as] the expressions of the success or failure experienced by the organism in its efforts to respond adaptively to environmental changes" (p. xvii). Here, the conditions of health and disease are expressions of bipolar thinking. In this context a given population's health is measured by its opposite, the population's morbidity and mortality statistics. These indexes of illness and death are used to appraise health and to direct interventions in specific aggregates. Persons suffering from disease were, and still are, ostracized by society. Social standards for health can lead to negative perceptions of persons with diseases that are in contradiction to these standards. Consider the treatment of persons with leprosy, disabling conditions, acquired immunodeficiency syndrome (AIDS), and drug addiction; they are often feared and viewed as not socially acceptable. Their condition or illness is contradictory to what is defined as healthy by society, and their presence threatens the perceived social order.

When health is defined as the absence of disease, evaluative statements about clients are made within the parameters of illness, using a system of disease signs and symptoms. "This definition of health has been largely the result of the domination of the biomedical sciences by a mechanistic conception of man. Man is viewed by physicians primarily as a physico-chemical system" (Smith, 1983, pp. 46–47). Health care professionals are prepared to make evaluative statements of illness by formulating a diagnostic statement from symptomatology and objective data. Such an evaluative statement requires comparisons to established norms. Illness becomes a deviation from these norms. Health then is a condition of the norm, whereas illness falls outside the range of normal. Rather than defining the components of health, the medical model, relying on illness identification, merely identifies health as the absence of disease. Thus being healthy is being within the range of normal, and more specific parameters are not identified. However, what falls within the medical norm may be nevertheless suboptimal. Then mediocrity becomes an acceptable definition of health, and because of this, the optimal conditions of normal may never be recognized, realized, or individualized.

Health as a Balanced State

The image of health as a balanced state incorporates epidemiology, which provides an important understanding of the relationships among host, agent, and environment in explaining health. *Epidemiology* is the study of patterns of health and the patterns of disease, disability, and death and other problems in populations of persons (Leavell & Clark, 1965). In a broad, widely accepted definition, epidemiology is stated to be "the study of the distribution and determinants of health-related states or events in specified populations and the application of this study to control of health problems" (Last, 1995, pp. 55–56). A major goal of epidemiology is to identify *aggregates,* or subpopulations, at high risk for disease or health-threatening conditions. The intent is to identify risk factors that put the aggregate at risk and then to modify or reduce those risks through preventive interventions. Efforts such as screening, case finding, and health education are geared toward populations most likely to gain from specific strategies developed for a particular disease (Gordis, 1996).

In the epidemiologic framework, health is identified along a health-illness-death continuum. The origins of health and illness are indicative of other processes that occur before the human being is affected. Key to these processes are the interactions of conditions in the environment, factors of the agent for disease, and predisposing genetic forces. "Heredity, social and economic factors, or physical environment may be creating a disease stimulus long before man and stimulus begin to interact to produce disease" (Leavell & Clark, 1965, p. 17). The preliminary interaction of the human host, potential disease agent, and environmental factors in disease production is referred to as the *period of prepathogenesis* (that is, the period before disease). Prepathogenesis is the period of health. The balance among the host, potential agent, and environment is reflective of the equilibrium inherent in the condition of health. It is not until the disease-provoking stimuli produce changes in the human system that the *period of pathogenesis,* or disease, results. The period of prepathogenesis can be thought of as the process in the environment, whereas the period of pathogenesis is the process in the human being, or human system.

Disease is a state of disequilibrium, or *dis-ease,* and health is a state of balance, or equilibrium. Equilibrium is achieved through the interaction of the multiple factors and forces that influence and contribute to health. The balance that is health is reflected in the nature and intensity of these interactions. Physical, physiological, psychological, social, cultural, spiritual, political, and economic forces interact and contribute to the unique image of health for each individual, family, group, and community. Health is a singular condition and a condition of society as well as a balance of these forces.

Cultural ideologies and traditions also influence the image of health as balance. For example, the harmony of yin and yang is balance. Yin and yang have been described as passive and active, feminine and masculine, nurturing and stimulating, and earthly and heavenly. Energy is balanced when these seemingly opposite forces work together. Imbalances between yin and yang are believed to be manifested in the ways internal organs function and can result in disturbances of vital energy, represented on the body's acupuncture meridians. Ayurveda, an ancient medical system that originated in India, emphasizes the equal importance of body, mind, and spirit (National Center for Complementary and Alternative Medicine [NCCAM], 2000). To a practitioner of Ayurveda, imbalances in *doshas*—physiological principles, or bodily humors—can lead to specific diseases. Various foods and emotions are believed to result in imbalances. Furthermore, the dominant medical system in Europe, from ancient Greek times to contemporary ones, emphasizes "the belief that ill health resulted from an imbalance of the body's four humors (blood, phlegm, yellow bile, and black bile)" (NCCAM, p. 8). "Habits and beliefs of people in a given community are not separate items but are the elements of a cultural system which determine their response to any disease. Each culture has its own ways of organizing experiences pertaining to health and disease" (Singh, 2001, p. 39).

Health as Growth

The foundation of the view that sees health as growth is found in the beliefs of noted developmental theorists (for example, Dewey, 1963; Piaget, 1963; Elkind, 1981; Erikson, 1963; Duvall, 1985; Havighurst, 1972). This image leads to a further view of health as the successful fulfillment of certain tasks appropriate to particular life stages. Persons are seen as having a capacity for growth that can be enhanced and supported; this development is seen as an ongoing process that occurs continuously and systematically throughout the life span. Growth is viewed as progressive. Health is seen as being intimately determined by individual lifestyle and behavioral choices. Interventions at critical life stages are believed to be the most effective and to foster optimal growth. Through identification of certain *transition points*, the unique needs, behaviors, and motivations of certain populations are targeted. In this framework, periods of transition involve restructuring and reorganization of both the inner and outer worlds of an individual. Frequently, these periods arise when there is an unfolding of events in which the status quo is challenged. Oftentimes this means new opportunities for enhancing growth and coping (Cowan & Cowan, 2003).

The concept that overall wellness in each life stage involves the achievement of certain cognitive, physiological, and psychological competencies is integral to a life-span approach to health as growth. Established norms are used to measure growth at each stage. Following an established pattern of expected progression through the stages is viewed as desirable and is anticipated. The movement from one stage of growth to another is predicated on some of the life skills and tasks accomplished in an earlier stage. The "failure" to achieve certain developmental skills during a particular stage may be viewed as impeding growth into the next stage.

The way the concept of aging is visualized in the framework of a life-span definition of health demands attention. In its most narrow definition, old age is delineated as the end stage of life, a time of anticipated decline when dependency and helplessness are expected outcomes. It is viewed as a time of final goal attainment, thus avoiding any need to establish health challenges for this population. From a broader viewpoint, aging is a complex cultural issue and is not defined merely by biological parameters. Although they may have altered physical abilities and changing expectations, aging persons retain the capacity for full participation in life. *Aging* in this view is an imprecise term that can be understood as both a loss and a goal. The process of aging is the process of life. Although older Americans today are considered healthier, wealthier, and better educated than the older members of previous generations (Federal Interagency Forum on Aging-Related Statistics, 2004), disparities exist, particularly among those with limited education, women, and minorities.

Over the course of the last three decades a body of literature has developed that is apart from the mainstream, disease-oriented framework and that has begun to describe the experiences of people who have coped successfully with traumatic events. Although much remains to be discovered about how people bounce back from negative events, this literature has explored trauma as an opportunity for psychological growth, which comes about through the challenge and struggle presented by the traumatic event itself (Tedeschi & Calhoun, 1995). Posttraumatic growth is variously seen as an outcome and as a process. A variety of terms have been identified to acknowledge the phenomenon in which growth and change develop and even advance beyond prior levels of adaptation after exposure to undesirable or extreme events. These terms include *resilience, hardiness,* and *thriving.*

When considering how some individuals, families, and larger social systems overcome crises and ongoing adversity while others become depleted and shattered, Walsh (2003) asserts that resilience is the key. From this strengths-oriented approach, life challenges become opportunities for growth. Resilience research has moved beyond considering it as a personal psychological trait and now sees it as a dynamic process (Masten, 1999). Resilience is the capacity to bounce back from adversity and grow through it as its effects are mitigated by protective and vulnerability factors (Luthar & Zelazo, 2003).

Hardiness has been described by Kobasa (1979) as a grouping of personality traits that includes control over life events, a life commitment, and a personal view of change as challenge. Hardiness is seen as a variable that influences the effects stress may have on an individual's physical and mental health. People who are hardy are perceived as having an increased ability to withstand stress (Low, 1996).

Thriving, which has been derived from resilience research, has been conceptualized as a dynamic process of adaptation whereby challenge provides an opportunity for growth and greater well-being. Thriving goes beyond coping and homeostasis to become transformative. It involves cognitive changes, a reexamination of self, and an ability to mobilize resources needed to deflect the impact of a threat or risk (O'Leary & Ickovics, 1995).

When one views *health-within-illness* (Moch, 1998) an opportunity unfolds to view illness as a potential growth catalyst. Health promotion efforts may have negated or ignored these opportunities in the past. However, if health and illness coexist, then within illness is the possibility of realizing health through a sense of meaningfulness, self-knowledge, positive change, and redefinition of life events. Likewise, at the end of life, efforts such as the hospice movement promote health when assisting individuals and families to find meaning in imminent death and to live well with terminal illness. "Our ultimate goal as a society and as members of communities surely is to maximize human development and the achievement of full human potential" (Hancock, Labonte, & Edwards, 1999, p. 522).

Health as Functionality

In the image of health as functionality, health is seen as the capacity to fulfill critical life functions. Functional health patterns for individuals include all activities that influence a person's relationship with the environment. Physiological functions include digestion, hydration, sleep, elimination, and circulation. Psychological functioning encompasses behavior, communication, and emotional development. Fulfillment of these functions defines a healthy individual. Likewise, families have functions to fulfill, including the capacity to nurture their members through physical, emotional, educational, and social support activities. Further, communities function to provide their members with resources to sustain themselves. A community is vital when members can meet their needs and in turn participate in the community's further development. At the global level, nations participate in achieving shared responsibility for mutual health goals for their respective and collective populations.

Functionality is viewed as the ability to carry out a given task. When the functional capacity of individuals, families, groups, and communities is limited, health is altered, and adaptation is necessary to adjust to the environment and fulfill functions. However, adaptation need not be viewed from such a narrow vantage point. It encompasses not only modification of the individual but also alteration of that individual's environment. From this perspective, disability is viewed as a *different ability,* one that requires an altered environment so that a person can achieve vital life functions (that is, the environment is made *accessible,* available to those with different abilities). Persons with disabling conditions then become equally able.

Rehabilitation, a level of prevention, focuses on recovering remaining capacity to maintain function. The strengths and capacities of the individual are realized differently to restore function, even if that function is modified. Recovering the capability to function as independently as possible enables the person, family, group, or community to depend less on other forms of support. Returning function, even if modified, enables social utility and a sense of purpose.

Participation in health activities depends on an individual's overall health function skills. Health literacy, for example, is a major skill necessary for comprehending information directed at improving health (Ratzan, 2001). Health literacy is the capacity to obtain, process, and understand basic health information and services needed to make appropriate health decisions (Ratzan & Parker, 2000). The National Adult Literacy Survey (NALS) has raised serious concerns about marginal health literacy skills among many Americans and about these individuals' ability to participate adequately in their health care (Ad Hoc Committee on Health Literacy for the Council on Scientific Affairs, American Medical Association, 1999). It is estimated that nearly half of all American adults, ninety million people, have difficulty understanding and acting on health information (Nielsen-Bohlman, Panzer, & Kindig, 2004). Health literacy therefore affects functional health.

Health as Goodness of Fit

The fit between the person and the surrounding environment is often imperceptible, as each is embedded in the other. It becomes impossible to distinguish the reciprocal relationship in this joining. The image of health as goodness of fit considers the meshing of the determining factors of health. Human biology, environment, health care, and lifestyle have been identified as the four major determinants of human health (Lalonde, 1974). Each of these determinants is important; however, special attention is now being given to the influence of individual lifestyle on personal health. This focus on lifestyle is inevitable given that the human life span is increasing, chronic disease has become a greater factor than communicable disease in morbidity and mortality, and the health care system has become increasingly focused on costs.

Lifestyle is about choosing. Individuals, families, groups, and communities choose options that set into motion unique interactions of factors and forces that have the potential to produce health or illness. Much progress in the overall major decline in death rates for the leading causes of death among Americans has been traced to reduction in risk factors. *Healthy People 2010* (U.S. Department of Health and Human Services, 2000) delineates health objectives for improving longevity and decreasing health disparities in our nation. Despite these advances resulting from preventive interventions, the United States continues to be burdened by preventable disease, injury, and disability. Focusing on lifestyle alone, however, rather than viewing health as an outcome of a multiplicity of determinants, can easily result in "blaming the victim." When the complex mix of biological, psychological, social, cultural, and political factors is underacknowledged and underestimated, the individual is held solely responsible for risk-taking behaviors and health outcomes.

Lifestyle is only one of the four major factors that determine health. Lifestyle is about choosing, to whatever extent possible. However, certain biological factors, although modifiable, are largely uncontrollable. In addition, environmental determinants of health are often negotiated at the public policy level, leaving individuals, families, groups, and communities without a sense of personal control. Environmental factors such as poverty, racism, and resource allocation challenge the individual's potential for health and limit choice. Also, the availability, accessibility, affordability, appropriateness, adequacy, and acceptability of health care (National Institute of Nursing Research, 1995) can enable or diminish health potential. No one factor alone determines an individual's health, which is shaped by the interlocking of these forces. Yet there is opportunity for change to occur at the point these factors interface.

The environment, a critical determinant of health, cannot be viewed in isolation any more than lifestyle can. The reciprocal relationship between people and their environment is emphasized in the ecological models of health. Recognition of the influences of intra- and interpersonal factors, community and organizational factors, and public policy is viewed as necessary to a full understanding of health-related behaviors and interventions (McLeroy, Bibeau, Steckler, & Glanz, 1988).

The preparation of public health professionals for addressing the public's health (Gebbie, Rosenstock, & Hernandez, 2003) relies on an understanding of the various determinants of health. The relationships and processes that link these forces are best described in an ecological model of health. Individual behavior; social, family, and community networks; living and working conditions; and broad social, economic, cultural, health, and environmental conditions at all levels of development and over the life span are linked in this model. The fit among these factors and forces shapes an understanding of the determinants of population health.

Health as Wholeness

A holistic image of health is central to healing and complementary health care delivery. Appreciating wholeness is enhanced by a framework that supports multiple interactions (Bertalanffy, 1968; Laszlo, 1972). The idea that every aspect of a human being, family, or community is linked and interacting arises from a systems theory orientation. A human being is constructed of subsystems that work together, and he or she is at the same time a subsystem of the family and community, which also are interacting parts of each other.

Each system is simultaneously a subsystem and a suprasystem. Boundaries define each system and allow, through their regulation, the flow of inputs and outputs that maintain energy and enable growth. In this framework, health can be viewed as system integrity and unity. Supporting the integrity of the human system is the focus for promoting and maintaining health.

Human beings are considered whole (that is, more than and different from the sum of their parts). "The whole has a unity, organization, and individuality that is not discoverable by means of the analysis of its parts. In fact, the analysis of the parts of the organism results in decreased perceptions of the qualities of the whole" (Blandino, 1969, quoted in Smith, 1983, p. 77). Employing the framework of Maslow (1968), Smith (1983) considers health to be the complete development of the individual's potential. Smith's eudaimonistic model focuses on the entirety of the organism, including the physical, social, aesthetic, and moral—not just the behavioral and physiological—aspects. In the eudaimonistic sense, health is wholeness. To be healthy is a goal toward which the human system strives.

Human systems are no longer viewed in isolation. Individual health is influenced by family health, and one member's health influences the health of other family members. Likewise, families are viewed within the contexts of groups, communities, and societies; families contribute to the health indicators of larger systems. Nations are viewed within the context of world health, contributing to and being influenced by the whole globe. No longer can health be solely determined by individual indicators. There is growing evidence that individual health and community health are interdependent. This awareness is reflected in the current understanding of population health. The key elements of population health assessment are aggregated health characteristics and disparities among groups; environmental, social, and economic health determinants; inequalities of opportunity; and community governance and the degree of distribution of power (Hancock, Labonte, & Edwards, 1999).

Health as Well-Being

Health is defined in the Preamble to the Constitution of the World Health Organization (WHO) (signed in 1946 and ratified in 1948) as follows: "Health is a state of complete physical, mental, and social well-being, and not merely the absence of disease or infirmity" (WHO, 1947). Freedom from disease and illness implies an ideal state among three significant sources of well-being—physical well-being, mental well-being, and social well-being. Referring to health as a "complete" state may mean that health requires no improvement and "that anything less than complete well-being is not health" (Buetow & Kerse, 2001, p. 74). Curiously, following this line of inquiry may result in the negation of health promotion efforts, because health cannot be improved. Bok (2004) asserts that defining health as "complete . . . well-being" may make the term unsuitable for either measuring or comparing states of health. "Even if someone did achieve such a state of complete health, it would be short-lived; and there would be no chance of finding members of any group, let alone inhabitants of a society or a region, enjoying such a felicitous state simultaneously" (p. 7).

Dunn (1961) uses this WHO definition to expand on the idea of *high-level wellness*, in which the term *health* implies being well not only in the body and mind but also within the family and community and having a compatible work interest. "High-level wellness for the individual is defined as an integrated method of functioning which is oriented toward maximizing the potential of which the individual is capable. It requires that the individual maintain a continuum of balance and purposeful direction within the environment where he is functioning" (pp. 4–5). In effect, health is viewed as balance along a goal-directed continuum within the context of the environment. The dynamic nature of health is implied as health potential is maximized. In other words, rather than being a complete static state, health involves maintaining completeness on an ongoing basis. Balance and dynamism are combined while a person, family, group, or community moves purposefully toward a goal.

Often what people describe as "feeling healthy" is a subjective sense of well-being—a subjective interpretation of personal indicators that produce a vague sense that everything is all right. Although the actual structure of general well-being is not clearly understood, it is thought to include the following contributors: emotions, beliefs, temperaments, behaviors, situations, experiences, and health

(Wheeler, 1991). *Well-being* is an imprecise term subsuming both subjective and objective definitions and methods of measurement. It may include self-reports of satisfaction and dissatisfaction, the presence or absence of a persistent mood level or transient emotional state, external environmental conditions, and biochemically related behavior (Kahn & Juster, 2002).

It is known that different individuals experience the sense of well-being in very different ways. The pursuit of well-being may include no formal definition, no clear-cut guidelines. However, the individual does know and understand some means for attaining this state. Perhaps it is not necessary or even possible to have a precise and objective definition of certain human experiences.

For many persons, humor is an important aspect of achieving well-being. In attempting to comprehend and live through the myriad of life experiences, people find that perceived reality can be altered through humor and its outward expressions. Humor is understood as a powerful tool, affecting both neurological and physiological transmissions in the body. It can reduce tension and frustration and startle a person out of complacency. Laughter and humor are powerful expressions that add vitality and "joy" (Cousins, 1979) to the experience of health and life.

Health as Transcendence

To view health as transcendence is to see the human potential for growth and development as limitless. Any boundaries of mind and body are believed to be self-imposed. According to this framework, human beings and intervention modalities are continuously evolving. Health is this process of self-discovery. Understanding on a cognitive level is not necessary for an intervention to be therapeutic. Some aspects of healing are experienced and understood by the client and health care professional at different levels of awareness. Persons are presented with a multitude of choices during their lifetimes. Moving outside personal comfort zones and stretching beyond these perceived boundaries can promote insecurity. Therefore, redefining health involves loosening boundaries and undergoing transformation. Support in this process is desirable and augmenting.

Health is seen as interrelated with the larger universe, integrating emotional and spiritual factors. The *self* is experienced and explored based on a definition that far transcends its ordinary definition; self becomes a "manifestation or expression of this much greater 'something' that is our deeper origin and destination" (Lawlis, 1996, p. 5). The process inherent in *body-mind-spirit* is understood as a unified whole that has great potential for experiencing, altering, and expressing health.

The perceived meaning that one attaches to an experience or event is recognized as having an integral connection to one's overall health experience. These perceived meanings affect both one's choices and the impacts of health interventions. When exploring the relationship between spirituality and health, it is generally acknowledged that the concept of spirituality lacks an accepted clear definition and is highly personal and contextualized (Coyle, 2001). However, it is also recognized that spirituality "motivates, enables, empowers, and provides hope" (p. 592). Spirituality has further been understood as "one's inward sense of something greater than the individual self or the meaning one perceives that transcends the immediate circumstances" (U.S. Office of Alternative Medicine, 1994, p. 8). It is this sense of meaning and purpose that supports an individual's ability to gain some control and mastery over his or her circumstances. A spiritual healing philosophy of health acknowledges the healing forces of modalities such as prayer, meditation, and focused thought (Institute of Medicine, 2005).

Health as Empowerment

A strong link between individuals' or communities' sense of power and the level of health they experience has been identified (Robertson & Minkler, 1994; Minkler, 1999). This power has been closely associated with the perceived degree of life *control* and *mastery*. Powerlessness has been identified as a broad-based risk factor for the development of disease. The empowerment process, as a health promotion intervention strategy, has been correlated with improving the health of populations (Wallerstein, 1992). Health professionals must respect and acknowledge the significance of clients' right to "name their own experience" as an integral part of the empowerment process. Without this, the professional risks subjectively overwhelming or affecting the lives of others by setting up a health agenda "for" clients that they "must" follow (Labonte, 1994).

Movement toward health evolves from a fully engaged sense of self. Definition and direction for health come from this strength. Change occurs as individuals and communities, in partnership with the health care professional and others, work toward the implementation of this personal vision of health.

Empowerment in its fullest meaning is context bound. It extends to include an awareness of all the forces that individuals, families, groups, and communities face as they attempt to transform their reality (Airhihenbuwa, 1994). Culture is one of these forces. Health experiences and choices originate within a cultural perspective. Cultural values, attitudes, and behaviors are seen as an integral part of a personal definition of health and disease. The empowerment process is expanded through actions that focus on improving the health of communities. Targeting only individual change dilutes the process. "Hence the empowerment process is maximized when community residents at large become mobilized around health concerns and initiate collective actions for well-being of the entire community"

(Braithwaite, Bianchi, & Taylor, 1994, p. 414). Owing to the interrelatedness of all people, health is a universal experience.

The view of health as empowerment includes the belief that individuals possess numerous and diverse self-care abilities that contribute to determining their health. Persons require certain self-care skills to feel in control and to direct their own life course, and community change depends on the ability of the community's members to self-direct. Self-care involves competency, which comes about as professionals transfer necessary skills and knowledge to individuals and communities. Much of the provision of health can now be seen as within the grasp of the consumer.

The ability to control and shape this vision is dependent on a redistribution of power within the health care system. Power is transferred as the client determines health actions and as the system of health care becomes accountable for providing client-focused care. With whom, then, does the responsibility for health lie? Although there is strong support for health promotion approaches stressing both personal and a broader social responsibility, it is actually the coalescing of these forces that permits "the creation of healthy public policies and health-promoting environments, within which individuals are better able to make choices conducive to health" (Minkler, 1999, p. 135).

Health as a Resource

In a discussion of health within the context of health promotion, the World Health Organization's Ottawa Charter broadened the conceptualization of health to include an understanding of the social, political, and economic determinants of health. In order to reach a state of health, "an individual or group must be able to identify and to realize aspirations, to satisfy needs, and to change or cope with the environment. Health, is therefore, seen as a resource for everyday life, not the objective of living. Health is a positive concept emphasizing social and personal resources, as well as physical capacities" (WHO, 1986, p. 1).

The idea of health as a resource for living expands the definition of health and its determinants to include the context in which health, or nonhealth, is considered and goes beyond an emphasis on individual lifestyle strategies to achieve health (Robertson & Minkler, 1994). As a resource for everyday living, health is not a state or absolute condition but rather the dynamic capability to deal with life's challenges and care for oneself. Health is competence; a well of strengths, some apparent and some unrecognized but all able to be cultivated and actualized. This resource embodies capacities that are usable, untapped, and potential. An inventory of strengths enables every human system to kindle its resource. Health is a life force for engaging in an evolving process of development.

This image of health as a resource for everyday living extends to community, society, and world proportions. "WHO and other UN-sponsored agencies such as the United Nations Development Program (UNDP) and the World Bank have recognized that health is central to human development, not only at the individual level, but also in terms of global macrosystems and social stability" (Shinn, 1999, p. 117). The editors of a Pan American Health Organization (PAHO) constitutional study on the right to health care have stated: "Health provides both the foundation for a just and productive society and the cornerstone of an individual's chance to develop his or her full potential. A population that is not healthy cannot learn, cannot work, cannot develop" (Fuenzalida-Puelma & Connors, 1989, p. xv). Health as a resource therefore integrates social, cultural, and political dimensions and includes equity (the right to equal and adequate access to health); integration of health measures across the continuum from promotion to prevention to recovery to survivorship; participation (mutual responsibility between systems and society); and efficiency (appropriate use of available resources) (adapted from WHO as cited in Shinn, 1999). Personal, community, societal, and global health are interconnected and inseparable resources.

Summary

There are many ways to envision health. Each frame of reference creates a different image. Images of health influence personal decision making as well as the establishment of health policies and programs at local, national, and global levels. The health care system, from the smallest unit of service to the entire system, reflects images of health. Health is dynamic. The possibilities for blending and exploring new images of health are endless. As health is redefined, people and communities have greater opportunities to expand its meaning and significance. Health care professionals protect the entitlement to health.

References

Ad Hoc Committee on Health Literacy for the Council on Scientific Affairs, American Medical Association. (1999). Health literacy: Report of the Council on Scientific Affairs. *JAMA, 28,* 552–557.

Airhihenbuwa, C. O. (1994). Health promotion and the discourse on culture: Implications for empowerment. *Health Education Quarterly, 21*(3), 345–353.

Bertalanffy, L. V. (1968). *General system theory.* New York: Braziller.

Bok, S. (2004, October). *Rethinking of the WHO definition of health* (Harvard Center for Population and Development Studies, Working Paper Series, Vol. 14, No. 7). Retrieved November 6, 2005, from http://www.hsph.harvard.edu/hcpds/wpweb/Bok_wp1407_2.pdf

Braithwaite, R. L., Bianchi, C., & Taylor, S. E. (1994). Ethnographic approach to community organization and health empowerment. *Health Education Quarterly, 21*(3), 407–416.

Buetow, S. A., & Kerse, N. M. (2001). Does reported health promotion activity neglect people with ill-health? *Health Promotion International, 16*(1), 73–78.

Cousins, N. (1979). *Anatomy of an illness as perceived by the patient: Reflections on healing and regeneration.* New York: Norton.

Cowan, P. A., & Cowan, C. P. (2003). Normative family transitions, normal family process, and healthy child development. In F. Walsh (Ed.), *Normal family processes* (3rd ed., pp. 424–459). New York: Guilford Press.

Coyle, J. (2001). Spirituality and health: Towards a framework for exploring the relationship between spirituality and health. *Journal of Advanced Nursing, 37*(6), 589–597.

Dewey, J. (1963). *Experience and education.* New York: Collier Books.

Dubos, R. (1965). *Man adapting.* New Haven, CT: Yale University Press.

Dunn, H. (1961). *High-level wellness.* Arlington, VA: Beatty.

Duvall, E.R.M. (1985). *Marriage and family development* (6th ed.). New York: HarperCollins.

Elkind, D. (1981). *Children and adolescents* (3rd ed.). New York: Oxford University Press.

Erikson, E. H. (1963). *Childhood and society* (2nd ed.). New York: Norton.

Federal Interagency Forum on Aging-Related Statistics. (2004). *Federal forum reports Americans aging well, but gaps remain.* Retrieved February 17, 2005, from http://www.agingstats.gov/chartbook2004/pr2004.html

Fuenzalida-Puelma, H., & Connors, S. (Eds.). (1989). *The right to health in the Americas.* Washington, DC: Pan American Health Organization.

Gebbie, K., Rosenstock, L., & Hernandez, L. M. (Eds.). (2003). *Who will keep the public healthy? Educating public health professionals for the 21st century.* Washington, DC: National Academies Press.

Gordis, L. (1996). *Epidemiology.* Philadelphia: Saunders.

Hancock, T., Labonte, R., & Edwards, R. (1999). Indicators that count! Measuring population health at the community level. *Canadian Journal of Public Health, 90* (Suppl. 1), 522–526.

Havighurst, R. J. (1972). *Developmental tasks and education* (3rd ed.). New York: McKay.

Institute of Medicine. (2005). *Complementary and alternative medicine in the United States.* Washington, DC: National Academies Press.

Kahn, R. L., & Juster, F. T. (2002). Well-being: Concepts and measures. *Journal of Social Issues, 58*(4), 627–644.

Kobasa, S. C. (1979). Stressful life events, personality and health: An inquiry into hardiness. *Journal of Personality and Social Psychology, 37*(1), 1–11.

Labonte, R. (1994). Health promotion and empowerment: Reflections on professional practice. *Health Education Quarterly, 21*(2), 253–268.

Lalonde, M. (1974). *A new perspective on the health of Canadians.* Ottawa: Government of Canada.

Last, J. M. (Ed.). (1995). *A dictionary of epidemiology* (3rd ed.). New York: Oxford University Press.

Laszlo, E. (1972). *The systems view of the world: The natural philosophy of the new developments in the sciences.* New York: Braziller.

Lawlis, G. F. (1996). *Transpersonal medicine: A new approach to healing the body-mind-spirit.* Boston: Shambhala.

Leavell, H. R., & Clark, E. G. (1965). *Preventive medicine for the doctor in his community: An epidemiologic approach.* New York: McGraw-Hill.

Low, J. (1996). The concept of hardiness: A brief but critical commentary. *Journal of Advanced Nursing, 24*(3), 588–590.

Luthar, S. S., & Zelazo, L. B. (2003). Research on resilience. In S. S. Luthar (Ed.), *Resilience and vulnerability: Adaptation in the context of childhood adversities* (pp. 510–549). New York: Cambridge University Press.

Maslow, A. H. (1968). *Toward a psychology of being* (2nd ed.). New York: Van Nostrand Reinhold.

Masten, A. S. (1999). Resilience comes of age: Reflections on the past and outlook for the next generation of research. In M. D. Glantz & J. L. Johnson (Eds.), *Resilience and development: Positive life adaptations* (pp. 281–296). New York: Kluwer Academic/Plenum.

McLeroy, K. R., Bibeau, D., Steckler, A., & Glanz, K. (1988). An ecological perspective on health promotion programs. *Health Education Quarterly, 15,* 351–378.

Minkler, M. (1999). Personal responsibility for health? A review of the arguments and the evidence at century's end. *Health Education & Behavior, 26*(1), 121–141.

Moch, S. D. (1998). Health-within-illness: Concept development through research and practice. *Journal of Advanced Nursing, 28*(2), 305–310.

National Center for Complementary and Alternative Medicine. (2000). *Expanding horizons of health care: Five-year strategic plan 2001–2005* (NIH Publication No. 01-5001). Washington, DC: U.S. Department of Health and Human Services, Public Health Service, National Institutes of Health.

National Institute of Nursing Research. (1995). *Community-based health care: Nursing strategies: National nursing research agenda.* Bethesda, MD: Author.

Nielsen-Bohlman, L., Panzer, A. M., & Kindig, D. A. (Eds.). (2004). *Health literacy: A prescription to end confusion.* Washington, DC: National Academies Press.

O'Leary, V. E., & Ickovics, J. R. (1995). Resilience and thriving in response to challenge: An opportunity for a paradigm shift in women's health. *Women's Health: Research on Gender, Behavior, and Policy, 1*(2), 121–142.

Piaget, J. (1963). *The origins of intelligence in children.* New York: Norton.

Ratzan, S. (2001). Health literacy: Communication for the public good. *Health Promotion International, 16*(2), 207–214.

Ratzan, S. C., & Parker, R. M. (2000). Introduction. In C. R. Selden, M. Zorn, S. C. Ratzan, & R. M. Parker (Comps.), *Current bibliographies in medicine: Health literacy* (NLM Publication No. CBM 2000–1). Bethesda, MD: U.S. Department of Health and Human Services, National Library of Medicine.

Robertson, A., & Minkler, M. (1994). New health promotion movement: A critical examination. *Health Education Quarterly, 21*(3), 295–312.

Shinn, C. (1999). The right to the highest attainable standard of health: Public health's opportunity to reframe a human rights debate in the United States. *Health and Human Rights, 4*(1), 114–133.

Singh, A. (2001). Women's illnesses: The Indian male perspective a search for linkage with Vedic concept of health & Hindu mythology. *Bulletin of the Indian Institute of History of Medicine, 31*(1), 39–56.

Smith, J. A. (1983). *The idea of health: Implications for the nursing professional.* New York: Teachers College.

Tedeschi, R. G., & Calhoun, L. G. (1995). *Trauma and transformation: Growing in the aftermath of suffering.* Thousand Oaks, CA: Sage.

U.S. Department of Health and Human Services. (2000). *Healthy people 2010: Understanding and improving health.* Washington, DC: U.S. Government Printing Office.

U.S. Office of Alternative Medicine. (1994). *Alternative medicine: Expanding medical horizons: A report to the National Institutes of Health on alternative medical systems and practices in the U.S.* Washington, DC: Author.

Wallerstein, N. (1992). Powerlessness, empowerment, and health: Implications for health promotion programs. *American Journal of Health Promotion, 6*(3), 197–205.

Walsh, F. (2003). Crisis, trauma, and challenge: A relational resilience approach for healing, transformation, and growth. *Smith College Studies in Social Work, 74*(1), 49–71.

Wheeler, R. J. (1991). The theoretical and empirical structure of general well-being. *Social Indicators Research, 24,* 71–79.

World Health Organization. (1947). Constitution of the World Health Organization. *Chronicle of the World Health Organization, 1*(1–2), 29–43.

World Health Organization. (1986). *Ottawa charter for health promotion* (WHO/HPR/HEP/95.1). Geneva: Author.

CHAPTER TWO

MODELS OF HEALTH PROMOTION

Sherri Sheinfeld Gorin

As discussed in Chapter One, health is an evolving concept. This chapter explains health promotion within the constraints of several dominant models in the field (global and national policies; the environmental approaches; the life course model; and the health attitude, belief, and behavioral change approaches) and details these models' implicit approaches to health. The loci of change are at either the microlevel (individual, family, group) or the macrolevel (societal, community, population) (Zaltman, Kotler, & Kaufman, 1972). (See Table 2.1.)

Models present a simplified picture of part of the health promotion phenomenon. Several of the models described in this chapter could also be characterized as theories of social relations. In general a theory (1) contains constructs (that is, mental images, such as *health*) that it seeks to explain or account for in some way; (2) describes relationships, often causal, among constructs; and (3) incorporates hypothesized relationships between the constructs and observable variables that can be used to measure the constructs (that is, *operationalized* constructs) (Judd, Smith, & Kidder, 1991). Several of these theories, such as that of social cognition, have been empirically verified and thus strong evidence for their veracity exists. Other models, even as they are guiding research and intervention development,

The author appreciates the helpful comments of Lawrence W. Green on this chapter.

TABLE 2.1. HEALTH PROMOTION MODELS AND HEALTH THEMES.

Model	Primary Health Theme	Focus (Macro or Micro)
Global policy	All themes but health as the antithesis of disease	Macro
National policy		
Health promotion	Health as a balanced state	Macro/micro
	Health as sense of well-being	
Health protection/disease prevention	Health as the antithesis of disease	Macro/micro
Environmental approaches		
Social ecology	Health as goodness of fit	Macro
	Health as wholeness	
Social network	Health as goodness of fit	Macro/micro
	Health as a resource	
Positive psychology	Health as sense of well-being	Micro
Social marketing	Health as sense of well-being	Macro
Political economy	Health as empowerment	Macro
Behavioral model of healthcare utilization	Health as a resource	Macro
PRECEDE[a]-PROCEED[b]	Health as functionality	Macro
Social responsibility	Health as empowerment	Macro
Life course models		
Innovation diffusion theory	Health as growth	Macro/micro
Stages of change[c]	Health as growth	Micro
Health attitude, belief, and behavioral change approaches		
Health belief model[c]	Health as functionality	Micro
Protection motivation theory	Health as the antithesis of disease	Micro
Cognitive-social health information–processing model	Health as functionality	Micro
Theory of planned behavior	Health as functionality	Micro
Prospect theory	Health as the antithesis of disease	Micro
Social learning theories		
Stimulus response theory	Health as functionality	Micro
Social cognitive theory[d]	Health as functionality	Micro

TABLE 2.1. HEALTH PROMOTION MODELS AND HEALTH THEMES, Cont'd.

Model	Primary Health Theme	Focus (Macro or Micro)
Health promotion matrix	Health as sense of well-being	Macro/micro
	Health as a resource	
Spirituality as a construct	Health as transcendence	Micro
Empowerment and community capacity building	Health as empowerment	Macro
	Health as a resource	

[a]PRECEDE: predisposing, reinforcing, and enabling constructs in ecosystem diagnosis and evaluation.

[b]PROCEED: policy, regulating or resourcing, and organizing for (I) health education, media, and advocacy; and (II) policy, regulation, resources, and organization; and (III) educational and environmental development and evaluation.

[c]Also considered part of the transtheoretical model.

[d]Also considered part of the transtheoretical and health belief models.

are at the same time undergoing verification and modification, through approaches similar to those outlined in the last part of this chapter.

Global Policy

Global health policy is often based on the World Health Organization's definition of *health,* which is currently the broadest, most inclusive definition of health and is designed for citizens of the world: "Health is a state of complete physical, mental, and social well-being, and not merely the absence of disease or infirmity" (WHO, 1946, p. 100).

In 1978, at Alma-Ata, Kazakhstan, representatives of nations throughout the world expressed the need for nations to develop access to primary health care that would enable their citizens to lead socially and economically productive lives. This meeting was followed by one in 1988 in Riga, Latvia, to identify the remaining gaps in health care, particularly for infants, children, and women of childbearing age. Strategies to achieve health for all persons by the year 2000 were drafted. They called for (1) empowering persons by providing information and decision-making opportunities, (2) strengthening local systems of primary health care, (3) improving education and training programs in health promotion and prevention for health care professionals, (4) applying science and technology to critical health problems, (5) using new approaches to health problems that have resisted solution, (6) providing special assistance to the least-developed countries, and (7) establishing a process for examination of the long-term challenges that must be addressed beyond the year 2000 in achieving health for all (World Health Organization [WHO], 1988). To implement the aim of the first conference and to develop the strategies of the second, WHO (1984) adopted the following five principles of health promotion:

1. Health promotion includes the population as a whole in the context of individuals' everyday lives, rather than focusing on persons at risk for specific diseases.
2. Health promotion is directed toward action on the causes or determinants of health.
3. Health promotion combines diverse but complementary methods or approaches, including communication, education, legislation, fiscal measures, organizational change, community development, and spontaneous local activities against health hazards.
4. Health promotion is particularly aimed at effective and concrete public participation.
5. While health promotion is basically an activity in the health and social fields and not a medical service, health care professionals—particularly in primary health care—have an important role in nurturing and enabling health promotion.

The WHO definition of health promotion offers a multidimensional characterization of health and incorporates a multitude of strategies, including individual and community change and legislation, under its rubric. The WHO definition assumes a person does not have sole control over his or her health. It does, however, allow people to take responsibility for their choices within a context of concomitant social responsibility for health. Further, on the philosophical level it implies that health is a means to an end—a *resource*—and an instrumental value, or good, for what it brings. Health, like power, is a resource differentially distributed in society (Gutiérrez, 1990). In the global policy model, health is not a good in and of itself or a value in its own right but a resource for living. Multisectoral cooperation—among public health, transportation, social welfare, and other systems—is necessary to the equitable distribution of health resources.

National Policy

It is estimated that in the United States unhealthy lifestyles are responsible for 54 percent of the years of life lost before the age of sixty-five years, environmental factors are responsible for 22 percent, and heredity for 16 percent (McGinnis & Foege, 1994). Thirty-three percent of all U.S. deaths can be attributed to three behaviors: tobacco use, physical inactivity, and poor eating habits (Mensah, 2005). Population-wide approaches to reduce the effects of behavioral and environmental factors, such as tobacco use, poor diet, inactivity, unsafe sexual behavior, microbial agent use, firearm use, drug and alcohol use, toxic agents, and motor vehicles, could decrease the 70 percent of early deaths for which these factors account (McGinnis & Foege, 1994).

Attention to influential scientific articles regarding environmental and behavioral health dangers and the federal interest in cost reduction of health care expenses led to the development of the *Healthy People 2010* document by the U.S. Department of Health and Human Services (2000). This monograph is the most recent of several national initiatives to develop health objectives for the country, and it has spawned a number of similar state initiatives. Details of the plan are found in Chapter Three; in general it provides a plan of action for the nation's health, with two major goals: to increase quality and years of healthy life and to eliminate health disparities. This document, like its predecessors, mixes both a health promotion and a disease prevention approach, although the implementation of many of the aims of Healthy People 2010 acknowledges the ecology of health promotion. Individuals, groups, organizations, and policymakers are considered active agents in shaping health practices and policies to optimize both individual wellness and collective well-being. For example, through *Steps to a Healthier US* (2005), funds were granted to the Cherokee nation to implement a statewide anti-tobacco abuse media effort, including instituting smoking bans and restrictions in schools and expanding the availability of smoking cessation programs to two local industries.

Health Promotion

The health promotion strategies developed in the Healthy People documents are related to individual lifestyle—personal choices made in a social context—that can have a powerful influence over one's health prospects. These strategies target issues such as physical activity; nutrition; sexuality; tobacco, alcohol, and other drug use; oral health; mental health and mental disorders; and violent and abusive behavior. Educational and community-based programs can address lifestyle choices in a cross-cutting fashion.

Health Protection

The health protection strategies set out in these documents are related to environmental or regulatory measures that confer protection on large population groups. These strategies address issues such as unintentional injuries, occupational safety and health, environmental health, food and drug safety, and fluoridation of water for oral health. Interventions applied to address these issues generally are not exclusively protective—they may provide a substantial health promotion element as well—and the principal approaches involve a community-wide, rather than individual, focus.

Disease Prevention

The disease prevention model in these documents focuses on the avoidance of illness and agents of illness as well as the identification and minimization of risk. This approach is found throughout the health promotion literature, most particularly in the work of the U.S. Preventive Services Task Force (USPSTF), as discussed further in Chapter Three. Epidemiologic data are the foundation for the development of this model. Epidemiology focuses on how diseases originate and spread in populations (Lilienfeld, 1976).

In a preventive approach the natural history of the disease at issue is examined to identify the interrelationship between the outside etiologic, or causal, agents and the biological response of the host and to determine the effects of environmental, social, and physical factors; community patterns of medical care; and the social and intellectual response of the host (Leavell & Clark, 1953). The target of the preventive intervention is selected based on the prevalence (proportion of the population affected) and the incidence (number of new cases per year) of the condition. In the USPSTF's work the target conditions selected are relatively common in the United States and are of major clinical significance. The natural history of a disease may depend on environmental conditions, like the prevalence of asthma in areas of high air pollution compared to areas of low air pollution. Similarly, the natural history of a disease may show variations related to sociodemographic characteristics of the affected individuals, such as their race or ethnicity, or the health service characteristics of their communities, such as access to care (Hutchison, 1969).

The traditional triad of primary, secondary, and tertiary prevention is often used to distinguish approaches. Primary preventive measures are those provided to individuals to prevent the onset of a targeted condition (for example, routine immunization of healthy children). Secondary preventive measures identify and treat asymptomatic persons who have already developed risk factors or preclinical disease but in whom the condition has not become clinically apparent (for example, screening for high blood pressure). Tertiary preventive measures are those directed toward persons as part of the treatment and management of their clinical and chronic diseases (for example, cholesterol reduction in clients with coronary heart disease or insulin therapy to prevent the complications of diabetes mellitus) (USPSTF, 1996).

Risk Assessment

In the disease prevention orientation, individuals and groups are characterized by their absolute, relative, or attributable *risk* for various diseases and disorders. According to the Royal Society (1983), "Risk is the probability that a particular adverse event occurs during a stated period of time, or results from a particular challenge." In the field of epidemiology, *absolute risk* measures the magnitude of the incidence of disease in a population, *relative risk* measures the strength of an association between a risk and a disease (for example, between smoking and lung cancer), and *attributable risk* is a measure of how much of the disease risk (for example, risk for coronary heart disease) is attributable to a particular exposure (for example, smoking) (Gordis, 2000). The *population attributable fraction* (PAF) refers to the fraction of disease cases (or deaths) in a population that is associated with an exposure (for example, obesity), generally by age groups. These metrics are generally less meaningful at the level of the individual than they are for populations (Goodman, 2005).

A critical clinical issue for health care professionals is how to portray risk of disease to a client. As posited by the health belief model (to be discussed later in this chapter), whether individuals respond to a health threat depends in part on how large they perceive their personal risk to be. Even though the definition of risk denotes that the risk taker's behavior is harmful, the real or perceived benefits of smoking, eating, and drinking may be seen differently by the person engaging in the activity and by an outsider. As discussed in Chapter Three, typical presentations of health risks (for example, in the news) may do little to inform these perceptions (Woloshin, Schwartz, & Welch, 2002). Generally, health care professionals and clients are poorly prepared for discussions of health risks (Schwartz, Woloshin, & Welch, 1999; Fong, Rempel, & Hall, 1999; Woloshin, Schwartz, & Welch, 2002; Lipkus & Hollands, 1999).

Three characteristics are important in the discussion of risk: (1) *clarity* (the discussion should answer these questions: What is the risk? What are the numbers? What is the time period? and, How dangerous is the disease?); (2) *context* (the discussion should present comparisons, looking at the risk in terms of the risk for an average person of similar diseases, of leading causes of death, and of all-cause mortality); and (3) *acknowledgment of uncertainty* (the discussion should address whether the risk factor changes the client's overall risk or causes disease and the precision of this risk estimate). A recent review has identified practical guidelines for the visual presentation of risk, including the use of a *risk ladder* (Lipkus & Hollands, 1999).

The discussion of risk should take place in the context of *informed decision making* (or IDM); shared decision making occurs when the client and the health care professional together discuss the risks and benefits of a proposed decision. Informed decision making occurs when an individual understands the disease or condition being addressed and also comprehends what the clinical service involves, including its benefits, risks, limitations, alternatives, and uncertainties. In IDM the client has considered his or her own preferences, believes that he or she has participated in decision making at a level that he or she desires, and makes a decision consistent with those preferences (Sheridan, Harris, & Woolf, 2004). Numerous decision aids are available to assist with IDM (for a review see O'Connor et al., 2004; also see Llewellyn-Thomas, 1995; BayesMendel Lab, 2004 [for a breast cancer diagnostic tool]; Harvard Center for Cancer Prevention, Harvard School of Public Health, 2004 [for a disease risk tool]).

Example of a Large Community Risk Prevention Program

The Framingham Heart Study, begun in 1948 in the town of Framingham, Massachusetts, and funded by the National Heart, Lung, and Blood Institute (NHLBI), is an exemplary epidemiologic study with ramifications for community-based risk modification. The data derived from study of the original cohort of 5,209 healthy residents between thirty and sixty years of age, 5,124 of their children and spouses, and 500 members of the Framingham minority community have been used to develop approaches to reduce heart disease, stroke, dementia, osteoporosis, arthritis, diabetes, eye disease, and cancer and to understand the genetic patterns of many common diseases (NHLBI, 2005).

Differences Among the Health Promotion, Health Protection, and Disease Prevention Concepts

The critical difference among these concepts lies in the underlying motivation they offer for a particular behavior on the part of individuals and populations (Pender, 2006). Health promotion encourages well-being and is oriented toward the actualizing of human potential and thus is positive in valence, or attractive to the client. Health protection, however, is directed toward a desire to actively avoid illness, to detect it early, or to maintain function within the constraints of illness, and holds a negative valence. Disease prevention is similar to health protection in that one is taking action to thwart the disease process by finding ways to modify the environment, behavior, and bodily defenses so that disease processes are eliminated, slowed, or changed (Parse, 1987).

Environmental Approaches

The ecological model focuses specifically on the components of health-promotive environments. Within this context, some national policies, such as those establishing acceptable levels of air quality, may highlight the role of the environment in optimizing states of well-being; further, policies may emphasize the connection between well-being and one's social and physical milieu (Stokols, 1992).

In the environmental approaches, healthfulness is seen as a multifaceted phenomenon incorporating physical health, emotional well-being, and social cohesion. Health may result from concurrent interventions in transactions between persons and environments over time (Stokols, 1992) and reflects the outcomes of joint approaches at multiple levels.

Social Ecology Model

Ecology pertains to the interrelationships between organisms and their environments (Hawley, 1950). The social ecology approach is grounded in a contextual view of human health and well-being (Moos, 1979). It attends to the social, institutional, and cultural contexts of person-environment relations. The model assumes that the healthfulness of a situation and the well-being of its participants are influenced by multiple aspects of the environment—both physical (geography, architecture, and technology) and social (culture, economics, and politics—or the "social determinants of health"; Green & Kreuter, 2005). Characteristics of the environment interact with features of the individual such as genetic heritage, psychological predispositions, and behavioral patterns; health is a result of that interplay. Environments may vary, for example, in their lighting, temperature, noise levels, and space arrangements; these are seen both as objective characteristics and as factors that can be perceived differently by each person (or subjective characteristics). The meshing of a unique environment and a particular person is unique.

The social ecology model incorporates components of systems theory, such as the dynamic states of interdependence, homeostasis, negative feedback, and derivation amplification (Cannon, 1932; Emery & Trist, 1972; Katz & Kahn, 1966; Maruyama, 1963). Person-environment interactions move through cycles of mutual influence, where each affects the other. The varied levels of human environments, such as worksites, are seen as complex systems in which each level is nested in more complex and distant levels. For example, the occupational health and safety of community work settings is directly influenced by state and local ordinances aimed at protecting public health and environmental quality (Stokols, 1992).

Environments differ in their relative scale and complexity, and the participants in these contexts may be studied as individuals, small groups, organizations, and populations. Interventions may be strengthened by the coordination of individuals and groups acting in different environments, such as corporate managers who shape organizational health policies alongside diverse teams of workers or health insurance companies (Green & Kreuter, 1991, 1999; Pelletier, 1984; Winett,

King, & Altman, 1989). Further, individuals' physical and emotional well-being is enhanced when environments are personally controllable and predictable (Karasek & Theorell, 1990). Environments that are *too* predictable and controllable, however, constrain opportunities for coping effectively with novel situations, thus impeding growth (Aldwin & Stokols, 1988).

The social ecology model recognizes the oftentimes contradictory influences of environments and persons. For example, a socially supportive family or organization may enable individuals to cope more effectively with physical constraints (for example, overcrowding, drab surroundings). A well-designed physical environment may not, however, spur much health promotion if interpersonal or intergroup relations result in conflict and stress.

Research deriving from social ecology models focuses on characteristics of an environment and differentiates health outcomes in terms of their severity, duration, and overall importance to individuals functioning in that setting. Research designed to optimize or enhance environmental quality and human well-being is central to these approaches.

Social Network Approach

The social network approach is consonant with the core concepts of the social ecology model (Eng, 1993; Sheinfeld Gorin, 1997; Gotay & Wilson, 1998). Within the context of nested systems—families, peer groups, organizations, and larger communities—the individual creates a network of unique relationships within which he or she exchanges with others emotional (for example, esteem, trust), appraisal (for example, affirmation, social comparison), informational (for example, advice, directives), and instrumental support (for example, money, time) (House, Landis, & Umberson, 1988; House & Kahn, 1985). These support sources form the most salient norms and values to which the individual responds and also form critical information convoys, subsequently influencing an individual's healthy behaviors. Health care professionals may also influence health promotion, particularly screening and risk assessment decisions and behaviors; their behaviors are similarly influenced by the social norms of their referent group, particularly other influential providers (Fox, Murata, & Stein, 1991; Lane & Brug, 1990; Ashford et al., 2000; Mandelblatt & Yabroff, 1999).

The influence of social support on health is well established (Cohen & Syme, 1985; Stroebe & Stroebe, 1996); social support is linked to lower mortality (Berkman, 1985), greater resistance to communicable diseases (Cohen, 1988), lower prevalence and incidence of coronary heart disease (Seeman & Syme, 1987), and faster recovery from heart disease and heart surgery (Ruberman, Weinblatt, Goldberg, & Chaudhary, 1984). In general, individuals who have minimal psychosocial resources appear to be more prone to illness and mood disturbances when faced with increased stress levels than do individuals with considerable social support (DeLongis, Folkman, & Lazarus, 1988).

There are two ways in which social support is posited to affect health (Cohen & Syme, 1985; Cohen & Wills, 1985; Stroebe & Stroebe, 1996). The *buffering* hypothesis argues that people benefit from social support only when they experience a stressful life event; the support leads them to experience a lesser degree of stress in the face of a challenging situation. The *direct effect* hypothesis argues that social relationships promote health and well-being regardless of the individual's stress level; the support allows the individual to feel secure in the knowledge that help will be provided when and if necessary or it keeps him or her from feeling lonely.

Social support is linked with the hedonic elements of positive psychology. Through the stability, predictability, and control that it provides, social support leads people to feel positively about themselves and their environment. These feelings, in turn, motivate people to want to take care of themselves, interact more positively with others, and demonstrate resilience in times of stress. Further, compared with those who are dour, individuals who are happy find it easier to develop a rich network of social support.

Although the preponderance of the evidence suggests that social networks positively influence health-promoting behaviors, among some population subgroups social norms may discourage these behaviors (Sheinfeld Gorin, 1997). For example, African American women may have social networks that are fearful of orthodox medical care and thus not able to encourage them to engage in health protective activities such as breast cancer screening (Burg & Seeman, 1994). Or, as individuals receive information about unpleasant aspects of cancer screening—pain, for example—from their friends and family members, they may reappraise their screening intentions (Honda & Sheinfeld Gorin, 2005).

Positive Psychology Perspective

The study of the relationship between valued subjective experiences such as contentment and satisfaction (in the past), hope and optimism (for the future), and flow and happiness (in the present), as well as civic virtues at the group level—the elements of a meaningful life—is called *positive psychology* (Seligman & Csikszentmihalyi, 2000, p. 6). The primary building block of positive psychology is the hedonic quality of current experience (Kahneman, 1999, p. 6), that which makes one moment "better" than another.

Positive emotion has been most fully studied in relation to physical health (Salovey, Rothman, Detweiler, & Steward, 2000; Taylor, Kemeny, Reed, Bower, &

Gruenewald, 2000), although the buffering function of resilience has been the focus of mental health prevention research (Masten, 2001). Taylor et al.'s work (2000) suggests that, although it is generally assumed that it is healthy to be rigorously objective about one's situation (Peterson, 2000; Schwartz, 2000; Vaillant, 2000), unrealistically optimistic beliefs about the future can protect people from illness, such as AIDS. The positive effects of optimism are mediated at the cognitive level, with optimistic individuals more likely than others to practice habits that enhance health and enlist social support.

In the face of life-threatening illnesses, positive illusions may be adaptive in part because they help people to find meaning in the experience (Taylor, 1983). Further, people who are optimistic and hopeful are actually more likely than others to provide themselves with unfavorable information about their disease, thereby preparing themselves to face up to diagnostic, treatment, and curative realities (even though their positive outcome estimates may be inflated). It is also possible that positive affective states, like happiness, may have a direct physiological effect that retards the course of illness (Seligman & Csikszentmihalyi, 2000; Salovey et al., 2000).

Many of the empirical studies derived from this approach offer considerable promise for the practice of health promotion; yet a number of conceptual and methodological challenges to the development of knowledge in this field remain. Perhaps the most important near-term contribution of this approach is the recognition that the health care professional can inspire hope in others. The health care professional's positive expectations (even when administering a placebo, a pharmacologically inert substance that yields symptom relief in about 35 percent of all patients; Hafen, Karren, Frandsen, & Smith, 1996) can have a concrete impact on the health of the client (Salovey et al., 2000).

Social Marketing Model

Social marketing is a framework frequently used in designing, targeting, refining, and implementing health promotion programs (Kotler & Roberto, 1989; Manoff, 1985). It adapts the approach used in commercial marketing to the arena of health behavior. The marketing framework revolves around four P's: product, price, place, and promotion. The *product* is generally the program (for example, weight reduction) and any attitudes, beliefs, ideas, additional behaviors, and practices connected with the program or the behavior (for example, health as a value). *Price* refers to any psychological or social effort, opportunity, or monetary cost associated with the adoption and use of the product. *Place* is the distribution point for the product (for example, an HMO). *Promotion* refers to the means of informing a target audience about the product and persuading them to use it (for example, videos, brochures, and television spots). A fifth variable is *positioning*, which refers to the unique niche occupied by the product (for example, a weight reduction program for seniors). Finally, a sixth variable, *politics*, describes the social and economic context (for example, the reimbursement policies for weight control counseling) that can facilitate or hinder the marketing process.

Political Economy Approach

The assumption of the political economy model is that the activities of organizations (as well as communities, groups, families, and individuals) are accounted for by the political context (a structure of rule) and economic system (an organized means for producing and exchanging goods and services) in which they are embedded (Sheinfeld Gorin & Weirich, 1995). Fundamental to the relationships between organizations and their contexts is an exchange of resources, such as money, persons, information, space, and social legitimacy (or reputation). These exchanges create a set of political and economic interdependencies both within the organization (among staff and workgroups) and within its context (its funders, regulators, accreditors, and clients). An organization tends to be influenced by those who hold the political and economic resources the organization needs. Thus the organization attempts to satisfy the demands of a given outside (or inside) group when that group holds a resource critical to organizational survival or has discretion over organizational use of the resource and when few alternative sources of that resource exist. For example, major accrediting organizations such as the Joint Commission on Accreditation of Healthcare Organizations (JCAHO) can demand significant changes in an organization by withholding a desired recognition or their "stamp of approval" (see Chapter Three).

Behavioral Model of Health Care Utilization

The behavioral model of utilization, developed by Andersen and Aday (1978), is frequently used to analyze the factors associated with patient use of health care services, to develop policies and programs to encourage appropriate use of services, and to promote cost-effective care (Aday, 1993). This model has been quite influential as a conceptual base for the burgeoning field of health services research. It suggests that health care use patterns at the individual level are influenced by predisposing, enabling, and need-related factors as well as environmental conditions.

Individuals are predisposed to use health care services by their genetic inheritance, sociodemographic factors such as age, social structure elements such as race or ethnicity, educational attainment, and knowledge of, beliefs about, or attitudes toward the use of health care. Factors that may enable or impede use of health care services include family income, health insurance coverage, a regular source of care, and travel and waiting times; at the community level they include the location, size, and number of providers or health care facilities, as well as provider characteristics such as gender and age (Phillips, Morrison, Andersen, & Aday, 1998). The individual's need for care may be influenced by both perceived and evaluated illness (for example, both self-rated health status and diagnosis).

Environmental variables such as health care delivery system characteristics, factors external to that system, and community-level enabling factors influence the individual's predisposing, enabling, and need factors (Andersen & Newman, 1973). Health care delivery system characteristics include policies, resources, organization, and financial arrangements influencing the accessibility, availability, and acceptability of medical care services (such as physician supply); these characteristics also reflect the economic climate, relative wealth, politics, level of stress and violence, and prevailing norms of the community.

PRECEDE-PROCEED Model

The PRECEDE-PROCEED model, developed by Lawrence Green (1974), was originally intended to influence the planning of health education programs. Over the past thirty years (and over 950 references to its use), the model has been expanded to include policy, regulatory, and organizational constructs in educational and environmental development that are generally regarded as central to the field of health promotion. The model seeks to address the question: "How do we best promote change in a powerful, coherent way?" (Best et al., 2003).

Health promotion planning proceeds in phases (Green & Kreuter, 1991, 2005), is ecological in orientation, and participatory in implementation. From the start, the health promotion plan is designed to follow a sequence of steps that are aligned with a logic model of causes and effects. In Phase I, the health care professional conducts a social assessment of the quality of life experienced by those whom the program might affect. For example, a program might focus on general social problems of concern to individuals or communities, such as alienation (social detachment or separation) among adolescents. The professional then evaluates specific health problems that appear to be contributing to the social problems (for example, the incidence of substance abuse among adolescents). In Phase II of the model, epidemiological, behavioral, and environmental assessment, specific behaviors that appear to be linked with the health problems are identified (for example, the frequency and duration of use of several kinds of drugs and alcohol). Both (qualitative) community self-study, using, for example, focus groups (Basch, 1987), and current, valid and reliable local epidemiologic data inform this step. (For detailed descriptions of common epidemiologic measures, see Gordis, 2000; Green & Kreuter, 2005, p. 90, also provide a simple comparison of these measures for planning purposes.)

As in the behavioral model of health care utilization, in the PRECEDE-PROCEED model, at Phase III, educational and ecological assessment, the health care professional identifies predisposing and enabling factors. In addition, in the PRECEDE-PROCEED model, because the focus is on those determinants of behavior over which educational and organizational strategy and policy could have a direct influence, *need* is replaced with *reinforcing factors*, and sociodemographic characteristics (such as gender) are removed from the predisposing influences on behavior (in this example, substance abuse). Predisposing factors that affect an individual's willingness to change include knowledge, attitudes, values, and perceptions, such as those identified previously and those discussed in relation to the health belief model later in this chapter. Enabling factors that may facilitate or present obstacles to change include the availability and accessibility of skills, resources, and barriers that help or hinder the desired behavior; the PRECEDE framework puts particular emphasis on barriers created by social forces or systems, such as insurance coverage, health care professional practices, and the location of or access to treatment resources. Reinforcing factors refer to rewards and feedback that are given to persons adopting and continuing a certain behavior. Reinforcements could include social support, advice, and feedback by health care providers, as well as images provided by the mass media. Proximal behaviors, or those that influence one's own or immediate others' health, are targets for change, as well as more distal policy or organizational change (Green & Kreuter, 2005).

In Phase IV, administrative and policy assessment and intervention alignment, the budgetary, personnel, and other resources; policies; abilities; and time necessary to make the program a reality are inventoried and examined. In this example, the health planner might link community members with funding sources to establish a school-based brief treatment center. In Phase V, a program to combat the problem is developed and implemented. While "evaluation is an integral and continuous part of planning that is separably tied to measurable objectives generated from the beginning of the first steps of the process" (Green & Kreuter, 2005, p. 16) at Phase VI, formal process evaluation is conducted, followed by impact and outcome evaluation in Phases VII and VIII. In this example the program is evaluated (for example, by clients and community members, who are provided with technical assistance from a university) as an integral and continuing part of program planning; both the short-term program or community and any longer-term societal effects are delineated (cf. Fawcet et al., 1995; Green & Kreuter, 1991, 2005).

Social Responsibility Model

The social responsibility model, so named because of the primacy attached to the value of government intervention on behalf of health and the model's focus on health as an end rather than as a means, is best expressed in the work of several British commissions (for example, the Black Report and the Acheson Report) and in the writings of Downie, Fyfe, and Tannahill (1990). The definition of health promotion in this model is expansive and assumes that health is a value to be pursued in its own right.

At the microlevel, these reports and writings argue, individuals have a moral duty to do what they can to improve their own health. Well-being is a value of its own; positive pleasures accrue to the healthy. At the macrolevel, they contend, health is a value that governments should promote and that access to health is a fundamental right that government must implement. Their approach has influenced recent WHO initiatives that view health as a multisectoral responsibility.

Life Course Models

Two general models are based on the concept of change over time: innovation diffusion and the stages of change. Life course is an appropriate metaphor for the patterns of change experienced by an individual, family, group, community, or populations over time. Transitions are met by social and cultural constructions around the meaning of health that change from one stage of life to another. For example, parenthood may be seen as a time when individuals reflect on "having no time" to keep healthy or physically fit (Backett & Davison, 1995, p. 635).

Demographics are also key to life course models. The relative proportions of the various groups in society can have enormous effects on societal definitions of health promotion and the value placed on them. This is evident in the demographic transitions developed nations are experiencing as a result of increases in the numbers of elderly individuals and in their proportion relative to other members of the population.

Health is a dynamic process that reflects cumulative experience and expression of genes over the life course (Susser & Terry, 2003). The framework highlights the influence of genetic, biological, behavioral, social, and economic contexts on development over the life span of individuals and populations, as well as intergenerational associations (Best et al., 2003; Halfon & Hochstein, 2002; Institute of Medicine, 2001; Ben-Shlomo & Kuh, 2002).

Four life course concepts hold particular promise for understanding health promotion. First, embedding, the process by which experiences are programmed into the structure and functioning of biological and behavioral systems (Hertzman, 1999; Best et al., 2003), suggests that there are critical and sensitive times to influence change. Critical times are those periods in development when changes are wholly or partially irreversible (for example, limb development in relation to maternal thalidomide use; Lynch & Davey Smith, 2005). Sensitive periods are also times of rapid change but there is more scope to modify or even reverse the changes outside of the temporal window (Ben-Shlomo & Kuh, 2002). For example, if exposure to human papillomavirus (HPV) through sexual intercourse occurs at an earlier rather than later age, the risk of infection leading to cervical cancer is increased (Munoz et al., 2003; Schiffman & Brinton, 1995).

Second, change over time is influenced by the net effect of risks and protective factors. Third, many early influences yield health outcomes later in life. The importance of early intervention on lifetime health has long been an axiom for students of human development. Fourth, it is important to examine changes over the life span rather than the short term (Best et al., 2003). In an example of these three points, historical cohort studies have found that through the influence of adverse maternal environments (malnutrition; stress; exposure to tobacco, drugs, and alcohol) birth weight, placenta size, and weight gain in the first years of life are associated with cardiovascular disease and other chronic diseases such as diabetes and hypertension in the fifth and sixth decades of life (Barker, 1998; Martyn, Barker, & Osmond, 1996; Rich-Edwards et al., 1997). Cholesterol, blood pressure, and overweight measured at young ages track, although imperfectly, into adulthood (Bao, Threefoot, Srinivasan, & Berenson, 1995; Kvaavik, Tell, & Klepp, 2003; Lauer & Clarke, 1990; Mahoney, Lauer, Lee, & Clarke, 1991), increasing risks for coronary heart disease, stroke, and type 2 diabetes. The age at smoking cessation is key to reducing risk for coronary heart disease, chronic obstructive pulmonary disease, and many cancers (detailed in Chapter Nine); risk declines fairly rapidly after cessation (Doll, Peto, Boreham, & Sutherland, 2004; Kawachi et al., 1994; Peto et al., 2000; Wannamethee, Shaper, Whincup, & Walker, 1995). More broadly, Keating and Hertzman (1999) speculate that the fundamental processes, such as neural sculpting, that affect brain and behavioral development interact with the growing chaos in the lives of children and adolescents with long-term effects on human capital and thus the wealth of nations. In short, this approach suggests that health represents the outcome of a trajectory of development over the life course.

Innovation Diffusion Theory

The innovation diffusion theory addresses the contexts within which innovations are adopted and used. *Innovations*—defined as new and qualitatively different ideas over time—require some conceptual reorientation among participants (Delbecq,

1978). Innovation adoption and use are influenced by three major factors: (1) the innovation itself, (2) the environment, and (3) the client system. For example, some clients may feel that the PACE exercise program described in Chapter Six is an innovation. The characteristics of the innovation itself (for example, its triability, relative advantage, observability, initial fit with the client's needs, ability to be reinvented to match or be adapted to changing needs, and simplicity) may affect its adoption and use. These characteristics emphasize the importance of tailoring an innovation's attributes to achieve its objectives.

According to innovation diffusion theory, one health care environment may differ from another in its affluence, complexity, rate of change, extent of conflict, and degree of cooperation—all of which influence the adoption and use of new ideas and programs (for example, local political support encourages the adoption of and use of health promotion programs, such as PACE). Finally, the client system itself (for example, the HMO within which the PACE program operates) may differ from that of other primary care settings in affluence; governance; structure; age; size; complexity; mission; degree of vulnerability; orientation toward, support of, and rate of change; cooperativeness; power; and extent of control over its members. These too affect the extent of adoption and use of innovations (Sheinfeld Gorin & Weirich, 1995).

When new, a health promotion program may move through the stages of adoption (from evaluation of the idea to initiation of the program to implementation and finally to routine use). Similarly, the use of a program may increase as the program continues (or decrease as it fails) to influence understanding among clients. Furthermore, persons exposed to a health promotion program may be classified, on the basis of their innovativeness, as innovators, early adopters, early majority, late majority, or late adopters. In community-based health promotion programs, new ideas, which are often first reported by the mass media, are mediated and modified through opinion leaders, who are often early adopters. The majority of persons are then influenced through interpersonal contact with opinion leaders, who are seen as credible sources of information. Collaboration among these leaders assists in both interpreting the needs of communities exposed to health promotion programs and encouraging the adoption of new ideas (Rogers, 1983). These leaders encourage adoption by eventually persuading the majority of persons, which may occur earlier or later in the process of adoption.

The introduction of new behaviors that diffuse through a client system is achieved by both mass and interpersonal communication. The success of mass communication depends on five factors: the credibility of the source, the content and design of the message, the delivery channel, the target audience, and the target behavior (McGuire, 1981). *Persuasion* refers to any type of social influence. For persuasion to take place, a message must be conveyed, the person(s) must receive and comprehend the message and be convinced by it, the message must be retained, and there must be behavioral manifestations that change has taken place. The aim of persuasion is to introduce inconsistency in two related beliefs; that, according to social adaptation theory, will lead to a reinterpretation of social reality (Fincham, 1992).

Stages of Change

The stages of change, or transtheoretical, model is based on the assumption that individuals move through a series of predictable stages when changing a behavior, such as stopping smoking or beginning an exercise program. These changes include the following stages (DiClemente, 1991; Prochaska & DiClemente, 1983; Prochaska, Velicer, Guadagnoli, Rossi, & DiClemente, 1991):

1. *Precontemplation* (considering the change)
2. *Contemplation* (starting to think about initiating change)
3. *Preparation* (seriously thinking about the change within a given time period [for example, the next six months] or taking early steps to change)
4. *Action* (making a change in or stopping the target behavior within a six-month period)
5. *Maintenance of change* (maintaining the target behavior change for more than six months; preventing relapse)

These stages are not necessarily linear. For example, the average smoker who quits reports at least several and often many relapses before achieving maintained abstinence (Fisher, Bishop, Goldmuntz, & Jacobs, 1988). The stages of change model may, however, suggest intervention points for different individuals at varied stages (Prochaska et al., 1991). In particular it has been used to explain smoking cessation and physical activity changes in individuals, as well as beginning cancer screening (Honda & Sheinfeld Gorin, 2006).

The mechanisms that drive movement through the stages are called the *processes of change* (Prochaska & DiClemente, 1983). These processes draw heavily on components of other models, such as the health belief model.

The transtheoretical model also addresses the general element of decision making regarding adoption of a behavior, using a decisional balance approach. Decisional balance compares the strength of the target behavior's perceived pros with that of the perceived cons. The relative weights persons assign to a behavior's pros and cons influences their decisions about behavioral change (Janis & Mann, 1977), such as continuing or ceasing to smoke.

Health Attitude, Belief, and Behavioral Change Approaches

The following four major theories—the health belief model, the theory of planned behavior, prospect theory, and social learning theory—along with their corollaries and derivative models identify different health-promotive paths for individuals or groups. Each model posits a trajectory for change in attitudes, beliefs, or behaviors.

Health Belief Model

The intention of one of the most prominent of these theories, the health belief model (modified by Becker, 1986), was to determine why some persons who are illness-free take actions to avoid illness, whereas others fail to take protective actions. Another aim of the health belief model was to predict the conditions under which people would engage in simple preventive behaviors, such as immunizations. The model was founded on the work of Kurt Lewin, who understood that the life space in which individuals live is composed of regions, some having a negative valence (one would seek to avoid), some a positive valence (one would seek to approach), and some a neutral valence (one would neither seek to approach nor avoid) (Lewin, Dembo, Festinger, & Sears, 1944).

The health belief model suggests that before an individual takes action, he or she must decide that the behavior, whether it be smoking, eating fatty foods, or engaging in unprotected sexual activity, creates a serious health problem; that he or she is personally susceptible to this health harm; and that moderating or stopping the behavior will be beneficial. The perceived barriers to undertaking a behavior are considered most salient to health-promotive efforts (Janz & Becker, 1984). A person's perceived susceptibility to a disease and perceived severity of harm are based to a great extent on that person's knowledge of the disease and its potential outcome. Although the combination of perceived susceptibility to harm and severity of harm provides the force for action and the perception of high benefits and low barriers provides a course of action, it is the *cues to action* that start the process of change (Rosenstock, 1974).

In an expansion of the health belief model, a separate construct of general health motivation was added. Motives are viewed as dispositions within which individuals approach certain categories of positive incentives. For example, the desire to maintain a state of good health is a component of health motivation (Becker, Drachman, & Kirscht, 1974; Maiman & Becker, 1984; Curry & Emmons, 1994). In the last ten years the health belief model has subsumed the self-efficacy construct from social cognitive theory to better explain health behaviors (Rosenstock, Strecher, & Becker, 1988).

Protection Motivation Theory

Protection motivation theory uses health threats, or fear appeals, to change behavior by highlighting the harmful personal consequences of health-damaging behaviors. For example, a program to encourage substance safety among teens might use pictures of dead addicts under white sheets in the morgue and explicit warnings against drug use. The model identifies two parallel processes in health behavior change: (1) cognitive processes involving representation of the health threat and the efficacy of available coping responses (for example, perceived risks of lung cancer and health benefits of quitting smoking) and (2) emotional or affective processes involving fear arousal (Orleans, Rotberg, Quade, & Lees, 1990; Velicer, DiClemente, Prochaska, & Brandenburg, 1985). The more personally salient the health risks are, the greater the motivational impact of the information. Empirical tests of protection motivation theory further suggest that threat appeals, rather than the emotional state of fear itself, strengthen long-sustained cognitive structures (that is, beliefs in the severity of the danger), as fear declines rapidly (Rogers, Deckner, & Mewborn, 1978). Generally, however, because of the difficulty of determining the appropriate timing and dose of fear, the promotion of healthy alternative behaviors is more effective (Job, 1988).

Cognitive-Social Health Information–Processing Model. The cognitive-social health information–processing model (C-SHIP) (Miller, Shoda, & Hurley, 1996) is a broad theoretical framework that incorporates both cognitive and affective responses to threats to health, primarily those responses related to cancer prevention and control (Leventhal, Safer, & Panagis, 1983; Miller, 1995; Shoda et al., 1998). According to the C-SHIP model, there are four distinctive cognitive-emotional processes that underlie the information processing of cancer risk information: (1) individuals' self-construals of their risk, including their knowledge levels and perceived risk; (2) their expectancies about the benefits and limitations of specific cancer-related actions; (3) their health values (for example, fatalistic attitudes about cancer); and (4) their cancer-specific emotional distress. A unique contribution of the model for health promotion is its description of *high monitors* (who scan for, and magnify, threatening cues) and *low monitors* (who distract from, and downgrade, threatening information) (Miller, 1995). Counseling strategies may be more effective when they are systematically tailored to the specific cognitive and affective profiles of individuals as they engage in health-promoting behaviors such as cancer screening (Miller, Shoda, & Hurley, 1996).

Theory of Planned Behavior

Ajzen and Fishbein (1980) developed the theory of reasoned action, later modified as the theory of planned behavior (TPB), which is a mathematical description of the relationship among beliefs (verbalized opinions), attitudes (judgments that a behavior is good or bad and that a person favors or is against performing the behavior), and intentions in determining action. The theory postulates that most volitional behavior can be predicted by beliefs, attitudes, and intentions; therefore efforts to change behavior should be directed at an individual's belief system. By altering the beliefs' underlying attitudes or norms, changes in behavioral intentions, and subsequently in behavior, can also be induced (Ajzen & Fishbein, 1980). According to the TPB (Ajzen, 2002), perceived behavioral control, even when not particularly realistic, can affect behavior indirectly by its impact on *intention*.

First, the health care provider identifies and measures the behavior to be changed. Once the behavior is defined, he or she may specify the determinants. A person's intention to perform (or not perform) a behavior is the immediate determinant of the action. Second, the person's intention is a function of two other determinants: (a) the person's attitude toward the behavior and (b) the person's subjective norm, or perception of the social pressures to perform or not perform the behavior in question (Ajzen & Fishbein, 1980). Individuals will intend to perform a behavior, such as brushing their teeth, when they evaluate it positively and when they believe that important others, such as parents, think they should perform it. The relative weights of the attitudinal and normative factors may vary from one person to another; thus one person may attach more weight to attitude; another to normative influences.

Further, attitudes are a function of behavioral and normative beliefs, perceived consequences of behavior, and the person's evaluation of these. The social or normative factor consists of the opinions of important referent individuals or groups (such as parents or peers). The person's motivation to comply with those opinions reflects a sense of the consequences of conforming (or not).

Specificity of intentions is highlighted in this theory. An action, such as exercising, is always performed with respect to a given target (for example, walking rather than running), in a particular context (for example, at work), and at a given time (for example, during lunch) (Ajzen & Fishbein, 1980). The theory also considers external variables (for example, access to family planning services for women using birth control) as influencing a person's beliefs or the relative importance a person attaches to attitudinal and normative considerations. Finally, the individual controls the relationship between the intention to act and the behavior. In a classic example, if a female maintains a positive attitude toward using birth control pills, is supported by a set of family and community norms supporting the use of contraception, and intends to use birth control pills, ultimately she will use them (Fishbein, Jaccard, Davidson, Ajzen, & Loken, 1980).

Prospect Theory

Prospect theory is a descriptive model that accounts for choice and decision-making strategies under conditions of risk (Kahneman & Tversky, 1984). The assumptions of the theory are threefold. First, risk decisions are influenced by subjective evaluations of relative gains and losses, as opposed to objective evaluations of absolute outcomes. Second, persons tend to make risk-averse choices for sure *gain* and to make risk-seeking choices for a gamble over a sure *loss*. Third, the theory states that the degree to which a choice (or behavior) is seen as a gain or a loss can vary depending on how the consequences of the behavior are presented, or *framed* (Curry & Emmons, 1994, p. 309).

When behavioral choices involve some risk or uncertainty, individuals will be more likely to take these risks when information is framed in terms of relative disadvantages (that is, losses or costs) of the outcomes. When behavioral choices involve little risk or uncertainty, individuals prefer options for which information is framed by relative advantages (that is, gains or benefits). Choosing to perform prevention behaviors (for example, wearing a condom) is a risk-averse option for maintaining good health; these behaviors should be promoted with gain-framed messages. For example, "using a condom during sexual intercourse can help to keep you healthy" (Salovey & Williams-Piehota, 2004). Behaviors involving an uncertain, potentially negative outcome (that is, risk), including detection behavior for HIV among asymptomatic or low-risk individuals, should be promoted with loss-framed messages. For example, "failing to use a condom during sexual intercourse exposes you to various sexually transmitted diseases such as HIV/AIDS" (Salovey & Williams-Piehota, 2004). Prospect theory has been applied to breast cancer screening, sunscreen use, HIV testing, condom use, and dental mouth washes. These approaches are distinguished from the fear appeals of protection motivation theory that do not frame messages by the salience of the risk.

Social Learning Theory

Social learning theory holds that behavior is determined by expectancies and incentives. Two approaches reflect this general theory: stimulus response theory and social cognitive theory. The role of cognition separates these two models. In social cognitive theory, expectancies are cognitive, or developed in the mind of the individual. Cognitive expectations (for example, feeling capable of stopping) influence the conduct of a behavior (for example, stopping smoking). In stimulus response theory, cognitive mediators are not present.

Stimulus Response Theory. Stimulus response theory rests on the belief that learning results from events (called reinforcements or consequences of behavior) that reduce physiological drives (for example, tension or anxiety) that activate behavior. Behavioral analysis relies on classic operant conditioning techniques. It involves objective definitions of the actions to be changed, measurable procedures for change, and an emphasis on antecedent and consequent events to change behavior. Over time, individuals may be conditioned to respond to cues in their environment by associating behaviors with them (for example, associating smoking with a stimulus such as a cup of coffee in the morning). To extinguish such conditioned responses, the individual must be exposed to the conditioned stimulus (for example, the coffee) without presentation of the unconditioned stimulus (for example, a cigarette) (Rachlin, 1991).

Similarly, several other principles of behavioral analysis (for example, the use of contingency management, feedback and goal setting, sharing and successive approximation, modeling, and prompting) may be applied successfully to encourage healthy behaviors. Contingency management involves a system of attaching rewards (for example, praise) to goal attainment (for example, losing weight). The initiation and maintenance of behavioral change may be accomplished by providing feedback and rewards so that the positive behavior itself becomes reinforcing. For example, healthy eating practices may be reinforced by teaching individuals to prepare appealing, simple, and quick meals (Kelly et al., 1992). The likelihood of the behavior itself becoming reinforcing is increased when successive approximations (intermediate goals) are used with shaping tactics (Kazdin, 1994). In these procedures, individuals performing behaviors that are within their repertoires take the next step on a goal attainment gradient, with each (subgoal) behavior having a higher likelihood of being reinforced. Programs teaching dieters how to lose weight begin with a low-fat variation of a meal dieters usually enjoy (such as vegetarian, rather than cheese, pizza). Further, such programs make strategic use of models, such as successful program graduates.

Social Cognitive Theory. Social cognitive theory developed from the stimulus response and earlier classical conditioning theories and extends its central concepts. The cornerstone of the model is the *reciprocal determinism* between cognition, behavior, and environment (Bandura, 1986, p. 22). Rather than focusing on the automatic shaping of behavior by environmental forces, social cognitive theory emphasizes the importance of intervening thought processes (for example, information acquisition, storage, and retrieval) and the importance of self-control for the performance of behavior. Most learning occurs through modeling, such as watching others prepare and eat meals, rather than trial and error. These vicarious and symbolic learning processes are affected by social influences. Self-regulatory processes, including self-generated inducements and consequences (for example, telling oneself to exercise daily so that one can climb a flight of stairs more easily) are highlighted in the theory. Social cognitive theory posits that the social environment, through the mechanism of social norms, affects a person's cognition and behavior.

Self-efficacy is a central concept in the application of social cognitive theory to health promotion. According to social cognitive theory (Bandura, 1986), both outcome and efficacy expectations are critical to behavioral change, such as modifying a diet. An outcome expectation is one's estimate that a given behavior (such as wearing the nicotine patch) can produce a given outcome, such as maintenance of smoking cessation. Self-efficacy is the conviction that one can execute this behavior successfully. Individuals high in self-efficacy, or more confident of their ability to maintain behavioral changes (for example, smoking cessation or ideal weight), will attempt to execute it more readily, with greater intensity, and with greater perseverance in response to initial failure than will individuals with comparatively lower self-efficacy (Baer & Lichtenstein, 1988; Devins, 1992).

Social cognitive theory posits that change occurs in phases: (1) promotion and motivation of persons toward changing a target behavior; (2) skills training so that individuals can acquire specific behavioral change skills; (3) development of support networks so that a new behavior can be maintained; (4) maintenance of the behavior through reinforcement; and (5) generalization to all levels of interaction, from the family to the community (Lefebvre, Lasater, Carleton, & Peterson, 1987).

Self-efficacy has been distinguished from locus of control, a similar concept. Locus of control is a generalized concept about the self, whereas self-efficacy is situation-specific (that is, it is focused on one's beliefs about one's personal abilities in specific settings).

Overlapping Constructs in the Theory of Planned Behavior, Social Cognition Theory, and the Stages of Change Model.

Several theories and models discussed so far have some overlapping constructs, suggesting the need for a more parsimonious understanding of the social psychological *pathways* by which beliefs, attitudes, values, and cognitions affect behavioral change. Perceived behavioral control, a feature of the theory of planned behavior, is considered conceptually similar to self-efficacy (Ajzen, 1991, 2002), also a concept in the stages of change (or transtheoretical) model and social cognitive theory. It may be that the nature of the influence of intention and the nature of the influence of stage of change on behavior are similar. Given that *self-efficacy* refers to "beliefs in one's capabilities to organize and execute the course of action required to produce given levels of attainment" (Bandura, 1998, p. 624), both perceived behavioral control and self-efficacy are similarly concerned with one's perceived ability to perform a sequence of behaviors (Ajzen, 2002). Further, pros and cons in the stages of change model are considered conceptually similar to the behavioral beliefs that shape attitude toward a behavior in the theory of planned behavior (Ajzen, 1991).

Health Promotion Matrix

A novel, as yet untested theory-based practice model for health promotion, the health promotion matrix (HPM) (Sheinfeld Gorin & Arnold, 1998; see Figure 2.1), provides an organizing framework for assessing client systems and guiding them toward health. The matrix equips the health care professional with an understanding of the client's images of health, a means for working with those images, and specific behaviors with which the professional and client may work. It gives the professional a means for understanding the client's view of health and a blueprint for maximizing health-promotive behaviors within varied contexts. Through the use of the matrix, the health care professional can assist the individual to modify his or her behavior, engage a group or family in altering a pattern of actions, or enlist the support of a community in changing health care policies.

At the core of the matrix is the notion of a health image. A *health image* is a picture, or concept, of health in the client's mind. The image is the client's representation of health, and as such, can serve as a motivating force for change. Health care professionals may examine the client's image of health from two per-

FIGURE 2.1. THE HEALTH PROMOTION MATRIX.

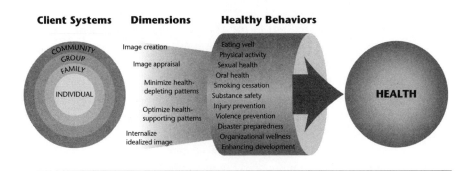

spectives: first, from the client's idealized picture of personal health and, second, relative to the client's current health. These two perspectives can then be juxtaposed in a dynamic comparison to reveal the discrepancies, or gaps, between them. Ultimately, the client's current health status will be altered through the adoption of health-promotive activities necessary to better realize the idealized picture.

The HPM is a multicomponent model, along whose dimensions, client systems, and positive, or healthy, behaviors (discussed in Chapters Five through Fifteen) each client may be located. To some extent all the models of change described earlier in this chapter form the basis for the HPM. Applied as part of the clinical process, the matrix assists health care professionals to individualize client care by identifying clients' unique health images, strengths, and capabilities and to focus on specific behaviors appropriate to each client's need. Further, the matrix assumes a reorientation of the health care professional's thinking toward the multiplicity of forces—biological, psychological, social, political, economic, cultural, and spiritual—impinging on clients as they begin the change process (Butterfield, 1990).

An intervention using the health promotion matrix involves the following five processes.

Image Creation

The concept of the health image is unique to this model. Entry into the HPM begins with the client picturing, or creating, an idealized image of health; it is the client's snapshot of his or her desired self. These images are often rich and varied and may emphasize the totality of being. The health care professional assists the client in clarifying or detailing his or her definition of health and the relative value health holds for him or her. In conjunction with the health care professional, the client crystallizes a positive and holistic image of health, one that is less encumbered by barriers and obstacles that he or she may have encountered in the past. This image becomes the aim of all subsequent intervention efforts.

For example, to assist the client in trying to create an image of himself or herself as a healthy person, the health care professional may ask the following: What do you see if you try to picture yourself as healthy? What would you like to be? or, How would you like to see yourself in relation to health? Questions such as these assist the client in visualizing an image of himself or herself as healthy. The sketch of one's healthy self may be made on paper or described verbally and may require more than one session to complete. The more specific and detailed the image, the more the health care professional can assist the client during image appraisal in recognizing what steps may be taken to achieve change.

Image Appraisal

During image appraisal the health care professional and the client define the client's current health status. As the health care professional and the client begin to examine the client's idealized view of health relative to the client's present state, a gap often emerges.

Beginning with an attempt to determine the client's motivation for change, the health care professional may ask about any change attempts, with questions such as these: Have you ever made any changes in yourself or your behavior? When did you make those changes? and, Were you able to sustain those changes? To assist the client in identifying the gap between the image and present health practices (in relation to the positive health behaviors described in Chapters Five through Fifteen), the health care professional may direct a series of queries to the client, starting with, for example: How do you feel about being a cigarette smoker? or, more specifically, Do you have a car seat for your baby? The image appraisal step often ends with the health care professional asking the client about changing present health practices to match those of the idealized image, with a question such as, Are you interested in an educational program about taking care of your teeth during pregnancy? Once the gap has been identified and, often, a commitment to change made, both client and professional begin the next steps in the process of change.

Minimize Health-Depleting Patterns

The health care professional may now assist the client in identifying depleting and supporting behaviors for one or more of the healthy behaviors. The matrix enables the client, in conjunction with the health care professional, to analyze patterns that are either health depleting or health promotive and to begin to change them. Often this proceeds in a problem-solving manner, moving from assessing the issues to developing choices, outlining alternatives, and evaluating each one, and then deciding on the optimal course of action.

Because the client may need assistance in altering a number of behaviors to narrow the gap between the ideal and the actual state, this process may take place over an extended time period. Together, the health care professional and the client prioritize the intervention areas.

To understand the depleting behaviors the health care professional may ask the client to list behaviors that are damaging, such as eating a high-fat, high-sugar diet or failing to engage in behaviors known to protect health, such as wearing a seat belt while driving. Barriers to behavioral change may rest in physiological forces, such as a craving; psychological attitudes, beliefs, or intentions toward change; social and cultural norms or patterns supporting certain behaviors; or economic, political, or spiritual factors. Lack of accessibility, few community resources, limited motivation to change, family members who support less healthy eating patterns, and a stressful job are examples of barriers that may prevent the client from taking the first step toward change. The health care professional seeks to specify the techniques or tools that may assist the client to change.

Optimize Health-Supportive Patterns

Optimizing supportive behaviors involves recognizing efforts toward undertaking healthy practices. Often clients are given recognition only when a health goal is reached, as though health itself were a static and absolute state of being. A client who envisions a healthy ideal of weighing fifty pounds less than his or her present weight could, however, receive praise and encouragement for every effort made toward altering eating patterns, regularly monitoring his or her weight, or redefining the meaning and purpose food holds in his or her life. Every instance of success is then recognized as a gain, and the client is rewarded with support and encouragement by the health care professional. Similarly, the health care professional and the client may identify other health-promotive beliefs, attitudes, and behaviors in which the client already engages. For example, a client may wear a seat belt on a regular basis, a family may join together for a balanced meal at least once a day, or a community may lobby for additional bike paths—all of which are health promotive and have the potential to optimize health. These positive health actions provide the energy necessary to contend with depleting behaviors (that is, to continue the process of change).

Internalize the Idealized Image

At this point in the change process the client has begun to close the gap between the idealized image and his or her real health status. The health care professional now assists the client to strive for greater consistency in daily actions relative to the pictured image of health. These new patterns no longer require constant surveillance. The no-longer-idealized-but-realized behaviors become part of the client's health status.

The health care professional continues to praise the client for the changed behaviors but also reviews the plan for further modifications so that the behaviors might be maintained indefinitely. Any problems with the intervention are noted, and supports are bolstered. The health care professional asks the client how she or he may be of further help and reaffirms the client's plan (for example, to remain at a healthy weight) for a specific length of time (for example, six months).

The health care professional's intent is to stabilize the altered health behaviors. As one set of behaviors is changed the health care professional and the client may review the idealized image of health and the new present state, using the HPM, to determine the next starting point for change.

The process of moving from image creation and image appraisal, through minimizing depleting patterns and optimizing supportive patterns, toward internalizing an idealized image of health is repetitive, involving reevaluations and reformulations of intervention foci. With the continued support of the health care professional, the client needs to periodically formulate alternative strategies to move again toward an idealized image of health. In addition, as a client grows and develops, his or her ideals could change. It is also possible that a client might never reach the idealized state; nonetheless the client may find success in the adoption of some health-sustaining patterns. The health care professional encounters clients in a multitude of states and contexts; the potential for supporting, protecting, and enhancing health is always a challenge.

Spirituality as a Health Promotion Construct

Many popular books, newspaper articles, and radio and television programs have been devoted to the concept of spirituality. Historically, spirituality, known as *spiritualism,* has been found within the purview of religion and has been fostered by religious groups and institutions. More recently, as some persons are returning to religious institutions to renew their spiritual sense, others are redefining their connections to traditional religions to create a spiritual dimension. Within the context of religion, *spirituality* may be defined as follows: "The spiritual core is the deepest center of the person. It is here that the person is open to the transcendent dimension; it is here that the person experiences ultimate reality. [Spirituality] explores the discovery of this core, the dynamics of its development, and its journey to the ultimate goal. It deals with prayer, spiritual direction, the various maps of the spiritual journey, and the methods of advancement in the spiritual ascent" (Cousins, 1987, p. x).

Spiritual support for health promotion may be defined as perceived support from a higher power (or powers), a sense of self-love, or a sense of connectedness to others in the experience of being human. Spirituality may be manifest in an individual's beliefs (for example, in a higher power or in the power of self-love), rituals (for example, setting out candles for dead relatives), or other practices (for example, attending a synagogue, church, or other religious institution; praying; meditating; or challenging injustice).

Several interventions that explicitly use spirituality to promote health are found in the health promotion field; they include therapeutic touch (*laying-on of hands*), directed healing (by healers), distant healing (intercessory prayer), and spiritism (*espiritismo*, a healing system used with the aid of a spiritist). To bring the body, mind, and spirit together, meditation (the attempt to achieve awareness without thought) is often practiced. Mindfulness, a moment-to-moment, nonjudgmental awareness, in the Zen tradition often obtained through meditation, has been applied to stress reduction, cognitive therapy, and eating interventions (Kabat-Zinn, 2005).

At present spirituality is considered a construct, or a mental image, rather than a fully developed model. It has been posited as a process through which hope affects health, for example. Two recent studies have demonstrated a more direct effect, however, showing that attendance at religious services is associated with reduced mortality (Hummer, Rogers, Nam, & Ellison, 1999; Oman & Reed, 1998). To form a model of spirituality in health promotion, more operational measures of the concept are necessary, and interventions designed to assess spirituality must be rigorously evaluated. The use of prayer in the practice of health care has been criticized as trivializing religion, however (Sloan et al., 2000). Yet health promotion practice often moves ahead of the evidence. For example, the American College of Physicians recently suggested four simple questions designed to elicit a *spiritual history*, with which health care professionals might ask seriously ill patients about their faith (Koening, 2000).

Empowerment and Community Capacity-Building: Cross-Cutting Constructs

The concepts of empowerment and community capacity-building, as central foundations of community health promotion, in addition to the development of evidence-based interventions and outcomes as described later in this chapter, traverse all the models. Both implement the principle of equity advanced in the World Health Organization agenda. Values, such as equity, are fundamental to these two constructs; to value something is to choose it for its own sake in preference to other alternatives.

Empowerment

Empowerment is a term with considerable weight and contested meanings. One's health is significantly affected by the extent to which one feels control or mastery over one's life or by the amount of power or powerlessness one feels (Wallerstein,

1992). From a political perspective, if health is seen as a resource, health promotion implies advocacy for its equitable distribution. At the core of empowerment is power, which is found in the process of increasing personal, interpersonal, or political exchanges (Gutiérrez, 1990). Community empowerment approaches value the process, rather than necessarily evidence-based interventions and outcomes or the structure of communities (Best et al., 2003).

A set of moral values underpins the empowerment construct in health promotion. Moral values may be defined as the "humanly caused benefits that human beings provide to others. . . . By way of illustration, we may say that love and justice are moral goods" (Kekes, 1993, p. 44). Moral values at the base of the empowerment construct include promoting human diversity (promoting respect and appreciation for diverse social entities) and self-determination (promoting the ability of clients to pursue their chosen goals without excessive frustration and in consideration of other persons' needs) for individuals and marginalized groups, especially communities.

The concept embodies the larger political aspects of power. "Empowerment theory is based on a conflict model that assumes that a society consists of separate groups possessing different levels of power and control over resources" (Gutiérrez, 1990, p. 150). Questions of power are key to empowerment (for example, Who has more power in a relationship? Are there attempts to share power?). Empowerment is thus attentive to rights and entitlements in relationships and to personal control over exchanges. Further, empowerment exists along a continuum—from personal power through community organization to political action (Labonte, 1986)—and implies potential conflict among differing views and interests.

Within the empowerment model of health promotion, however, Becker (1986) cautions that health may become a moral imperative. The pursuit of health may become more important than the pursuit of any other values, including distributive justice (Rawls, 1971). Health could become more important as a value than seeking opportunities for the more vulnerable members of society to attain it.

Community Capacity-Building

Community, although an evolving concept subject to numerous interpretations, may be defined concretely as "a group of people living in the same defined area sharing the same basic values and organization," or abstractly as "a group of people sharing the same basic interests" (Rifkin, Muller, & Bichman, 1988, p. 933).

McKnight (1986) highlights the sense of connectedness among members of a community in describing its characteristics: (1) capacity- rather than deficiency-oriented; (2) informal; (3) rich in stories that "allow people to reach back into their common history and their individual experience for knowledge about truth and direction for the future"; and (4) incorporating celebration, tragedy, and fallibility "into the life of the community" (p. 58).

The emphasis health promotion puts on the community is explicitly political, in that the community becomes a mediating structure between the domain of individuals' everyday life (microlevel) and the larger social, political, and economic context within which individuals live (macrolevel). Capacity is built as communities increase their abilities to participate in economic and political decisions, thereby enhancing health at the macrolevel (McKnight, 1990). Therefore community health promotion often stresses the importance of structures and effective governance, service integration, efficiency and accountability, and information and management systems (Best et al., 2003).

Health care professionals must consider under what conditions individuals should sacrifice their personal uniqueness for the good of the community as well as how many resources the community should provide to promote the health of a few. Further, it is important that as communities become more responsible for health promotion and confront complex, often multisectoral problems, such as mental illness, the broader health services continue to support them both politically and economically.

Evidence for the Effectiveness of Health Promotion

The development of evidence for the effectiveness of health promotion has become more important as the push for evidence-based practice in medicine, nursing, and other health professions has grown (see Chapter Three for more discussion of this topic). Evidence can be considered a fact or datum that is used, or could be used, in making a decision or judgment or in solving a problem. Such evidence, when used alongside good reasoning and principles of valuation, answers the question *why* (Butcher, 1998). Some consider evidence a culturally or geographically biased notion, borne of logical positivism, as delineated by such philosophers as Bertrand Russell and Ludwig Wittgenstein. In the philosophical tradition of logical positivism, meaning is verifiable only through rigorous observation and experiment. The randomized clinical trial and the quasi-experiment rest within this tradition. Anthropology and some branches of sociology have alternative approaches to assessing evidence and the effectiveness of interventions (see the section "Evaluation as Social Research" later in this chapter) that some feel are more relevant to health promotion in non-Western countries.

Health promotion is eclectic, multidisciplinary, and practice oriented. Many of its principal activities relate to advocacy, partnerships, and coalition building, functions that require more art than science; effectiveness studies may fail to capture the holistic focus of many health promotion activities (McQueen, 2001). Yet practitioners and advocates of health promotion need to demonstrate that health promotion is a field with tangible benefits to offer the public.

A key challenge in health promotion is to foster and develop high-quality, widely recognized and acceptable standards for evidence-based evaluation. Several approaches to developing evidence for the effectiveness of health promotion are described in detail in Chapter Three, including the work of the U.S. Preventive Services Task Force and the Task Force on Community Preventive Services. These efforts have been joined by those of the International Union for Health Promotion and Education (IUHPE), an advisory group that produced an influential report for the European Commission on the evidence of health promotion effectiveness (IUHPE, 1999). Finally, evidence of economic benefits from health promotion are important to many of these advisory groups; cost-effectiveness evaluation is described further in Chapter Sixteen. In this chapter the program evaluation approach is applied to the development of evidence for the effectiveness of health promotion.

Approaches to Building Evidence for Health Promotion: Program Evaluation

Program evaluation, or evaluation research, is the systematic application of social research procedures for assessing the conceptualization, design, implementation, and utility of social intervention and human service programs (Rossi & Freeman, 1993). Program evaluation generally is used for assessing program effectiveness and efficiency, for improving program and service delivery, and for guiding resource allocation and policy development.

The program evaluation process is shaped in part by a program's goals and is embedded in a definition of health promotion and a unique concept of health. To move from a concept of health to a theory of health promotion and finally to a test of one or more aspects of that model in an operating program, one must be able to measure key constructs.

Health may be measured subjectively (from the person's or community's own experience or sense of feeling *well, in touch,* or *empowered*). Yet health may also be measured objectively (for example, by measuring resting heart rate or muscular strength). The data derived from interviews with clients or listening to their stories may be combined with data obtained from physical measures of client physiological functioning, observations of client behavior, or psychometrically sound assessments of clients' attitudes, beliefs, and behaviors. Qualitative and quantitative measures may together refine a more perfect picture of health.

The experience of health may vary both within and among clients. Yet consensus has developed around the use of several general instruments to measure health-related quality of life. One of the more widely used and translated instruments, now considered a "classic," the Short Form Health Survey (SF-36), addresses six factors: physical, social, and role abilities; general mental health; general health perceptions; and symptoms (Fylkesnes & Forde, 1992; McHorney, Ware, & Raczek, 1993; Ware & Sherbourne, 1992). The instrument is composed of a series of questions, is easy to administer, and is comprehensible. Its psychometric, or measurement, properties are known and highly regarded.

Program evaluation, as an assessment of the processes and effects of a health promotion program or its components, begins with setting an evaluation agenda, including examining health promotion models and the program focus and design. The agenda generally is set in consideration of or in conjunction with those who will use the research and those who will be affected by it. Next, the research is formulated, planned, and implemented. As with other forms of social research, this process is systematic to ensure maximal construct validity (a strong relationship between the constructs and their measures) and reliability (constancy or consistency of measures over time, place, and person). Finally, the results are disseminated so that they may be used for program change. Generally, the findings are shared with key decision makers or client groups, or both.

Within this general framework the health care professional may adopt one of the following four main models of evaluation, each of which implies a different understanding of the relationship between the program and its stakeholders (those with an interest in the program's processes and effects). The four models are evaluation as synonymous with applied research; evaluation as part of systems management, as an aid to program administration; evaluation as professional judgment; and evaluation as politics (Smith & Glass, 1987). Each is discussed in turn.

Evaluation as Social Research

The first model considers evaluation a form of social research, with the concomitant use of the scientific method, either in the positivist or a constructivist tradition. The positivist scientific tradition assumes relationships within causal models. For example, the impacts of an intervention to reduce smoking among adolescents (the *cause*) are assessed relative to the effects on quit rates. Program goals are well specified and measurable. Rigorously designed comparative studies, true field experiments, randomized clinical trials, and quasi-experiments are implemented. Methodological rigor, including both internal validity—in testing for causality—and external validity—or the generalizability of the evaluation—is critical. The evaluation is primarily summative (conducted at the outcome of the effort), comparative, and quantitative. Program success is judged relative to a comparison group in an experimentally controlled setting.

Ideally, the program evaluator working in the experimental tradition seeks to recruit as homogeneous a population as possible, to systematically administer a well-defined protocol to participants, to randomize the participants to their test or placebo condition, to *blind* the researchers and the participants to condition(s), and to reduce participant attrition. By so doing, the program evaluator may understand efficacy—that is, the benefit that a program (for example, a mass media, legislative, and taxation campaign for smoking cessation) or its component interventions (for example, a mass media message) produces under ideal conditions, often using carefully defined participants in a research setting. Pragmatic trials, however, generally measure effectiveness or the benefit the program or the intervention produces in routine clinical practice (Roland & Torgerson, 1998, p. 285). They compare new approaches to the best current program or intervention and may administer different protocols to participants and assess a full range of health gains, for example, a reduction in stroke or an improvement of quality of life rather than just a reduction of blood pressure.

By contrast, the constructivist tradition, as part of ethnomethodology, focuses on persons' lived experiences, with those experiences understood as being located in a particular sociohistorical context. In this methodology the evaluator is a research instrument himself or herself and produces a type of narrative, text, or case report for the evaluation (Schwandt, 1990). For example, in a study of programs to increase community empowerment, the evaluator might use focus groups, intensive interviewing, and case studies. Program evaluators might also use content analysis, the systematic independent reading of a body of texts, images, and symbolic matter. The evaluator is seeking to understand multiple discourses on how people experience becoming healthy (Labonte & Robertson, 1996; Marlett, 1994). The evaluation may be either formative (providing information before the program is complete) or summative and qualitative.

Ideally, rigorous criteria for the systematic collection and interpretation of data collected using qualitative methods are applied, including a conceptual model that allows comparisons and contrasts, unitizing (relying on unitizing schemes—in context analysis, systematically distinguishing segments of texts; Krippendorff, 2004); purposive sampling of the population or the texts; recording or coding based on instructions; reducing data to manageable representations and summarizing or simplifying them; abductively inferring contextual phenomena (in content analysis, bridging the gap between descriptive accounts of text and what they refer to, entail, provoke, or cause; Krippendorff, 2004) or inferring constructs from the data; and narrating the answer to the research question. In accepting the results of qualitative analyses, rather than reliability and validity as criteria, trustworthiness, credibility, transferability, embodiment, accountability, reflexivity, and emancipatory aims have been advanced as alternatives (Denzin & Lincoln, 2000, p. 13).

Program success is also judged by criteria developed by the stakeholders or relative to other similar programs.

Evaluation as a Contributor to Systems Management

The second model incorporates evaluation into systems management, with the organization being viewed as an interrelated set of inputs, processes, and outputs. The evaluator describes these system parts and relates them to each other, relative to the stated goals. The program manager can then make decisions to regulate and improve the functions of the system. Research methods include program audits, performance appraisals, cost analyses, client satisfaction surveys, and continuous quality improvement programs. The evaluator is interested in the level of attainment on performance indicators of the given goals and in discrepancies between the stated objectives and performance (Thompson, 1992). The evaluation tends to be formative, in that information is conveyed to program administrators during the assessment process and is designed to be produced in a technically proficient manner.

Evaluation as Professional Judgment

A third model, evaluation as professional judgment, considers experts to be the appropriate persons to make judgments about the quality of a program. This model is found in accreditation approaches and assumes that peer review is objective, reliable, and valid. The experts' methods include direct observation, often using checklists and interviews with clients. Of late these approaches have been integrated with evidence-based (using social research methods) standards of practice. The experts judge the program data against established standards, and program administrators and others in the profession generally are the audience for the evaluation. Other groups with an interest in the evaluation are generally not considered.

Evaluation as Politics

Evaluation as politics, the fourth general model, highlights the proposition that evaluation and politics are inextricably intertwined. Evaluation studies are not directed simply toward one decision maker but toward all major stakeholders who play a role in maintaining, modifying, or eliminating the program. In the evaluation-as-politics approach each program has stakeholders and active partisans competing with each other for a greater share of authority over resources and social affairs. "At every stage, evaluation is only one ingredient in an inherently political process" (Rossi & Freeman, 1993, p. 417). The model uses a variety of methodological approaches, from controlled experiments to naturalistic case studies. Different reports or presentations are prepared for different audiences. The credible evaluation report is comprehensible, correct, complete, and reasonable to partisans on all sides (Cronbach, 1982).

Summary

The numerous health promotion models explored in this chapter differ in their view of health, the outcome they wish to describe or explain. Each varies in its intended target, whether micro (individuals, groups, families) or macro (communities or populations). Further, the moral values implied by the cross-cutting constructs of empowerment and community capacity-building suggest different uses of these theoretical approaches. Each question asked about the process and outcome of health promotion calls for evidence, born of varied evaluation models and measurement approaches.

References

Aday, L. A. (1993). Indicators and predictors of health services utilization. In S. Williams & P. Torrens (Eds.), *Introduction to health services* (chap. 3). Albany, NY: Delmar.

Ajzen, I. (1991). The theory of planned behavior. *Organizational Behavior and Human Decision Processes, 50*, 179–211.

Ajzen, I. (2002). Perceived behavioral control, self-efficacy, locus of control, and the theory of planned behavior. *Journal of Applied Social Psychology, 32*, 665–683.

Ajzen, I., & Fishbein, M. (Eds.). (1980). *Understanding attitudes and predicting social behavior.* Upper Saddle River, NJ: Prentice Hall.

Aldwin, C., & Stokols, D. (1988). The effects of environmental change on individuals and groups: Some neglected issues in stress research. *Journal of Environmental Psychology, 8,* 57–75.

Andersen, R. M., & Aday, L. A. (1978). Access to medical care in the U.S.: Realized and potential. *Medical Care, 16,* 533–546.

Andersen, R. M., & Newman, J. F. (1973). Societal and individual determinants of medical care utilization in the United States. *Milbank Memorial Fund Quarterly, 51,* 95–124.

Ashford, A., Gemson, D., Sheinfeld Gorin, S., Bloch, S., Lantigua, R., Ahsan, H., et al. (2000). Cancer screening and prevention practices of inner city physicians. *American Journal of Preventive Medicine, 19,* 59–62.

Backett, K. C., & Davison, C. (1995). Lifecourse and lifestyle: The social and cultural location of health behaviors. *Social Science and Medicine, 40*(5), 629–638.

Baer, J. S., & Lichtenstein, E. (1988). Cognitive assessment. In D. M. Donovan & G. A. Marlatt (Eds.), *Assessment of addictive behaviors* (pp. 189–213). New York: Guilford Press.

Bandura, A. (1986). *Social foundations of thought and action.* Upper Saddle River, NJ: Prentice Hall.

Bandura, A. (1998). Health promotion from the perspective of the Social Cognitive Theory. *Psychological Health, 13,* 623–649.

Bao, W., Threefoot, S. A., Srinivasan, S. R., & Berenson, G. S. (1995). Essential hypertension predicted by tracking of elevated blood pressure from childhood to adulthood: The Bogalusa Heart Study. *American Journal of Hypertension, 8,* 657–665.

Barker, D.J.P. (1998). *Mothers, babies, and health in later life.* London: Latimer Trend.

Basch, C. E. (1987). Focus group interview: An underutilized research technique for improving theory and practice in health education. *Health Education Quarterly, 14,* 411–448.

BayesMendel Lab, Sidney Kimmel Comprehensive Cancer Center at Johns Hopkins University. (2004). *BRCAPRO.* Retrieved September 2005 from http://astor.som.jhmi.edu/BayesMendel/brcapro.html

Becker, M. (1986). The tyranny of health promotion. *Public Health Review, 14,* 15–23.

Becker, M. H., Drachman, R. H., & Kirscht, J. P. (1974). A new approach to explaining sick-role behavior in low-income populations. *American Journal of Public Health, 64,* 205–216.

Bell, D. (1993). *Communitarianism and its critics.* Oxford, England: Oxford University Press, Clarendon Press.

Ben-Shlomo, Y., & Kuh, D. (2002). A lifecourse approach to chronic disease epidemiology: Conceptual models, empirical challenges and interdisciplinary perspectives. *International Journal of Epidemiology, 31,* 285–293.

Berkman, L. F. (1985). The relationship of social networks and social support to morbidity and mortality. In S. Cohen & S. L. Syme (Eds.), *Social support and health* (pp. 243–262). San Diego, CA: Academic Press.

Best, A., Stokols, D., Green, L. W., Leischow, S., Holmes, B., & Buchholz, K. (2003). An integrative framework for community partnering to translate theory into effective health promotion strategy. *American Journal of Health Promotion, 18,* 168–176.

Burg, M. M., & Seeman, T. E. (1994). Families and health: The negative side of social ties. *Annals of Behavioral Medicine, 16*(2), 109–115.

Butcher, R. B. (1998). Foundations for evidence-based decision making. In National Forum on Health, *Canada health action: Building on the legacy* (Vol. 5, pp. 259–290). Quebec: Éditions MultiMondes.

Butterfield, P. G. (1990). Thinking upstream: Nurturing a conceptual understanding of the societal context of health behavior. *Advances in Nursing Science, 12*(2), 1–8.

Cannon, W. B. (1932). *The wisdom of the body.* New York: Norton.

Cohen, S. (1988). Psychosocial models of the role of social support in the etiology of physical disease. *Health Psychology, 7,* 269–297.

Cohen, S., & Syme S. L. (1985). Issues in the study and application of social support. In S. Cohen & S. L. Syme (Eds.), *Social support and health* (pp. 3–22). San Diego, CA: Academic Press.

Cohen, S., & Wills, T. A. (1985). Stress, social support, and the buffering hypothesis. *Psychological Bulletin, 98,* 310–357.

Cousins, E. (1987). Jewish spirituality: From the sixteenth-century revival to the present. In A. Green (Ed.), *World spirituality: An encyclopedic history of the religious quest* (Vol. 14, pp. ix–x). New York: Crossroad.

Cronbach, L. J. (1982). *Designing evaluations of educational and social programs.* San Francisco: Jossey-Bass.

Curry, S. J., & Emmons, K. M. (1994). Theoretical models for predicting and improving compliance with breast cancer screening. *Annals of Behavioral Medicine, 16*(4), 302–316.

Delbecq, A. L. (1978). The social political process of introducing innovation in human services. In R. Sarri & Y. Hasenfeld (Eds.), *The management of human services* (pp. 309–339). New York: Columbia University Press.

DeLongis, A., Folkman, S., & Lazarus, R. S. (1988). The impact of daily stress on health and mood: Psychological and social resources as mediators. *Journal of Personality and Social Psychology, 54,* 486–495.

Denzin, N. K., & Lincoln, Y. S. (2000). Introduction: The discipline and practice of qualitative research. In N. K. Denzin & Y. S. Lincoln (Eds.), *Handbook of qualitative research* (pp. 1–28). Thousand Oaks, CA: Sage.

Devins, G. M. (1992). Social cognitive analysis of recovery from a lapse after smoking cessation: Comment on Haaga and Stewart. *Journal of Consulting and Clinical Psychology, 60*(1), 29–31.

DiClemente, C. C. (1991). Motivational interviewing and the stages of change. In W. Miller & S. Rollnick (Eds.), *Motivational interviewing* (pp. 191–203). New York: Guilford Press.

Doll, R., Peto, R., Boreham, J., & Sutherland, I. (2004). Mortality in relation to smoking: 50 years' observations on male British doctors. *British Medical Journal, 328,* 1519–1528.

Downie, R. S., Fyfe, C., & Tannahill, A. (1990). *Health promotion: Models and values.* New York: Oxford University Press.

Emery, F. E., & Trist, E. L. (1972). *Towards a social ecology: Contextual appreciations of the future in the present.* New York: Plenum.

Eng, E. (1993). Save Our Sisters Project. *Cancer, 72,* 1071–1077.

Fawcet, S. B., Paine-Andrews, A., Francisco, V. T., Schultz, J. A., Richter, K. B., Lewis, R. K., et al. (1995). Using empowerment theory in collaborative partnerships for community health and development. *American Journal of Community Psychology, 23*(5), 677–697.

Fincham, S. (1992). Community health promotion programs. *Social Science and Medicine, 35*(3), 239–249.

Fishbein, M., Jaccard, J. J., Davidson, A. R., Ajzen, I., & Loken, B. (1980). Predicting and understanding family planning behaviors: Beliefs, attitudes, and intentions. In I. Ajzen & M. Fishbein (Eds.), *Understanding attitudes and predicting social behavior* (pp. 131–147). Upper Saddle River, NJ: Prentice Hall.

Fisher, E. B., Bishop, D. B., Goldmuntz, J., & Jacobs, A. (1988). Implications for the practicing physician of the psychosocial dimensions of smoking. *Chest, 38,* 194–212.

Fong, G. T., Rempel, L. A., & Hall, P. A. (1999). Challenges to improving health risk communication in the 21st century: A discussion. *Journal of the National Cancer Institute Monographs, 25,* 173–176.

Fox, S. A., Murata, P. J., & Stein, J. A. (1991). The impact of physician compliance on screening mammography by women. *Annals of Behavioral Medicine, 151,* 50–56.

Fylkesnes, K., & Forde, H. (1992). Determinants and dimensions involved in self-evaluation of health. *Social Science and Medicine, 35*(3), 271–279.

Goodman, S. (2005). Attributable risk in epidemiology: Interpreting and calculating population attributable fractions. In IOM Board on Population Health and Public Health Practice, *Estimating the contributions of lifestyle-related factors to preventable death: A workshop summary.* Washington, DC: National Academies Press.

Gordis, L. (2000). *Epidemiology.* Philadelphia: Saunders.

Gotay, C. C., & Wilson, M. E. (1998). Social support and cancer screening in African American, Hispanic, and Native American women. *Cancer Practice, 6,* 31–37.

Green, L. (1974). Toward cost-benefit evaluations of health education: Some concepts, methods, and examples. *Health Education Monographs, 2* (Suppl. 1), 34–64. (Reprinted in *Supplement to the Report of the President's Committee on Health Education,* 1974, New York: National Health Council, and in U.S. Congress, 1975, *Disease control and health education and promotion,* pp. 939–965, Washington, DC: Author.)

Green, L. W., & Kreuter, M. W. (1991). *Health promotion planning: An educational and environmental approach* (2nd ed.). Palo Alto, CA: Mayfield.

Green, L. W., & Kreuter, M. W. (1999). *Health program planning.* New York: McGraw-Hill.

Green, L. W., & Kreuter, M. W. (2005). *Health program planning: An educational and ecological approach with PowerWeb bind-in card.* New York: McGraw-Hill.

Green, L. W., Nathan, R., & Mercer, S. (2001). The health of health promotion in public policy: Drawing inspiration from tobacco control. *Health Promotion Journal of Australia, 12*(2), 110–116.

Gutiérrez, L. (1990). Working with women of color: An empowerment perspective. *Social Work, 35,* 149–154.

Hafen, B. Q., Karren, K. J., Frandsen, K. J., & Smith, N. L. (1996). *Mind/body health: The effects of attitudes, emotions, and relationships.* Needham Heights, MA: Allyn & Bacon.

Halfon, N., & Hochstein, M. (2002). Life course health development: An integrated framework for developing health, policy, and research. *Milbank Memorial Quarterly, 80,* 433–479.

Harvard Center for Cancer Prevention, Harvard School of Public Health. (2004). *Your disease risk.* Retrieved September 2005 from http://www.yourdiseaserisk.harvard.edu/index.htm

Hawley, A. H. (1950). *Human ecology: A theory of community structure.* New York: Ronald Press.

Hertzman, C. (1999). Population health and human experiences. In D. P. Keating & C. Hertzman (Eds.), *Developmental health and the wealth of nations: Social, biological and educational dynamics* (pp. 21–40). New York: Guilford Press.

Honda, K., & Sheinfeld Gorin, S. (2005). Modeling pathways to affective barriers on colorectal cancer screening among Japanese Americans. *Journal of Behavioral Medicine, 28,* 115–124.

Honda, K., & Sheinfeld Gorin, S. (2006). A model of stage of change to recommend colonoscopy. *Health Psychology, 25,* 65–73.

House, J. S., & Kahn, R. I. (1985). Measures and concepts of social supports. In S. Cohen & S. L. Syme (Eds.), *Social support and health* (pp. 83–108). San Diego, CA: Academic Press.

House, J. S., & Landis, K. R., & Umberson, D. (1988). Social relationships and health. *Science, 241,* 540–545.

Hummer, R. A., Rogers, R. G., Nam, C. B., & Ellison, C. G. (1999). Religious involvement and U.S. adult mortality. *Demography, 36,* 273–285.

Hutchison, G. B. (1969). Evaluation of preventive services. In H. C. Schulberg, A. Sheldon, & F. Baker (Eds.), *Program evaluation in the health fields* (Vol. 1, pp. 59–72). New York: Human Sciences Press.

Institute of Medicine. (2001). *Health and behavior: The interplay of biological, behavioral, and societal influences.* Washington, DC: National Academies Press.

International Union for Health Promotion and Education. (1999). *The evidence of health promotion effectiveness: A report for the European Commission by the International Union for Health Promotion and Education.* Brussels, Luxembourg: ES-EC-EAEC.

Janis, I. L., & Mann, L. (1977). *Decision making: A psychological analysis of conflict, choice and commitment.* New York: Free Press.

Janz, N. K., & Becker, M. H. (1984). The health belief model: A decade later. *Health Education Quarterly, 11,* 1–47.

Job, R.F.S. (1988). Effective and ineffective use of fear in health promotion campaigns. *American Journal of Public Health, 78,* 163–167.

Judd, C. M., Smith, E. K., & Kidder, L. H. (1991). *Research methods in social relations* (6th ed.). Austin, TX: Holt, Rinehart & Winston.

Kabat-Zinn, J. (2005). Conversations with Jon Kabat-Zinn: Bringing mindfulness to medicine (Interview by Karolyn A. Gazella). *Alternative Therapies, 11,* 57–64.

Kahneman, D. (1999). Objective happiness. In D. Kahnemann, E. Diener, & N. Schwartz (Eds.), *Well-being: The foundations of hedonic psychology* (pp. 3–25). New York: Russell Sage Foundation.

Kahneman, D., & Tversky, A. (1984). Choices, values, and frames. *American Psychologist, 39,* 341–350.

Karasek, R., & Theorell, T. (Eds.). (1990). *Healthy work: Stress, productivity, and the reconstruction of working life.* New York: Basic Books.

Katz, D., & Kahn, R. L. (1966). *The social psychology of organizations.* New York: Wiley.

Kawachi, I., Colditz, G. A., Stampfer, M. J., Willett, W. C., Manson, J. E., Rosner, B., et al. (1994). Smoking cessation and time course of decreased risks of coronary heart disease in middle-aged women. *Archives of Internal Medicine, 154,* 169–175.

Kazdin, A. E. (1994). *Behavior modification in applied settings* (5th ed.). Pacific Grove, CA: Brooks/Cole.

Keating, D. P., & Hertzman, C. (Eds.). (1999). *Developmental health and the wealth of nations: Social, biological and educational dynamics.* New York: Guilford Press.

Kekes, J. (1993). *The morality of pluralism.* Princeton, NJ: Princeton University Press.

Kelly, J. A., St. Lawrence, J. S., Stevenson, L. Y., Houth, A. C., Kuliehman, A. C., Diaz, Y. E., et al. (1992). Community AIDS/HIV risk reduction: The effects of endorsements by popular people in three cities. *American Journal of Public Health, 2,* 1483–1489.

Koening, H. G. (2000). Religion, spirituality, and medicine: Application to clinical practice. *JAMA, 284,* 1708.

Kotler, P., & Roberto, E. (1989). *Social marketing: Strategies for changing public behavior.* New York: Free Press.

Krippendorff, K. (2004). *Content analysis: An introduction to its methodology.* Thousand Oaks, CA: Sage.

Kvaavik, E., Tell, G. S., & Klepp, K. I. (2003). Predictors and tracking of body mass index from adolescence into adulthood: Followup of 18 to 20 years in the Oslo Youth Study. *Archives of Pediatrics and Adolescent Medicine, 157,* 1212–1218.

Labonte, R. (1986). Social inequality and healthy public policy. *Health Promotion, 1*(3), 341–351.

Labonte, R., & Robertson, A. (1996). Delivering our goods, showing our stuff: The case for a constructivist paradigm for health promotion research and practice. *Health Education Quarterly, 23*(4), 431–447.

Lane, D. S., & Brug, M. A. (1990). Breast cancer screening: Changing physician practices and specialty variation. *New York State Journal of Medicine, 90,* 288–292.

Lauer, R. M., & Clarke, W. R. (1990). Use of cholesterol measurements in childhood for the prediction of adult hypercholesterolemia: The Muscatine Study. *JAMA, 264,* 3034–3038.

Leavell, H. R., & Clark, E. G. (1953). *Textbook of preventive medicine.* New York: McGraw-Hill.

Lefebvre, R. C., Lasater, T. M., Carleton, R. A., & Peterson, G. (1987). Theory and delivery of health programming in the community: The Pawtucket Heart Health Program. *Preventive Medicine, 16,* 80–95.

Leventhal, H., Safer, M. A., & Panagis, D. M. (1983). The impact of communications on the self-regulation of health beliefs, decisions, and behavior. *Health Education Quarterly, 10,* 3–29.

Lewin, K., Dembo, T., Festinger, L., & Sears, P. S. (1944). Level of aspiration. In J. Hunt (Ed.), *Personality and the behavioral disorders: A handbook based on experimental and clinical research* (pp. 333–378). New York: Ronald Press.

Lilienfeld, A. M. (1976). *Foundations of epidemiology.* New York: Oxford University Press.

Lipkus, I. M., & Hollands, J. G. (1999). The visual communication of risk. *Journal of the National Cancer Institute Monographs, 25,* 149–163.

Llewellyn-Thomas, H. (1995). Patients' health-care decision making: A framework for descriptive and experimental investigations. *Medical Decision Making, 15,* 101–106.

Lynch, J., & Davey Smith, G. (2005). A life course approach to chronic disease epidemiology. *Annual Review of Public Health, 26,* 1–35.

Mahoney, L. T., Lauer, R. M., Lee, J., & Clarke, W. R. (1991). Factors affecting tracking of coronary heart disease risk factors in children: The Muscatine Study. *Annals of the New York Academy of Sciences, 623,* 120–132.

Maiman, L. A., & Becker, M. H. (1984). The health belief model: Origins and correlates in psychological theory. In M. H. Becker (Ed.), *The health belief model and personal health behavior* (pp. 9–26). Thorofare, NJ: Slack.

Mandelblatt, J. S., & Yabroff, K. R. (1999). Effectiveness of interventions designed to increase mammography use: A meta-analysis of provider-targeted strategies. *Cancer Epidemiology, Biomarkers, and Prevention, 8,* 759–767.

Manoff, R. K. (1985). *Social marketing: Imperative for public health.* New York: Praeger.

Marlett, N. (1994). *Partnerships and communication in health promotion research.* Paper presented at the Third Annual Health Promotion Research Conference, Calgary, Alberta, Canada.

Martyn, C. N., Barker, D.J.P., & Osmond, C. (1996). Mothers' pelvic size, fetal growth, and coronary heart disease in men in the UK. *Lancet, 348,* 1264–1268.

Maruyama, M. (1963). The second cybernetics: Decision-amplifying mutual causal processes. *American Scientist, 51,* 164–179.

Masten, A. S. (2001). Ordinary magic: Resilience processes in development. *American Psychologist, 56,* 227–238.

McGinnis, J. M., & Foege, W. H. (1994). Actual causes of death in the United States. *JAMA, 270,* 2207.

McGuire, W. (1981). Theoretical foundations of campaigns. In R. E. Rice & W. J. Paisley (Eds.), *Public communication campaigns* (pp. 41–70). Thousand Oaks, CA: Sage.

McHorney, C. A., Ware, J. E., & Raczek, A. E. (1993). The MOS 36-Item Short-Form Health Survey (SF-36): Psychometric and clinical tests of validity in measuring physical and mental constructs. *Medical Care, 31,* 247–263.

McKnight, J. L. (1986). Well-being: The new threshold of the old medicine. *Health Promotion, 1,* 75–80.

McKnight, J. (1990). Politicizing health care. In P. Conrad & R. Kern (Eds.), *The sociology of health and illness: Critical perspectives* (pp. 432–436). New York: St. Martins Press.

McQueen, D. V. (2001). Strengthening the evidence base for health promotion. *Health Promotion International, 16,* 261–268.

Mensah, G. A. (2005). Attributing risks in preventable death: What metrics best inform health policy? In Institute of Medicine, *Estimating the contributions of lifestyle-related factors to preventable death: A workshop summary.* Washington, DC: National Academies Press.

Miller, S. M. (1995). Monitoring versus blunting styles of coping with cancer influence the information patients want and need about their disease (implications for cancer screening and management). *Cancer, 76,* 167–177.

Miller, S. M., Shoda, Y., & Hurley, K. (1996). Applying cognitive-social theory to health-protective behavior: Breast self-examination in cancer screening. *Psychological Bulletin, 119,* 70–94.

Moos, R. H. (1979). Social ecological perspectives on health. In G. C. Stone, F. Cohen, & N. E. Adler (Eds.), *Health psychology: A handbook* (pp. 523–547). San Francisco: Jossey-Bass.

Munoz, N., Bosch, F. X., deSanjose, S., Herrero, R., Castellsague, X., Shah, K. V., et al. (2003). Epidemiologic classification of human papillomavirus types associated with cervical cancer. *New England Journal of Medicine, 348,* 518–527.

National Heart, Lung, and Blood Institute. *Framingham Heart Study: 50 Years of research success.* Retrieved September 2005 from http://www.nhlbi.nih.gov/about/framingham/index.html

O'Connor, A. M., Stacey, D., Entwistle, V., Llewellyn-Thomas, H., Rovner, D., Holmes-Rovner, M., et al. (2004). Decision aids for people facing health treatment or screening decisions (Cochrane Review). *Cochrane Library, 2.*

Oman, D., & Reed, D. (1998). Religion and mortality among the community-dwelling elderly. *American Journal of Public Health, 88,* 1469–1475.

Orleans, C. T., Rotberg, H. L., Quade, D., & Lees, P. (1990). A hospital quit-smoking consult service: Clinical report and intervention guidelines. *Preventative Medicine, 19*(2), 198–212.

Parse, R. (1987). *Nursing science: Major paradigms, theories and critiques.* Philadelphia: Saunders.

Pelletier, K. R. (1984). *Healthy people in unhealthy places: Stress and fitness at work.* New York: Dell.

Pender, N., Murdaugh, C. L., & Parsons, M. A. (2006). *Health promotion in nursing practice* (5th ed.). Upper Saddle River, NJ: Pearson Prentice-Hall.

Peterson, C. (2000). The future of optimism. *American Psychologist, 55,* 68–78.

Peto, R., Darby, S., Deo, H., Silcocks, P., Whitley, E., & Doll, R. (2000). Smoking, smoking cessation, and lung cancer in the UK since 1950: Combination of national statistics with two case-control studies. *British Medical Journal, 321,* 323–329.

Phillips, K. A., Morrison, K. R., Andersen, R., & Aday, L. A. (1998). Understanding the context of healthcare utilization: Assessing environmental and provider-related variables in the behavioral model of utilization. *Health Services Research, 33,* 571–596.

Prilleltensky, I. (1997). Values, assumptions, and practices: Assessing the moral implications of psychological discourse and action. *American Psychologist, 52*(5), 517–535.

Prilleltensky, I., & Gonick, L. (1996). Politics change, oppression remains: On the psychology and practice of oppression. *Political Psychology, 17,* 127–147.

Prochaska, J. O., & DiClemente, C. C. (1983). Stages and processes of self-change of smoking: Toward an integrative model. *Journal of Consulting and Clinical Psychology, 51,* 390–395.

Prochaska, J. O., Velicer, W. F., Gaudagnoli, E., Rossi, J. S., & DiClemente, C. C. (1991). Patterns of change: Dynamic typology applied to smoking cessation. *Multivariate Behavioral Research, 26,* 83–107.

Rachlin, H. (1991). *Introduction to modern behaviorism* (3rd ed.). San Francisco: Freeman.

Rawls, J. (1971). *A theory of justice.* Cambridge, MA: Harvard University Press, Belknap Press.

Rich-Edwards, J. S., Stamfer, M. J., Manson, J. E., Rosner, B., Hankinson, S. E., Colditz, G. A., et al. (1997). Birth weight and risk of cardiovascular disease in a cohort of women followed up since 1976. *British Medical Journal, 315,* 396–400.

Rifkin, S. B., Muller, F., & Bichman, W. (1988). Primary health care: On measuring participation. *Social Science in Medicine, 29,* 931–940.

Rogers, E. (1983). *Diffusion of innovation.* New York: Free Press.

Rogers, R. W., Deckner, C. W., & Mewborn, C. R. (1978). An expectancy-value theory approach
to the long-term modification of smoking behavior. *Journal of Clinical Psychology, 34,* 562–566.

Roland, M., & Torgerson, D. J. (1998). Understanding controlled trials: What are pragmatic
trials? *British Medical Journal, 316,* 285.

Rosenstock, I. M. (1974). The health belief model and preventive health behavior. In M. H.
Becker (Ed.), *The health belief model and personal health behavior* (pp. 27–59). Thorofare, NJ: Slack.

Rosenstock, I. M., Strecher, V. J., & Becker, M. H. (1988). Social learning theory and the
health belief model. *Health Education Quarterly, 15*(2), 175–183.

Rossi, P. H., & Freeman, I. E. (1993). *Evaluation: A systematic approach* (5th ed.). Thousand Oaks,
CA: Sage.

The Royal Society. (1983). *Risk assessment: Report of a Royal Society study group.* London: The
Royal Society.

Ruberman, W., Weinblatt, E., Goldberg, J. D., & Chaudhary, B. (1984). Psychosocial influences
on mortality after myocardial infarction. *New England Journal of Medicine, 311,* 552–559.

Salovey, P., Rothman, A. J., Detweiler, J. B., & Steward, W. T. (2000). Emotional sates and
physical health. *American Psychologist, 55,* 68–78.

Salovey, P., & Williams-Piehota, P. (2004). Field experiments in social psychology: Message
framing and the promotion of health protective behaviors. *American Behavioral Scientist, 47,*
488–505.

Schiffman, M. H., & Brinton, L. A. (1995). The epidemiology of cervical carcinogenesis.
Cancer, 76, 1888–1901.

Schwandt, T. (1990). Paths to inquiry in the social disciplines. In E. Guba (Ed.), *The paradigm
dialog* (pp. 258–276). Thousand Oaks, CA: Sage.

Schwartz, B. (2000). Self determination: The tyranny of freedom. *American Psychologist, 55,* 79–88.

Schwartz, L. M., Woloshin, S., & Welch, H. G. (1999). Risk communication in clinical practice:
Putting cancer in context. *Journal of the National Cancer Institute Monographs, 25,* 124–133.

Seeman, T. E., & Syme, S. L. (1987). Social networks and coronary artery disease: A comparison of the structure and function of social relations as predictors of disease. *Psychosomatic
Medicine, 49*(4), 341–354.

Seligman, M.E.P., & Csikszentmihalyi, M. (2000). Positive psychology: An introduction. *American Psychologist, 55,* 5–14.

Sheinfeld Gorin, S. (1997). Outcomes of social support for women survivors of breast cancer.
In E. J. Mullen & J. L. Magnabosco (Eds.), *Outcomes measurement in the human services: Cross-
cutting issues and methods* (pp. 276–289). Washington, DC: NASW Press.

Sheinfeld Gorin, S., & Arnold, J. (1998). *The health promotion handbook.* St. Louis, MO: Mosby.

Sheinfeld Gorin, S., & Weirich, T. (1995). Innovation use: Performance assessment in a community mental health center. *Human Relations, 48*(12), 1427–1453.

Sheridan, S. L., Harris, R. P., & Woolf, S. H. (2004). Shared decision making about screening
and chemoprevention: A suggested approach from the US Preventive Services Task Force.
American Journal of Preventive Medicine, 26, 56–66.

Shoda, Y., Mischel, W., Miller, S. M., Diefenbach, M., Daly, M. B., & Engstrom, P. F. (1998).
Psychological interventions and genetic testing: Facilitating informed decisions about
BRCA1/2 cancer susceptibility. *Journal of Clinical Psychology in Medical Settings, 5,* 3–17.

Sloan, R. P., Bagiella, E., VandeCreek, L., Hover, M., Casalone, C., Hirsch, T. J., et al. (2000).
Should physicians prescribe religious activities? *New England Journal of Medicine, 342,* 1913–1916.

Smith, M. L., & Glass, G. V. (1987). *Research and evaluation in education and the social sciences.* Upper Saddle River, NJ: Prentice Hall.

Steps to a healthier US. Retrieved July 2005 from http://www.healthierus.gov/steps/grantees/2004/cherokee.html

Stokols, D. (1992). Establishing and maintaining healthy environments: Toward a social ecology of health promotion. *American Psychologist, 47*(1), 6–22.

Stroebe, M., & Stroebe, W. (1996). The role of loneliness and social support in adjustment to loss: A test of attachment versus stress theory. *Journal of Personality and Social Psychology, 70*(6), 1241–1249.

Susser, E., & Terry, M. B. (2003). A conception-to-death cohort. *Lancet, 361,* 797–798.

Taylor, S. E. (1983). Adjustment to threatening events: A theory of cognitive adaptation. *American Psychologist, 38,* 1161–1173.

Taylor, S. E., Kemeny, M. E., Reed, G. M., Bower, J. E., & Gruenewald, T. L. (2000). Psychological resources, positive illusions, and health. *American Psychologist, 55,* 99–109.

Thompson, J. C. (1992). Program evaluation within a health promotion framework. *Canadian Journal of Public Health, 83*(Suppl. 1), 567–571.

U.S. Department of Health and Human Services. (2000). *Healthy People 2010* (2nd ed.). Retrieved August 2005 from http://www.healthypeople.gov

U.S. Preventive Services Task Force. (1996). *Guide to clinical preventive services.* Baltimore: Williams & Wilkins.

Vaillant, G. E. (2000). Adaptive mental mechanisms: Their role in a positive psychology. *American Psychologist, 55,* 89–98.

Velicer, W. F., DiClemente, C. C., Prochaska, J. O., & Brandenburg, N. (1985). Decisional balance measure for assessing and predicting smoking status. *Journal of Personality and Social Psychology, 48*(5), 1279–1289.

Wallerstein, N. (1992). Powerlessness, empowerment, and health: Implications for health promotion programs. *American Journal of Health Promotion, 6*(30), 197–205.

Wannamethee, S. G., Shaper, A. G., Whincup, P. H., & Walker, M. (1995). Smoking cessation and the risk of stroke in middle-aged men. *JAMA, 274,* 155–160.

Ware, J. E., & Sherbourne, C. D. (1992). The MOS 36-Item Short Form Health Survey (SF-36): Conceptual framework and item selection. *Medical Care, 30,* 473–483.

Winett, R. A., King, A. C., & Altman, D. G. (1989). *Health psychology and public health: An integrative approach.* New York: Pergamon Press.

Woloshin, S., Schwartz, L. M., & Welch, H. G. (2002). Risk charts: Putting cancer in context. *Journal of the National Cancer Institute, 94,* 799–804.

World Health Organization. (1946). *Preamble* to the Constitution of The World Health Organization as adopted by the International Health Conference, New York, June 19–22, 1946; signed on July 22, 1946, by the representatives of 61 states (Official records of the World Health Organization, no. 2, p. 100) and entered into force on April 7, 1948.

World Health Organization. (1984). *Health promotion: A discussion document on the concepts and principles.* Copenhagen: WHO Regional Office for Europe.

World Health Organization. (1988). *From Alma-Ata to the year 2000: Reflections at midpoint.* Geneva: Author.

Zaltman, G., Kotler, P., & Kaufman, I. (1972). *Creating social change.* Austin, TX: Holt, Rinehart & Winston.

CHAPTER THREE

CONTEXTS FOR HEALTH PROMOTION

Aaron P. Gorin
Sherri Sheinfeld Gorin

Health promotion between the client and the health care professional emerges in a context of policies, influential groups, and monetary exchanges. Healthy public policy provides the overall framework in which health promotion can occur. Public policy is established when government authorities and particular social groups define their intentions to influence the behavior of citizens by the use of positive or negative sanctions (Lowi, 1972; Mayer & Greenwood, 1980). Public policy provides both a framework to which practitioners react and a target for advocates to change. Ultimately, through its influence on community norms and values, policy may effect change in client behaviors through laws, rules or regulations, operational decisions, or judicial decrees. This chapter details both the political and economic contexts for health promotion and the unique steps practitioners may take to change these conditions.

The Political Economy Framework

As introduced in Chapter Two, conceptually, health promotion may be characterized as a political economy: that is, a political system (a structure of rule) and an economy (a system for producing and exchanging goods and services) (Wamsley & Zald, 1967; Gargiulo, 1993). In the United States, political support for health promotion is defined by the degree to which important actors at the federal, state, and local levels take an interest in health promotion, have the power and resources to influence it, and communicate their expectations and demands about it to concerned communities, organizations, groups, health care professionals, families, and individuals (Longest, 2002).

From the perspective of the health care professional, the major economic actors in the field of health promotion are the varied payers who reimburse providers for services and programs (for example, commercial insurance companies) and the general types of health-promotive activities they support (for example, smoking cessation counseling). (In Chapter Sixteen other aspects of the economy of health promotion are explored.)

The political economy perspective limits both the contexts and targets for health promotion. Further, although one can separate the political and economic contexts conceptually by their major intent or strategy—health improvement or cost reduction—their aims and tactics may overlap. For example, the content of the U.S. Department of Health and Human Services (2000a) *Healthy People 2010* report, although oriented toward health-promotive goals, is embedded in a legislative context that emphasizes cost reductions, and these reductions are implicit in the suggested preventive actions. Another example is managed care systems, which are designed to reduce costs, in part through the use of preventive services.

Political Contexts for Health Promotion

The primary political contexts for health promotion are defined by legislation, influential actors, and organizational policy (see Table 3.1).

Legislation

U.S. legislation for health promotion may be enacted at the federal, state, or local level. We also briefly consider international legislation.

Federal Legislation. Traditionally, public health law has been concerned with the protection and preservation of the public's health and the processes of administrative regulation and rule making resulting from the implementation of these aims. Because of its broad statutory authority, the federal government possesses several powers regarding health care: individuals may be denied the right to decide whether or not to submit to a medical examination or treatment, the state may collect sensitive health care information about a person or his or her sexual associates, and if a disease is contagious, compulsory hospitalization or segregation from the community may be imposed. The exercise of these public health powers requires

TABLE 3.1. MAJOR POLITICAL INFLUENCES ON HEALTH PROMOTION.

Influence	Focus	Examples
Omnibus federal legislation for health promotion	Defines health promotion for AIDS awareness.	PL 104-146, Ryan White CARE Act Amendments, 1996.
	Creates federal agency.	PL 106-129, Healthcare Research and Quality Act, 1999.
Other nations	Integrates health promotion into health care system.	Polish hospital legislation, August 27, 2004.
State legislation	Specifies laws for nutrition, safety, physical exercise.	California's Latino Childhood Obesity Prevention Initiative demonstration project, 2004.
	Passes limited omnibus legislation.	
Local legislation	Implements ordinances for protection of public health.	Get Fit North Carolina program, 2004.
U.S. Preventive Services Task Force	Reviews evidence of effectiveness of clinical preventive services.	*Guide to Clinical Preventive Services.*
	Issues clinical practice guidelines.	
Federal agencies		
U.S. Department of Health and Human Services	Establishes goals for national health promotion.	Healthy People 2010 initiative.
	Encourages the development of legislation, policies, and state programs.	
Federal Drug Administration	Monitors and assesses specific drugs (especially tobacco).	Mandate for Safer Childhood Vaccines, 42 U.S.C. § 300aa-27 (2005).
U.S. Department of Agriculture	Monitors and assesses nutritional programs.	Iowa's EFNEP (Expanded Food & Nutrition Education Program) for schools, 1998–2002.
World Health Organization	Develops health promotion policies and programs.	Health for All in the Year 2000.
	Encourages development of national legislation for health promotion.	Healthy Cities projects.

TABLE 3.1. MAJOR POLITICAL INFLUENCES ON HEALTH PROMOTION, Cont'd.

Influence	Focus	Examples
First International Conference on Health Promotion	Defined aims of health promotion internationally.	Ottawa Charter for Health Promotion. Achieving Health for All.
Voluntary and professional organizations	Encourage inclusion of health promotion on national, state, local political agendas; research monies for health promotion.	American Public Health Association. American Cancer Society.
Accreditors	Establish standards for health promotion. Monitor and assess compliance with standards.	National Commission for Quality Assurance. Joint Commission for Accreditation of Healthcare Organizations.
Media	Report and examine emerging issues in health promotion. Increase attention to health promotion.	Specialized columns in newspapers, television news reports and specials, radio news and talk shows, Internet sites for health, Web logs (*blogs*).
Community advocacy groups and coalitions	Advocate for legislation, policies, monies, and political attention to specific health promotion issues.	Mothers Against Drunk Driving. Doctors Ought to Care (antismoking). Smoking or Health.
School districts and schools	Develop, implement, and evaluate educational health promotion programs for children and youth.	45 state-required comprehensive school health education programs exist. 93% of local school districts have antismoking education in elementary schools.
Worksites	Develop, implement, evaluate, and consult on cost-effective health promotion programs to enhance productivity.	95% of employers with 50 or more employees offer at least one health promotion activity.
Public health departments and health care facilities	Implement public health laws and develop policies. Develop, implement, and evaluate clinical and population-based, cost-effective health promotion.	One-half of public health departments provide clinical preventive care and blood pressure measurements. Screening tests performed in 75% of all emergency room visits.

a delicate balancing of the state's power to act for the community's common good and the individual's rights to liberty, autonomy, and privacy (Gostin, 1986).

The Nixon administration created the President's Committee on Health Education by declaring that "it is in the interest of our entire country to educate and encourage each of our citizens to develop sensible health practices" (Guinta & Allegrante, 1992, p. 1033). The committee's report recommended the creation of public and private organizations to stimulate, coordinate, and evaluate health education programs. The administration believed it could preserve the health of Americans, control escalating health care costs, and present a less costly alternative to national health insurance than was being proposed at the time (Guinta & Allegrante, 1992).

As a result of this initial interest, the National Consumer Health Information and Health Promotion Act of 1976 was passed during the Ford administration; it was the first legislation to address health promotion comprehensively. In amending the Public Health Service Act, it established the Office of Consumer Health Education and Promotion and the Center for Health Education and Promotion, set forth national goals for health information and promotion, and developed a systematic strategy for goal achievement. It also established the federal Office of Disease Prevention and Health Promotion in the Office of the Assistant Secretary for Health to coordinate prevention-related activities of the Department of Health and Human Services, to serve as a liaison with the private sector, and to operate a national health information clearinghouse. The Act defined health education and promotion as follows: "A process that favorably influences understandings, attitudes and conduct, including cultural awareness and sensitivity, in regard to individual and community health." Specifically, it affects and influences individual and community health behavior and attitudes in order to moderate self-imposed risks, maintain and promote physical and mental health and efficiency, and reduce preventable illness, disability, and death (National Consumer Health Information and Health Promotion Act of 1976, § 4).

A Report of the Senate Committee on Labor and Public Welfare that addressed this Act stressed the influence of "activated patients," who were more involved in decision making; community programs, specifically in schools; and (in conjunction with the Occupational Safety and Health Administration [OSHA]) union and industry initiatives for worksites. Nutrition to educate the "misnourished"—those who lack the knowledge to choose which foods are best for them—was of particular import to the committee, as were the role of the media and the federal programs to monitor these efforts. The report addressed health education "manpower" and asserted the importance of specialists in this area and the critical role nurses, in particular, should continue to play. The report also stressed the need to evaluate the effectiveness of community programs.

This Act was amended by a number of subsequent acts, including the Preventive Health Amendments of 1993, which addressed breast and cervical cancer screening, injury prevention, prevention and control of sexually transmitted diseases, and production of biennial reports on nutrition and health. This legislation reflects the enormous influence advocates for women's health—particularly in the area of breast cancer screening and treatment—and advocates focused on AIDS have had on the legislative process. More current legislation reflects continued congressional legislative interest in nutrition (see Table 3.2).

Within the broad context of public health law, recent federal legislation concerning health promotion has reflected a newly sophisticated understanding of the scientific bases for the transmission of disease. Thus this legislation has focused on the most efficacious and least intrusive intervention approaches, such as counseling for long-standing, relatively intractable behaviors, such as smoking. Nonetheless, we found comparatively little omnibus legislation concerned with health promotion (that is, legislation that addresses health promotion explicitly and comprehensively) at either the state or federal levels through a search of the Congressional Index, the THOMAS system, and Internet listings of recent federal and state legislative activity, such as listings by the National Conference of State Legislatures. Recent omnibus legislation has focused primarily on children's health and on eliminating minority health disparities through Acts enabling greater access to health care and greater quality control for health systems, pharmaceuticals, and treatment programs (see Table 3.2).

State Legislation. States in the United States play a major role in policy areas ranging from welfare and health insurance to gambling and lotteries. As a result of these multiple interests some states adopt laws relevant to health promotion and others choose not to. Similarly, some states adopt strict laws whereas others adopt more lenient ones (Shipan & Volden, 2005). Public health law consonant with the federal statutes, particularly to impede the spread of infectious and venereal diseases, is found in all states, however (Gostin, 1986).

There is no omnibus state legislation concerning health promotion comparable to that at the federal level, perhaps, in part, because sections of federal legislation limit state actions. Legislation that addresses specific aspects of health promotion, from tobacco control and safety (for example, the use of motor vehicle seat belts and bicycle helmets) to minority disparity reduction and nutrition and obesity counseling, has passed in numerous states. Smoking control has emerged as important in both state and local legislation, and from 1975 to 2000, forty states adopted laws restricting or banning smoking in government buildings, and thirty-two enacted laws that placed similar restrictions on smoking in restaurants (Shipan

TABLE 3.2. EXAMPLES OF HEALTH PROMOTION LEGISLATION.

Common Name	Public Law Number	U.S. Code Title and Section Numbers
Ryan White CARE Act Amendments, 1996	PL 104-146	42 U.S.C. §§ 201 et seq.
Mammography Quality Standards Reauthorization Act, 1998	PL 105-248	42 U.S.C. §§ 201 note, 354 et seq.
Healthcare Research and Quality Act, 1999	PL 106-129	42 U.S.C. §§ 201 note, 299
Children's Health Act, 2000	PL 106-310	42 U.S.C. § 01 note
Public Health Improvement Act, 2000	PL 106-505	42 U.S.C. § 01 note
Minority Health and Health Disparities Research and Education Act, 2000	PL 106-525	42 U.S.C. § 02 note
Best Pharmaceuticals for Children Act, 2003	PL 107-109	21 U.S.C. § 55a 42 U.S.C. §§ 284 et seq.
Hematological Cancer Research Investment and Education Act, 2002	PL 107-172	42 U.S.C. § 201 note 42 U.S.C. § 285a-10 note
Rare Diseases Act, 2002	PL 107-280	42 U.S.C. § 201 note 42 U.S.C. § 283h
United States Leadership Against HIV/AIDS, Tuberculosis, and Malaria Act, 2003	PL 108-25	22 U.S.C. § 7601 note
Mosquito Abatement for Safety and Health Act, 2003	PL 108-75	42 U.S.C. § 201 note 42 U.S.C. §§ 243 et seq.
Garrett Lee Smith Memorial Act, 2004	PL 108-355	42 U.S.C. § 201 note 42 U.S.C. § 290bb-36 note

& Volden, 2005). In addition, nutrition and obesity counseling is addressed in numerous state statutes, such as Arkansas Act 1220 of 2003, which creates the Arkansas Child Health Advisory Committee that is responsible for the development of nutritional and physical activity standards and recommendations on food served to children, and Colorado H.R. 1016 of 2003, which supports effective nutrition programs that promote long-term health and lifelong physical wellness for Colorado citizens (National Conference of State Legislatures, 2005).

Local Legislation. Numerous city governments, including those of New York City, Los Angeles, San Francisco, and Houston, have historically instituted legislation concerning the protection of public health, particularly laws dealing with infectious and venereal diseases (Gostin, 1986). Of the 663 U.S. cities and towns with populations exceeding 50,000 in the year 2000, about one-half have adopted some form of smoking control regulations in the past quarter century (Schroeder, 2004). For example, in 2003, New York state prohibited smoking at work, in bars, food service areas, enclosed swimming pools, and on all mass transportation ("Clean Indoor Air Act," NYSDOH, Section 1399). Nutrition too has been a focus of local municipalities. For example, the North Carolina Division of Public Health (2005) is sponsoring the Eat Smart Move More . . . North Carolina program, a statewide initiative that promotes increased opportunities for physical fitness and healthy eating through both policy and environmental changes. Additionally, the state of Alaska has started the Take Heart Alaska program, a cardiovascular disease prevention plan that attempts to institute a comprehensive cardiovascular health status report in each local municipality (State of Alaska, 2005).

Legislation in Other Nations. Most U.S. health promotion initiatives conducted to date have targeted behavioral change primarily at the level of the individual (Green, Nathan, & Mercer, 2001). In contrast many European countries have not regarded omnibus legislation on health promotion as necessary because health promotion activities are integrated into their health care systems; further, many general health laws already make health care professionals responsible for health promotion and health education (Leenen, Pinet, & Prims, 1985). Sweden's Health and Medical Services Act of 1982, for example, emphasizes preventive activities and states that all forms of health and medical care are expected to include information and health education. In some eastern European and former Soviet bloc countries, turbulent political changes have impeded any unified legislative movement on health promotion. Many other countries rely on voluntary agreements with industry, thus limiting the role of national government (Roemer, 1982, 1986; World Health Organization, 1988).

Beyond Europe, countries have looked to the World Health Organization (WHO) and its Health for All by the Year 2000 initiative, launched by the Alma-Ata International Conference on Primary Health Care in 1978, which renewed the emphasis on community participation and on more equitable access to basic health resources (WHO, 1978). Article 25 of the seminal United Nations' Universal Declaration of Human Rights (United Nations, 1948) establishes health promotion as a priority for mothers, children, and the elderly, and serves as the basis for international health-promotive efforts. Such efforts include tobacco cessation programs in Australia enforced by statutory and judicial edicts such as restrictions and prohibitions on the marketing and advertising of the product (Reynolds, 1994; Green et al., 2001). In Belgium the Flemish Institute for Health Promotion (2005) seeks to provide health promotion services and local health consultation groups to serve as a portal to preventive health care resources for its citizens. In Poland legislation passed in 2004 will provide more funds to assist health promotive efforts in struggling state hospitals and clinics ("Poland's Lawmakers Pass Legislation . . . ," 2004).

Influential Actors

Public education campaigns and commercial advertising have increased interest in low-fat diets, physical exercise, and weight management. New screening technologies, such as the controversial computed tomography (CT) for the early detection of lung cancer (Henschke et al., 1999; Mulshine & Henschke, 2000), and new interventions, such as a vaccine against the human papillomavirus (HPV) to reduce the risk of cervical cancer (Franco & Harper, 2005), are emerging alongside increased public interest. With the growth of the Internet and other information technologies, many clients have become more knowledgeable about prevention and professional guidelines for screening. Health plans too have begun to realize that offering comprehensive health promotion and disease prevention is a valuable marketing tool for attracting new members.

The most influential actors in the health promotion field include the U.S. Preventive Services Task Force and selected federal agencies, world health agencies, voluntary and professional organizations, accreditors, media, and community advocacy groups and coalitions.

U.S. Preventive Services Task Force. Evidence-based medicine—that is, clinical practice based on accepted scientific findings, which are generally reviewed by a professional or scientific body—has become a critical influence on health care providers. One of the key actors in this arena is the U.S. Preventive Services Task Force (USPSTF), established by the U.S. Public Health Service in 1984. It is an independent panel of mostly nonfederal experts in primary care and prevention that uses a systematic methodology to review the evidence for the effectiveness of clinical preventive services (for example, screening tests, counseling interventions, immunizations, and chemoprevention); assigns ratings to the quality of the data; and issues clinical practice recommendations reflecting the strength of the supporting evidence (Woolf, Jonas, & Lawrence, 1996). The USPSTF has collaborated with medical subspecialties committed to the evidence-based policy, such as the American College of Physicians and the American Academy of Family Physicians, as well as with its Canadian counterparts. Task force findings have often varied from those of advocacy groups that have relied on older, opinion-based methods of review.

The first USPSTF assessed sixty topic areas in its *Guide to Clinical Preventive Services*, published in 1989. That USPSTF was disbanded with the publication of the guide; with the growth in scientific evidence, a second USPSTF was convened in 1990. In 1996, it published a second edition of the *Guide to Clinical Preventive Services* (USPSTF, 1996), comprising evaluations of 200 interventions in seventy areas. This 1996 guide accompanied the *Prevention Guidelines* of the Centers for Disease Control and Prevention (CDC) (Friede, O'Carroll, Nicola, Oberle, & Teutsch, 1997). In 1998, the *Clinicians' Handbook of Preventive Services* and the Put Prevention into Practice national implementation program were released.

In late 1998, the Agency for Healthcare Research and Quality (AHRQ) convened the current USPSTF. The USPSTF's guidelines are based on systematic evidence reviews conducted by two AHRQ-supported Evidence-Based Practice Centers (one at Oregon Health and Science University and the other at Research Triangle Institute-University of North Carolina), and advice from varied government and private panels of reviewers. The final recommendations balance the relative harms and benefits, including cost, by rating the quality of the evidence as "good," "fair, " or "poor," and the net benefit as "substantial," "moderate," "small," or "zero/negative" (Sheridan, Harris, & Woolf, 2003). The third edition of the *Guide to Clinical Preventive Services* (USPSTF, 2004) provides the latest available recommendations on preventive interventions, screening tests, counseling, immunizations, and medication regimens for more than eighty conditions. The USPSTF recommendations have founded performance measures that are used to judge quality by the National Committee for Quality Assurance (NCQA), peer review organizations (PROs), and the Joint Commission for Accreditation of Healthcare Organizations (JCAHO), holding providers and health care systems accountable for delivering effective health care.

For some health problems, such as secondhand smoke exposure, community-based interventions are more likely to decrease the problem behavior than are health care provider interventions. In 1996, the CDC thus formed the Task Force on Community Preventive Services to address a broad range of interventions, targeting communities and health care systems rather than individual clients. This task force's *Guide to Community Preventive Services* (Zaza, Briss, Harris; Task Force on Community Preventive Services, 2005) also provides public health decision makers with recommendations on population-based interventions to promote health and to prevent disease, injury, disability, and premature death at the state and local levels.

Yet identifying effective interventions can be difficult in prevention, where randomized controlled trials are often difficult to conduct. There is strong evidence for the effectiveness of brief clinician counseling in smoking cessation (Sheinfeld Gorin & Heck, 2004) and in reducing problem drinking. Intensive dietary counseling can lead to reduced dietary fat and cholesterol intake and increased fruit and vegetable consumption. Effective primary care–based interventions to increase physical activity have been more difficult to identify, although the PACE approach described in Chapter Six of this volume holds significant promise. Some studies suggest that provider counseling can increase the use of seat belts, child safety seats, and bicycle helmets, particularly when this counseling is delivered to parents of infants and young children. Brief counseling interventions aimed at high-risk individuals can increase condom use and prevent the spread of sexually transmitted diseases. Health provider recommendation is central to compliance with cancer screening tests, such as those for the breast, colon, and cervix (see Mandelblatt & Yabroff, 1999, for a review).

Barriers to the Dissemination of the USPSTF Guidelines. In practice, health care professionals vary in their use of counseling to change client behaviors. These variations are one contributor to the disparities in health care quality among ethnic and racial subgroups of the population.

Provider-level barriers to counseling include limited time, lack of training in prevention, lack of perceived effectiveness of selected preventive services, and practice environments that fail to facilitate prevention (Ashford et al., 2000; Sheinfeld Gorin et al., 2000; Hulscher, Wensing, van der Weijden, & Grol, 2002). Physicians find counseling time consuming and difficult to track and to charge; in fact physician time for counseling clients about health promotion is relatively short, often from two to six minutes (Mullen & Holcomb, 1990; Kushner, 1995; Ockene et al., 1995; Patton, Kolasa, West, & Irons, 1995; Burton et al., 1995; Price, Clause, & Everett, 1995; Schectman, Stoy, & Elinsky, 1994; Thompson, Schwankovsky, & Pitts, 1993; Ammerman et al., 1993; Cushman, James, & Waclawik, 1991; Logsdon, Lazaro, & Meier, 1989).

In addition to the barriers at the provider level, patient factors limit access to counseling (as well as to health care in general). Patient-related barriers include limited or no health insurance; limited literacy; delay in symptom recognition, diagnosis, and treatment; poor cultural matches between patients and providers; mistrust, low awareness, or limited knowledge of health care services; misunderstanding of provider instructions; and poor prior interactions with the health care system (reviewed in Institute of Medicine [IOM], 2003). Patient psychosocial barriers to care include fear, overestimation of personal disease risks, and a sense of fatalism (Sheinfeld Gorin, 2005; Sheinfeld Gorin & Albert, 2003; Honda & Sheinfeld Gorin, 2005; Sheinfeld Gorin & Heck, 2005) and also limited social support (Berkman & Syme, 1979; Berkman, 1995).

Similarly, provider-patient process factors, such as poor communication and uncertainty, may limit access to health care and health-promoting counseling, particularly for racial and ethnic subgroups. Within the time pressures exerted by the demands of modern health care and the beliefs about the likely cause of a patient's condition that are inculcated in medical students through their training, even bias and stereotyping may limit access to health care, particularly among minority patients (IOM, 2003)

Finally, system-level barriers—such as language barriers, differences in the geographic availability of health care institutions (including pharmacies) and in the distribution of health-promoting environments (for example, grocery stores selling healthful foods, Diez-Roux, 2003; parks; and bike and walking paths for physical activity), and enrollments of Medicaid patients in managed care systems that disrupt existing community-based provider practices and care networks (IOM, 2003)—may influence access to and the provision of quality care. Thus substantial gaps in the delivery of preventive health care remain.

Other Influences on Evidence-Based Practice. Internationally, the Cochrane Collaboration, a voluntary association of academics and clinicians, supports the development and publication of systematic reviews of rigorous studies in health. These reviews are widely available on the Web and through standard bibliographical search engines, such as MedLine. Although, in general, association members' interest rests more in treatment evaluations than in health promotion, the Australasian Cochrane Center in Melborne, Australia, is starting to support systematic reviews in health promotion and disease prevention, and a review group has been formed to examine the evidence for screening tests. Efforts are under way to form an evidence-based behavioral health review group. The Campbell Collaboration similarly supports systematic reviews of studies in health, as does the National Institute for Clinical Excellence (NICE) in the United Kingdom, and the Health Evidence Network (HEN) sponsored by the WHO Regional Office for Europe. Generally, the findings of these international collaborations have less influence on health care practice in the United States than do the findings of national groups, such as the USPSTF.

Selected Federal Agencies. Although health promotion policies are housed in several federal agencies, only the actions of the U.S. surgeon general and the CDC, which are functions of the U.S. Department of Health and Human Services (USDHHS) and, more specifically, the U.S. Public Health Service, are described at any length in this text. In particular the *Healthy People* documents, presented under the auspices of the surgeon general, have had unprecedented influence on the health promotion field because of the extent of participation that the health care community had in their preparation, their credibility, and the form and content of their texts. These documents are credited with beginning the second revolution in public health.

The First Public Health Revolution. The *first public health revolution* began with the watershed 1848 Public Health Act in Britain, and from that point forward the principle of state intervention in the lives of individuals to promote outcomes of social value was established. In particular this nineteenth-century revolution sought to improve the social and physical environment to decrease health hazards. This Act, as well as the two that preceded it (the English Towns Improvement Act of 1847 and the Liverpool Sanitary Act of 1846), provided a remedy for particular problems, designated *nuisances,* and allowed public authorities to order their removal. These nuisances were largely seen as things that smelled offensively, supporting the *miasmatic* idea that bad smells were a sign of disease. The Act authorized the undertaking of public health works, such as controls over slaughterhouses, common lodging houses, and offensive trades. It contained requirements for all new houses to be built with drains that connected to sewage systems where possible or to a cesspit. It also created a public health structure, the General Board of Health, which functioned as a national public health authority, and local boards of health, which consisted of supervisors of local surveyors and inspectors of nuisances. Responsibility for sewers was vested in the local boards, which had powers to control and cleanse (Reynolds, 1994).

The Second Public Health Revolution. The *second public health revolution,* reflected in *Healthy People: The Surgeon General's Report on Health Promotion and Disease Prevention* (U.S. Department of Health, Education and Welfare, Public Health Service, 1979), heralded the importance of lifestyle changes to health promotion and the importance of the reduction of chronic disease and the achievement of a better quality of life for all.

Early criticisms of the 1979 document and the second public health revolution were myriad (Neubauer & Pratt, 1981; Tesh, 1981). These criticisms focused on the importance attached to promoting individual lifestyle and behavioral change rather than to making policy recommendations to alter the social and economic factors that determine health (Neubauer & Pratt, 1981). The lifestyle hypothesis of the 1979 document approached disease as though ill health were the result of personal failure—a "victim-blaming" strategy—rather than placing disease causes and "solutions" in larger social and economic contexts (Navarro, 1976). The community response to this strategy was considerable, and concomitant changes in the health promotion field led to changes in subsequent publications of the Surgeon General.

The 1979 document was expanded in 1980, under the title *Promoting Health/Preventing Disease: Objectives for the Nation*. This document was followed by *Healthy People 2000* (USDHHS, 1991); *Healthy People 2000: Midcourse Review and 1995 Revisions* (USDHHS, 1995); *Healthy People 2000: Final Review;* and most recently, *Healthy People 2010*.

Healthy People 2010. *Healthy People 2010* (USDHHS, 2000a) provides a plan of action for the nation's health, with two major goals, to increase quality and years of healthy life and to eliminate health disparities. As did its forerunners, it establishes a set of specific *objectives*, 467 in number, organized into twenty-eight *focus areas*, as a basis for coordinated efforts to improve public health on the national, state, and local levels, and to be used as a teaching tool. Twenty-one of these objectives are found within ten *leading indicators*, which involve physical activity, overweight and obesity, tobacco use, substance abuse, responsible sexual behavior, mental health, injury and violence, environmental quality, immunization, and access to health care. The twenty-eight focus areas traverse the three broad categories of public health that were found in *Healthy People 2000:* health promotion, health protection, and preventive services. An interactive, online database, DATA2010, updated quarterly (CDC, 2005b), is available to track the *Healthy People 2010* objectives.

Unlike all previous national documents of this type, *Healthy People 2010* places the reduction of health disparities, improving life expectancy, and improving quality of life at its core. It also reflects a more integrated approach to health promotion, from lifestyle to environmental approaches, than previous documents do. In consonance with the *Health 21* document from WHO, and at variance with the individual risk orientation of *Healthy People 2000, Healthy People 2010* also reflects goals and objectives related to supportive environments.

Centers for Disease Control and Prevention. The Centers for Disease Control and Prevention is unique in the extent of its influence on the health promotion field because it is one of the few (and the oldest) agencies devoted to the singular mission of promoting health and quality of life, by preventing and controlling disease, injury, and disability. Through its twelve centers, institutes, and offices, it stewards a wide range of activities involving chronic disease prevention and health promotion, environmental health, infectious disease (for example, human immunodeficiency virus [HIV], sexually transmitted disease [STD], and tuberculosis [TB]) prevention, injury prevention and control, occupational safety and health, the national immunization program, epidemiology, and health statistics. Its scope is international and ranges from the review of privatization efforts to work with state and local health agencies. Few health promotion efforts fall outside its auspices (CDC, 2005a).

Other National Agencies. Several other national agencies are also active in health promotion. The Food and Drug Administration safeguards the nation's food supply (with the exception of meat and poultry products), dietary supplements (only postmarketing; see Chapter Ten), drugs and devices used for animals, cosmetic products, medical devides, radiation-emitting electronic products, and biologics by helping safe and effective products reach the market in a timely way and monitoring them for continued safety after they are in use. Recently, it was unsuccessful in its attempt to regulate nicotine as a drug. The Occupational Safety and Health Administration of the U.S. Department of Labor has established guidelines on workplace violence and initiatives in ergonomics that have been important to health promotion of late. The U.S. Department of Agriculture has been particularly influential through the nutritional programs it administers: the food stamps program for low-income Americans; the Special Supplemental Nutrition Program for Women, Infants, and Children (WIC); and child nutrition programs. Last, the Environmental Protection Agency enforces the removal of toxic wastes and monitors toxic air pollution and pesticide use, a key component of health promotion.

National Voluntary and Professional Organizations. Numerous singularly focused voluntary organizations such as the American Cancer Society, the American Heart Association, and the American Lung Association have advanced the health promotion agenda nationally and internationally and have educated clients. Similarly, professional groups such as the American Public Health Association and the American College of Preventive Medicine, in pursuing their members' interests, have either directly influenced omnibus health promotion legislation or specific legislation (for example, concerning nutrition) and have provided direct service to clients.

The more than 300 professional associations contributing to health promotion in this country have assisted in the development of a national agenda for health promotion; have influenced legislation; and have engaged in education, screening, and other preventive services for clients. These associations include the

American Public Health Association, Society for Public Health Education, American Nurses Association, American Academy of Family Physicians, American College of Physicians, American College of Preventive Medicine, American College of Nutrition, American Dietetic Association, American Physical Therapy Association, American Dental Association, and National Association of Social Workers. Many of these organizations and groups are represented by some of the 18,000 registered lobbyists who incurred roughly $3 billion in 2003 expenses (Mike Scott, director of Government Affairs, American Society of Anesthesiologists, personal communication, January 19, 2004) to influence legislation and national, state, and local agendas.

Multilateral Organizations: WHO. The World Health Organization (WHO), formed in 1948 as a function of the United Nations, is the most influential worldwide actor in health promotion. Its guiding principles were first articulated in the Alma-Ata Declaration on Primary Health Care of 1978, emphasizing that health is a fundamental right, to be guaranteed by the state; that people should be prime movers in shaping their health services, using and enlarging upon the capacities developed in their societies; that health services should operate as an integral whole, with promotive, preventive, curative, and rehabilitation components; and that any Western medical technology used in non-Western societies must conform to the cultural, social, economic, and epidemiologic conditions of the individual countries. The Alma-Ata declaration was endorsed by every country in the world (WHO, 1978).

WHO's orientation toward health promotion was developed in 1986 during the First International Conference on Health Promotion, held in Ottawa, Canada (Canadian Public Health Association, 1986). After the Ottawa conference, WHO convened a series of global conferences to explore healthy public policy (in Adelaide, Australia, in 1988), supportive environments for health (in Sundsvall, Sweden, in 1991), and determinants of health in the twenty-first century (in Jakarta, Indonesia, in 1997). At the fifth conference (in Mexico City in 2000), the Mexico Ministerial Statement on Health Promotion yielded the most recent health promotion framework, which focuses on bridging the equity gap through promoting health. The sixth conference (in Bangkok, Thailand, in 2005) produced the Bangkok Charter for Health Promotion, with frameworks and strategies for sustainable and integrated health promotion. Of late, WHO has begun to recognize the importance of health promotion among the growing number of aging individuals worldwide, as reflected in its structural integration of its Chronic Diseases and Health Promotion functions into a single department and in its Ageing and Life Course initiative.

Over time, WHO has altered its definition of health and health promotion, moving from an individual risk factor modification model to a model that embodies a social resource orientation, as found in its *Health for All* report. *Health for All*, similar in intent to *Healthy People 2000*, embodies thirty-eight regional targets within six themes; its adoption by the member states of the European region of WHO in 1984 was key to the widespread recognition of health promotion. It includes targets for modifying individual lifestyles for disease risk reduction (the focus of *Healthy People 2000*), alongside the goal to promote a "social model of health," which grew from a European tradition linking social reform and public health (Kickbusch, 2003).

The *Health for All* document describes five lifestyle and health targets, grouped as a *package*, that address healthy public policy, social support systems, knowledge and motivation, positive health behavior, and health-damaging behavior. In WHO's subsequent revisions of the targets in 1991 and 1998, it has highlighted the complex political and social processes necessary to achieve changes in health. The *Health for All* targets (1) focus on primary health care; (2) emphasize the role of the health care system emphasis in the promotion of health and the prevention of disease; (3) highlight effective cooperation among all sectors of government and society; (4) rely on a well-informed, motivated, and actively participating community (as a key element for attaining common goals); (5) strengthen international cooperation (as health problems transcend national frontiers); and (6) emphasize the reduction of health inequalities as far as possible (WHO, 1985). Equity is a key concern of *Health for All*; the principles assert that people need social and economic opportunities to maintain and develop their health. Unlike *Healthy People 2000*, which was primarily concerned with lifestyle changes, more than one-half of the *Health for All* targets require changes in legislation (Pinet, 1986). To date, twenty-seven European countries have formulated targets using the WHO policy as a starting point, as have regions, provinces, and cities (Kickbusch, 2003). A report published in 2001 by the Swedish National Committee for Public Health (a parliamentary committee) is a notable example, focusing on both health determinants and health promotion rather than health behaviors.

The most recent WHO target documents (notably *Health 21*, a revision of *Health for All*, WHO, 1999) have reinforced the commitment to address health determinants and to seek strategic entry points outside the health care system (Kickbusch, 2003). "Health is a powerful political platform" (WHO, 1999).

A European document (WHO, 1998) derived from *Health 21* has strengthened the commitment to the values of equity, participation, solidarity, sustainability, and accountability. These values, with their humanist orientation, stand in contrast to the population-health orientation and economic rationales of many other health promotion documents.

Examples of WHO Health Promotion Initiatives. WHO member states have recently agreed to the impressive *Framework Convention on Tobacco Control* (WHO,
2004b), with 164 signatories, that may serve as a mandate for tobacco control programs throughout the world (see Chapter Nine for more discussion). WHO has
also prepared the WHO *Global Strategy on Diet, Physical Activity and Health* (2004a),
to direct member states' attention to this emerging health promotion area.

Yet another example of a WHO health promotion activity is the Healthy
Cities project. This project began in Canada in 1984 and in Europe in 1986. The
explicit aim of the WHO Healthy Cities project is to localize the *Health for All* strategy in designated cities by involving political decision makers and by building a
strong local lobby for public health interests. The qualities of a healthy city developed by the project were thought to be related to residents' well-being and quality of life (Hancock & Duhl, 1988). In 2003, the WHO Healthy Cities network
launched its fourth phase (WHO, 2005). These projects, still in development, stress
a municipal approach to health promotion through extensive community participation, intersectoral cooperation, partnerships at all levels, good urban governance, and the implementation of comprehensive city plans for health promotion.

These projects have expanded throughout Europe, in other French- and
Spanish-speaking regions of the world, in the Asian Pacific region (for example,
Australia, Japan, and New Zealand), and in an increasing number of developing
countries (for example, Iran and Ghana). The Pan American Health Organization has created a strong *healthy municipalities network* that includes hundreds of cities.

In the United States, the Coalition for Healthy Cities and Communities has
based its work on the WHO approach (Association for Community Health Improvement, 2005; Kickbusch, 2003). For example, California Healthy Cities and
Communities has funded community-based nutrition and physical activity programs in several cities, and these programs have included the enactment of policies for land and complementary water use, improved access to produce, elevated
public consciousness about health, culturally appropriate educational and training materials, and strengthened community-building skills (Twiss et al., 2003). The
active role of citizens and the community is central to this settings approach.

Some of these projects have been assessed by systematically evaluating their impact on social and political processes. Some "promising interventions" (IOM, 2000a)
have helped to frame health in terms of relevance to people and communities.

Canadian Leadership and the Third Public Health Revolution. Canada has
been a leader in promoting health, both nationally and internationally. In 1974,
A New Perspective on the Health of Canadians, also known as the Lalonde Report (after
the Canadian Minister of Health at that time), assessed priorities for improving
the health status of the Canadian population and was instrumental in bringing

attention to the health promotion movement (Lalonde, 1974). The report describes the relationships between access to health care services, human biology, environment, and individual behaviors, and estimates the relative contribution to outcomes that progress in each of these areas might make (USPSTF, 1996). In 1986, Canada's Public Health Association and Health and Welfare Canada played a significant role in the development of health promotion internationally through their cosponsorship (with the World Health Organization) of the First International Conference on Health Promotion, where the Ottawa Charter for Health Promotion was produced, and nationally through the release of *Achieving Health for All: A Framework for Health Promotion* (also known as the Epp report) (Epp, 1986). Analyses of *Achieving Health for All* revealed its attention to individual responsibilities and rights, health promotion, and broad health determinants, as well as its consonance with a more cost-contained health care delivery system (Iannantuono & Eyles, 1997). The Ottawa Charter's conceptualization of health as a "resource for living" and its shift in focus from disease prevention to "capacity building for health" initiated the *third public health revolution* by concomitantly committing health promotion to social reform and equity (Kickbusch, 2003; Breslow, 1985). In the third public health revolution, health is recognized as a key dimension of the quality of life. The Ottawa Charter seeks to move health out of the professional action frame into organizations and the community (the "context of everyday life"). Health promotion is produced in the dynamic exchange between people and their environments; the process of involvement is considered health promoting in that it creates self-esteem, a sense of worth, and social capital (Kickbusch, 2003). The charter outlines five key action areas that reinforce each other, with the goal of improving the health of populations: (1) build healthy public policies (policies supportive of health in sectors other than health), (2) create environments supportive of health, (3) develop personal skills, (4) strengthen community actions, and (5) reorient health services for health promotion. Health professionals are to "enable, advocate, and mediate."

Similarly, in 1976 the Canadian government undertook one of the first comprehensive efforts to examine the effectiveness of clinical preventive care when it convened the Canadian Task Force on the Periodic Health Examination, now called the Canadian Task Force on Preventive Health Care (CTFPHC). Using explicit criteria to judge empirical research on clinical preventive services, the CTFPHC examined preventive services for seventy-eight target conditions, releasing its report in 1979. Between 1979 and 1994, it published a series of updates and revisions to the original report, released in 1994 as the *Canadian Guide to Clinical Preventive Health Care*. Called "the red brick," because of its 1,009 pages and its color, this guide has been considered a standard reference tool for Canadian primary care physicians (USPSTF, 1996; Canadian Task Force on the Periodic

Health Examination, 1994; Canadian Task Force on Preventive Health Care, 2000). Presently, the CTFPHC continues to publish its evidence reviews and recommendations, in English and in French, in major Canadian journals and online. As discussed earlier in this chapter in relation to the USPSTF's work, several challenges remain in the clinical implementation of the CTFPHC guidelines.

Accreditors. Accreditation is a self-assessment and external peer review process used by health care organizations to accurately assess their level of performance in relation to established standards and to implement ways to continuously improve the health care system (Tregloan, 1998). In particular, patient safety is a major issue for health care professionals, payers, and patients. Over the past five years, dozens of bills have been submitted to the U.S. Congress addressing patient safety and the need to ensure quality health care delivery systems, including the Patient Safety and Quality Improvement Act of 2003. The need to provide health service accountability has never been greater.

In some countries there is one main accreditation program for health services (for example, the Health Quality Service in the United Kingdom and Quality Health in New Zealand), whereas in the United States two major accrediting groups—the National Commission for Quality Assurance (NCQA) and the Joint Commission on Accreditation of Healthcare Organizations (JCAHO)—maintain standards for the quality of organizations' structured health promotion activities. Other organizations, such as the National Association for Healthcare Quality and the American Society of Health-System Pharmacists, may monitor medication safety, and prestigious scientific groups, such as the Institute of Medicine and the nonprofit Institute for Healthcare Improvement, may document the overall quality of health care through their focus on seminal issues, such as health disparities, without issuing certifications. Additionally, rapidly growing groups such as the Utilization Review Accreditation Committee (URAC) serve to promote continuous improvement in the quality and efficiency of health care delivery services by streamlining the processes used to determine whether health care is medically necessary, helping to keep health care costs down for both payers and providers.

Accreditors use a combination of on-site expert surveys of an organization and reviews of written materials to determine whether an organization has met preestablished guidelines for health care. Accreditation indicates that an entity has adopted a set of quality standards and that its performance is continually reviewed. Accreditation, although voluntary, is critical to a health care center's continued receipt of insurance funds, competition for employer health care contracts, and licensure for Medicare certification through *deemed status* (as a home health agency or hospice). Often, accreditation by major accreditors serves as an adjunct to federal or state inspection of health care facilities. These external accreditations are important adjuncts to the continuous quality improvement (CQI) systems that monitor, correct, and enhance the services of many agencies.

NCQA is a private, not-for-profit organization dedicated to improving health care quality and is frequently referred to as a watchdog for the managed care industry. Thirty states now recognize NCQA accreditation as meeting certain regulatory requirements for health plans, eliminating the need for a separate state review. NCQA evaluates health plans in the areas of patient safety, confidentiality, consumer protection, access, service, and continuous improvement; its Health Plan Employer Data and Information Set (HEDIS) *report card* requirements guide the managed care industry.

Since 1997, NCQA has produced an annual *State of Health Care Quality* report that provides an overall assessment of the performance of the health care system. These findings are issued before the annual open enrollment season, when most Americans choose their health plan for the following year. In compiling these data, NCQA requires an organization to evaluate the use of preventive services among those at risk, including cholesterol measurement; exercise promotion; smoking cessation; and counseling for prevention of motor vehicle injury, sexually transmitted diseases, and alcohol and other drug abuse (NCQA, 2004). The evaluation process includes looking at both the groups at risk and the population as a whole.

Under the guidance of NCQA, consumers, insurance purchasers, and health maintenance organizations (HMOs) developed the HEDIS measures for HMOs to evaluate the quality of services and care they provide. HEDIS addresses a broad range of important health issues including childhood and adolescent immunization status, high blood pressure control, asthma medication use, antidepressant medication management, breast cancer screening, and smoking cessation counseling. Using the HEDIS findings, NCQA has recently created the Quality Compass,® which allows users to compare health plans side by side and to make health care coverage decisions based on quality and value as well as provider network and price (NCQA, 2005).

JCAHO is the predominant standards setting and accrediting body in the United States, with more than 15,000 health care organizations and programs under its supervision, including ambulatory care centers, home health care centers, behavioral health care organizations, health care networks, corporate health services, long-term care organizations, hospitals, and pathology and clinical laboratory services. Since 1994, JCAHO has enumerated health promotion and disease prevention guidelines for health care networks, including HMOs, preferred provider organizations (PPOs), and other managed care entities that are performance or outcome focused. It addresses each organization's level of performance in areas such as patient rights, patient treatment, and infection control and the organization's performance with respect to health promotion and disease prevention.

For behavioral health care organizations, including those that provide mental health and addiction services, JCAHO has developed draft standards for behavioral health promotion and illness prevention (JCAHO, 2005).

JCAHO also awards disease-specific care certification to health plans, hospitals, and other service delivery settings that provide disease management and chronic care services. In 1997, JCAHO launched its ORYX® initiative, which integrates outcomes and other performance measures into the accreditation process, affording a flexible approach that can support quality improvement efforts across all health delivery systems; by 2004, almost all hospitals were expected to comply with new standards and submit data across several core components (JCAHO, 2005).

Efforts to standardize accreditation procedures were helped when, in 2003, NCQA and JCAHO formed a partnership for the purpose of establishing an accreditation program for efforts to protect human subjects in research. This union also realizes one aim of behavioral health advocates by allaying fears about how informed consent for research participation is obtained from individuals with serious mental illnesses.

The Media. The media provide illumination and a focus of attention that is enormously powerful, particularly when the spotlight can be held in place. When governments, advocates, and others are setting their health care agendas, the mass media may provide the first step in public awareness and change; conversely, by withholding attention, they can leave issues in the dark (Wallack, Dorfman, Jernigan, & Themba, 1993). Even though the media recently have begun to expand their coverage of health-promotive lifestyles, communication challenges remain.

The American public depends on the news media for reliable health information. Yet many health care professionals meet with difficulties when sharing science news with the public through the mass media (Rowan, 2005). For example, the media may not always report health threats accurately. These inaccuracies may contribute to the public's overestimation of mortality from causes that are actually infrequent (for example, deaths resulting from illicit drugs) and underestimation of mortality from causes that are frequent (for example, heart disease) (Adams, 1992–1993; Frost, Frank, & Mailbach, 1997). (There is considerable confusion about how best to discuss health risks in numerical terms, however, even in clinical settings; Woloshin, Schwartz, & Welch, 2002.) Moreover, the media may, at the same time, promote healthful eating through public service announcements and promote high-fat, high-sugar foods through paid advertising.

Health care providers may enhance their communication with the mass media by using several evidence-based strategies from the CAUSE model (Rowan, Bethea, Pecchioni, & Villagran, 2003). This model involves earning the *c*onfidence of respected journalists, creating awareness of health issues, deepening under-standing, gaining the satisfaction of news coverage, and motivating enactment or behavioral change. (For a bibliography of works on health risk communication see U.S. National Library of Medicine, 2003.)

Mass media interventions can be more cost effective for a large target group relative to individual clinical interventions. Successful media interventions tend to share several characteristics: (1) they use a multimedia approach with ties to community interventions, such as support groups (Hastings, 1989; McAlister, 1982); (2) they concentrate on knowledge or awareness rather than attitude and behavioral change (Hastings, 1989; Roberts & Maccoby, 1985); and (3) they at-tempt to change the more tractable behaviors, such as understanding one's prob-lems, rather than, for example, altering one's genetic predispositions (Barker, Pistrang, Shapiro, Davies, & Shaw, 1993). A 2004 University of Vermont and Baylor College of Medicine study, for instance, found that a carefully tailored mass media program had reduced cigarette smoking by over 30 percent six years after the program's initiation (Baylor College of Medicine, 2004).

To evaluate media interventions, one must specify the type of changes de-sired, the population subgroups in which the changes are desired, and the cir-cumstances under which they are desired (Barker et al., 1993). The use of long time frames, such as a period of years, is also recommended in the measurement of change (Lorion, 1983).

From an advocacy perspective (that is, when seeking to use the media to in-fluence those who can change the social environment), several approaches appear important. Media advocates frame issues in terms of root causes and focus on pol-icy concerns rather than personal behaviors. They use the dramatic story, with characters, plots, villains, and heroes. Advocates take advantage of opportunities to respond to breaking news, such as a decision in a tobacco company trial, to cre-ate news of their own. Media advocates know what their adversaries' reactions to a story will be, and they maintain controlled communication with the press. They seek to understand their topic, plan their goals, and understand how the media work (Wallack et al., 1993).

The explosion of the Internet with its Web communities and individual Web logs, or blogs, allows for rapid dissemination of information to the consumer seek-ing quick and easy advice regarding health habits. Blogs are quickly becoming fo-rums for the rapid exchange of ideas on all topics, with the Pew Center indicating that one in nine Web viewers frequents blogs, translating to about fifty million readers worldwide (MarketingVOX News, 2004). These forums can be used to generate dialogue, but they can also be dominated by those with commercial in-terests or competing claims, increasing decision conflict. Anonymous Internet por-tals managed by reputable health care organizations, such as the CDC, may be an effective vehicle for channeling essential messages to consumers who may find it difficult to parse conflicting information in TV, radio, or print media.

Community Advocacy Groups and Coalitions. Community groups, such as Mothers Against Drunk Driving (MADD) and the National Alliance of Breast Cancer Organizations (NABCO), have been effective advocates for change in laws concerning drinking and driving (MADD) and breast cancer (NABCO). In the case of tobacco use, for example, community and professional groups have organized coalitions to lobby successfully for legislation that outlaws smoking in public buildings, workplaces, restaurants, schools, and sporting events across the country and, in conjunction with international partners such as the World Health Organization, in many parts of the developed world. They have influenced schools of medicine to teach smoker counseling, they have provided consultation for clinical trials in community settings (for example, COMMIT and ASSIST, as described in Chapter Nine), and they have galvanized community attitudes toward favoring smoking control.

Organizational Policy

Organizations such as schools, workplaces, public health departments, and health care facilities are central to the implementation of health promotion legislation, regulations, and policies and are essential to the formation of new initiatives. These organizations wield considerable influence on community, group, and individual behavior and, as community-based programs, are the focus of many of the objectives of *Healthy People 2010.*

School Districts and Schools. Lifetime patterns of diet, exercise, smoking, and coping with stress may be established in childhood. Because the roughly sixty million children and youths in America spend much of their days in school, the school has become an important context in which to change these patterns, through legislation, policies, and regulation. Children may learn about their bodies and the effects of different lifestyle behaviors in this context. Children may also gain access to necessary preventive services, such as age-appropriate immunizations, nutritious meals, and regular, organized physical activity. The school also may connect families to health insurance programs, potentially through state waiver funding or through Medicaid aid packages, thus enriching a family's ability to continue to receive preventive services.

Many schools have adopted the CDC's Healthy Youth program eight-component model for a coordinated school health program. This model encourages schools to use health education, physical education, health services, nutritional services, health promotion for staff, counseling and psychological services, a healthy school environment, and parent and community involvement to motivate and assist students to maintain and improve their health, prevent disease, and reduce health-related risk behaviors (CDC, 2005c). The number of school-based health centers (SBHCs) that have implemented this program has grown substantially, from 200 in 1990 to 1,498 in 2002, representing a 650 percent increase in twelve years. School-based health centers can be found in forty-five states plus the District of Columbia, with sixteen of these states providing full grant support to these centers.

Health-related coursework and programs vary across schools, state by state. In 2002, the percentage of schools in each state that required health education for students in grades 6 through 12 ranged from 32.7 percent to 100 percent, with a median of 92.3 percent. Most schools (median, 93.7 percent) taught one or more separate required health education courses (CDC, 2002), almost all (95 percent) local school districts had antismoking education in elementary schools. Although most schools (93 percent) provided some instruction concerning alcohol and other drug use, only about 51 percent provided related counseling services (CDC, 2002). In 2002, only 6.5 percent of middle and junior high schools and 5.8 percent of senior high schools met the recommended standard of daily physical education for all students. This percentage must be increased to comply with the *Healthy People 2010* objectives that call for daily physical education as a comprehensive approach to promoting health among young people.

Healthy People 2010 has extended the mandate for educating students about health in middle, junior, and high schools to colleges and universities. This document emphasizes six priority areas; injuries, both intentional and unintentional; tobacco use; alcohol and illicit drug use; sexual behaviors that cause unintended pregnancies and sexually transmitted diseases; dietary patterns that cause disease; and inadequate physical activity. According to *Healthy People 2010*, only 6 percent of college and university students have received information in all six priority areas. Thus, engaging university trustees and administrations, college health services, student groups, parents, and community groups in increasing health promotion awareness and literacy among these young adults is key.

The State Children's Health Insurance Program (SCHIP) gives grants to states to provide health insurance coverage to the approximately ten million uninsured children in families with incomes up to 200 percent of the federal poverty level. This program, enacted under Public Law 105-33 (passed in 1997), and Title XXI of the Social Security Act, allows states to expand Medicaid or to create their own children's health insurance programs and provides an alternative to employer-based health insurance by using schools as the grouping mechanism to negotiate group health insurance policies. The program also increases health care stability because coverage is not disrupted if a parent changes or loses his or her job. States are allowed to impose premiums, deductibles, or fees, but no copayments can be charged for pediatric preventative care, including immunizations. Through this cost-sharing method, states can match federal funds provided through the SCHIP program to cover children who otherwise would receive no coverage for a variety of services (American Academy of Pediatrics, 2005).

Worksites and Unions. Over 148 million adult persons go to work every day; individuals spend more than one-third of their waking hours at work (Bureau of Labor Statistics, 2005a; Gomel, Oldenburg, Simpson, & Owen, 1993). Fourteen out of every 100 U.S. workers belong to a labor union (Bureau of Labor Statistics, 2005b) and generally have access to medical care through their benefit plans. As a result, worksites and unions are important components of community-wide health promotion efforts. Further, traditional worksite-based health promotion programs are seen as an employee benefit that increases employee morale and attracts and retains good workers at relatively little cost. In 1999, 95 percent of employers with fifty employees or more reported offering at least one health promotion activity (Association for Worksite Health Promotion, 1999).

Workplaces oriented toward promoting good health for employees in order to decrease costs of absenteeism, increase productivity, or create more effective organizations may offer multifaceted supportive programs, employee assistance programs (EAPs) for behavioral health promotion, and health insurance. Since the 1990s, under the Drug-Free Workplace Act of 1988, EAPs have become the linchpin of many workplace-based substance abuse programs, alongside drug-free workplace policies, training and educational programs, and the identification of illegal drug users (Glemigani, 1998; Hoffman, Larison, & Sanderson, 1997; Greenberg & Grunberg, 1995; Delaney & Ames, 1995; Galvin, 2000). In addition, under Occupational Safety and Health Administration (OSHA) regulations, worksites integrate the protection of employee health through setting and enforcing safety standards, training workers, and offering safety education. As described in Chapter Fourteen, the more progressive worksites may see the creation of healthful work as an aim in itself.

Although worksite-based health promotion programs are generally well accepted (Johansson & Partanen, 2002), have been found effective in reducing employees' health risks (Wilson, Holman, & Hammock, 1996; Heaney & Goetzel, 1997), and have the potential to reduce health costs to employers (Edington, Yen, & Witting, 1997), recruiting participants remains a challenge. Of the employees who reported access to such programs in the National Health Interview Survey, only 4.6 percent participated in smoking cessation programs, 34.7 percent in stress management programs, 27.6 percent in nutrition programs, and 39.4 percent in cancer screening programs (Grosch, Alterman, Petersen, & Murphy, 1998). Participation was highest among those with a college education or greater (48.8 percent, compared to 24.6 percent among those with less than a high school diploma).

Although many worksite-based health promotion programs attempt to maximize participation, some encourage participation according to employees' health risk profiles (Breslow, 1999). This *population health management* approach attempts to lower the risks of high-risk employees while maintaining the status of lower-risk employees (Serxner, Anderson, & Gold, 2004), matching the health message and the program component (for example, newsletters, help lines, workshops, or printed information) to the employee's readiness to change (Prochaska & Velicer, 1997).

Union-based health promotion projects may have access to blue-collar workers who may be otherwise difficult to reach and who have higher rates of smoking and poorer health outcomes than workers in white-collar positions do (Albertsen, Hannerz, Borg, & Burr, 2003; Barbeau, Krieger, & Soobader, 2004; Turrell, Hewitt, Patterson, Oldenburg, & Gould, 2002). There is some evidence to suggest that unions are amenable to worksite risk modification programs, such as smoking cessation interventions that include systematic prevention messages as well as policy changes (Sorensen et al., 2000), and comprehensive programs designed to change dietary behaviors (Heimendinger et al., 1995).

Smaller worksites are often unable to offer employee assistance programs; smaller firms are also less likely to offer their workers comprehensive health insurance that includes preventive services. Outsourcing, using existing community services, and collaborating with unions and trade or professional organizations may enhance employees' access to traditional worksite health promotion programs, particularly for employees of smaller organizations.

Public Health Departments and Health Care Facilities. Public health departments and other health care facilities are influential contexts for the process of health promotion. Created by statute, public health departments reflect the interests of state and local advocacy groups and government officials (Gebbie, 2000). *Healthy People 2010,* alongside the need to develop the public health infrastructure and to strengthen the public health workforce (see Chapter Four), data, systems, and resources, presented the development of a model public health statute as an objective. *Public Health in America* (Public Health Functions Steering Committee, 1994), a consensus document, reflects a recent initiative also designed to strengthen the nation's public health infrastructure.

Public health departments, oriented toward optimizing the health of the entire community, have traditionally been concerned with ensuring health through the control of communicable diseases; health education; environmental sanitation;

consumer protection; and the provision of medical and nursing services for the diagnosis, treatment, and prevention of diseases in hard-to-reach populations (McCaig, 1994b). Health departments are, however, changing rapidly under the pressure to improve early detection of disease, as part of disaster preparedness (and thus also to improve their rapid, real-time information sharing; Broome & Loonsk, 2004; also see Chapter Thirteen). They are also under pressure to increase access to health care for the culturally and linguistically diverse populations in the communities they serve (Liao et al., 2004). Public health activities are generally coordinated by a network of municipal, state, and federal agencies and are quite diverse (CDC & the National Association of County and City Health Officials, 1994).

More than forty million Americans receive one or more clinical services through public health departments, and about one-half of these agencies provide clinical preventive care (CDC & the National Association of County and City Health Officials, 1994). In many of these departments, services are offered in a *package*, including immunizations, health education, tuberculosis screening and treatment, well-child visits, nutritional services for women and children, sexually transmitted disease screening, partner identification and treatment, and HIV testing and counseling. Often, preventive care is built into the medical protocols departments must follow; many of these protocols are derived from state or federal statutes.

Hospitals, and particularly hospital emergency rooms (ERs), provide another context for health promotion. They are the primary sites for clinical care among vulnerable members of the population, such as the homeless, the uninsured, and the working poor. More than 120 million persons visit an emergency room each year, generally for the treatment of a presenting illness or injury, possibly from their occupations. Blood pressure measurement, a screening test, is performed in most ER visits (Frew, 1991). Nonurgent problems, often among the more vulnerable in the population, account for many ER visits, thus enabling health care professionals to screen for hypertension, hypercholesterolemia, cervical and other cancers, and syphilis and to conduct other forms of early detection (Chernow & Iserson, 1987; Burns, Stoy, Feied, Nash, & Smith, 1991; Hogness, Engelstad, Linck, & Schorr, 1992; Hibbs, Ceglowski, Goldberg, & Kauffman, 1993). ER staff have an opportunity to counsel patients on injury prevention (McCaig, 1994a) and smoking cessation. Although preventive care is provided in this setting and the ER serves as the primary clinical site for many in the population, this usage is not without problems. The waits are often long; elevations in blood pressure may be a result of anxiety, thus leading to misdiagnoses; and follow-up—critical to prevention of sexually transmitted diseases, for example—is rare (Avner, 1992).

Economic Contexts for Health Promotion

In 2004, the United States spent $1.8 trillion dollars on health, 95 percent of which went for direct medical services. Only 5 percent was allocated to preventing and promoting health (Centers for Medicare and Medicaid Services, Office of the Actuary, 2005). Approximately 15.3 percent of the 2003 gross domestic product (GDP) was earmarked for health expenditures, a figure that has been rising steadily over the past decade. Additionally, according to the Centers for Medicare and Medicaid Services (CMS) (formerly the Health Care Financing Administration [HCFA]), per capita expenditure will increase at an annual rate of 7.3 percent, from $4,637 in 2000 to $9,216 by 2011 (CMS, Office of the Actuary, 2005). Despite this generous national expenditure, the United States consistently ranks below many industrialized nations in population wellness, ranking thirty-seventh in the most recent WHO survey of longevity and quality of life (WHO, 2004c).

Commercial insurance companies, Blue Cross Blue Shield and other health plans, federal insurance programs, and managed care are the major sources of monies for health promotion services. About 85 percent of Americans are covered by health insurance through these insurers and employer self-insurance, including administrative service contracts. Importantly, however, forty-four million persons, including 11.2 million children, are without any health insurance because they are employed by firms that do not offer coverage or because their incomes are below the poverty line and they cannot afford it (U.S. Census Bureau, 2004). Uninsured children are more likely than the insured to lack a usual source of health care, to go without needed care, and to experience worse health outcomes (IOM, 2002). Thirty percent of children without coverage are under six years old, and one in three uninsured children lives in a family below the poverty line (Mills & Bhandari, 2003).

More and better insurance coverage for health screening and counseling would encourage wider use of preventive services, but it is difficult for commercial insurers to develop a financially viable market for them. Because health insurance was initially developed to protect individuals from the largely unpredictable and high costs of hospitalization and catastrophic illness, by definition it is generally limited to services that are deemed *medically necessary* to diagnose and treat illness rather than for prevention (Garland & Stull, 2004). For example, the use of health promotion programs such as nutrition counseling is predictable (based on the presence of specific risk factors) and relatively low in cost, so such programs have never been considered medically necessary (Riedel, 1987). Further, commercial insurers have increasingly been criticized for failing to curtail the rapid health care cost increases that might accompany new programs and that are outpacing worker earnings increases and inflation rates.

The World Bank, another source of funds for government programs, has a significant influence on international economies, so its recent designation of health as an indicator of national development will affect the health promotion field. Additionally, through their efforts to bring curative medicines to market, the pharmacological, botanical, and biotechnology industries are briefly discussed in this text as contributors to the economy of health promotion (see Table 3.3).

Commercial Insurance Companies

Since the 1930s, commercial insurance companies have reimbursed the insured patient, or *beneficiary*, with stipulated sums of money to be applied against expenditures for the insured risks. Subscribers bear sole responsibility for identifying their need for health care, locating the providers of care, and paying for the care. The insurer reimburses them for their *reasonable and customary* expenses (Shouldice, 1991). In the face of escalating costs, employers have begun to shift costs to employees and to expand the types of insurance plans offered as consumers react to the cost-cutting measures of the HMO-dominated 1990s and seek greater flexibility for their health dollar. Many of today's employer groups are self-insured (that is, they bear the entire risk for their employees internally); a commercial insurance company may then simply administer an employer's plans, without the attribution of risk.

Health insurers plans and policies are driven largely by concerns over rising health care costs. A 2003 survey of New Jersey insurance plans (New Jersey Business & Industry Association, 2003a, 2003b) found that health insurance costs increased by an average of 13 percent in 2003, after a 15 percent spike in 2002. Survey respondents reported paying an average of $6,692 per covered employee for policies in 2003, up $781 from 2002, and up over 53 percent from 1998. A Kaiser Family Foundation survey of 2,800 companies conducted in the fall of 2004 found that for companies with fewer than 200 employees, insurance premiums increased 15.5 percent, compared with 13.2 percent for larger companies. The study also found that erosion of retiree health care benefits is a growing concern as employers are forced to scale back because of rising costs (Kaiser Family Foundation and Health Research and Educational Trust, 2004).

Among employer groups, any employee demand for preventive services encounters pressures to control costs. Employees, too, may tend to resist raising premiums to pay for additional benefits (Steckler, Dawson, Goodman, & Epstein, 1987). Faced with increasing competition for the business of healthy employer

TABLE 3.3. COMPONENTS OF MAJOR ECONOMIC PROGRAMS FOR HEALTH PROMOTION.

Program	Focus	Examples of Components
Commercial insurance companies[a]	Reimburse client with fixed sum for expenses of insured risks. May manage self-insurance by companies.	91% offer colorectal, prostate, breast, and cervical cancer screening. 90% offer mammograms. 87% offer HIV/AIDS education. 76% offer nutrition counseling. 98% offer diabetes screening. 99% offer smoking cessation.
Blue Cross Blue Shield[b]	Offers nonprofit medical contracts for medical services to members; generally reimburses on preset schedule. Insurer of last resort to many.	Preventive screenings offered. Smoking cessation offered. Offers coverage to 1 in 3 Americans through managed care programs such as HMOs, PPOs, POS plans, Medicare managed care, integrated delivery systems.
Federal insurance programs		
Medicare[c]	Provides health insurance to 97% of those older than 65 years: Part A (compulsory hospitalization insurance); Part B (supplementary medical insurance).	14% of population enrolled in managed care plans. Covers pneumococcal vaccines, hepatitis A vaccine, pap smears, mammography.
Medicare supplemental insurance	Supplements basic Medicare coverage.	
Medicaid[d]	Provides health insurance to low-income population and to disabled population.	40% of beneficiaries enrolled in managed care. Mandated preventive services of periodic screening; family planning for children younger than 21 years.
Federal Employees Health Benefits Program (FEHB)[e]	Provides voluntary health insurance coverage for 88% of 8.6 million active and retired federal employees.	Risk plans cover eyeglasses. Dental X-rays, cleaning covered.

TABLE 3.3. COMPONENTS OF MAJOR
ECONOMIC PROGRAMS FOR HEALTH PROMOTION, Cont'd.

Program	Focus	Examples of Components
TRICARE/CHAMPUS (Civilian Health and Medical Program for the Uniformed Services)[f]	Provides a comprehensive managed health care delivery system for active members of the armed forces, their dependents, and retirees; coordinates care in military hospitals and clinics with services from civilian health care professionals.	Extensive clinical health promotion and disease prevention examinations (for example, health risk appraisals, laboratory tests) and counseling (for example, tobacco, diet, physical activity, safe sex).
Veterans Health Administration medical care[g]	Operates 1,300 sites of care for individuals who served honorably in armed forces.	May choose managed care for preventive care.
Indian Health Service[h]	Provides medical care and health services for 1.5 million Native Americans, including Alaska Natives.	Smoking cessation policies and programs offered. May choose managed care plan for preventive care.
Managed care organizations (MCOs)	Integrate financing and delivery of appropriate medical services to covered individuals.	Techniques employed to manage health of a defined population. 59% of plans provide full coverage for at least one type of pharmacotherapy used for smoking cessation, such as bupropion or nicotine replacement therapy (NRT).
Health maintenance organizations (HMOs)[i]	Offer prepaid health care arrangements. Subject to capitation.	Health promotion programs most likely to be offered are weight control, stress management, smoking cessation.
Preferred provider organizations (PPOs)[j]	Contract with providers to deliver covered services for discounted fee.	88% cover adult physical examinations.
Exclusive provider organizations (EPOs)[k]	Similar to the HMO, but members must remain within the network to receive services.	Similar to HMOs.

TABLE 3.3. COMPONENTS OF MAJOR ECONOMIC PROGRAMS FOR HEALTH PROMOTION, Cont'd.

Program	Focus	Examples of Components
Point-of-service (POS) plans[l]	Combine HMO and PPO features; network of contracted MDs.	89% cover physical examinations.
Health savings accounts (HSAs)[m]	Consumer-directed health care products.	Requires high-deductible health insurance plan.
Managed behavioral health care[n]	Mental health and substance abuse benefit package.	Offers individual health risk assessments, self-help groups, outreach programs.
Workers' compensation[o]	Provides health insurance coverage for employees injured or ill on the job.	Supports safe environments, safety inspections, counseling.
World Bank[p]	Supports development for international economies.	*World Development Report 2002* supports intersectoral actions for health.
Pharmaceutical, botanical, and biotechnology industries[q]	Applies to gene mapping, the manufacture and production of drugs and botanicals, recombinant DNA technology, and compounds acting in the cell for commercial purposes.	Provides anticholesterol drugs, vitamins, minerals.

[a]American Health Insurance Plans (AHIP), 2002.

[b]Blue Cross Blue Shield, 2005.

[c]De Lew, 2000.

[d]De Lew, 2000.

[e]Office of Personnel Management, 2005.

[f]U.S. Department of Defense, 2004.

[g]U.S. Department of Veterans Affairs, 2005.

[h]USDHHS, 2005a; Hodge, 1999.

[i]U.S. Preventive Services Task Force, 2004.

[j]AHIP, 2002.

[k]AHIP, 2002.

[l]AHIP, 2002.

[m]Freudenheim, 2005.

[n]Freedman & Trabin, 1994.

[o]Shouldice, 1991.

[p]World Bank, 1993.

[q]IMS Global, 2003.

groups, insurers are less likely to add any benefits that increase their costs relative to competitors' costs, unless a clear demand exists. Insurers who elect to cover preventive services, such as smoking cessation programs, may put themselves at risk of adverse selection relative to their competitors—for example, by attracting smokers, who are likely to use proportionately more medical care (Milliman and Robertson Inc., 1987). Although much is known about the impact of health insurance coverage on access to and the outcomes of preventive interventions, such as smoking cessation programs, it remains difficult for insurers to price them and for employers to finance them.

Finally, insurers tend to look at whether any benefits of preventive care will be realized over the time period the insurer covers the policyholder. Many of the benefits that accrue after a person quits smoking, for example, may not be realized by the health insurer if the policyholder switches plans, which is likely to occur within five years of going to work for a company. As a result, most insurance companies limit their time frame for realizable benefits from smoking cessation to three to five years; the reimbursable health care costs for the smoker receiving the benefits must be lower at the end of two years than they are for the smoker not receiving these benefits (USDHHS, 2000b). Health care providers are especially attuned to this time frame and may structure health promotion programs to allow insurance companies to realize short-term benefits while concomitantly allowing government purchasers to reap the vastly larger long-term benefits as well. Since the passing of the Health Insurance Portability and Accountability Act (HIPAA) of 1996, individual rights to information privacy have hindered attempts to monitor patients to assess long-term benefits of wellness promotion programs, thus confounding attempts at achieving accurate cost-benefit analyses of program effectiveness.

Despite these barriers, recently, to maintain a competitive advantage and to reduce costs, particularly among self-insured employers, commercial insurance companies have begun to focus on health promotion. Health promotion programs have tended to enhance enrollee retention through enriched satisfaction—an increasingly important concern in the brutally competitive health care insurance market.

In fact, 100 percent of small, medium, and large health care plans offered a wellness or health promotion plan as of 2002. Almost all (96 percent) insurance companies cover a general disease self-management program with a twenty-four-hour nurse phone line as part of a basic benefit. According to the 2002 American Health Insurance Plans (AHIP) Survey of Health Insurance Plans, major health insurers offer a range of additional health-promotive programs, including colorectal, prostate, breast, and cervical cancer screening (91 percent), mammography (90 percent), diabetes screening (98 percent), HIV/AIDS counseling (87 percent), nutrition counseling (76 percent), and back care and injury prevention activities (73 percent). Since the 1980s, many insurers have offered rate advantages for nonsmokers and individuals who maintain a healthy weight.

In addition, 79 percent of insurers cover fitness center activities, 68 percent cover stress reduction programs, and 64 percent offer health risk appraisal initiatives (AHIP, 2002). Some insurers also cover alternative healing methods, such as chiropractic care, massage therapy, or acupuncture (the insertion of hair-thin needles into specific points on the body to prevent or to treat disease), when prescribed by a physician. A recent study (Kaiser Family Foundation and Health Research and Educational Trust, 2004) found that employer coverage for acupuncture increased 14 percent from 2002 to 2004, with 47 percent of all employers surveyed offering acupuncture as a covered health benefit, up from 33 percent in 2002. The components of these programs vary, however, as does their effectiveness.

Health Plans: Blue Cross and Blue Shield

Health plans, such as Blue Cross and Blue Shield or Group Health Cooperative of Puget Sound, are organizations that insure the health care for a defined population, usually by employing managed care techniques. These techniques are designed to improve the health of a defined population and the health care quality and to coordinate medical care and its costs. Managed care approaches used by health plans include benefit design, prevention and early treatment programs, provider credentialing and network design, health care quality improvements, coordination of care across multiple providers, disease management programs, utilization review, and restricted formularies and generic drug substitution programs (Manley, Griffin, Foldes, Link, & Sechrist, 2003). According to the 1997 and 2000 national surveys of a random sample of health plans conducted by the American Association of Health Plans, impressive gains have been made in encouraging tobacco cessation, including community-based tobacco control, as described further in Chapter Nine. For example, 59 percent of plans provide full coverage for at least one type of pharmacotherapy used for smoking cessation, such as bupropion or nicotine replacement therapy (NRT). These gains have been supported by the collection of HEDIS measures on tobacco counseling.

Blue Cross and Blue Shield are nonprofit health plans that have loosely affiliated with one another (and are known collectively as Blue Cross Blue Shield [BCBS]). BCBS governs a network of more than eighty-eight million people, one out of every three Americans; offers forty plans in fifty states, the District of Columbia, and Puerto Rico; processes the majority of Medicare claims, at an estimated $200 billion dollars per year; and contracts with more hospitals and physicians than any other insurer (Blue Cross Blue Shield, 2005). The BCBS federal health plan is the largest privately underwritten health insurance contract in the world, with more than 50 percent of all federal employees and retirees enrolled (Blue Cross Blue Shield, 2005). In response to cost pressures, since 1993 BCBS plans in twenty-eight states have begun to join together to form single corporations to pool resources, creating for-profit subsidiaries, forming alliances with for-profit enterprises, or dropping their nonprofit status altogether and going public (Consumers Union, 2001).

To many, Blue Cross and Blue Shield plans are the insurers of last resort. Blue Cross contracts with local hospitals to cover members at a set reimbursement schedule. To the client, Blue Cross provides *first dollar, first day* coverage. Blue Shield plans are nonprofit medical contracts for physician services. Members are reimbursed for those services according to a preset schedule. The two plans complement each other.

Blue Cross Blue Shield has formed HMOs, preferred provider organizations (PPOs), point-of-service (POS) plans, health savings accounts, and government health care plans, including a Medicare managed care network, and offers free health care benefits to eligible uninsured children through the "Caring Program for Children," which is financed through matching funds from forty BCBS plans (Blue Cross Blue Shield, 2005). BCBS has developed integrated delivery systems to partner with hospitals and physicians so that clients may move more easily from one level of care to another.

BCBS has in some cases developed model benefits for preventive screenings, as well as disease and chronic case management initiatives that promote education to improve consumers' ability to make informed health care decisions. Because so large a percentage of health care costs result from lifestyle behaviors (McGinnis & Foege, 1993), personal health practice changes can serve as cost regulators for the majority of preventive care dollars. Preventive services covered by BCBS in full (not subject to a deductible), include well-child visits, adult routine physicals, immunizations, mammograms, pap smears, and prostate cancer screening. Health programs may also offer discounts on gym memberships, nutrition and fitness programs, or health fairs and community events promoting wellness as an adjunct to Web-based health assessment tools and personalized support for individuals with chronic conditions such as diabetes, heart conditions, or cancer.

Federal Insurance Programs

The federal government's health insurance programs include Medicare; Medicaid; the Federal Employees Health Benefits Program; TRICARE, for the armed services; Veterans Health Administration medical care; and the Indian Health Service. The Centers for Medicare and Medicaid Services is responsible for managing Medicare and Medicaid and also the State Children's Health Insurance

Program, spending over $360 billion a year buying health care services for these beneficiaries (USDHHS, 2005b).

Medicare is a federally administered program that provides hospital and medical insurance protection to 97 percent of persons age sixty-five years of age and older, disabled persons younger than age sixty-five who receive cash benefits under Social Security or Railroad Retirement programs, persons of all ages with chronic kidney disease, and some aliens and federal civil service employees who pay a monthly premium. The benefit package, administration, and payment methods were modeled on the private sector insurance plans prevalent in the 1960s, such as Blue Cross Blue Shield and Aetna's Plan for Federal Employees (Ball, 1995). In 2003, Medicare financed about 17 percent of the nation's health care spending (CMS, Office of the Actuary, 2003). For the portion of the working population covered by Social Security, Medicare provides compulsory hospitalization insurance (Part A) and voluntary supplementary medical insurance (Part B); Part B helps to pay for physicians' services, other medical services, and supplies not covered by the hospitalization plan.

Managed care plans serve Medicare beneficiaries through three types of contracts: *risk* plans, *cost* plans, and health care *prepayment* plans (HCPPs). Medicare pays risk plans a per capita (per person) premium set at approximately 95 percent of the projected average expenses for a fee-for-service beneficiary living in the same county as the Medicare beneficiary. Risk plans must provide all Medicare-covered services, and most plans offer additional services, such as prescription drugs and eyeglasses. Risk plans have enrolled about 75 percent of Medicare managed care participants (De Lew, 2000). Cost plans are paid a predetermined monthly amount per beneficiary, based on a total estimated budget. Cost plans must provide all Medicare-covered services but do not provide the additional services that most risk plans offer. HCPPs are paid similarly to cost plans but cover only a part of the Medicare benefit package, excluding inpatient hospital care, skilled nursing, hospice, and some home health care.

From 1990 to 2000, enrollment increased in Medicare HMOs, from 1.82 million to 6.19 million (about 16 percent of the Medicare population), paralleling a similar trend toward increased HMO enrollment among non-Medicare enrollees (De Lew, 2000). Enrollment has declined over the past several years as the appeal of managed care has diminished.

Since its inception in 1965, the Medicare program has been reluctant to reimburse for preventive services because they are generally seen as predictable and do not lower reimbursement costs (Schauffler, 1993); however, at present it covers a one-time preventive physical exam; mammography and colorectal, cervical, and prostate cancer screening; cardiovascular screening (for cholesterol and other blood lipid levels); flu, pneumococcal, and hepatitis B vaccinations; bone mass measurements (for those at risk for osteoporosis); diabetes screening; and glaucoma tests. Some of these services require payments of a deductible, however (CMS, 2005d). To fill the gaps in preventive services, 29 percent of fee-for-service Medicare beneficiaries supplement their Medicare benefits with private insurance (usually known as MedSup or Medigap policies), whereas only 7 percent of risk HMO beneficiaries have a Medigap policy (De Lew, 2000). Among the most common forms of Medicare supplemental insurance (disability income insurance, long-term care insurance, and dental expense insurance), only dental insurance supplies and encourages preventive care (such as X-rays and cleanings). Yet Medicare's involvement in quality assurance for hospitals, nursing homes, and other health care settings allows it to play an important role in setting the agenda for health education as a preventive tool for disease avoidance in at-risk populations (De Lew, 2000).

Medicaid, administered by each state according to federal requirements and guidelines, is financed by both state and federal funds. Over its forty-year history it has provided medical assistance to persons who are eligible for cash assistance programs, such as Aid to Families with Dependent Children (AFDC) and Supplemental Security Income (SSI). Medicaid benefits may also be available to persons who have enough income for basic living expenses but cannot afford to pay for their medical care. Today it continues to be a safety net for the health and long-term care needs of forty million low-income, elderly, or disabled Americans. It is a source of insurance for more than one in seven Americans, and accounts for 15 percent of national health care spending. It is the major source of federal financial assistance to the states, accounting for 40 percent of all federal grant-in-aid payments (Urban Institute, 2000). Adults and children in low-income families make up 73 percent of Medicaid enrollees but absorb only 25 percent of Medicaid spending. The elderly and disabled account for the majority of spending, largely due to their intensive use of acute care services and the costliness of long-term care in institutional settings.

The majority of Medicaid spending is for beneficiaries with modest incomes: 33 percent of the program spending is on behalf of those with incomes of $10,000 or less (Mulligan, 2005). Spending for enrollees therefore has important ramifications for the health system as a whole. Special payments for rural, inner-city, and teaching hospitals and other safety net providers help to guarantee access to care for all the population groups who live in medically underserved areas. Mandated preventive services include periodic screening and family planning for children younger than twenty-one years of age, as well as cancer screenings (for example, of the cervix).

The Federal Employees Health Benefits Program (FEHB) provides voluntary health insurance coverage for about 88 percent of all 8.6 million active and retired federal employees (Office of Personnel Management, 2005). Employees choose among three competing types of health plan: (1) government-wide plans, (2) employee organization plans sponsored by employee organizations or unions, and (3) comprehensive medical plans, or HMOs. FEHB is jointly financed by the government, which covers 72 to 75 percent of premium costs, and by enrollees, who pay the remaining 25 to 28 percent.

TRICARE (formerly CHAMPUS) provides health care for active duty military personnel whose orders do not specify a period of thirty days or less and their dependents, retired and former military personnel entitled to retainer or retirement pay or the equivalent and their dependents, and dependents of deceased members of the U.S. armed forces.

The Veterans Health Administration of the U.S. Department of Veterans Affairs (VA) (2005) operates 1,300 sites of care for individuals who served honorably in the armed forces. Under the Veterans' Health Care Eligibility Reform Act of 1996, Veterans Health Administration medical centers may negotiate with managed care entities to provide health services, thus increasing the options for preventive services. Under Public Law 104-262 provisions, the VA has the authority to furnish health promotion and disease prevention services and primary care and has flexibility to provide outpatient treatment, hospital care, and other means of care in the most efficient way possible.

The Indian Health Service, an agency within the Department of Health and Human Services, provides medical care and health services for approximately 1.5 million American Indians, including Alaska Natives, who belong to more than 562 federally recognized tribes in thirty-five states (USDHHS, 2005a). The Indian Health Service was among the earliest entities to enact smoke-free health care settings, finding that daily cigarette consumption among clients decreased after implementation of the policy (Hodge, 1999).

Worksite-Based Health Insurance

Three out of every five nonelderly Americans receive employer-based health insurance, often including preventive health care, either from their own or another family member's job. Economic downturns, combined with less workplace insurance coverage of workers' families, however, can reduce that coverage, with serious consequences for the health of employees and their families. Between 1999 and 2002, a period of economic downturn, the share of Americans with employer-provided health insurance from either their own or a family member's job fell, from 71.7 percent to 61.6 percent. In 2002, employer-based insurance covered fewer low-wage workers than high-wage workers (47.3 percent and 89.7 percent, respectively) and fewer workers in small firms than workers in large firms (65.5 percent versus

77.9 percent). Among low wage workers, fewer than two in five had employer-provided health insurance. Some families live without health insurance; others turn to the Medicaid system, SCHIP in particular, to cover their children. The health consequences for the uninsured are particularly acute for low-wage African American and Latino families (Center for Economic and Policy Research, 2004).

Managed Care

Managed care is a system that integrates the financing and delivery of appropriate health care services to covered individuals; it has served as an important recent influence on the provision of preventive services. Generally, as described earlier in this chapter, it includes four elements: (1) arrangements with selected providers to furnish a comprehensive set of health care services to members, (2) explicit standards for the selection of health care providers, (3) formal programs for ongoing quality assurance and utilization review, and (4) significant financial incentives for members to use providers and procedures covered by the plan (AHIP, 2002). The two broadest arrangements for financing and delivery are fee-for-service indemnity arrangements and prepaid health care. Under fee-for-service indemnity arrangements the consumer incurs expenses for health care from providers whom she or he selects. The provider is reimbursed for covered services in part by the insurer and in part by the consumer, who is responsible for the amount not paid by the insurer. Under indemnity arrangements the provider and the insurer have no relationship beyond adjudication of the claim presented for payment, nor is there a mechanism for integrating the care the consumer may receive from multiple providers (CDC, 2002).

Although the field is changing rapidly, four traditional and one emerging managed care forms predominate: (1) health maintenance organizations (HMOs), (2) preferred provider organizations (PPOs), (3) exclusive provider organizations (EPOs), (4) point-of-service (POS) plans, and (5) health savings account, or flexible savings account, plans. Managed care structures are financed under either *risk* or *capitation* approaches. A risk contract is generally negotiated between an HMO (or a *competitive medical plan*, a federal designation for a plan that operates similarly to an HMO) and an entity such as the CMS or an employer. The HMO agrees to provide all services to enrolled members on an at-risk basis for a fixed monthly fee. Capitation is a negotiated amount that an entity such as an HMO pays monthly to a provider whom the enrollee has selected as a primary care physician.

HMOs. The Health Maintenance Organization Act of 1973 committed the federal government to a time-limited demonstration of effort toward and support of HMO development. The Act defines HMOs as entities that provide basic health services to their enrollees, using prepaid enrollment fees that are fixed uniformly under a community-rating system, without regard to the medical history of any individual or family. The HMO provides comprehensive and preventive health care benefits for a defined population, and the consumer of an HMO agrees to use the HMO's providers for all covered health care services. The HMO agrees to provide all covered health care services for a set price—the per person premium fee. The consumer must pay any additional fees (*copayments*) for office visits and other services used. The HMO also organizes the delivery of this care through the infrastructure it builds of providers and through the implementation of systems to monitor and influence the cost and quality of care.

HMOs generally are also subject to capitation. The provider is responsible for delivering or arranging for the delivery of health care services required by an enrollee. However, the capitation is paid whether or not the physician has provided services to an enrollee. In this way the health care provider shares with the HMO a portion of the financial risk for the cost of care provided to enrollees (CDC, 1995).

An HMO is generally arranged as one of five kinds of service structures: (1) staff (the HMO contracts with solo salaried physician practices), (2) group (the HMO pays a per capita rate to a physician group), (3) network (the HMO contracts with two or more independent group practices, paying a fixed monthly fee per enrollee), (4) independent practice association (IPA) (the HMO contracts with individual physicians or associations of private physicians on a per capita rate, flat retainer system, or negotiated fee-for-service rate), or (5) mixed (the HMO uses a combination of two or more of these models).

In the current U.S. health care system, the HMO is the insurance vehicle best structured to encourage prevention. Over 95 percent of HMOs cover health-promotive services, including health education about diet, physical activity, and medication use (AHIP, 2002). Persons enrolled in staff-model health maintenance organizations are more likely to be offered health promotion programs—such as cholesterol or blood pressure screening, weight control, stress management, and smoking control—by their plan or physician than are persons enrolled in an independent practice association or indemnity plan (IOM, 2000b).

PPOs. The preferred provider organization is a variant of the fee-for-service indemnity arrangement, wherein the PPO contracts with providers in the community to deliver covered services for a discounted fee. Providers under contract are referred to as *preferred providers*. The PPO gives consumers greater freedom than the HMO does in choosing providers, but like the HMO, it tries to achieve savings by directing clients to providers who are committed to cost-effective delivery of care. PPOs have contracts with networks or panels of providers who agree to provide medical services and to be paid according to a negotiated fee schedule. Enrollees generally experience a financial penalty if they choose to get care from a nonaffiliated provider, but that option is available.

EPOs. The exclusive provider organization, too, is similar to the HMO, but the member must remain within the network to receive benefits. It uses primary physicians as gatekeepers, often capitates providers, has a limited provider panel, and uses an authorization system and other features of the HMO. EPOs are regulated under insurance statutes and are not governed by most state and federal HMO regulations in states where they are allowed to operate (Kongstvedt, 1993). As a result, certain health conditions may not be covered by an EPO.

POS Plans. Point-of-service plans combine characteristics of both HMOs and PPOs and use a network of contracted participating providers. Enrollees select a primary care physician who controls referrals to medical specialists. If care is received from a plan provider, the plan member pays little or nothing out of pocket; care provided by nonplan providers is reimbursed by fee-for-service or capitation arrangements, and members pay higher copayments and deductibles. Financial incentives are used to avoid provider overuse. About 89 percent of POS plans cover adult physical examinations (AHIP, 2002).

HSAs and FSAs Health savings accounts (HSAs), or flexible savings accounts (FSAs), are the latest in a continually expanding portfolio of consumer-directed health care products. They are becoming increasingly popular with consumers who demand flexibility to fit their particular health care needs. These plans were created by the 2003 Medicare Modernization Act (CMS, 2003) to allow consumers to save money tax free and apply withdrawals to health expenses. The accounts may require the purchase of a high-deductible health insurance plan; money in the accounts may be used for health expenses subject to the deductible. Many employers consider these accounts a way of shifting more of the rapidly rising medical costs to workers; generally, younger and healthier workers contribute to these accounts.

Managed Behavioral Health Care. The mental health and substance abuse benefit packages that cover most privately insured Americans typically involve some form of managed care. A majority of conventional PPO and HMO plans cover mental health and substance abuse treatment programs (AHIP, 2002). Approximately 170 million Americans who have either commercial or public insurance coverage for mental health and substance abuse have this coverage through a managed behavioral health care organization (American Managed Behavioral Healthcare Association, 2005).

Some insurance companies are devoted to this area and other insurers offer *carve-out* behavioral health care insurance to their clients in addition to their regular insurance offerings. The response to these carve-outs has been positive, leading to considerable growth in this field. Three core methods are used to manage behavioral health care. In principle these methods are similar to those used to manage medical care; however, because of unique characteristics of the client groups served, their implementation differs. The three methods are (1) managed benefits, which are designed to control care use and expenditures through, for example, gatekeepers who authorize care; (2) managed care, which limits the authorization of benefits for reimbursement to necessary and appropriate care delivered in the least restrictive, least intrusive setting by a qualified provider; and (3) managed health, which offers health advisers, individual health risk assessments, self-help groups, crisis debriefing services, and outreach programs to frequent users of health care services (Freedman & Trabin, 1994). A series of rigorous, federally funded studies has begun to develop best practices for managed care organizations and worksites to use when integrating their behavioral health (particularly substance abuse) and health promotion programs (Galvin, 2000).

Workers' Compensation

All state legislatures have enacted workers' compensation, or statuary disability benefits—laws that provide health insurance coverage for employees who are injured or become ill while on the job during the course of employment (Shouldice, 1991). Benefits are established by state laws and include all reasonable medical care, rehabilitation services necessary to return the injured employee to work, and partial repayment of lost wages. Funds for workers' compensation come from employers and state and local taxes. To promote health and therefore save money, safe environments—for example, those with educational programs, safety inspections, and counseling on safe work practices—are emphasized. Workers' compensation stress-related claim prevention and management is another emerging area for managed behavioral health care.

World Bank

The World Bank, the name by which the International Bank for Reconstruction and Development has come to be known, is a specialized agency of the United Nations that provides loans to countries for development projects. Its affiliate, the International Development Association, makes loans to less developed member countries on a long-term basis at no interest.

The World Bank, concerned with the worldwide increases in the cost of health care and the inequities in access, has devoted one of its annual world development reports to health (World Bank, 1993). The report highlights the importance of intersectoral actions to improve the enabling environment (for example, the educational system) for health. It stresses the need for greater efficiency in the distribution of resources within the health care sector, emphasizing the most cost-effective interventions for conditions responsible for the greatest burden of suffering in each country. It also encourages reform to improve the efficiency of interventions that had passed the test for effectiveness. Importantly, the report stresses that good health, sound nutrition, reproductive policies, and effective health services are critical links in the chain of events that allow countries to break out of low economic growth and the vicious cycle of poverty, poor health, and declining health. These findings could have considerable influence on the developing economies of the world.

Pharmacological, Botanical, and Biotechnological Industries

The pharmacological industry is a major force in health care, with a worldwide market of $491.8 billion in sales (IMS Global, 2004). The largest U.S. firms include: Pfizer, Johnson & Johnson, Merck, Abbott, and Bristol-Myers Squibb. Additionally, generic biologics, a category that includes vaccines, blood products, biotechnology products, and gene therapy, are estimated to have reached $30 million in sales in 2003, with growth expected at 135 percent to 2010, at which point the market will be $12 billion worldwide (Datamonitor, 2004). The top-selling therapeutic categories in the United States in 2004 were cardiovascular ($6.179 billion in pharmaceutical sales), central nervous system ($5.792 billion), alimentary ($4.66 billion), and respiratory ($2.82 billion) (IMS Global, 2004). Although mainly oriented toward tertiary prevention, the pharmaceutical industry does contribute to primary prevention through the development of drugs for such conditions such as hypercholesterolemia and osteoporosis and needs such as weight reduction.

The entry of pharmaceuticals into the market is restricted by the Food and Drug Administration (FDA) in the United States and by equivalent agencies in other countries. The FDA's ability to conduct postmarketing surveillance of pharmaceuticals' effects has been a source of considerable contention of late, with the forced removal from the market of several popular drugs.

The estimated $70 billion worldwide biotechnology market (IMS Global, 2003) is also growing. Biotechnology is a collection of technologies that focus on the cellular and molecular processes of living organisms. To date, more than 200 million people worldwide have received more than ninety biotechnology drug products and vaccines approved by the FDA, with more than 400 biotechnology drug products currently in trials and thousands more in clinical development each year (Frost & Sullivan, 2005). Companies in this industry produce genetic screening tests (for example, for locating mutations in the breast cancer suscepti-bility genes BRCA1 and BRCA2 or mismatch repair genes), detection and diag-nostic products (for example, for detecting cervical cancer), and pharmaceuticals (oftentimes using recombinant DNA technology or developing compounds that act within the cell) (Weber, 1997).

The United States continues to dominate the biotechnology market, in terms of both the number of companies in the sector and research and development spending. The latest data (IMS Global, 2003) show that 63 percent of biophar-maceutical development work is done in the United States, compared with 25 per-cent in Europe and 7 percent in Japan.

Biotechnology companies are also discovering the functions of human genes, as is the U.S. Human Genome Project. The genetic testing products produced by this industry in particular pose ethical quandaries for health care professionals. Questions about the sharing of genetic information with health and life insurance companies and managed care companies are the most pressing at present. The optimal process a health care professional might use to share genetic information with clients, and how that process might encourage behavioral change, also re-mains uncertain, as discussed further in Chapter Seventeen.

Complementary and Alternative Medicine

More than 40 percent of U.S. adults report using some form of complementary and alternative medicine (CAM), including prayer for health reasons, deep breath-ing exercises, chiropractic, and acupuncture (described further in Chapter Four). Although prayer for health reasons is the most commonly used CAM (53 percent of all women and 36.4 percent of all men; Barnes, Powell-Griner, McFann, & Nahin, 2004), an estimated fifteen million adults take herbal remedies or high-dose vitamins along with prescription drugs. Total visits to CAM providers each year exceed those to primary care physicians, adding up to an annual out-of-pocket cost for CAM exceeding $27 billion. Many hospitals, managed care plans, and conventional practitioners are incorporating CAM therapies into their prac-tices, and schools of medicine, nursing, and pharmacy are beginning to teach about CAM (IOM, 2005, p. 1).

Medicinal herbs (plants used for their effects on the body) are central to CAM approaches. Some medicinal herbs (defined here more generally as useful plants) that have been assessed for their effects on health include chili peppers (Capsicum), cranberries (Vaccinium macrocarpon), evening primrose oil (Oenothera biennis), garlic (Allium sativum), onion (Allium cepa), ginger (Zingiber officinale), licorice (Glycyrrhiza glabra), St. John's wort (Hypericum perforatum), and valerian (Valeriana officinalis) (Fugh-Berman, 1996).

Considerable controversy exists, however, about the methodological strength of the evidence supporting the effects of herbal and other complementary medical approaches on health promotion and their cost effectiveness relative to conventional medical protocols (Joyce, 1994; Ernst, 1994; Sewing, 1994). The Institute of Medicine has thus recommended that investigators use and develop as necessary common methods, measures, and standards for the generation and interpretation of evidence necessary for making decisions about the use of CAM. This challenge will require considerable monetary investment by federal agencies such as the National Center for Complementary and Alternative Medicine. Additionally, the IOM suggests strengthening the Dietary Supplement Health and Education Act of 1994 (in which the FDA is authorized to establish good manufacturing practice regulations specific to dietary supplements); increasing the integration of CAM with conventional medicine in research, training, credentialing, and practice; training scientists and clinicians in CAM; and developing infrastructure (for example, within the Department of Veterans Affairs) (IOM, 2005).

Strategies for Health Promotion in the Policy Context

Health care professionals may adopt a variety of strategies to promote the health of populations. A strategy of policy change, the context of which was explored in this chapter, may be pursued concomitantly with or subsequent to other strategies discussed throughout this book.

In its most rational form the policymaking process proceeds from goal determination to needs assessment and the specification of objectives, to the design of alternative courses of action, to the estimation of consequences of alternative actions, to the selection of a course of action, and to implementation and evaluation, with a feedback loop to the goal-setting stage (see Mayer & Greenwood, 1980, for a summary). Concurrently, the policy process may be seen as a "general course of action or inaction rather than specific decisions" (Heclo, 1972, p. 85), ruled by forces that are fluid and unpredictable (Hacker, 1996). The strategies designed to influence policy must therefore consider both its rational and its emergent processes.

The various tactics the health care professional undertakes are also part of a dynamic process, both directing—in pursuit of a larger aim—and directed—by those affected or potentially affected by the policy change. The first step in this process is building agendas, identifying problems in terms of pressing social issues, and developing a solution that incorporates the interests of affected groups. Second, the problems are defined by their prevalence, location in society, and importance. Their causes are detailed, and appropriate interventions are developed to ameliorate them. In this context the use of social science methodology is central. Policy options are selected, and proposals advocating particular choices are advanced to an involved policy leader. Methods of policy persuasion, critical to influencing a choice, include determining the objectives of the persuasion (in written or oral form), diagnosing the audience (particularly gauging the degree of hostility to the idea), and tailoring the objectives to the audience. Concomitantly, health care professionals develop a political strategy grounded in current realities through contact with interest groups, legislators, and others who wield power over the decision-making process and who can assist in the successful development and implementation of policy and its evaluation.

The target of the health care professional's influence determines the role the professional chooses to play in effecting this change. These roles include indirect involvement, such as identifying and communicating information from different sources; consultation through advocacy, such as citizen participation and coalition organization; and direct involvement, such as passing referenda and citizen initiatives and seeking political appointment and public office (Mico, 1978; Simonds, 1978).

Summary

Given the varied contexts, both political and economic, for health promotion, the health care professional has a number of avenues along which to press for change, particularly for policy change. Within these complex contexts, where interests and exchanges are multiple, the health care professional may seek to affect one or several interrelated levels.

He or she may seek to advocate for changes in federal, state, local, or international legislation; in a regulation or a policy; or in accreditation standards. He or she may consider organizing coalitions with other voluntary or professional groups to push for change in the definition and practice of health promotion or to increase health-promotive practice in underserved community groups. He or she may share information with others about strategies for implementing *Healthy People 2010*. He or she may organize client groups to advocate for change in Medicare or Medicaid reimbursement policies for health-promotive care. He or she may run for political office on a platform supporting both quality and cost outcomes in health care or backing provisions to protect the findings of genetic testing. The contexts for health promotion are rich with possibilities for change. Further discussion of these roles is found in the next chapters.

References

Adams, W. C. (1992–1993). The role of media relations in risk communication. *Public Relations Quarterly, 37*, 28–32.

Albertsen, K., Hannerz, H., Borg, V., & Burr, H. (2003). The effect of work environment and heavy smoking on the social inequalities in smoking cessation. *Public Health, 117*(6), 383–388.

American Academy of Pediatrics. (2005). *Children's health insurance status*. Retrieved September 2005 from http://www.aap.org/advocacy/schipsum.htm

American Health Insurance Plans. (2002). *AHIP Survey of Health Insurance Plans: Chart book of findings*. Retrieved November 2005 from http://www.ahipresearch.org/pdfs/2_2002Surv ChartBook.pdf

American Managed Behavioral Healthcare Association. (2005). Home page. Retrieved November 2005 from http://www.ambha.org

Ammerman, A. S., DeVellis, R. F., Carey, T. S., Keyserling, T. C., Strogatz, D. S., Haines, P. S., et al. (1993). Physician-based diet counseling for cholesterol reduction: Current practices, determinants and strategies for improvement. *Preventive Medicine, 22*(1), 96–109.

Ashford, A., et al. (2000). Cancer screening and prevention practices of inner city physicians. *American Journal of Preventive Medicine, 19*, 59–62.

Association for Community Health Improvement. (2005). Home page. Retrieved September 2005 from http://www.healthycommunities.org

Association for Worksite Health Promotion. (1999). *1999 National Worksite Health Promotion Survey: Report of survey findings* (Survey conducted by Association for Worksite Health Promotion, William Mercer, Inc., & U.S. Department of Health and Human Services). Northbrook, IL: Author.

Avner, J. R. (1992). The difficulties in providing primary care in the emergency department. *Pediatric Emergency Care, 8*, 101–102.

Ball, R. (1995). What Medicare's architects had in mind. *Health Affairs, 14*(4), 62–72.

Barbeau, E. M., Krieger, N., & Soobader, M. J. (2004). Working class matters: Socioeconomic disadvantage, race/ethnicity, gender, and smoking in NHIS 2000. *American Journal of Public Health, 94*(2), 269–278.

Barker, C., Pistrang, N., Shapiro, D. A., Davies, S., & Shaw, I. (1993). You in mind: A preventive mental health television series. *British Journal of Clinical Psychology, 32*, 281–293.

Barnes, P. M., Powell-Griner, E., McFann, K., & Nahin, R. L. (2004). Complementary and alternative medicine use among adults: United States, 2002. *Advance Data, 343*. Retrieved September 2005 from http://nccam.nih.gov/news/camstats.htm

Baylor College of Medicine. (2004). *Tobacco prevention and control*. Retrieved September 2005 from http://saludenaccion.org/tobacco/tobacco-mass-media.html

Berkman, L. F. (1995). The role of social relations in health promotion. *Psychosomatic Medicine, 57*, 245–254.

Berkman, L. F., & Syme, S. L. (1979). Social networks, host resistance, and mortality: A nine year follow-up study of Alameda County. *American Journal of Epidemiology, 109*(2), 186–204.

Blue Cross Blue Shield. (2005). *Covering America: 75 years and counting*. Retrieved November 2005 from http://www.bcbs.com

Breslow, L. (1999). From disease prevention to health promotion. *JAMA, 281*, 1030–1033.

Broome, C. V., & Loonsk, J. (2004). Public health information network: Improving early detection by using a standards-based approach to connecting public health and clinical medicine. *Morbidity and Mortality Weekly Report, 53* (Suppl.), 199–202.

Bureau of Labor Statistics. (2005a). *Labor force statistics from the Current Population Survey.* Retrieved November 2005 from http://www.bls.census.gov/cps/cpsmain.htm

Bureau of Labor Statistics. (2005b). *Union membership shows distinct geographic patterns.* Retrieved April 1, 2005, from http://www.bls.gov/opub/ted/2000/Oct/wk5/art04.htm

Burns, R. B., Stoy, D. B., Feied, C. F., Nash, E., & Smith, M. (1991). Cholesterol screening in the emergency department. *Journal of General Internal Medicine, 6*(3), 210–215.

Burton, L. C., Paqlia, M. J., German, P. S., Shapiro, S., Damiano, A. M., & the Medicare Preventive Services Research Team. (1995). The effect among older persons of general preventive visits on three health behaviors: Smoking, excessive alcohol drinking, and sedentary lifestyle. *Preventive Medicine, 24*(5, Special Issue), 492–497.

Canadian Public Health Association. (1986). Ottawa Charter for Health Promotion. *Health Promotion, 1*(4), iii–v.

Canadian Task Force on Preventive Health Care. (2000). *Evidence-based clinical prevention.* Retrieved September 2005 from http://www.ctfphc.org

Canadian Task Force on the Periodic Health Examination. (1994). *The Canadian guide to clinical preventive health care.* Ottawa: Canada Communication Group.

Center for Economic and Policy Research. (2004). *Health insurance data briefs #5: Public versus private health insurance.* Retrieved November 2005 from http://www.cepr.net/health_insurance/hi_5.html

Centers for Disease Control and Prevention. (1995, November 17). Prevention and managed care: Opportunities for managed care organizations, purchasers of health care, and public health agencies. *Morbidity and Mortality Weekly Report, 44*(RR-14), 1–12.

Centers for Disease Control and Prevention. (2002). *School health profiles.* Retrieved November 2005 from http://www.cdc.gov/HealthyYouth/profiles

Centers for Disease Control and Prevention (2005a). *About us.* Retrieved November 2005 from http://www.cdc.gov/aboutcdc.htm

Centers for Disease Control and Prevention. (2005b). *CDC Wonder* [Database]. Available at http://wonder.cdc.gov

Centers for Disease Control and Prevention. (2005c). *Healthy Youth! Coordinated school health program.* Retrieved September 2005 from http://www.cdc.gov/HealthyYouth/CSHP/index.htm

Centers for Disease Control and Prevention & the National Association of County Health Officials. (1994). *Blueprint for a healthy community: A guide for local health departments.* Washington, DC: National Association of County Health Officials.

Centers for Medicare and Medicaid Services. (2003). *Medicare Modernization Act.* Retrieved November 2005 from http://www.cms.hhs.gov/medicarereform

Centers for Medicare and Medicaid Services. (2005a). *About us.* Retrieved November 2005 from http://www.cms.hhs.gov

Centers for Medicare and Medicaid Services. (2005b). *Health care spending in the United States slows for the first time in seven years.* Retrieved October 2005 from http://www.cms.hhs.gov/media/press/release.asp?Counter=1314

Centers for Medicare and Medicaid Services. (2005c). *Medicare information resource.* Retrieved October 2005 from http://www.cms.hhs.gov/medicare

Centers for Medicare and Medicaid Services. (2005d). *Stay healthy.* Retrieved September 2005 from http://www.medicare.gov/health/overview.asp

Centers for Medicare and Medicaid Services, Office of the Actuary. (2003). *The nation's health dollar: 2003—Where it came from/where it went.* Retrieved November 2005 from http://www.cms.hhs.gov/statistics/nhe/default.asp

Centers for Medicare and Medicaid Services, Office of the Actuary. (2005). Retrieved November 2005 from http://www.cms.hhs.gov/statistics/nhe/projections-200/t.2.asp

Chernow, S. M., & Iserson, K. V. (1987). Use of the emergency department for hypertension screening: A prospective study. *Annals of Emergency Medicine, 16,* 180–182.

Consumers Union. (2001). *Blue Cross, Blue Shield conversion update: September 2001.* Retrieved November 2005 from http://www.consumersunion.org/health/bcbs-update901.htm

Cushman, R., James, W., & Waclawik, H. (1991). Physicians promoting bicycle helmets for children: A randomized trial. *American Journal of Public Health, 81*(8), 1044–1046.

Datamonitor. (2004). *Biotechnology: Global industry guide* (Reference Code OHEC4534). Retrieved November 2005 from http://www.datamonitor.com

De Lew, N. (2000). Medicare: 35 Years of Service. *Health Care Financing Review, 22*(1), 75–103.

Delaney, W. P., & Ames, G. (1995). Team attitudes, drinking norms and workplace drinking. *Journal of Drug Issues, 25,* 275–290.

Diez-Roux, A. (2003). Residential factors and cardiovascular risk. *Journal of Urban Health, 80,* 569–589.

Edington, D. W., Yen, L. T., & Witting, P. (1997). The financial impact of changes in personal health practices. *Journal of Occupational and Environmental Medicine, 39*(11), 1037–1046.

Epp, L. (1986). *Achieving health for all: A framework for health promotion.* Ottawa: Health and Welfare Canada.

Ernst, E. (1994). Placebos in medicine: Comment. *Lancet, 345,* 65.

Flemish Institute for Health Promotion. (2005). *Flemish Institute for Health Promotion introduction.* Retrieved November 2005 from http://www.vig.be/content/html/VIG_english.htm

Franco, E. L., & Harper, D. M. (2005). Vaccination against human papillomavirus infection: A new paradigm in cervical cancer control. *Vaccine, 23*(17–18), 2388–2394.

Freedman, M. A., & Trabin, T. (1994). *Managed behavioral healthcare: History, models, key issues, and future course.* Washington, DC: U.S. Center for Mental Health Services.

Freudenheim, M. (2005, January 11). Health savings accounts off to slow start. *New York Times,* p. C17.

Frew, S. A. (1991). *Patient transfers: How to comply with the law.* Dallas, TX: American College of Emergency Physicians.

Friede, A., O'Carroll, P. W., Nicola, R. M., Oberle, M. W., & Teutsch, S. M. (1997). *CDC prevention guidelines: A guide to action.* Baltimore: Williams & Wilkins.

Frost & Sullivan. (2005). *Biotech and drug discovery industry: Biotechnology today and tomorrow.* Retrieved (proprietary access) November 2005 from http://www.frost.com.prod/prod/servlet/vp-further-info.pag?mode=open&sid=2845386

Frost, K., Frank, E., & Mailbach, E. (1997). Relative risk in the news media: A quantification of misrepresentation. *American Journal of Public Health, 87,* 842–845.

Fugh-Berman, A. (1996). *Alternative medicine—What works: A comprehensive easy-to-read review of the scientific evidence, pro and con.* Tucson, AZ: Odion Press.

Galvin, D. M. (2000). Workplace managed care: Collaboration for substance abuse prevention. *Journal of Behavioral Health Services and Research, 27,* 125–130.

Gargiulo, M. (1993). Two-step leverage: Managing constraint in organizational politics. *Administrative Science Quarterly, 38*(1), 1–19.

Garland, M., & Stull, J. (2004). *Module 9: Public health and health system reform: Access, priority setting, and allocation of resources.* Association of Schools of Public Health. Retrieved November 2005 from http://www.asph.org/UserFiles/Module9.pdf

Gebbie, K. M. (2000). State public health laws: An expression of constituency expectations. *Journal of Public Health Management and Practice, 6*(2), 46–54.

Glemigani, J. (1998, March). Best practices that boost productivity. *Business and Health,* pp. 37–42.

Gomel, M., Oldenburg, B., Simpson, J., & Owen, N. (1993). Work-site cardiovascular risk reduction: A randomized trial of health risk assessment, education, counseling, and incentives. *American Journal of Public Health, 83*(9), 1231–1238.

Gostin, L. O. (1986). The future of public health law. *American Journal of Law and Medicine, 12*(3 & 4), 461–490.

Green, L., Nathan, R., & Mercer, S. (2001). The health of health promotion in public policy: Drawing inspiration from the tobacco control movement. *Health Promotion Journal of Australia, 12*(2), 12–18.

Greenberg, E. S., & Grunberg, L. (1995). Work alienation and problem alcohol behavior. *Journal of Health and Social Behavior, 36,* 83–102.

Grosch, J. W., Alterman, T., Petersen, M. R., & Murphy, L. R. (1998). Worksite health promotion programs in the U.S.: Factors associated with availability and participation. *American Journal of Health Promotion, 13*(1), 36–45.

Guinta, M. A., & Allegrante, J. P. (1992). The President's Committee on Health Education: A 20-year retrospective on its politics and policy impact. *American Journal of Public Health, 82*(7), 1033–1041.

Hacker, J. S. (1996). National health care reform: An idea whose time came and went. *Journal of Health Politics, Policy and Law, 21*(4), 647–696.

Hancock, T., & Duhl, I. (1988). *Promoting health in the urban context.* Copenhagen: World Health Organization.

Hastings, G. B. (1989, September). *The mass media in health promotion: Ten golden rules.* Paper presented at the BPS International Conference on Health Psychology, Cardiff, Wales.

Health and Medical Services Act of 1982 [Sweden], SFS (Svensk forfattningssamling)-1982-736 (Effective 1/1/83).

Health Maintenance Organization Act of 1973, 42 U.S.C. §§ 201 notes et seq. (1994).

Heaney, C. A., & Goetzel, R. Z. (1997). A review of health-related outcomes of multi-component worksite health promotion programs. *American Journal of Health Promotion, 11*(4), 290–307.

Heclo, H. (1972). Policy analysis. *British Journal of Policy Sciences, 2,* 83–108.

Heimendinger, J., Feng, Z., Emmons, K., Stoddard, A., Kinne, S., Biener, L., et al. (1995). The Working Well trial: Baseline dietary and smoking behaviors of employees and related worksite characteristics. *Preventive Medicine, 24,* 180–193.

Henschke, C. I., McCauley, D. I., Yankelevitz, D. F., Naidich, D. P., McGuinness, G., Miettinen, O. S., et al. (1999). Early lung cancer action project: Overall design and findings from baseline screening. *Lancet, 354,* 99–105.

Hibbs, J. R., Ceglowski, W. S., Goldberg, M., & Kauffman, F. (1993). Emergency department–based surveillance for syphilis during an outbreak in Philadelphia. *Annals of Emergency Medicine, 22*(8), 1286–1290.

Hodge, F. (1999). *Center for American Indian Research and Education* (PowerPoint presentation). Retrieved November 2005 from http://www.cmh.pitt.edu/PPT/Hodge1999.ppt

Hoffman, J. P., Larison, C., & Sanderson, A. (1997). *An analysis of worker drug use and workplace policies and programs.* Rockville, MD: SAMHSA Office of Applied Studies.

Honda, K., & Sheinfeld Gorin, S. (2005). Modeling pathways to affective barriers on colorectal cancer screening among Japanese Americans. *Journal of Behavioral Medicine, 28,* 115–124.

Hogness, C. G., Engelstad, L. P., Linck, L. M., & Schorr, K. A. (1992). Cervical cancer screening in an urban emergency department. *Annals of Emergency Medicine, 21,* 933–939.

Hulscher, M. E., Wensing, M., van der Weijden, T., & Grol, R. (2002). Interventions to implement prevention in primary care (Cochrane Review). *Cochrane Library, 2.*

Iannantuono, A., & Eyles, J. (1997). Meanings in policy: A textual analysis of Canada's "Achieving Health for All" document. *Social Science in Medicine, 44*(11), 1611–1621.

IMS Global. (2003). *US innovation will drive domination.* Retrieved November 2005 from http://www.ims-global.com/insight/news_story/0103

IMS Global (2004). *IMS health.* Retrieved November 2005 from http://www.ims-global.com

Institute of Medicine. (2000a). *Promoting Health: Intervention strategies from social and behavioral research.* Washington, DC: Author.

Institute of Medicine. (2000b). *The role of nutrition in maintaining health in the nation's elderly: Evaluating coverage of nutrition services for the Medicare population.* Retrieved November 2005 from http:/www.nap.edu/openbook/0309068460/html/1.html

Institute of Medicine. (2002). *Health insurance is a family matter.* Washington, DC: National Academies Press.

Institute of Medicine. (2003). *Unequal treatment: Confronting racial and ethnic disparities in health care.* Washington, DC: National Academies Press.

Institute of Medicine. (2005). *Complementary and alternative medicine in the United States.* Washington, DC: National Academies Press.

Johansson, M., & Partanen, T. (2002). Role of trade unions in workplace health promotion. *International Journal of Health Services, 32*(1), 179–193.

Joint Commission on Accreditation of Healthcare Organizations. (2005). *Facts about behavioral health care accreditation.* Retrieved November 2005 from http://www.jcaho.org/htba/behavioral+health+care/facts.htm

Joyce, C.R.B. (1994). Placebo and complementary medicine. *Lancet, 344,* 1279–1281.

Kaiser Family Foundation and Health Research and Educational Trust. (2004). *Employer health benefits 2004 annual survey.* Retrieved September 2005 from http://www.kff.org/insurance/7148/index.cfm

Kickbusch, I. (2003). The contribution of the World Health Organization to a new public health and health promotion. *American Journal of Public Health, 93*(3), 383–388.

Kongstvedt, P. R. (1993). *The managed health care handbook* (2nd ed.). Gaithersburg, MD: Aspen.

Kushner, R. F. (1995). Barriers to providing nutrition counseling by physicians: A survey of primary care practitioners. *Preventive Medicine 24*(6), 546–552.

Lalonde, M. (1974). *A new perspective on the health of Canadians.* Ottawa: Information Canada.

Leenen, J. J., Pinet, G., & Prims, A. V. (1985). *Trends in health legislation in Europe* (EURO Doc. ICP/HLE 101 E). Copenhagen: WHO Regional Office for Europe.

Liao, Y., Tucker, P., Okoro, C. A., Giles, W. H., Mokdad, A. H., & Harris, V. B. (2004). REACH 2010 surveillance for health status in minority communities—United States, 2001–2002. *Morbidity and Mortality Weekly Report, 53*(SS06), 1–36.

Logsdon, D. N., Lazaro, C. M., & Meier, R. V. (1989). The feasibility of behavioral risk re-
    duction in primary medical care. *American Journal of Preventive Medicine, 5*(5), 249–256.

Longest, B. B., Jr. (2002). *Health policymaking in the United States* (3rd ed.). Chicago: AUPHA/HAP.

Lorion, R. P. (1983). Evaluating preventive interventions: Guidelines for the serious social
    change agent. In R. D. Felner, L. A. Jason, J. N. Moritsugu, & S. S. Farber (Eds.), *Preventive
    psychology: Theory, research and practice* (pp. 251–272). Oxford, England: Pergamon.

Lowi, T. J. (1972). Population policies and the American political system. In R. L. Clinton,
    W. S. Flash, & R. K. Godwin (Eds.), *Political science in population studies* (pp. 25–53). Lexing-
    ton, MA: Heath.

Mandelblatt, J. S., & Yabroff, K. R. (1999). Effectiveness of interventions designed to
    increase mammography use: A meta-analysis of provider-targeted strategies. *Cancer
    Epidemiology, Biomarkers, and Prevention, 8,* 759–767.

Manley, M. W., Griffin, T., Foldes, S. S., Link, C. C., & Sechrist, R.A.J. (2003). The role of
    health plans in tobacco control. *Annual Review of Public Health, 24,* 247–266.

MarketingVOX News. (2004). *Blog stats redux.* Retrieved November 2005 from http://www.
    marketingvox.com/archives/2004/11/23/blog_stats_redux

Mayer, R. R., & Greenwood, E. (1980). *The design of social policy.* Upper Saddle River, NJ:
    Prentice Hall.

McAlister, A. (1982). Mass and community organization for prevention programs. In
    A. M. Jeger & R. S. Slotnick (Eds.), *Community mental health and behavioral ecology: A handbook
    of theory, research and practice* (pp. 243–256). New York: Plenum.

McCaig, L. F. (1994a). National Ambulatory Medical Care Survey: 1992 emergency depart-
    ment summary. *Advance Data, 245,* 1–12.

McCaig, L. F. (1994b). National Hospital Ambulatory Medical Care Survey: 1992 outpatient
    department summary. *Advance Data, 248,* 1–12.

McGinnis, J. M., & Foege, W. H. (1993). Actual causes of death in the United States. *JAMA,
    270,* 2207–2212.

Mico, P. R. (1978). An introduction to policy for health educators. *Health Education Mono-
    graphs, 6* (Suppl. 1), 7–17.

Milliman and Robertson, Inc. (1987). *Health risks and behavior: The impact on medical costs.* Brook-
    field, WI: Author.

Mills, R. J., & Bhandari, S. (2003). *Health insurance coverage in the United States: 2002* (Current
    Population Reports). Washington, DC: U.S. Census Bureau.

Mullen, P. D., & Holcomb, J. D. (1990). Selected predictors of health promotion counseling by
    three groups of allied health professionals. *American Journal of Preventive Medicine, 6*(3), 153–160.

Mulligan, C. (2005). *Medicaid eligible populations* (Presentation by Charles Mulligan to the
    Medicaid Commission Meeting, October 26–27, 2005). Retrieved November 2005 from
    http://www.cms.hhs.gov/faca/mc/milligan_module1.pdf

Mulshine, J. L., & Henschke, C. I. (2000). Prospects for lung-cancer screening. *Lancet, 355,* 592–593.

National Committee for Quality Assurance. (2004). *The state of health care quality 2004: Industry
    trends and analysis.* Retrieved November 2005 from http://www.ncqa.org/communica-
    tions/SOMC/SOHC2004.pdf

National Committee for Quality Assurance. (2005). *About NCQA.* Retrieved November 2005
    from http://www.ncqa.org/about/about.htm

National Conference of State Legislatures. (2005). *Health promotion: State legislation and statutes
    database.* Retrieved November 2005 from http://www.ncsl.org/programs/health/pp/
    healthpromo.cfm

National Consumer Health Information and Health Promotion Act of 1976, 42 U.S.C. §§ 301 et seq. (1994).

Navarro, V. (1976). *Medicine under capitalism.* New York: Prodist.

Neubauer, D., & Pratt, R. (1981). The second public health revolution: A critical appraisal. *Journal of Health Politics, Policy and Law, 6*(2), 205–228.

New Jersey Business & Industry Association. (2003a). *NJ employers hit with 15% increase in health costs, high inflation expected to continue, survey finds.* Retrieved November 12, 2005, from http://www.njbia.org/mar3103.htm

New Jersey Business & Industry Association. (2003b). *Statement of Philip Kirschner, executive vice president, New Jersey Business & Industry Association, 2003 Health Benefits Survey, March 31, 2003.* Retrieved November 12, 2005, from http://www.njbia.org/news_newsr_030331_statement.asp

North Carolina Division of Public Health. (2005). *Eat Smart Move More program.* Retrieved November 2005 from http://www.eatsmartmovemorenc.com/aboutus.htm

Ockene, J. K., Ockene, I. S., Quirk, M. E., Hebert, J. R., Saperia, G. M., Luippold, R. S., et al. (1995). Physician training for patient-centered nutrition counseling in a lipid intervention trial. *Preventive Medicine, 24*(6), 563–570.

Office of Personnel Management. (2005). *Federal Employees Health Benefits Program.* Retrieved November 2005 from http://www.opm.gov/insure/health/about/fehb.asp

Patton, D., Kolasa, K., West, S., & Irons, T. (1995). Sexual abstinence counseling of adolescents by physicians. *Adolescence, 30*(120), 963–969.

Pinet, G. (1986). The WHO European Program. *American Journal of Law and Medicine, 12*(3 & 4), 441–460.

Poland's lawmakers pass legislation meant to stave off bankruptcy of hospitals. (2004, September 10). *AP News Wire.* Retrieved November 2005 from http://www.NewsRx.net

Preventive Health Amendments of 1993, PL 103-183 (42 U.S.C. §§ 233 et seq. [1993]).

Price, J. H., Clause, M., & Everett, S. A. (1995). Patients' attitudes about the role of physicians in counseling about firearms. *Patient Education and Counseling, 25*(2), 163–170.

Prochaska, J. O., & Velicer, W. F. (1997). The transtheoretical model of health behavior change. *American Journal of Health Promotion, 12*(1), 38–48.

Public Health Functions Steering Committee. (1994). *Public health in America.* Washington, DC: U.S. Public Health Service, Office of Disease Prevention and Health Promotion.

Reynolds, C. (1994). The promise of public health law. *Journal of Law and Medicine, 1,* 212–222.

Riedel, J. E. (1987). Employee health promotion: Blue Cross and Blue Shield plan activities. *American Journal of Health Promotion, 1*(4), 28–32.

Roberts, D. F., & Maccoby, N. (1985). Effects of mass communication. In G. Lindzy & E. Aronson (Eds.), *Handbook of social psychology: Vol. 2. Special fields and applications* (pp. 539–598). New York: Random House.

Roemer, M. I. (1982). Market failure and health care policy. *Journal of Public Health Policy, 3*(4), 419–431.

Roemer, M. I. (1986). *An introduction to the U.S. health care system.* New York: Springer.

Rowan, K. E. (2005). Communication challenges. In Institute of Medicine, *Estimating the contributions of lifestyle-related factors to preventable death: A workshop summary* (pp. 47–48). Washington, DC: National Academies Press.

Rowan, K. E., Bethea, L. S., Pecchioni, L., & Villagran, M. (2003). A research-based-guide for physicians communicating cancer risk. *Health Communication, 15,* 239–252.

Schauffler, H. H. (1993). Disease prevention policy under Medicare: A historical and political analysis. *American Journal of Preventive Medicine, 9*(2), 71–77.

Schectman, J. M., Stoy, D. B., & Elinsky, E. G. (1994). Association between physician counseling for hypercholesterolemia and patient dietary knowledge. *American Journal of Preventive Medicine, 10*(3), 136–139.

Schroeder, S. A. (2004). Tobacco control in the wake of the 1998 master settlement agreement. *New England Journal of Medicine, 350*(3), 293–301.

Serxner, S., Anderson, D. R., & Gold, D. (2004). Building program participation: Strategies for recruitment and retention in worksite health promotion programs. *American Journal of Health Promotion, 18*(4), 1–6.

Sewing, K.-Fr. (1994). Placebos in medicine: Comment. *Lancet, 345*, 65–66.

Sheinfeld Gorin, S. (2005). Colorectal cancer screening compliance among urban Hispanics. *Journal of Behavioral Medicine, 28*, 125–137.

Sheinfeld Gorin, S., & Albert, S. M. (2003). The meaning of risk to first degree relatives of women with breast cancer. *Women and Health, 37*, 97–117.

Sheinfeld Gorin, S., & Heck, J. (2004). Meta-analysis of the efficacy of tobacco cessation counseling: A comparison of physicians, nurses, and dentists. *Cancer Epidemiology, Biomarkers, and Prevention, 13*, 2012–2022.

Sheinfeld Gorin, S., & Heck, J. (2005). Cancer screening among Latino subgroups in the United States. *Preventive Medicine, 40*, 515–526.

Sheinfeld Gorin, S., et al. (2000). Cancer education among primary care physicians in an underserved community. *American Journal of Preventive Medicine, 19*, 53–58.

Sheridan, S. L., Harris, R. P., & Woolf, S. H. (2003). *Shared decision-making about screening and chemoprevention: A suggested approach from the U.S. Preventive Services Task Force* (AHRQ Publication No. 04-0529). Rockville, MD: Agency for Healthcare Research and Quality.

Shipan, C. R., & Volden, C. (2005). *Policy diffusion from cities to states: Antismoking laws in the US.* Presented at the Law, Economics, and Organization Workshop, Yale University.

Shouldice, R. G. (1991). *Introduction to managed care: Health maintenance organizations, preferred provider organizations, and competitive medical plans.* Arlington, VA: Information Resources Press.

Simonds, S. K. (1978). Health education: Facing issues of policy, ethics, and social justice. *Health Education Monographs, 6* (Suppl. 1), 17–27.

Sorensen, G., Stoddard, A. M., Youngstrom, R., Emmons, K., Barbeau, E., Khoransanizadeh, F., et al. (2000). Local labor unions' positions on worksite tobacco control. *American Journal of Public Health, 90*, 618–620.

State of Alaska. (2005). *Health promotion unit.* Retrieved November 2005 from http://health.hss.state.ak.us/dph/chems/health_promotion

Steckler, A., Dawson, L., Goodman, R. M., & Epstein, N. (1987). Policy advocacy: Three emerging roles for health education. *Advances in Health Education and Promotion, 2*, 5–27.

Tesh, S. (1981). Disease causality and politics. *Journal of Health Politics, Policy and Law, 6*(3), 369–390.

Thompson, S. C., Schwankovsky, L., & Pitts, J. (1993). Counseling patients to make lifestyle changes: The role of physician self-efficacy, training and beliefs about causes. *Family Practice, 10*(1), 70–75.

Tregloan, M. L. (1998). "Defining and assessing health care standards: An international picture." *Healthcare and Informatics Review, 4*(6). Retrieved November 2005 from http://hcro.enigma.co.nz/website/index.cfm?fuseaction=articledisplay&FeatureID=109

Turrell, G., Hewitt, B., Patterson, C., Oldenburg, B., & Gould, T. (2002). Socioeconomic differences in food purchasing behaviour and suggested implications for diet-related health promotion. *Journal of Human Nutrition and Dietetics, 15*(5), 355–364.

Twiss, J., Dickinson, J., Duma, S., Kleinman, T., Paulsen, H., & Rilveria, L. (2003). Community gardens: Lessons learned from California Healthy Cities and Communities. *American Journal of Public Health, 93*(9), 1435–1438.

United Nations. (1948). *Universal declaration of human rights.* Retrieved November 2005 from http://www.un.org/Overview/rights.html

Urban Institute. (2000). *Analysis of Medicaid enrollees and expenditures.* Prepared for the Kaiser Commission on Medicaid and the Uninsured. Unpublished report.

U.S. Census Bureau. (2004). *Health insurance statistics: Low income uninsured by state.* Retrieved November 2005 from http://www.census.gov/hhes/hlthins/liuc03.html

U.S. Department of Defense. (2004). *TRICARE Handbook.* Retrieved September 2005 from http://www.tricare.osd.mil/TricareHandbook

U.S. Department of Health and Human Services. (1991). *Healthy people 2000: National health promotion and disease prevention objectives* (DHHS Publication No. [PHS] 91-50213). Washington, DC: U.S. Government Printing Office.

U.S. Department of Health and Human Services. (1995). *Healthy people 2000: Midcourse review and 1995 revisions.* Washington, DC: U.S. Government Printing Office.

U.S. Department of Health and Human Services. (2000a). *Healthy people 2010: Understanding and improving health.* Washington, DC: Government Printing Office.

U.S. Department of Health and Human Services. (2000b). A historical review of efforts to reduce smoking in the United States. In *Reducing tobacco use: A report of the surgeon general* (chap. 2). Retrieved November 2005 from http://www.cdc.gov/tobacco/sgr/sgr_2000/chapter2.pdf

U.S. Department of Health and Human Services. (2005a). *Indian Health Service introduction.* Retrieved November 2005 from http://www.ihs.gov/PublicInfo/PublicAffairs/Welcome_Info/IHSintro.asp

U.S. Department of Health and Human Services. (2005b). *Topic 3.2.7: Centers for Medicare and Medicaid Services (CMS).* Retrieved November 2005 from http://knownet.hhs.gov/grants/orientDR/hcfa2.htm

U.S. Department of Health, Education and Welfare (now U.S. Department of Health and Human Services). (1979). *Healthy people: The surgeon general's report on health promotion and disease prevention* (PHS Publication No. 79-55071). Washington, DC: Author.

U.S. Department of Veterans Affairs, Veterans Health Administration. (2005). *Department of Veteran Affairs fact sheet.* Retrieved November 12, 2005, from http://www1.va.gov/opa/facts/docs/vafacts.doc

U.S. Government Printing Office. (1997). *Public and private laws.* Retrieved November 2005 from http://www.access.gpo.gov/nara/publaw/104publ.html

U.S. National Library of Medicine. (2003). *Current bibliographies in medicine 2000-7: Health risk communication.* Retrieved September 2005 from http://www.nlm.nih.gov/pubs/cbm/health_risk_communication.html

U.S. Preventive Services Task Force. (1996). *Guide to clinical preventive services* (2nd ed.). Baltimore: Williams & Wilkins.

U.S. Preventive Services Task Force. (2004). *Guide to clinical preventive services* (3rd ed.). Retrieved September 2005 from http://www.ahrq.gov/clinic/uspstfix.htm

Veterans' Health Care Reform Eligibility Act of 1996, PL 104-262, 38 U.S.C.A. §§ 101 note et seq. (1994).

Wallack, L., Dorfman, L., Jernigan, D., & Themba, M. (1993). *Media advocacy and public health: Power for prevention.* Thousand Oaks, CA: Sage.

Wamsley, G., & Zald, M. (1967). *The political economy of public organizations: A critique and approach to the study of public administration.* Bloomington: Indiana University Press.

Weber, J. (1997, January 13). Drugs and biotech. *Business Week,* p. 110.

Wilson, M. G., Holman, P. B., & Hammock, A. (1996). A comprehensive review of the effects of worksite health promotion on health-related outcomes. *American Journal of Health Promotion, 10*(6), 429–435.

Woloshin, S., Schwartz, L. M., & Welch, G. (2002). Risk charts: Putting cancer in context. *Journal of the National Cancer Institute, 94*(11), 799–804.

Woolf, S. H., Jonas, S., & Lawrence, R. S. (Eds.). (1996). *Health promotion and disease prevention in clinical practice.* Baltimore: Williams & Wilkins.

World Bank. (1993). *World development report 1993: Investing in health.* New York: Oxford University Press.

World Bank (2002). *World development report 2002: Building institutions for markets.* Retrieved November 2005 from http://www.worldbank.org/wdr/2001/fulltext/fulltext2002.htm

World Health Organization. (1978). *Alma-Ata 1978: Primary health care: Report of the international conference on primary health care, Alma-Ata, USSR, September 6–12, 1978.* Geneva: Author.

World Health Organization. (1985). *Targets for health for all.* Copenhagen: WHO Regional Office for Europe.

World Health Organization. (1988, April 5–9). *Report on the Adelaide Conference: Healthy public policy: Second International Conference on Health Promotion.* Adelaide, South Australia: Author.

World Health Organization. (1998, May). *Health 21: An introduction to the health for all policy framework for the WHO European Region* (European Health for All Series, No. 5). Geneva: Author.

World Health Organization. (1999). *Health 21: Health for all in the 21st century.* Copenhagen: Author.

World Health Organization. (2004a). *Global strategy on diet, physical activity and health.* Retrieved September 2005 from http://www.who.int/dietphysicalactivity/goals/en

World Health Organization. (2004b). *WHO Framework Convention on Tobacco Control* (Report No. WHA56.1). http://www.who.int/gb/EB.WHA/PDF/WHA56/ea56r1.pdf

World Health Organization. (2004c). *World health report 2004: Changing history.* Geneva: Author.

World Health Organization. (2005, September 19). *Introduction to healthy cities.* Retrieved November 2005 from http://www.who.dk/healthy-cities/introducing/20050202_1

Zaza, S., Briss, P. A., & Harris, K. W.; Task Force on Community Preventive Services (Eds.). (2005). *The guide to community preventive services: What works to promote health?* New York: Oxford University Press.

CHAPTER FOUR

AGENTS FOR HEALTH PROMOTION

Laurel Janssen Breen
Joan Arnold

We are confronted by the inability of our current health care system to address the needs of our diverse public. While recognizing failed attempts to recreate a system to provide health care for all, we are mindful of the profound disparities that persist and deepen, isolating groups from each other; the ever increasing diversity of our population; the capacities of our health care system to advance care through technology; and the complexities of seeking appropriate and acceptable care. The challenges of new roles, altered relationships, and changes in the power structure continue. The unanswered questions become more frustrating as the gap between those who have and those who have not widens. Health care professionals are redefining themselves within a system of care where the key terms are *competence, outcomes, regulation, cost containment,* and *care management.* A commentary by Ed O'Neil (2005), director of the Center for Health Professions, points out five trends that have been noted for years but that health care futurists must still consider in realizing a newly configured system: individual responsibility for the financing of health care, consumer revolution for reform, mass customization of care, embracing of technology, and a radically different utilization of the health care workforce. With little expectation that a national health insurance program will come to be, and with the burden on employers caused by the current reliance on employer-supplied health insurance, other approaches, like health savings accounts, for financing health care will take precedence. Given this forecast of a greater reliance on direct financial contributions from individuals for health care, it is expected that consumers who pay more for their health care benefits will demand more control over how these resources are spent for what they want. The current failures of our individualized but yet highly variable approach to the delivery of health care have resulted in "making American health care expensive, unsafe and unsatisfying" (O'Neil, 2005). Mass customization of care would focus on greater efficiency, innovation, and customer input. The history of health care delivery includes a varied relationship with the public. Despite our many successes, it is suggested that in some of our past attempts to affect the health behavior of others, health care professionals have created or exacerbated a number of undesirable developments. Care management technology will require the merging of biotechnology (biotech) and information technology (infotech) to meet the new health care arrangements demanded by consumers. Finally, a radically different configuration of the workforce will be used to carry out these trends in the future.

Although the evolving health environment requires the maintenance of clinical excellence, it also beckons us to examine our professional responsibilities, cultural proficiencies, ethical standards, personal biases, outreach skills, and community-based strategies for service. As a community of health care professionals, how well-equipped are we to personally and collectively participate in the process of our own behavioral change? Are we capable of approaching a restructuring of power collaboratively, with our clients and with each other?

In redefining the health care system we are also reshaping the goal of health care to embrace health promotion. As we redefine health, are we able to embrace diversity in our approach to health promotion? As health care professionals still embedded in an illness-oriented system, we may find the challenge of redefinition in this new environment an onerous task.

The Next Generation of Agents for Health Promotion

Our paradigm of health promotion will shift when we move from an illness-oriented perspective of care delivery to a perspective that supports health as an ideal. Each health care professional reckons with the impact of having been reared in an educational framework that often understood health as the antithesis of illness. Health in this view is defined as the state that can be restored and maintained when illness is treated effectively by the intervention skills of providers. When it has not been seen as the opposite of illness, health has been viewed as part of an illness continuum and defined by illness parameters. Shifting to a health promotion continuum requires a new view of health and illness. The health care professional becomes a provider of *health* care, having synthesized health as the new framework for practice. The provider views client systems through the lens of health promotion, allowing for a different interpretation of client patterns, needs, and system responses. Needs are interpreted from knowledge, skills, and standards that promote health.

Defining indicators of health necessitates an understanding of the complexity and diversity of the human condition. Research to define and substantiate indicators of health is emerging. Outcome measures are becoming established. The focus and philosophy underlying the use of skills learned in the disease framework will not support the provider in the delivery of health promotion care. Health promotion requires a practice that supports the strengths and capabilities of the client, who also defines and determines health care decisions. The provider remains a resource and facilitator in this partnership. The client is the expert, and the provider offers useful and meaningful information and skills that aids the client in realizing health.

Clients may be experiencing frustration, confusion, alienation, and invalidation when they look toward health care professionals for help in using available services to optimize their health. Some health services may be unfamiliar to clients. Yet, many clients come to providers with an openness to learn and choose for themselves. Others, however, may still seek direction from the professional. Creating paths for direct access to health care professionals and responding to their varied needs and preferences enables clients to truly be consumers of *health* care.

Defining Health Care Agents

Who are health care professionals? The Bureau of Labor Statistics (BLS) (2004–2005b), of the U.S. Department of Labor, compiles the numbers of employed providers in the health diagnosing and treating occupations (see Table 4.1).

Health services was the largest industry in the United States in 2002, providing 12.9 million jobs according to the BLS (2004–2005a), including 12.5 million jobs for wage and salary workers and about 382,000 jobs for the self-employed. Further, ten out of the twenty occupations projected to grow the fastest are concentrated in health services. In terms of new wage and salary jobs created between 2002–2012, about 16 percent, or 3.5 million jobs, will be in health services, more than in any other industry.

The health service facilities in which health care professionals are employed fall into nine segments: hospitals, nursing and residential care facilities, physician offices, dentist offices, home health care services, offices of other health practitioners, outpatient care centers, other ambulatory health care services, and medical and diagnostic laboratories. About 518,000 establishments make up the

TABLE 4.1. HEALTH DIAGNOSING AND TREATING OCCUPATIONS, 2002.

Profession	Number Employed
Audiologists	11,000
Chiropractors	49,000
Dentists	153,000
Dietitians and nutritionists	49,000
Occupational therapists	82,000
Optometrists	32,000
Pharmacists	230,000
Physical therapists	137,000
Physician assistants	63,000
Physicians and surgeons	583,000
Podiatrists	13,000
Recreational therapists	27,000
Registered nurses	2,300,000
Respiratory therapists	112,000
Speech-language pathologists	94,000

Source: Data from BLS, 2004–2005b.

health services industry. The offices of physicians, dentists, and other health practitioners make up 75 percent of health service establishments. Hospitals, as the largest employer, make up only 2 percent of all health service establishments but employ 41 percent of the health care workforce (BLS, 2004–2005a). Table 4.2 describes how wages and salaries vary among these nine segments of the health services industry.

Cost containment is surely influencing the health services industry, as evidenced by the increasing emphasis on outpatient ambulatory care, the growing limitations on services considered unnecessary or low priority, and the simultaneous stress on preventive care. This focus on preventive care is expected to reduce the inevitable cost of undiagnosed, untreated conditions. In the meantime, enrollment in various forms of managed care programs, including preferred provider organizations, health maintenance organizations, and point-of-service plans, continues to burgeon. Key to the functioning of these programs is controlling costs through an emphasis on preventive care. Cost effectiveness is also a force behind

TABLE 4.2. PERCENTAGE DISTRIBUTION OF WAGE AND SALARY EMPLOYMENT AND OF HEALTH SERVICES ESTABLISHMENTS.

Establishment Type	Establishments (%)	Employment (%)
Health services, total	100.0	100.0
Hospitals, public and private	1.9	40.9
Nursing and residential care facilities	11.7	22.1
Offices of physicians	37.3	15.5
Offices of dentists	21.6	5.9
Home health care services	2.8	5.5
Offices of other health practitioners	18.2	3.9
Outpatient care centers	3.1	3.3
Other ambulatory health care services	1.5	1.5
Medical and diagnostic laboratories	1.9	1.4

Source: BLS, 2004–2005a.

the ongoing integration of delivery systems, mergers, and the combining and streamlining of financial and managerial functions. A 2002 Deloitte & Touche survey of hospitals revealed that the number of stand-alone, independent facilities hospitals is expected to decrease (BLS, 2004–2005a). These myriad changes will continue to be forces that reshape not only the manner in which health services are provided but also the disposition of the health care workforce.

Employment in health services continues to grow for many reasons. The demand for health services, especially home health care and nursing and residential care, will increase as the number of people in the older age groups expands. As health care technology continues to advance, the survival rate of those affected by severe illnesses and injuries will increase. New technologies will make it possible for illnesses previously not identifiable and treatable to be treated. Integrated health systems and group practices will grow in size and complexity, requiring additional jobs in office and administrative support. Industry growth will continue, resulting from the shift from inpatient care to less expensive outpatient care, influenced by technological advances and consumer demand. Surely, health service workers, prepared at all levels of education and training, will continue to be in demand, with emphasis on specialized clinical and administrative positions (BLS, 2004–2005a).

The Challenge of Collaborative Partnerships for Health Promotion

Whereas the basic ideas and philosophy of cross-disciplinary work are nothing new, the acceptance of goals as shared challenges may be. Historically, an uneven distribution of power has existed among health care professionals, limiting their capacity to collaborate effectively not only with other providers but also with consumers. Collaboration rests on the knowledge, skills, and capabilities of each discipline, and collaborators should be willing to combine efforts for the greater good of clients, whether individuals, families, groups, communities, nations, or the global society. Reform of the health care system through collaboration requires steadfast determination and reexamination of the way health care professionals relate to each other and with clients, of the values of each discipline, and of the expectations of the public. At this pivotal point in its history, health promotion must reposition and align itself in *the new public health* (Kickbusch & Payne, 2003), identify the objectives it has in common with the complementary and alternative medicine movement (Hill, 2003), and share power with the public it serves.

In his discussion of how to ground empowering health promotion in day-to-day practice, Labonte (1994) outlined a series of guidelines, or characteristics, that can serve as a basis for a collaborative practice. These characteristics involve legitimacy/power sharing, self-knowledge, respect, and commitment (Exhibit 4.1). They reflect the necessity for participating partners to explore, expand, and question their relationship to personal needs and responsibilities in each partnership. For a list of inquiries supportive of collaborative partnerships, see Exhibit 4.2.

The New Public Health

As discussed in Chapter Three, Kickbusch (2003) refers to three revolutions in the new public health. The first revolution addressed sanitary conditions and was directed at fighting infectious disease. The second focused on the health behavior of the individual, specifically on risks associated with noncommunicable disease and premature death. The third and most current revolution challenges us to discover the forces and influences that make people healthy. This perspective expands our concern to the level of health policy, social conditions, and population health. Awofeso (2004) questions what is really new about the new public health and challenges current public health workers to learn from the past, be activists in dealing with emerging threats, and work to reform the health promotion framework.

EXHIBIT 4.1. CHARACTERISTICS
OF A COLLABORATIVE PARTNERSHIP.

Legitimacy/Power Sharing

Each partner brings an established identity and accountability that is recognized by all. All partners must know and acknowledge their relationship to overall power. Differences in power and status are noted and able to be discussed. Negotiating a transfer of power and resources takes skill and trust. Some conflict is inevitable and must be confronted. This redistribution of power is part of the process and a desired outcome.

Self-Knowledge

Individual partners must know who they are and what they can provide independently and in partnership with others. This self-awareness can support the capacity for continued growth and expanded identity.

Respect

The individual autonomy of all partners is recognized. Differences are explored within an environment of support. Existing boundaries between partners can be examined. All partners value the benefits that can be derived from a cooperative relationship. Effective communication and negotiation can flow from this core of esteem.

Commitment

There is inquiry into the objectives of all the partners, but a vision of a shared goal is able to replace independent goals. There is an investment in maximizing impact through joint efforts. From this position comes the motivation and ability to delineate responsibilities and to build in purposeful, ongoing evaluation. All persons feel responsible for goal attainment. One measure of success is the level of cooperation that is achieved.

Source: Adapted from Labonte, 1994, 1999.

The Institute of Medicine's Committee on Educating Public Health Professionals for the 21st Century has been charged "to develop a framework for how, over the next 5 to 10 years, education, training, and research in schools of public health could be strengthened to meet the needs of future public health professionals to improve population-level health" (Gebbie, Rosenstock, & Hernandez, 2003, p. 3), and to make recommendations for overall improvement in public health professional education, training, research, and leadership. Public health professionals represent diverse professional disciplines and are employed to improve health through taking a population focus. Their diversity is reflected not only in the variety of their disciplines but also in their varied work settings and in

EXHIBIT 4.2. INQUIRIES THAT
SUPPORT COLLABORATIVE PARTNERSHIPS.

- Am I able to take an objective inventory of the skills I possess?

- What specific advantages might I gain from entering a collaborative relationship?

- Do I consistently and nonjudgmentally ask my clients about their use of other therapies?

- Do I feel threatened at the prospect of collaborative work?

- At what point along the "power continuum" do I view my profession residing?

- Do I look toward collaboration as a means to increase legitimacy?

- Do I feel I would have more to give than to get from collaboration?

- Do I feel others have a good understanding of my capabilities?

- Is it difficult for me to participate in mutual goal setting?

- Do I enjoy the role of being a resource and consultant?

- When consulting with others, do I feel patronized or talked down to?

- How frequently am I asked to consult outside my discipline?

- Have my past experiences with collaboration been positive?

- In which areas do I consider myself an expert?

- How consistently do I meet the expectations of my clients?

- Am I adaptable to changing circumstances?

- Do I seek out objective evaluations of my work?

- How capable am I of integrating the feedback obtained from these evaluations?

- Am I often impatient when working in a group?

- Do I frequently refer outside my discipline?

- Do I view myself as a risk taker?

- Am I comfortable with the role of advocacy?

- Which professions am I most comfortable using as resources?

- Am I constantly updating my referral resources?

- How do I view my responsibilities in the area of forming public policy about health promotion?

- What are my concerns regarding comanaging a client who is using other therapies?

the numerous kinds of professional activities they perform. Relying predominantly on an ecological view of health, adapted from the work of Dahlgren and White-head (1991), the committee designed a guide to thinking about the determinants of population health (see Figure 4.1).

The committee's report asserts that an understanding of the theoretical underpinnings of the ecological model is needed to develop research that explains the pathways for and the interrelationships of the multiple determinants of health. Once these are understood the public health professional will be able to "address the challenges of globalization, scientific and medical technologies, and demographic transformations" more effectively (Gebbie et al., 2003, p. 6). As discussed in Chapter Two, the ecological approach to health permits the development of multiple strategies for influencing health determinants relevant to the desired health outcomes. The committee recommends a framework based on the ecological model for strengthening public health education, training, research, and practice. Simply put, the model recognizes that "the health of individuals and the community is determined by multiple factors and by their interrelationships" (p. 25) and that the future

FIGURE 4.1. APPROACH AND RATIONALE: A GUIDE TO THINKING ABOUT THE DETERMINANTS OF POPULATION HEALTH.

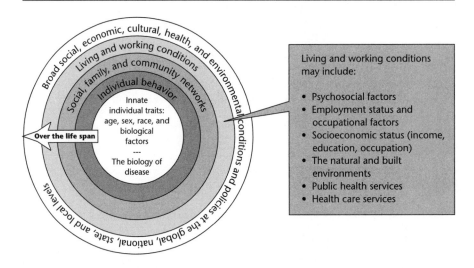

Source: Gebbie, Rosenstock, & Hernandez, 2003. Adapted from Dahlgren and Whitehead, 1991. The dotted lines denote interaction effects between and among the various levels of health determinants; Worthman, 1999.

of public health relies on the education of public health professionals who will be prepared to shape programs and policies for improving population health.

In addition to the traditional core areas of knowledge—namely, epidemiology, biostatistics, environmental health, health services administration, and social and behavioral sciences—the committee detailed eight content areas that have become or will become significant to public health and public health education: informatics, genomics, communication, cultural competence, community-based participatory research, global health, policy and law, and public health ethics (Gebbie et al., 2003). Further, the future direction of public health education will require the fulfillment of six major responsibilities (p. 9):

1. Educate the educators, practitioners, and researchers as well as to prepare public health leaders and managers.
2. Serve as a focal point for multi-school transdisciplinary research as well as traditional public health research to improve the health of the public.
3. Contribute to policy that advances the health of the public.
4. Work collaboratively with other professional schools to assure quality public health content in their programs.
5. Assure access to life-long learning for the public health workforce.
6. Engage actively with various communities to improve the public's health.

Integrative Medicine

The Committee on the Use of Complementary and Alternative Medicine by the American Public (Institute of Medicine [IOM], 2005) acknowledges that *integrative medicine* is now most frequently defined as health care that integrates conventional medicine and complementary and alternative medicine (CAM) therapies. The goal of integrative medicine is the delivery of safe and effective care that is collaborative, interdisciplinary, and respectful of diverse sources of interventions. As the public is taking a more critical view of conventional health care, CAM has grown in both popularity and usage. As many as 42 percent of the people in America are seeking out CAM modalities to address their health concerns, however, fewer than 40 percent of this group have disclosed that usage to their primary care providers (p. 13). Although both health care consumers and mainstream health care professionals have demonstrated interest in using some forms of CAM, there is little evidence of strong collaborative work between health promotion and complementary and alternative medicine (Hill, 2003).

In 1992, the U.S. Congress formally established the Office of Unconventional Therapies; this later evolved into the Office of Alternative Medicine (OAM), under the direction of the National Institutes of Health (NIH), to link the alternative health care community with federally sponsored research and regulations and to reduce barriers to bridging alternative therapies to the public. It was anticipated that to gain total integration, with full provider rights and privileges, complementary and traditional providers needed to become interrelated parts of one system of health care. Further, the safety, efficacy, mechanism of action, and cost effectiveness of individual alternative treatments would need to be more fully explored (Eisenberg, 1997). In 1998, the OAM was expanded by Congress, becoming the National Center for Complementary and Alternative Medicine (NCCAM). Since that time, Congressional support for NCCAM's goals has been evident in ongoing budgetary support. NCCAM is dedicated to "exploring complementary and alternative healing practices in the context of rigorous science, training researchers, and disseminating authoritative information" (NCCAM, 2000, p. 11).

In the absence of a single recognized definition of CAM, the Committee on the Use of Complementary and Alternative Medicine by the American Public chose the following definition to reflect the scope and essence of CAM as used by the American public: "Complementary and alternative medicine (CAM) is a broad domain of resources that encompass health systems, modalities, and practices and their accompanying theories and beliefs, other than those intrinsic to the dominant health system of a particular society or culture in a given historical period. CAM includes such resources perceived by their users as associated with positive health outcomes. Boundaries within CAM and between the CAM domain and the domain of the dominant system are not always sharp or fixed" (IOM, 2005, p. 19).

Although no definitive CAM classification system exists, the most widely recognized taxonomy, proposed by NCCAM (2000), specifies five categories:

1. Alternative medical systems
2. Mind-body interventions
3. Biologically based treatments
4. Manipulative and body-based methods
5. Energy therapies

Alternative medical systems refer to entire systems of theory and practice that developed apart from conventional medicine, such as Ayurvedic medicine, Chinese medicine, homeopathy, and naturopathy. Mind-body interventions include practices such as meditation and mental healing. These practices, even though based in the human mind, affect the human body and physical health. Biologically based treatments include diets, herbal preparations, and other "natural" products such as minerals, hormones, and other biologicals. Examples are

St. John's wort and fish oil and specialized diets addressing risk reduction for certain diseases. The fourth CAM category includes therapies that involve movement or manipulation of the body, including massage therapy and chiropractic. The final category, energy therapy, rests on an understanding of interacting biofields. Energy fields within the body and the surrounding electromagnetic fields outside the body can be manipulated.

A second approach to classifying alternative modalities, put forth by Kaptchuk and Eisenberg (2001), is a descriptive taxonomy based on derived philosophy and underlying theory. Their first category, CAM, consists of professionalized or distinct medical systems (chiropractic, acupuncture, homeopathy), popular health reform (specialized diets and dietary supplements), New Age healing methods (qi gong, Reiki, magnets), psychological interventions, and the use of conventional therapies in unconventional ways. The second category is made up of population-specific practices, such as the unique religious or ethnic practices of a cultural group (Native American traditional medicine, Puerto Rican spirits, folk medicine, or religious healing) (IOM, 2005).

Partnering with Clients

Most definitions of health promotion include the concept of empowerment, a concept legitimized by the Ottawa Charter for Health Promotion (WHO, 1986). Central to all these definitions is the direct relationship between an individual's level of health and the amount of perceived control the individual has in life situations. The scope of the term *empowerment* has grown beyond individual power to include an understanding that empowerment is a multifaceted dynamic interchange occurring on many levels (Airhihenbuwa, 1994; Labonte, 1994; Wallerstein, 1992). As we move into the twenty-first century, one focus of public health is the need to make this concept of empowerment operational (Laverack & Labonte, 2000).

In its broadest definition, empowerment is a multilevel construct that involves people assuming control and mastery over their lives in the context of their social and political environment; they gain a sense of control and purposefulness that enables them to exert political power as they participate in the democratic life of their community for social change (Wallerstein, 1992, p. 198). Further, the idea of the "multidimensionality of empowerment" has led to visualizing empowerment as a continuum. This *empowerment continuum* acknowledges that interventions at every level (individual, family, group, community, organizational, and political) have the innate potential to be empowering (Robertson & Minkler, 1994, p. 302).

Empowerment is not limited or defined by the level at which it occurs. The visualization of empowerment as a continuum can be seen as both a validation and a focus for practitioners. It frees up an understanding of the boundless potential of health promotion work. It acknowledges the diversity of approaches that practitioners at all points in the health-illness continuum use. Interventions at both the microlevel and macrolevel have the capacity to promote system change and to affect the overall well-being and health of communities. Any level can be the starting point for this change process. At a time when the goal is collective action and community-based care delivery for the purpose of maximum impact and cost effectiveness, it seems important to not diminish the empowering effects of individual-based care. The empowered teenager who seeks out and correctly uses birth control gains mastery and control over personal destiny. At a different level on the same empowerment continuum lie the community education and political action work needed to secure the clinic this teenager and other classmates may feel comfortable enough to visit.

In our attempt to incorporate an expanded notion of empowerment, we must also struggle with reengineering the provider-client relationship. There is a recognition that this new definition of empowerment brings an entirely new set of expectations. Behaviors and terminologies from a past paradigm are no longer useful. Beyond the generalized discussions regarding the philosophy of a shared power base and community partnership comes the real task of operationalizing this new construct of empowerment. In moving empowerment beyond a theoretical focus into an operational agenda, partnerships for health are essential, and it is necessary to ensure that systems of care and care management are culturally competent and proficient (Goode & Harrison, 2000). Empowerment, one of central tenets of health promotion, requires both health care agents and clients to develop a new skill set. The skills of cultural and linguistic competence and health literacy assist the agent in navigating the new landscape of health services. Client health is facilitated through the acquisition of learned skills for self-care management. The client, cognizant of health as a personal resource, integrates therapeutic health care actions to improve his or her quality of life.

The Health Care System as Context for Health Promotion

The term *health care system* is a misnomer. The U.S. health care system did not develop *systematically*, and it essentially does not address the *health* needs of the nation or is it always caring. There is no overarching framework or identification of values and assumptions that organizes the settings for care and the delivery of health services. The ability to pay has been a significant factor in the ability to secure care, leaving those without insurance and overqualified for publicly funded programs out of the picture. Health care is not for all. Special needs and categories dictate eligibility for care. Fragmentation is regarded as the "central feature of the U.S. health care system" (Shortell, Gillies, Anderson, Erickson, & Mitchell, 1996, p. 1). The dream of seamless care addressing the trajectory of human needs across the life span is far from a reality because fragmentation and specialization force clients to direct their own care. Others are simply alienated from health care services. Health care, rather than being valued as a basic human right and fundamental entitlement, is episodically provided within a cost-conscious context. This illness-driven nonsystem reveals the serious contradictions in the term *health care system* and begs rethinking. Rethinking health care means reformulating the focus of care so that it aims for health and transforming the organization of care delivery to a more integrated system of health care.

System change is accomplished through individual efforts and social policy. The individual provider possesses power, and power is enhanced through an effective partnership with clients. The health care system can be altered to become more humane, responsive to human needs, and supportive of health—the health of clients and providers. Creating a dignified environment in which to receive care, one that is free from smoke, radiation, asbestos, allergens, and other toxic agents, is an important start. Ensuring that health care is available, accessible, affordable, appropriate, adequate, and acceptable is a challenge for providers and recipients of care (National Institute of Nursing Research, 1995). The findings of the U.S. Preventive Services Task Force (1996) suggest that interventions must address clients' personal health practices and that providers and clients should share in decision making. Further, the task force urges that every opportunity must be made to deliver preventive services, especially to persons with limited access to care, and recognizes that community-level interventions must take place. The health care delivery system can be altered to become the context for health promotion. A collaborative model for changing the health system is recommended.

The health care professional is at the heart of change; the health care professional is an agent for change. Health care professionals are ideally positioned to collaborate with each other and to form alliances with clients to make a positive impact on the delivery system and on the pressing health care issues of our time. Functioning as an advocate for health means assuming an empowering role. The health care advocate strives to improve and protect health care and to create an environment for the promotion of health. At the crossroads of quality and effective care management, the health care professional advocates efficiency in care management as well as responsiveness to human needs. The system for care must become a system for health care, emphasizing the value and necessity of promoting health as well as representing health through the system's own image and actions.

This challenge does not deny the importance of autonomy and individuality; rather, it calls for an increase in solidarity, support for the common good, the fostering of other-directedness, and the development of community. Reform means the promotion and protection of health for all—a health care delivery system that enables health care professionals to become *health* care professionals and is in fact a system for *health* care. Central to this set of beliefs is the idea that the system is centered on persons and communities, not developed for providers and organizations. Clients are engaged as full partners with health care professionals in the mutual process of re-creating health care.

The present health care delivery system must be altered to provide the context for health promotion. Health cannot be a realistic goal without a system to support it. Health care for all will remain an unfulfilled dream unless the practice environment supports the providers of health care in delivering health promotion services.

Changing Systems for Health Promotion

The health promotion movement has emphasized an eclectic and multidisciplinary approach (WHO, 1984), and it has been difficult to establish benchmarks for evidence-based health promotion practices. The current research milieu emphasizes traditional, or Western, research standards, which involve studying outcomes, but it is often difficult to isolate the outcomes of health promotion. Health promotion is about change that occurs on a continuum from individuals to populations, and mixed approaches to practice are commonplace. McQueen's (2001) solution for this dilemma is that "rather than retreating to limited rules for what constitutes evidence, there is a need to look toward analytical frameworks that recognize the complexity of the field" (p. 266). In order to demonstrate its effectiveness the health promotion movement must develop standards for evidence-based practice that more fairly evaluate health promotion on its own terms.

Traditionally, health care professionals have been the acknowledged *gatekeepers* for the health care system. As identified experts they possess the necessary education, skills, and language to successfully negotiate the complexities of the system. They start from inside the system and can take an insider's view. From this vantage point, health care professionals have become comfortable with a concept of empowerment in which they are the ones doing the empowering. The timing and the conditions of sharing power with clients have remained within the active control of the provider. Past emphasis has fostered the continuation of this arrangement. "Professionals, as the empowering agent, the subject of the relationship, remain the controlling actor, defining the terms of the interaction" (Labonte, 1994, p. 255). The client remains the receiver of this act. Almost automatically, our language reflects this passive client role. When speaking of a community, we address its need to "be empowered." Yet, empowerment has been difficult to define in terms of outcomes, because it is most easily recognized in its absence, as powerlessness (Wallerstein, 1992).

Moving beyond this provider-centered view of empowerment means refocusing. It means stretching beyond what may be professional validation to true acceptance of the client as the expert in his or her own experience. Thus it means a transfer of knowledge, skills, resources, access, and language, but it extends far beyond that. Empowerment can occur only in an environment that supports its existence. "Empowerment is not something that can be given; it must be taken" (Rappaport, 1985, p. 18). Health care professionals need to learn how to establish and maintain this empowering environment—an environment in which the client at all levels sees the potential and value in seizing power.

Organizational Self-Assessment

Health care organizations recognize the necessity of ensuring services for culturally and linguistically diverse populations. This commitment must be based on a thoughtful organizational self-assessment, including an analysis of attitudes and beliefs, practices, policies, and structures, if the organization is to incorporate cultural competence within itself. A determination of client needs, interests, and preferences is required. Some strategies are detailed in Chapter Two. Ultimately, the goal is the implementation of culturally competent policies, practices, and procedures and, ideally, a strategic organizational plan with "defined short-term and long-term goals, measurable objectives, identified fiscal and personnel resources, and enhanced consumer and community partnerships. Self-assessment can also provide a vehicle to measure outcomes for personnel, organizations, population groups and the community at large" (Goode, Jones, & Mason, 2002, p. 2). The values and principles that guide successful self-assessment activities include the following (Goode et al., 2002, pp. 2–3):

- Self-assessment is a strengths-based model.
- A safe and non-judgmental environment is essential to the self-assessment process.
- A fundamental aspect of self-assessment assures the meaningful involvement of consumers, community stakeholders and key constituency groups.
- The results of self-assessment are used to enhance and build capacity.
- Diverse dissemination strategies are essential to the self-assessment process.

Strengths-Based Approaches. An orientation toward maximizing strengths can be used to "create targeted policy responses that can identify, enhance, and sustain strengths; follow long-term goals; and prioritize integrated strategies that have effects that cut across individual, family, and community levels of functioning and across several specific adversities" (Leadbeater, Schellenbach, Maton, & Dodgen, 2004, p. 25). The characteristics of strengths-based approaches are outlined in Table 4.3 and contrasted with problem-based approaches.

Cultural Competence and Proficiency. Organization-level change requires significant alterations in infrastructure as well as policies and procedures. Cultural competence at the organization level, just as at the individual level, is an ongoing developmental process. Exhibit 4.3 displays selected activities of health care organizations striving to achieve cultural competence and cultural proficiency, two stages on the cultural competence continuum.

Given the need to carefully consider the values and principles governing health care organization participation in community engagement, the National Center for Cultural Competence has designed a checklist (Exhibit 4.4) to guide cultural and linguistic competence in community engagement. Also, because health care organizations have structures and policies to govern their participation in research, few mandate the incorporation of culturally competent and participatory action designs; therefore the National Center for Cultural Competence has designed a checklist for a culturally competent research agenda (see Exhibit 4.5).

TABLE 4.3. PROBLEM-FOCUSED VERSUS STRENGTHS-BASED APPROACHES.

Problem-Focused Approaches	Strengths-Based Approaches
Correct deficits	Build strengths and resources
Have a short-term impact	Have a long-term impact
Provide crisis intervention	Provide primary prevention
Involve reactive planning	Involve proactive planning
Seek end points	Incorporate ongoing assessment
Target risks in populations	Target variations in risks and strengths of populations

Adapted from Leadbeater, Schellenbach, Maton, & Dodgen, 2004, p. 25.

EXHIBIT 4.3. SELECTED ACTIVITIES OF HEALTH CARE ORGANIZATIONS STRIVING TO ACHIEVE CULTURAL COMPETENCE AND CULTURAL PROFICIENCY.

Cultural Competence

- Create a mission statement that articulates principles, rationale and values for culturally competent service delivery.
- Implement policies and procedures that support practice models which incorporate culture in the delivery of services.
- Develop structures that allow consumers and other community members to plan, deliver and evaluate services.
- Implement policies and procedures to recruit, hire and maintain a diverse and culturally competent workforce.
- Provide fiscal support and incentives for improving cultural competence at the broad, program and staff levels.
- Dedicate resources to conduct organizational self-assessment.

Cultural Proficiency

- Continue to add to the knowledge base of culturally and linguistically competent practice by conducting research and developing new treatments, interventions and approaches for health education.
- Employ staff and consultants with expertise in culturally and linguistically competent health care practice, health education and research.
- Publish and disseminate promising and proven health care practices and interventions and health education materials.
- Actively pursue resource development to continue to enhance and expand the organization's current capacities.
- Advocate with and on behalf of individuals, children, and families from traditionally underserved populations.
- Establish and maintain partnerships with diverse constituency groups, which span the boundaries of the health care arena.

Source: Goode & Harrison, 2000, p. 5.

Health Literacy. As we attempt to advance health promotion in an environment of rapid change and chaos, effective communication will lead the advance of health. "Health literacy ought to be the common 21st century currency we all share that values health as a central tenet of individual and community life" (Ratzan, 2001, p. 214). In its narrowest sense, health literacy has been thought of as the ability of an individual to follow prescribed care directives. However, broader definitions have now acknowledged that health literacy is a composite of

EXHIBIT 4.4. CHECKLIST TO FACILITATE
CULTURAL COMPETENCE IN COMMUNITY ENGAGEMENT.

Does the health care organization have

- A mission that values communities as essential allies in achieving its overall goals?

- A policy and structures that delineate community and consumer participation in planning, implementing and evaluating the delivery of services and supports?

- A policy that facilitates employment and exchange of goods and services from local communities?

- A policy and structures that provide a mechanism for the provision of fiscal resources and in-kind contributions to community partners, agencies or organizations?

- Position descriptions and personnel performance measures that include areas of knowledge and skill sets related to community engagement?

- A policy, structures and resources for in-service training, continuing education and professional development that increase capacity for collaboration and partnerships within culturally and linguistically diverse communities?

- A policy that supports the use of diverse communication modalities and technologies for sharing information with communities?

- A policy and structures to periodically review current and emergent demographic trends to

  determine whether community partners are representative of the diverse population in the geographic or service area?

  identify new collaborators and potential opportunities for community engagement?

- A policy, structures and resources to support community engagement in languages other than English?

Source: Goode, 2001, p. 6.

individual and social factors. Health literacy is now believed to comprise a complex mix of reading, writing, numeracy, listening, conceptual knowledge, and oral speaking skills that are affected by the culture and context of the individual. Furthermore, this expanded vision of health literacy reflects the interrelationship of health care provider skills and overall societal factors.

The definition of health literacy accepted by both the Institute of Medicine and *Healthy People 2010* is, "the degree to which individuals have the capacity to obtain, process and understand basic health information and services needed to make appropriate health decisions" (Ratzan & Parker, 2000; USDHHS, 2000). In this view, health literacy is acknowledged as those individual and population-based capacities that foster and empower actions to achieve greater independence

EXHIBIT 4.5. CHECKLIST TO FACILITATE THE DEVELOPMENT OF POLICIES, STRUCTURES, AND PARTNERSHIPS THAT SUPPORT A CULTURALLY COMPETENT RESEARCH AGENDA IN PRIMARY HEALTH CARE.

If the primary health care organization/program conducts or participates in research, does it have

- A policy that requires research initiatives to use culturally competent and participatory action methodologies that include the active involvement of consumers/key stakeholders in all aspects of research process (e.g. design, sampling, instrumentation, data collection and analysis, and dissemination)?

- A policy that delineates ethical consideration for conducting or participating in research initiatives?

- Organizational structures and resources to participate in and/or convene coalitions concerned with the broad range of health, social and environmental issues impacting racially, ethnically and culturally diverse populations?

- A policy and structures to meet with members of diverse communities and advocate to determine priority health issues and needs as a basis to develop collaborative research initiatives?

- A policy, structures and procedures to systematically collect, maintain and analyze health data specific to the racial, ethnic and cultural groups served?

- A policy and practices that support personnel to participate on review boards within universities, colleges and other organizations engaged in primary health care research?

- A policy, procedures and practices that support reciprocity within a given community that partners in research initiatives (e.g. economic benefits, employment and other resources)?

- A policy, structures and resources to pursue grants/contracts or collaborate with other organizations to conduct research initiatives concerned with eliminating health disparities?

- A policy to hire personnel or employ consultants with expertise in conducting research that uses culturally competent and participatory action methodologies?

- Resources, policies and practices to provide information to consumers and communities about the benefits of participating or collaborating in research initiatives?

- Policies and structures to help bridge the gap between current research as it impacts racially, ethnically and culturally diverse groups and clinical practice, including

    personnel who periodically survey research studies and emerging bodies of evidence?

    a mechanism to examine research findings and their implications for policy development, clinical protocols and health education?

    policy, structures and practices to conduct health education for consumers on research findings that impact them and the communities in which they live?

Source: Goode & Harrison, 2000, p. 6.

in health activities and to triumph over barriers to health (Nutbeam, 2000). The challenges within health promotion are how to improve our measurement of and response to health literacy needs for all Americans (Berkman et al., 2004).

The extent of low health literacy is only beginning to be realized. It is estimated that "nearly half of all American adults—90 million people—have difficulty understanding and acting upon health information" (Nielsen-Bohlman, Panzer, & Kindig, 2004, p. 1). The scope of the problem is evident in varied aspects of health care and limits participation and understanding of health transactions. Although the Institute of Medicine report titled *Health Literacy: A Prescription to End Confusion* (Nielsen-Bohlman et al., 2004), emphasizes that people with limited health literacy come from diverse backgrounds, limited health literacy is most prevalent among older adults, people with limited education, and those with limited English proficiency (LEP). Low health literacy is further complicated by health professionals' use of specialized terminology. When limited literacy and low socioeconomic status are coupled, the capacity to become empowered and engage in health promotion strategies is severely diminished.

Evidence of the relationship between health literacy and health outcomes is burgeoning. Further, the IOM report on health literacy points to illustrations of disparity: people with limited health literacy have decreased ability to share in health care decision making, exhibit lower levels of adherence to plans of care, and self-report lower health status. These data suggest an association between health literacy, health care utilization, and health care costs ((Nielsen-Bohlman et al., 2004, p. 7) at the system level. To illustrate, compared to adequate health literacy, low health literacy is correlated with higher rates of hospitalization (Baker et al., 2002).

Although the challenge of achieving the vision of a health literate America is considerable, the IOM believes such achievement is possible: "We envision a society within which people have the skills they need to obtain, interpret, and use health information appropriately and in meaningful ways. We envision a society in which a variety of health systems structures and institutions take responsibility for providing clear communication and adequate support to facilitate health-promoting actions based on understanding" (Nielsen-Bohlman et al., 2004, p. 13).

The U.S. Department of Health and Human Services' Office of Minority Health (OMH) has developed recommendations for national standards for culturally and linguistically appropriate services (CLAS) in health care, in order to ensure that all people entering the health care system receive equitable and effective treatment (see Exhibit 4.6). The intention of these CLAS standards is to correct inequities that currently exist in the provision of health services and to make services more responsive to the individual needs of consumers. Although

EXHIBIT 4.6. CULTURALLY AND LINGUISTICALLY APPROPRIATE SERVICES (CLAS STANDARDS).

1. Health care organizations should ensure that patients/consumers receive from all staff members effective, understandable, and respectful care that is provided in a manner compatible with their cultural health beliefs and practices and preferred language.

2. Health care organizations should implement strategies to recruit, retain, and promote at all levels of the organization a diverse staff and leadership that are representative of the demographic characteristics of the service area.

3. Health care organizations should ensure that staff at all levels and across all disciplines receive ongoing education and training in culturally and linguistically appropriate service delivery.

4. Health care organizations must offer and provide language assistance services, including bilingual staff and interpreter services, at no cost to each patient/consumer with limited English proficiency at all points of contact, in a timely manner during all hours of operation.

5. Health care organizations must provide to patients/consumers in their preferred language both verbal offers and written notices informing them of their right to receive language assistance services.

6. Health care organizations must assure the competence of language assistance provided to limited English proficient patients/consumers by interpreters and bilingual staff. Family and friends should not be used to provide interpretation services (except on request by the patient/consumer).

7. Health care organizations must make available easily understood patient-related materials and post signage in the languages of the commonly encountered groups and/or groups represented in the service area.

8. Health care organizations should develop, implement, and promote a written strategic plan that outlines clear goals, policies, operational plans, and management accountability/oversight mechanisms to provide culturally and linguistically appropriate services.

9. Health care organizations should conduct initial and ongoing organizational self-assessments of CLAS-related activities and are encouraged to integrate cultural and linguistic competence-related measures into their internal audits, performance improvement programs, patient satisfaction assessments, and outcomes-based evaluations.

10. Health care organizations should ensure that data on the individual patient's/consumer's race, ethnicity, and spoken and written language are collected in health records, integrated into the organization's management information systems, and periodically updated.

11. Health care organizations should maintain a current demographic, cultural, and epidemiological profile of the community as well as a needs assessment to accurately plan for and implement services that respond to the cultural and linguistic characteristics of the service area.

EXHIBIT 4.6. CULTURALLY AND LINGUISTICALLY APPROPRIATE SERVICES (CLAS STANDARDS), Cont'd.

12. Health care organizations should develop participatory, collaborative partnerships with communities and utilize a variety of formal and informal mechanisms to facilitate community and patient/consumer involvement in designing and implementing CLAS-related activities.

13. Health care organizations should ensure that conflict and grievance resolution processes are culturally and linguistically sensitive and capable of identifying, preventing, and resolving cross-cultural conflicts or complaints by patients/consumers.

14. Health care organizations are encouraged to regularly make available to the public information about their progress and successful innovations in implementing the CLAS standards and to provide public notice in their communities about the availability of this information.

Source: U.S. Public Health Service, Office of Minority Health, 2000.

designed to address all populations, they also specifically target the needs of those who experience unequal access to health services.

Given that health care organizations have been slow to develop and implement policies and structures to guide the provision of interpretation and translation services, placing the burden of providing such services at the practitioner and consumer level, a checklist has been designed by the National Center for Cultural Competence specifically to support linguistic competence (Exhibit 4.7).

Policy Development and Implementation

Creating a health care system for health promotion requires collaboration among the disciplines and with clients. System change is a process. The process of change can include instituting policies for health. Developing a new policy, implementing that policy, and evaluating the impact of that policy are phases in the process of system change (see Exhibit 4.8). The entire process rests on collaboration from all levels of the system—with individuals working toward a common, beneficial goal.

Step 1: Approach the Problem. The critical decision to adopt and support a health promotion environment is the first and most important hurdle. Because the underlying structure and values of an institution are being challenged, the change will take time. However, every effort to move toward a healthy system is significant.

EXHIBIT 4.7. CHECKLIST TO FACILITATE THE DEVELOPMENT OF LINGUISTIC COMPETENCE IN PRIMARY HEALTH CARE ORGANIZATIONS.

Does the primary health care organization or program have

- A mission statement that articulates its principles, rationale and values for providing linguistically and culturally competent health care services?

- Policies and procedures that support staff recruitment, hiring and retention to achieve the goal of a diverse and linguistically competent staff?

- Position descriptions and personnel/performance measures that include skill sets related to linguistic competence?

- Policies and resources to support ongoing professional development and in service training (at all levels) related to linguistic competence?

- Policies, procedures and fiscal planning to ensure the provision of translation and interpretation services?

- Policies and procedures regarding the translation of patient consent forms, educational materials and other information in formats that meet the literacy needs of patients?

- Policies and procedures to evaluate the quality and appropriateness of interpretation and translation services?

- Policies and procedures to periodically evaluate consumer and personnel satisfaction with interpretation and translation services that are provided?

- Policies and resources that support community outreach initiatives to persons with limited English proficiency?

- Policies and procedures to periodically review the current and emergent demographic trends for the geographic area served in order to determine interpretation and translation services needed?

Source: Goode, Sockalingam, Brown, & Jones, 2001, p. 4.

During this step it is most important to become familiar with the facts about health promotion. Studies that relate to the cost savings from promotion of health are critical to approaching the problem. Summarizing findings, especially of evaluation studies on the significance of health promotion interventions, creates a body of knowledge supportive of shifting an institution's mission to valuing health. The health care professional becomes a resource for health promotion and informs other providers at the institution about the efficacy of health promotion interventions and the significance of improved health for individuals, families, groups, and communities. It is helpful during this step to hold discussions and conferences on organizational wellness. Health promotion may be the topic of grand rounds,

EXHIBIT 4.8. STEPS FOR POLICY CHANGE
IN HEALTH PROMOTION.

1. Approach the problem.

2. Develop new policy.

   a. Encourage institutional participation.

   b. Gather information.

   c. Prepare a written policy.

   d. Plan an implementation strategy.

3. Implement the policy.

   a. Communicate the policy.

   b. Carry out the policy.

4. Evaluate the impact of the policy.

Source: Adapted from Sheinfeld Gorin, 1989, pp. 41–49.

the focus of an institution's newsletter, or the organizing theme for case conferencing. Every opportunity to bring health promotion to the forefront of systems thinking assists in creating excitement about shifting institutional emphasis and generating enthusiasm among health care professionals for becoming agents of health promotion.

Step 2: Develop New Policy. Developing a policy requires health care professionals to participate with the public and to move from receptivity to responsiveness. Those willing to appreciate the data generated through step 1 of the process of system change now respond to the call to develop policy. Policy development focuses on altering the mission of the institution to support health promotion actions. The participants in conferences, rounds, and any other forums in which health promotion was discussed become the critical mass for a more action-oriented step 2. Recruiting the support of key participants is critical to policy development.

Success during this step is contingent on the best possible representation of participants. Consumers and providers form an alliance that pressures the institution to realign its mission to support health promotion activities. During this step it is important to determine whether representatives of all the institution's key components are involved. The communication network of the institution is activated to link as many professionals as possible, thereby connecting the divisions they represent. Change is an organic process; the whole institution must be considered. Leaving out any vital component will weaken the process of change.

Moving from receptivity to responsiveness requires that participants learn to value change. Key to valuing health promotion is the recognition that health promotion interventions really make a difference. The most significant differences are the decreased cost of providing services, recipients' increased quality of life, and recipients' positive evaluation of rendered care. Highlighting the care-related costs of an illness by comparing costs incurred with and without a health promotion perspective makes the case even more convincing. Savings in health care costs coupled with consumer satisfaction provide definitive arguments for the institutionalization of health promotion (see Chapter Sixteen).

Encourage Institutional Participation. To involve those affected in the change process, a task force may be formed. If diverse aspects of the institution are represented and if the capability of participants to expedite decisions is recognized, the task force will manifest the possibility for change. Representatives from all levels of the organization should be included. The activities of the task force may include gathering information from those affected in order to identify behaviors and attitudes about health promotion, reviewing and revising any existing policies, compiling information into a list of recommendations or developing a single policy, designing a health promotion policy implementation plan, and developing a budget for the change efforts.

If the task force is to fulfill its role, it should be given real authority by the top-level administration and should have public support. The groundwork for creating trust and meaningful responsibility is cultivated during this stage. A sense of responsibility reduces resistance to policy changes and promotes trust among those involved. Early involvement and an educational thrust prepare the organization for system change.

Gather Information. The first activity of the task force is to gather information from those who would be affected by a change in the care system: providers, consumers, and other staff. The task force explores their attitudes toward change and commitment to health promotion.

The task force should complete the following activities:

1. Gather research on health promotion.
2. Contact representatives of other health promotion programs, and review the strategies for change that were successful for their systems.
3. Survey all those who will be affected by a shift to a health promotion environment; a questionnaire or focus group may be used, with the goals of

identifying support for the health promotion policy, identifying opposition, and determining the issues of most concern to the organization.

4. Gather data on the impact of creating a health promotion environment; the patterns of morbidity, mortality, sick days, disability claims, medical leaves of absence, productivity, and efficiency should be examined.
5. Develop baseline measures of the organization's standing in the community (that is, determine what kind of *health image* the institution has); consumers and visitors may complete questionnaires, or focus groups or a town hall meeting may be held to examine the organization's image in the community.
6. Evaluate union contracts as they relate to health benefits and health insurance.

Prepare a Written Policy. After reviewing surveys and other data, the task force should prepare a written report as the background for system change. The governing board will review the policy for board approval. The best policy is brief, specific, and simple. The component parts of a policy are the policy statement, the rationale for the policy, the statement of who will be affected, the effective date of implementation, and any enforcement procedures, if applicable.

Plan an Implementation Strategy. The following activities should be part of implementing a strategy for a health promotion policy:

1. Create an implementation timetable.
2. Decide on a promotional campaign for communicating the policy to staff, clients, and the community.
3. Plan an effective communication method.
4. Decide on enforcement procedures, if applicable.
5. Plan staff education sessions.
6. Develop a plan to evaluate the policy.

Step 3: Implement the Policy. The task force and the organization administration set a target date for implementing a health promotion policy.

Communicate the Policy. A clear presentation of a health promotion policy increases the likelihood of a good reception, because uncertainty is a major source of resistance to change. To minimize uncertainty, all parties affected should be informed about the change and provided with the reasons for it and the intended benefits. This kind of awareness building should be part of every stage of the process of system change. The amount of time it takes to change a policy should not be underestimated. Three months to one year or more may be required, depending on the institution's size and the effectiveness of its communication network.

A public relations campaign should emphasize ways the institution will be strengthened by developing a health promotion environment. It is beneficial to employ a variety of approaches to communicate the new policy to the community, providers, and clients.

Carry Out the Policy. While the health promotion policy statement is being distributed, the task force may develop a timetable for implementation. Time is a critical element for persons who are preparing for change. Having a time buffer usually gives persons time to adjust.

A date for the policy to take effect is then set. It is important to consider choosing a date that is of significance to the institution or that is associated with the intended purpose of the policy change. If any restrictions will apply, they should be phased in gradually so that no person feels alienated. During the transition period, educational sessions about health promotion may be planned. Giving incentives helps ease the adjustment and compensates for any changes that are viewed as restrictive.

Because system change takes time, it is unreasonable to expect that creating a health promotion environment will happen instantly. Although the goal should be clear from the outset, hasty implementation reduces the support of persons who believe their right to smoke or to remain physically inactive, for example, is being limited or taken away. Implementing the policy before there is sufficient readiness can result in frustration, discouragement, and failure. It is crucial to prepare adequately and realize that acceptance requires time.

If a step-by-step approach to phasing in health promotion occurs, a commitment to the strategies on a defined timetable should be communicated, so that people know when each change will occur.

Step Four: Evaluate the Impact of the Policy. In this stage the administration, working with the task force, makes minor adjustments to the policy for health promotion, firmly establishes the health promotion environment, and evaluates the results.

Persons tend to resist change, especially system change that affects personal behavior and choice. A carefully designed plan can reduce resistance while enhancing cooperation, acceptance, and support for health promotion change.

Individuals enforcing the health promotion policy should keep the message positive and focused. The position of the institution on health promotion should be clearly stated.

The task force should plan an evaluation to determine the effectiveness of a health promotion environment and to provide information about any problems. The evaluation can measure immediate changes in attitudes and behavior or long-term outcomes, such as statistics on the number of sick days, productivity measures, and patterns of morbidity and mortality.

Short-term assessments using surveys can be undertaken three to six months after the policy has been implemented. The results of the initial survey may be used as a baseline. These follow-up surveys will measure the impact of the policy. Measurements of short-term outcomes may answer the following questions:

- Are persons complying with the policy?
- What are their attitudes?
- Have those affected persons implemented health promotion strategies?

Long-term effects are more difficult to measure. Long-term changes require at least one year to become stabilized. Examples of long-term outcomes include answers to the following questions:

- Have there been any changes in the use of sick time, requests for medical leaves of absence, or disability claims?
- Have morbidity and mortality decreased?
- Is the institution known in the community as an agency for health promotion through its actions?

This collaborative model for change is critical to the success of system change. Changes require the support of an institution's top administration and governing board. Change agents help set the agenda for a health promotion environment. They educate top decision makers about the positive impact of a health promotion policy environment on employee productivity, provider and client health, and the institution's public image.

Summary

Health promotion has always incorporated the central ideas of change, development, and improvement. Within this environment, major issues arise regarding the process of planning and participating in change. As health professionals we are faced with the responsibility of articulating a consistent philosophy of practice that can be put into operation effectively. Our relationships to ourselves, our peers, and our clients come under examination. The tools and approaches we use in our daily practice are explored and tested for their ongoing viability and inclusiveness.

Redefining the health care professional as an intervention agent, within a traditional illness-oriented, provider-driven health care system, is not an easy task. Yet the future of health promotion in a reformed health care system relies on the active participation of health care agents in this massive reorganization process. Realigned client-provider relationships, cross-disciplinary partnerships, and the impact of consumer demands are shaping health care reform in communities, nations, and global society. This reshaping has been thrust upon health care professionals and has been greeted with skepticism, but it also has presented health care professionals with new opportunities for redefinition never before possible. Health care reform presents challenges and opportunities. Accepting, valuing, and understanding how to participate in change guarantees a role in shaping the future of health care. Change, from simple to complex, emerges through systematic collaborative planning. The steps for system change and the characteristics of shared empowerment detailed in this chapter will inform health care agents concerned about health promotion. Health care agents must understand the past, thoughtfully examine the present, and acknowledge that the future is a shared one.

References

Airhihenbuwa, C. O. (1994). Health promotion and the discourse on culture: Implications for empowerment. *Health Education Quarterly, 21*(3), 345–353.

Awofeso, N. (2004). What's new about the "new public health"? *American Journal of Public Health, 94*(5), 705–709.

Baker, D. W., Gazmararian, J. A., Williams, M. V., Scott, T., Parker, R. M., Green, D., et al. (2002). Functional health literacy and the risk of hospital admission among Medicare managed care enrollees. *American Journal of Public Health, 92*(8), 1278–1283.

Berkman, N. D., DeWalt, D. A., Pignone, M. P., Sheridan, S. L., Lohr, K. N., Lux, L., et al. (2004, January). *Literacy and health outcomes: Summary* (Evidence Report/Technology Assessment No. 87; AHRQ Publication No. 04-E007-1). Rockville, MD: Agency for Healthcare Research and Quality.

Bureau of Labor Statistics. (2004–2005a). *Career guide to industries, health services.* Retrieved November 1, 2004, from http://www.bls.gov/oco/cg/cgs035.htm

Bureau of Labor Statistics. (2004–2005b). *Occupational outlook handbook.* Retrieved November 1, 2004, from http://www.bls.gov/oco/home.htm

Dahlgren, G., & Whitehead, M. (1991). *Policies and strategies to promote social equity in health.* Stockholm: Institute for Future Studies.

Eisenberg, D. M. (1997). Advising patients who seek alternative medical therapies. *Annals of Internal Medicine, 127,* 61–69.

Gebbie, K., Rosenstock, L., & Hernandez, L. M. (Eds.). (2003). *Who will keep the public healthy? Educating public health professionals for the 21st century.* Washington, DC: National Academies Press.

Goode, T. D. (2001). *Engaging communities to realize the vision of one hundred percent access and zero health disparities: A culturally competent approach.* Washington DC: Georgetown University Child Development Center, National Center for Cultural Competence.

Goode, T. D., & Harrison, S. (2000). *Cultural competence in primary health care: Partnerships for a research agenda.* Washington, DC: Georgetown University Child Development Center, National Center for Cultural Competence.

Goode, T. D., Jones, W., & Mason, J. (2002). *A guide to planning and implementing cultural competence: Organizational self-assessment.* Washington, DC: Georgetown University Child Development Center, National Center for Cultural Competence.

Goode, T., Sockalingam, S., Brown, M., & Jones, W. (2001, January). *Linguistic competence in primary health care delivery systems: Implications for policy makers.* Washington, DC: Georgetown University Child Development Center, National Center for Cultural Competence.

Hill, F. J. (2003). Complementary and alternative medicine: The next generation of health promotion? *Health Promotion International, 18*(3), 265–272.

Institute of Medicine. (2005). *Complementary and alternative medicine in the United States.* Washington, DC: National Academies Press.

Kaptchuk, T. J., & Eisenberg, D. M. (2001). Varieties of healing: 2. A taxonomy of unconventional healing practices. *Annals of Internal Medicine, 135*(3), 196–204.

Kickbusch, I. (2003). The contribution of the World Health Organization to a new public health and health promotion. *American Journal of Public Health, 93*(3), 383–388.

Kickbusch, I., & Payne, L. (2003). Twenty-first century health promotion: The public health revolution meets the wellness revolution. *Health Promotion International, 18*(4), 275–278.

Labonte, R. (1994). Health promotion and empowerment: Reflections on professional practice. *Health Education Quarterly, 21*(2), 253–268.

Labonte, R. (1999). Mutual accountability in partnerships: Health agencies and community groups. *Promotion & Education, 6*(1), 3–8, 36.

Laverack, G., & Labonte, R. (2000). A planning framework for community empowerment goals within health promotion. *Health Policy and Planning, 15*(3), 255–262.

Leadbeater, B., Schellenbach, C. J., Maton, K. I., & Dodgen, D. W. (2004). Research and policy development for building strengths: Processes and contexts of individual, family and community development. In K. I. Maton, C. J. Schellenbach, B. J. Leadbeater, & A. L. Solarz (Eds.), *Investing in children, youth, families, and communities* (pp. 13–30). Washington, DC: American Psychological Association.

McQueen, D. V. (2001). Strengthening the evidence base for health promotion. *Health Promotion International, 16*(3), 261–268.

National Center for Complementary and Alternative Medicine. (2000). Expanding horizons of health care: Five-year strategic plan 2001–2005 (NIH Publication No. 01-5001). Washington, DC: U.S. Department of Health and Human Services.

National Institute of Nursing Research. (1995). *Community-based health care: Nursing strategies.* Washington, DC: U.S. Department of Health and Human Services.

Nielsen-Bohlman, L., Panzer, A., & Kindig, D. A. (2004). *Health literacy: A prescription to end confusion* (Executive Summary). Retrieved January 17, 2005, from http://www.nap.edu/catalog/10883.html

Nutbeam, D. (2000). Health literacy as a public health goal: A challenge for contemporary health education and communication strategies into the 21st century. *Health Promotion International, 15*(3), 259–267.

O'Neil, E. (2005). *Five old trends for a new year.* The Center for the Health Professions. Retrieved January 5, 2005, from http://www.futurehealth.ucsf.edu/from_the_director_0105.html

Rappaport, J. (1985, Fall). The power of empowerment language. *Social Policy, 16,* 15–21.

Ratzan, S. C. (2001). Health literacy: Communication for the public good. *Health Promotion International, 16*(2), 207–214.

Ratzan, S. C., & Parker, R. M. (2000). Introduction. In C. R. Selden, M. Zorn, S. C. Ratzan, & R. M. Parker (Comps.), *Current bibliographies in medicine: Health literacy* (NLM Publication No. CBM 2000-1). Bethesda, MD: U.S. Department of Health and Human Services, National Library of Medicine.

Robertson, A., & Minkler, M. (1994). New health promotion movement: A critical examination. *Health Education Quarterly, 21*(3), 295–312.

Sheinfeld Gorin, S. (1989). *Stopping smoking: A nurse's guide.* New York: American Health Foundation.

Shortell, S. M., Gillies, R. R., Anderson, D. A., Erickson, K. M., & Mitchell, J. B. (1996). *Remaking health care in America: Building organized delivery systems.* San Francisco: Jossey-Bass.

U.S. Department of Health and Human Services. (2000). *Healthy people 2010: Understanding and improving health.* Washington, DC: U.S. Government Printing Office.

U.S. Preventive Services Task Force. (1996). *Guide to clinical preventive services* (2nd ed.). Baltimore: Williams & Wilkins.

U.S. Public Health Service, Office of Minority Health. (2000). *Assuring cultural competence in health care: Recommendations for national standards and an outcomes-focused research agenda.* Retrieved November 2005 from http://www.omhrc.gov/clas/finalcultural1a.htm

Wallerstein, N. (1992). Powerlessness, empowerment, and health: Implications for health promotion programs. *American Journal of Health Promotion, 6*(3), 197–205.

World Health Organization. (1984). *Health promotion: A discussion document on the concepts and principles.* Copenhagen: WHO Regional Office for Europe.

World Health Organization. (1986). *Ottawa Charter for Health Promotion* (WHO/HPR/HEP/95.1). Geneva: Author.

Worthman, C. M. (1999). Epidemiology of human development. In C. Panter-Brick & C. M. Worthman (Eds.), *Hormones, health, and behavior: A socio-ecological and lifespan perspective* (pp. 47–104). New York: Cambridge University Press.

PART TWO

PRACTICE FRAMEWORKS
FOR HEALTH PROMOTION

CHAPTER FIVE

EATING WELL

Lorraine E. Matthews

Ask almost any American and she or he will affirm that a good diet is essential for good health; however, most Americans also state that their diet could be better (International Food Information Counsel, 2003). And even though they are bombarded with health information across the various media outlets, and even though they continue to spend billions of dollars on a variety of dietary supplements, weight loss products, and low-carbohydrate snack foods, Americans continue to get heavier.

Of the ten leading causes of death among Americans, four are directly related to diet: coronary heart disease, cancer, stroke, and diabetes mellitus (McGinnis & Foege, 1993). Over the past decade the federal government, along with a number of other groups, has introduced a major series of prevention programs that focus on weight loss, increased activity, increased consumption of fruits and vegetables, and related programs (U.S. Department of Agriculture [USDA], 1992; USDA & U.S. Department of Health and Human Services [USDHHS], 1995; USDHHS, 2001). However, since the beginning of this century anyway, the overwhelming emphasis has been on weight control. According to the 2001 USDHHS report *The Surgeon General's Call to Action to Prevent and Decrease Overweight and Obesity*, more than half of all Americans are either overweight or obese. The report added that if not addressed, overweight and obesity may soon cause as much preventable disease and death as cigarette smoking. Another recent study (Finkelstein, Fiebelkorn,

& Wang, 2003) found that America's extra weight costs the nation as much as $93 billion in annual medical bills, and the government pays about half that amount. This cost is comparable to the annual medical bills resulting from smoking, an amount estimated at about $75 billion a few years ago. Overall, the annual medical costs for an obese person are about 37.4 percent more, or $732 higher, than the costs for someone of normal weight (Finkelstein et al., 2003). Exact numbers are sometimes difficult to determine, however. In March 2004, the Centers for Disease Control and Prevention (CDC) announced that poor diet and physical inactivity were responsible for 400,000 deaths in 2000, a 33 percent jump from 1990. However, in December 2004, the CDC announced that the study behind the March report contained statistical errors and might have overstated the problem and that the CDC might thus have overstated the figure by 80,000, representing an increase of less than 10 percent over the 1990 statistic, although the agency was still recalculating the figure (American Dietetic Association, 2004). Edge (2004) points out that based on the federal government's Healthy Eating Index, a survey of American food habits that was last published in 1996, almost 88 percent of American diets fell into the "poor" or "needs improvement" categories in 1996. She argues that even though we know a great deal about what a healthful diet is, what we do not know is how to get that 88 percent of Americans to choose one.

A particular concern, and one that has grabbed the attention of the media and state and local governments, is the especially rapid increase in overweight among children. It is estimated that 15 percent of both children (aged six to eleven) and adolescents (aged twelve to nineteen) in the United Stated are overweight (CDC, 2002). The associated health conditions and financial burden have caused this emerging epidemic to become a major public health concern (Barlow, Dietz, Klish, & Trowbridge, 2002; Ball et al., 2003; CDC, 2002) in part because a number of medical conditions that were once prevalent only among adults are now emerging in young people. These include hyperlipidemia, glucose intolerance, hypertension, and diabetes (CDC, 2002). Also of concern is that when compared to adolescents who maintain healthy weights, overweight adolescents have a greater chance of becoming overweight adults (Binns & Ariza, 2004).

How did we arrive at this point? Edge (2004) points out that the United States has a long history of food assistance programs, which began largely during the Great Depression, and for most of the twentieth century the primary priority was eliminating hunger. Over time, food distribution policies have evolved into three principle components: food stamp programs, school lunch programs, and the Special Supplemental Nutrition Program for Women, Infants, and Children (WIC). Over approximately the same span of time, the federal government has put increasingly more emphasis on nutrition education and healthy eating. However, Nestle (2003), in her book *Food Politics,* details the tactics that the food industry has used to shape government food and nutrition policies and to convince Americans to eat more. She describes the intense lobbying that went into crafting the USDA's Dietary Guidelines and the Food Guide Pyramid. The published versions are much less stringent than those originally proposed, because of intense pressure from key members of the food industry. She also details the intense effort of the food industry to market to children of all ages through television advertising and exclusive contracts with schools. Edge (2004) argues that the federal government sends mixed messages. She points out that even though the U.S. surgeon general has referred to obesity as "the terror within" and even though obesity has been estimated to cost taxpayers $117 billion annually, current legislation being considered by Congress authorizes a mere $60 million in funding to state and local entities for promotion of healthy eating and physical activity, particularly to school-age children and adolescents. Nevertheless, many states have implemented programs that seek to improve the food and nutrition environment in public schools—eliminating or changing products in vending machines, preventing schools from signing exclusive beverage contracts with major soft drink companies (known as *pouring contracts*), increasing nutrition and physical activity education for children and teens, and helping local school districts to develop and implement guidelines for school-based food advertising (Public Health Institute, 2004; Pennsylvania Advocates for Nutrition and Activity, 2003).

The Dilemma of Food, Nutrition, and Health

Given the statistics this chapter has provided so far, it would seem logical that Americans would simply recognize that changes need to be made and implement them. The information is readily available and the message is relatively simple—eat less and exercise more. Yet they don't. Millions of Americans struggle with this message and continue to search desperately for ways to improve their health and their appearance without having to sacrifice any of their favorite foods and related behaviors.

It is important to understand that the role of food and nutrition in the promotion of health and well-being is unique. Unlike a person who must stop and avoid certain behaviors completely when they become problems, the person with eating issues must still continue to eat. For example, the person who abuses alcohol must come to grips with the fact that he or she can no longer use this product, and he or she can have some success in avoiding places where alcohol is served;

however, the person who abuses food must somehow learn to make changes in the use of this substance that even though it creates problems is essential for continued life; moreover, food is everywhere.

Consumers, adults and children, are faced with choosing among tens of thousands of food items in the average supermarket, and many of these markets now sport ready-to-serve foods and an array of fresh baked goods. National and local fast-food restaurants abound, not only as stand-alone stores but also within other locations such as department stores, recreation facilities, and even health care facilities. An increasing array of food items is also found in the national chain super department stores, in pharmacies, in stationery stores, and in a wide variety of other commercial establishments. Even the various dollar store chains sell a wide variety of foods, most of them readily available, nonperishable, and highly processed. The problem is, of course, that many of these relatively inexpensive foods are high in fat, salt, and calories but low in essential nutrients. Nestle (2003) argues that this is due in part to the food industry's ability to take surpluses of some basic food stuffs and process them into cheap foods with few nutrients and then dump them on the U.S. food market. Interestingly, the low-carbohydrate craze that has swept this nation has created a whole new family of *low-carb*, high-fat snack bars that are touted as healthy. (Check any large pharmacy, and you will find at least one aisle stocked with rather expensive, low-carbohydrate snack foods, perhaps over one hundred different kinds.)

An important reality that must be remembered is that to most people most of these foods *taste good*. Fast-food menu items are popular because people like them. Although many of the major fast-food restaurants have added lighter fare to their menus, the big sellers remain the high-calorie, high-fat sandwiches and meals.

These facts are important because health care professionals who are trying to move consumers toward a more healthful diet have to somehow convince them to decrease their intake of the readily accessible, relatively inexpensive foods that they have come to like.

Developing a Dietary Intervention Model

As health care professionals struggle with how to change unhealthy eating behaviors, it is necessary to look at the various health behavior models that have been developed to try to explain why people do what they do and what, if anything, will bring about change. A detailed discussion of the various theoretical models to explain health behavior change can be found in Chapter Two. The focus here will be on models that help us identify key issues in behaviors surrounding eating and issues that seem to be the most effective in helping people change how they eat.

The health belief model (HBM) is one of the most frequently used models to explain change in eating behavior. It was developed in the 1950s by a group of psychologists to help explain why people would or would not use health services (Rosenstock, 1966). The HBM hypothesizes that health-related action depends on the simultaneous occurrence of three classes of factors:

- The existence of sufficient motivation (or health concern) to make health issues salient or relevant.
- The belief that one is susceptible (vulnerable) to a serious health problem or to the sequelae of that illness or condition. (This susceptibility is often termed a *perceived threat.*)
- The belief that following a particular health recommendation will be beneficial in reducing the perceived threat and will do so at a subjectively acceptable cost. (*Cost* refers to what it will take to overcome *perceived barriers* in order to follow the health recommendation; McKenzie & Smeltzer, 2001.)

This seems to be an appropriate model to use to examine whether individuals will even consider making positive changes in eating decisions. To illustrate, consider the case of two men: one who is aged fifty, about twenty-five pounds overweight, and with a diagnosis of elevated cholesterol levels and related problems; the other is aged twenty-five and also about twenty-five pounds overweight but with no other apparent problems. If both men receive the same information about the benefits of lowering their fat intake and increasing their fruit and vegetable intake, it is possible that they will react to the message differently. On the one hand the fifty-year-old may recognize that he is at risk for heart disease (perceived susceptibility) and that his health condition could deteriorate rapidly if he does not make changes (perceived threat). However, because making these changes will require him to stop eating daily lunches at his favorite take-out restaurant, he will have to consider the cost (perceived barrier) of bringing his own lunch or making healthier selections. Because he knows that making these changes could reduce his risk of heart disease (perceived benefit), he is more likely to weigh the benefit and the barrier and make a positive decision to change his diet. On the other hand the young man with no apparent symptoms may consider the cost too great and may not follow through with the suggested changes.

The HBM also contains the construct of *self-efficacy,* which is defined as an individual's confidence in his or her ability to take action or execute the behavior that produces the desired outcome (Janz, Champion, & Strecher, 2002). Even when environment and social network are considered, they are usually defined within the context of the individual's perception. If the fifty-year-old man described earlier is a widower with limited shopping and cooking skills, he may lack the confidence to make the necessary changes in his diet even if he clearly understands the need to make these changes. Therefore, it is incumbent on the health care provider to offer this client support and opportunities to learn new skills and increase his self-confidence so that he can improve his diet. Perhaps a referral to a class on cooking for singles that is provided at a nearby community center will help him improve.

Bandura's social cognitive theory (SCT) has been applied to both health education and health behavior programs because it not only takes into account the individual but also incorporates the environment for the behavior. Social cognitive theory evaluates behavior by considering the competing forces of the person, the behavior, and environmental influences. First, it brings together different concepts—cognitive, emotional, and behavioral—of behavioral change. Second, fresh behavioral research and practice can be formulated from the various constructs and processes that make up SCT (Baranowski, Perry, & Parcel, 2002). Reinforcement is an integral part of learning, but emphasize the role of subjective hypotheses or expectations held by the individual (McKenzie & Smeltzer, 2001). In addition, the interaction between a person and his or her environment is continuous and can influence the person's opportunity to change. Family members, peers, the neighborhood, and the availability of particular foods all shape a person's external environment, which can in turn affect the ability to change eating behavior. If, on the one hand, the fifty-year-old man with high cholesterol has a family that encourages him and supports his effort to change, he will likely have some success. On the other hand, if a thirteen-year-old boy with diabetes is afraid that his friends will make fun of him because he limits his food choices in the cafeteria line, he is less likely to actively make positive changes in his eating habits, even if he understands that it may make him feel better.

An interesting study on weight management for postpartum women employed the transtheoretical model of stages of change to gauge the women's readiness to participate in the program (Krummel, Semmens, Boury, Gordan, & Larkin, 2004). In the transtheoretical model the stages of change dimension reflects a person's readiness to change behavior, or the person's engagement in behavioral change, at a given point in time. The first two stages represent people who are least ready to change (precontemplation) or are ambivalent about change (contemplation); the third state represents people who are preparing to change in the next month (preparation); the last two stages represent active behavioral change if the change is recent (action) or sustained behavioral change if the change has been maintained for more than six months (maintenance). Movement through the stages is fluid and cyclical as people try to change their behavior (Nigg et al., 1999). This study looked at 151 postpartum WIC recipients who were all over eighteen years old and had a child younger than two years old. They were sorted at random into different weight management programs. At the conclusion of the study, 55 percent of the women were found to be in the action stage for weight loss, but fewer were in the action stage for the following weight management behaviors: avoiding high-fat foods (24 percent), increasing fiber (19 percent), and exercising three times per week (29 percent). The authors concluded that by emphasizing the pros and decreasing the cons for weight management, women may be able to change their behaviors to promote better weight management. Several strategies such as training in selecting low-fat restaurant choices, reading food labels, and group discussion helped the women move into the action stage.

What does this mean in terms of working with clients? The key for the health care professional is to realize that the client sitting in front of him or her is not one dimensional and neither is the health behavior in question. Cartright, commenting on the Krummel et al. study, points out that the stages of change model contends that behavioral change is more likely to occur when one reaches the later stages. She adds that given this model, the health care professional should determine a client's level of readiness before beginning education (Cartright, 2004). Another very important mantra to remember is that "one size does not fit all." No two clients will have exactly the same problems or issues when it comes to intervention in the way they eat. The health care professional needs to be able to select from various models to most effectively understand and provide assistance to a client.

The Physiology of Eating

The science of nutrition is an interdisciplinary field that focuses on the study of foods, nutrients, and health (Brown, 2002). Most of what is known in the field of nutrition has come after 1900, with a particularly rapid increase in knowledge over the last decade. This ever-increasing body of knowledge is also changing views on what constitutes the best nutritional advice. Indeed, this exploding body of information has contributed to consumer confusion about health and optimal diet. To set the stage for a discussion of diet and nutrition, a brief overview of the basics is provided.

A person's diet must include foods that provide the nutrients required to sustain life and for his or her body to grow and maintain itself. The body requires six types of essential nutrients, which can be defined as families of molecules that are indispensable to the body's functioning and that the body cannot make for itself. Without any one of these six, the body's overall health will be impaired.

Although water provides no energy and essentially no other nutrients, it is the most abundant nutrient. It is constantly lost from the body and must constantly be replaced. An important point to remember in terms of public health is that as adults age, the percentage of total body water declines, so adequate fluid intake is especially important in older adults (Chernoff, 1999, pp. 18–19).

The only energy-producing nutrients are proteins, carbohydrates, and fats. Proteins also provide essential building materials that form body structures and are the basis for many essential compounds. Some protein is found in almost all foods, but the primary food sources are meats, eggs, dairy products, and legumes. Carbohydrates and fats also provide basic components for a number of essential compounds and structures required by the body, although to a lesser degree than proteins. With the exception of milk and honey, carbohydrates are found only in plant products. Carbohydrates are generally categorized into two groups—simple sugars, which are usually are found naturally in fruits and some vegetables, and complex carbohydrates, or starches, which are abundant in grain products and starchy vegetables. Fat is also present in varying amounts in almost all foods. Its primary animal sources are meat, meat products, and dairy products made from milk, and its primary vegetable source is the germ of most seeds, grains, and many nuts. As a rule, animal fats tend to be more highly saturated and vegetable fats tend to be more unsaturated. A key point to remember about fat is that due to its chemical structure, fat yields over twice as many calories (nine calories per gram) as protein and carbohydrate (four calories per gram each).

Included in the general category of fats are a number of complex organic compounds that are not used for energy production but rather as building blocks of various essential compounds in the body. Only one of these complex compounds, cholesterol, will be discussed here. Found only in animal tissues, cholesterol is an essential sterol that is part of a number of structures and compounds in the body. The human body makes cholesterol even when it is completely absent from the diet. Although some is necessary, too much cholesterol in the body can cause clogged arteries and is a major risk factor for cardiovascular disease.

Even though they have been recognized for many years, *trans fats* have recently received a lot of publicity and have begun to appear on food labels. Briefly, oils can be made solid by adding hydrogen to the double bonds of their fatty acids. This process, called hydrogenation, makes some of the fatty acids in oils saturated and generally enhances shelf life and baking qualities, but it also changes the structure of the fatty acids. Trans fats do occur naturally in a few foods, but the primary dietary sources are products made from hydrogenated fats, a category that includes most baked and fried food and many butter substitutes. The reason they are of concern is that diets high in trans fats are related to an increased risk of heart disease, at a rate similar to that in people eating diets high in saturated fats (Hu et al., 1999).

The last two groups of essential nutrients are vitamins and minerals, which are found in a wide variety of foods. They do not provide any energy, and all but a few are needed in very minute amounts in the body. A few minerals serve as parts of body structures (for example, calcium and phosphorus in bones and teeth), but the primary role of vitamins and minerals is to regulate body processes. These processes include digesting foods, moving muscles, disposing of wastes, growing new tissue, healing wounds, and obtaining energy from carbohydrates, fats, and proteins (Brown, 2002).

Extensive research and improved technology have also allowed medical science to focus on selected vitamins and minerals for prevention of specific conditions. For example, folic acid has been found to be a key element in the normal development of the fetal neural tube, which is the precursor to the spinal cord and the brain. A woman who has subclinical levels of folic acid very early in her pregnancy is at increased risk of having a child with spina bifida or a similar condition (Brown, 2002). Neural tube defects (NTDs) are among the most common birth defects, affecting about 4,000 pregnancies annually in the United States. Approximately 70 percent of NTDs can be prevented by consumption of adequate folic acid before and during early pregnancy (CDC, 2000).

There are also substances in foods in addition to nutrients that affect health. Two that have received considerable attention are antioxidants and phytochemicals. The former are chemical substances that prevent or repair damage to cells caused by exposure to oxidizing agents, both in the environment and in the body. Many different antioxidants are found in food, but some are made in the body. Phytochemicals are chemical substances in plants, some of which affect body processes in humans in ways that may benefit health. Consumption of foods rich in various phytochemicals may help to prevent certain types of cancer, infections, and heart disease (Brown, 2002).

A few other key concepts regarding nutrition that health care professionals need to understand and convey to clients include the following:

- The body is like a large chemistry laboratory that functions effectively and with much regularity. Although how it works may be considered miraculous, the body does not function through magic; there is an ordered purpose for the reactions, even if health care professionals do not completely understand them.

- The foods that humans eat are also chemicals, and they interact with the chemicals in the body—also in an ordered manner. There are no magic foods; however, some have higher concentrations of the nutrients and other substances that humans need.
- The nutrient fat is unique in that it cannot be excreted or eliminated from the body. The only way to remove it is through oxidation, or burning. The loss (burning) of one pound of fat requires the person to use approximately 3,500 more calories than the calories taken in from food (Brown, 2002). Most people can reduce their body fat by a maximum of two to three pounds in one week. Although weight loss may be more rapid initially when someone significantly reduces caloric intake, most of that loss is in the form of water and some muscle tissue but very little fat. Therefore, diet plans that promise significant loss of several pounds a week are deceptive.
- Human bodies require regular exercise. If exercise is not a part of a person's regular activities (for example, his or her work), then it should be planned into the day. Attempts at weight reduction through changes in eating habits are marginally effective when there is no physical activity component (National Heart, Lung, and Blood Institute [NHLBI] & North American Association for the Study of Obesity, 2000). However, as discussed in the next chapter, the need for exercise goes well beyond weight control. For individuals to make lasting changes in their eating behaviors, they must understand that diet and physical activity have complementary beneficial effects in relation to the major chronic diseases.

For optimal health the processes just described must occur with efficiency and regularity. This requires an adequate, consistent supply of nutrients. Some nutrients, such as vitamin C, are almost completely used up on a daily basis, with little being stored in the body. Thus symptoms of deficiency can be seen in a matter of weeks in a susceptible person who does not ingest the vitamin. Other nutrients, such as calcium, phosphorus, protein, and fat, are normally stored in the body, so an overt deficiency takes much longer to manifest itself. In reality, however, the classic deficiency diseases of scurvy (inadequate vitamin C), beriberi (inadequate thiamin), and similar conditions are rarely seen today in this country, thanks to almost universal enrichment and fortification of commonly eaten foods. In the United States these conditions are primarily seen in high-risk groups, such as persons who abuse alcohol, persons with specific diseases such as cancer or acquired immunodeficiency syndrome (AIDS), and persons who chronically ingest highly restricted diets. These same high-risk individuals are often on a regimen of medications that can also interfere with the efficacy of certain nutrients (Brown, 2002).

The Changing Focus of Nutrition and Health

As the major causes of death have shifted from infectious to chronic diseases, emphasis is now focused on the maintenance of health and the reduction of the risk for chronic diseases such as heart disease, hypertension, stroke, diabetes mellitus, and some types of cancer. However, a major concern today is that these conditions once found primarily in middle-aged adults are now occurring in with some frequency in children and adolescents (Ball et al., 2003). It is now well documented that improved nutritional behaviors will lower the at-risk person's potential for developing these diseases. The federal government has mounted a major national effort to reduce the rate of chronic diseases such as heart disease and diabetes through an emphasis on a healthier lifestyle, including dietary change and increased physical activity (USDHHS, 2001).

This initiative poses novel challenges to the health care professional—challenges even more complicated today than they were a few years ago. Today consumers are exposed to a barrage of diet and health information on a variety of fronts—the traditional media sources, infomercials, Internet Web sites, and direct-mail materials—and much of it is conflicting and confusing. Among the most controversial dietary issues are high-protein and very low carbohydrate diets. Versions of these diets have been around for decades, but they have been popularized recently by books for the lay reader and lots of marketing. Three of the better-known ones are the Zone diet, the South Beach diet, and the Atkins diet, all of which focus on a high-protein diet with very limited carbohydrate intake. The first two are based on an eating plan that is 40 percent carbohydrate, 30 percent protein, and 30 percent fat, whereas the Atkins plan doesn't really place any restrictions on fat. Proponents of these diets state that the 40-30-30 ratio of macronutrient intake allows the body to more efficiently burn calories, leading to loss of weight, reduction of body fat, and increases in lean body mass. Another argument supporting this type of diet is the claim that it reduces high insulin levels and insulin resistance, problems that proponents claim result from consuming high-carbohydrate meals (Brown, 2002).

At the other extreme are proponents of very low fat diets, which of necessity restrict protein and include ample amounts of complex carbohydrates. The best-known diet of this type comes from Dean Ornish (1994, 2004). Ornish argues that even though the high-protein, very low carbohydrate diet may cause some temporary weight loss, it can increase the risk of heart disease and related conditions because of its increased fat content and very low fiber content. One point that all these plans agree on is that there must be a significant reduction in simple and highly processed carbohydrates—sugar and other sweeteners, soft drinks and other sweetened beverages, and prepared foods that contain large of amounts of highly refined grains. Of concern is that many consumers do not know how to differentiate between factual and false information and how to sort out what they should be eating. As noted earlier, the low-carbohydrate craze has spawned a wide variety of snack foods and energy bars that may have one-fourth to one-third fewer simple sugars than ordinary snack foods do. However, this is due mainly to the use of sugar substitutes, and these foods are not low calorie and usually contain a lot of fat. The promotion of these items is reminiscent of the heavy marketing of fat-free desserts and snack foods about a decade ago. Although fat free, they were very high in calories and had greater amounts of simple carbohydrates than ordinary desserts do. It is not surprising that consumers get confused. The thing that consumers often don't understand regarding either of these two extremes is that even though the specialty foods they are purchasing are labeled "low fat" or "low carbohydrate," they still usually have a lot of calories.

Of greater concern is that this information overload is also confusing many health care professionals, causing them to give incorrect or incomplete information to their clients. An example of this is the effort by some health care professionals to promote low-carbohydrate diets to the majority of their patients, without really understanding the ramifications for some people of omitting an entire food group. Growing children, even those that are overweight, should not be deprived of the nutrients found in an essential food group. Although it is quite appropriate to restrict foods with high concentrations of simple sugars (candy, soft drinks, and so forth), it is not a good idea to eliminate whole and enriched grain products and starchy vegetables for growing children and most adults.

Consumers do feel the tension between what they believe they should eat and what they do eat. For example, women participating in focus groups in two urban community health centers in Philadelphia stated that they had made some changes in their diets because of health concerns. Their major concern was preventing heart disease, strokes, and diabetes, although a few discussed diet and cancer. They acknowledged that their time for food preparation was limited and that their families ate take-out food more often then they would have liked (Opoku-Boateng, 2004). These same women voiced concern about their children's health and the foods that they ate; however, over half did not feel they could really control their children's food selections.

Defining a Healthy Diet

Defining a healthy diet is difficult. Most people have their own vision of what constitutes a healthy diet, even if they don't always follow it. Comments from participants in parent and child focus groups in a community health center indicated that most had very specific ideas about what foods should be included in a healthy diet, even if they didn't necessarily use those foods on a regular basis (Opoku-Boateng, 2004). Further, there are some differences in the types and amounts of food required at different stages of life and in the presence of certain chronic diseases.

In 2005, the federal government released the latest version of *Dietary Guidelines for Americans* (USDHHS & USDA, 2005). The guidelines contain forty-one key recommendations: twenty-three of them are for the general public, and eighteen are for certain populations, such as children or older adults. They are summarized here:

- To maintain a healthy body weight, balance calories taken in with calories expended.
- To reduce the risk of chronic disease in adulthood, engage in a moderate-intensity physical activity at least thirty minutes a day on most days of the week.
- To prevent gradual weight gain in adulthood, engage in about sixty minutes of moderate to vigorous activity on most days of the week while keeping calories constant.
- To maintain weight loss in adulthood, do sixty to ninety minutes of daily moderate-intensity physical activity while keeping calories constant.
- Limit intake of saturated and trans fats, cholesterol, added sugar, salt, and alcohol.
- On a 2,000-calorie diet, eat two cups of fruit and two and one-half cups of vegetables each day.
- Eat three or more one-ounce equivalents of whole-grain products each day, with the rest of the recommended grains coming from enriched or whole-grain products.
- Consume three cups a day of fat-free or low-fat milk or equivalent milk products.
- Consume less than 10 percent of total calories from saturated fatty acids and less than 300 milligrams a day of cholesterol, while keeping trans fatty acid consumption as low as possible.
- Keep total fat intake between 20 percent and 35 percent of calories, with most fats coming from sources of polyunsaturated and monounsaturated fatty acids.
- Eat lean, low-fat, or fat-free meat, poultry, dry beans, and milk or milk products.
- Consume less than 2,300 milligrams of sodium—about one teaspoon of salt—per day.
- Increase potassium intake with fruits and vegetables.
- Limit alcoholic beverages to one (women) or two (men) drinks per day. Some individuals, including pregnant women, should not drink alcohol.

Although these recommendations remain general guidelines that can be adapted to a variety of food preferences for different ethnic groups and cultures, they are more comprehensive than the previous USDA guidelines. Consumers will need help trying to put them into practice.

Most Americans are familiar with the Food Guide Pyramid (USDA & USDHHS, 1995) of the last decade, which is widely found on food packages, in advertisements, and in numerous health and nutrition education materials (see Figure 5.1). As an adjunct to the new Dietary Guidelines, a revised Food Guide Pyramid was introduced in April 2005 (USDA, 2005). The new pyramid (see Figure 5.2) is called MyPyramid, Steps to a Healthier You and is designed to be interactive. Consumers are asked to go online (at www.mypyramid.gov) and enter their age, gender, and activity level. Then they get a food plan for their appropriate calorie level. Each individual food plan includes daily amounts to eat from each food group and a limit for intake of discretionary calories: added fat, added

FIGURE 5.1. FOOD GUIDE PYRAMID.

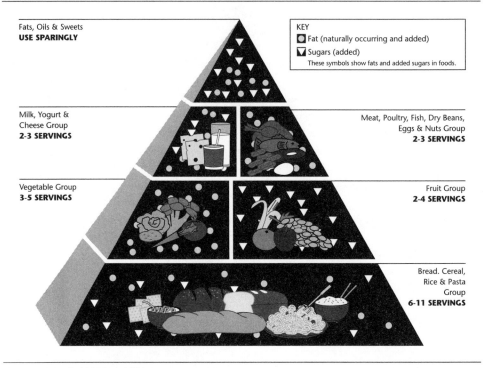

Source: USDA & USDHHS, 1995.

FIGURE 5.2. MYPYRAMID: STEPS TO A HEALTHIER YOU.

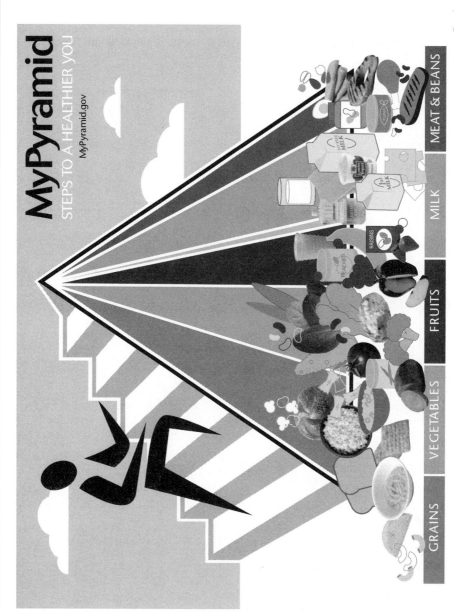

(Continued)

FIGURE 5.2. MYPYRAMID: STEPS TO A HEALTHIER YOU, Cont'd.

GRAINS	VEGETABLES	FRUITS	MILK	MEAT & BEANS
Make half your grains whole	Vary your veggies	Focus on fruits	Get your calcium-rich foods	Go lean with protein
Eat at least 3 oz. of whole-grain cereals, breads, crackers, rice, or pasta every day 1 oz. is about 1 slice of bread, about 1 cup of breakfast cereal, or ½ cup of cooked rice, cereal, or pasta	Eat more dark-green veggies like broccoli, spinach, and other dark leafy greens Eat more orange vegetables like carrots and sweet potatoes Eat more dry beans and peas like pinto beans, kidney beans, and lentils	Eat a variety of fruit Choose fresh, frozen, canned, or dried fruit Go easy on fruit juices	Go low-fat or fat-free when you choose milk, yogurt, and other milk products If you don't or can't consume milk, choose lactose-free products or other calcium sources such as fortified foods and beverages	Choose low-fat or lean meats and poultry Bake it, broil it, or grill it Vary your protein routine – choose more fish, beans, peas, nuts, and seeds

For a 2,000-calorie diet, you need the amounts below from each food group. To find the amounts that are right for you, go to MyPyramid.gov.

Eat 6 oz. every day	Eat 2½ cups every day	Eat 2 cups every day	Get 3 cups every day, for kids aged 2 to 8, it's 2	Eat 5½ oz. every day

Find your balance between food and physical activity

- Be sure to stay within your daily calorie needs.
- Be physically active for at least 30 minutes most days of the week.
- About 60 minutes a day of physical activity may be needed to prevent weight gain.
- For sustaining weight loss, at least 60 to 90 minutes a day of physical activity may be required.
- Children and teenagers should be physically active for 60 minutes every day, or most days.

Know the limits on fats, sugars, and salt (sodium)

- Make most of your fat sources from fish, nuts, and vegetable oils.
- Limit solid fats like butter, stick margarine, shortening, and lard, as well as foods that contain these.
- Check the Nutrition Facts label to keep saturated fats, trans fats, and sodium low.
- Choose food and beverages low in added sugars. Added sugars contribute calories with few, if any, nutrients.

MyPyramid.gov
STEPS TO A HEALTHIER YOU

USDA

U.S. Department of Agriculture
Center for Nutrition Policy and Promotion
April 2005
CNPP-15

USDA is an equal opportunity provider and employer.

Source: USDA, 2005.

sugar, and alcohol (Ferroli, 2005). What concerns a number of nutrition and health educators is that to use MyPyramid one must use the Internet, which isn't always readily available to consumers. Further, because MyPyramid focuses on individual needs, it is more difficult than the previous Food Guide Pyramid to use in group educational programs and in printed educational materials. Nutrition and research professionals at the federal level are currently addressing these issues, however, and appropriate guidance materials are expected to become available directly from USDA or from state extension agencies (Lynn James, nutrition consultant, Extension Service, The Pennsylvania State University, personal communication, 2005).

Another major difference is that the previous Food Guide Pyramid promoted choosing a recommended number of daily servings from each of the five major food groups, with the range in the number of servings generally based on age and gender, whereas MyPyramid lists the recommended daily amounts of foods in cups or ounces. This was done primarily because of the nearly universal concern about American caloric intake. There has also been much concern about the public's lack of understanding about portion sizes, however. Many consumers have been confused about both the number of servings and the serving sizes. The majority of serving sizes listed on the previous pyramid are from one-half to three-fourths of one cup, which is a lot less than most Americans eat. For example, most persons who eat rice or pasta with a meal eat at least one cup, which translates into two servings. *Portion distortion* is a major concern among nutrition professionals, as the size of commercially available food portions has grown considerably in recent years. Consumers seem to be convinced that "more for less" is preferable, and manufacturers have obliged by increasing the portion sizes of a variety of commonly eaten foods and beverages—bagels, french fries, soft drinks, and a variety of snack foods. Although a few manufacturers of retail food products have started making some products in smaller sizes, it is essential for health care professionals to continue to educate consumers on the need to dish up smaller portions (Callahan, 2004). The change in format for MyPyramid is an attempt to help consumers do this. Finally, in terms of presentation, the previous pyramid listed the food groups in horizontal blocks, but MyPyramid displays the food groups vertically, in bands of different colors, with a runner racing up the side. Again, consumers and health professionals will need some assistance in navigating the new pyramid.

Health care professionals should be aware that the Food Guide Pyramid has had its detractors since its inception, but it remains the model that is most commonly used. Nestle (2003) details some of the battles joined and compromises made for its first version. Some food industry interest groups complained about their particular location on the pyramid—for example, the dairy and egg industry thought

that being located on the upper tiers diminished these foods' perceived importance. Groups representing people who follow strict vegetarian diets complained
of being left out of consideration.

Most recently, some researchers have called for a complete reorganization.
Willet (2003) and colleagues proposed changing the base of the original pyramid
to include whole-grain products and monounsaturated fats such as olive oil and
nut oils. Simple sugars and most processed carbohydrates are then placed on the
top. Modified versions have been devised for a number of different groups, including vegetarians, Asian Americans, Hispanic Americans, African Americans, pregnant women, and older adults.

Health care professionals should keep in mind that although there have been
significant changes in the presentation of this national eating guide, there is much
information that remains the same. Table 5.1 summarizes the differences between
the two guides.

- *Grain group.* Breads, cereals, and pasta form the base of the previous pyramid
  and the first vertical tier of MyPyramid. Consumers need to make half of their
  total grain intake whole grains and to consume three or more one-ounce equivalents (based on a 2,000-calorie diet). An ounce-equivalent of grains is about
  one slice of bread, one cup of ready-to-eat cereal, or one-half cup of cooked
  pasta or rice or cooked cereal. The rationale behind this recommendation is
  that the phytonutrients in whole grains are important in reducing the risk of
  cardiovascular disease, cancer, and other chronic diseases, when whole grains
  are eaten as part of an overall healthy diet (Ferroli, 2005). Whole grains also
  provide dietary fiber, which helps keep the gastrointestinal tract healthy and
  maintains adequate laxation. Also, commercially baked products that are high
  in fat should be discouraged because they are sources of saturated fats and trans
  fats, which should be very limited. It is also reasonable to include here some of
  the starchier vegetables, such as yams and sweet potatoes, that are staples in
  many cultures, as they are rich in fiber, vitamins, and minerals and are very low
  in fat.
- *Vegetable group.* In the previous pyramid vegetables and fruits were grouped together on the second horizontal tier; however, MyPyramid splits them into the
  second and third vertical tiers. For a 2,000 calorie diet, the recommendation is five servings of vegetables, or two and one-half cups. MyPyramid also
  recommends consuming a variety of vegetables, with the emphasis on dark-
  green vegetables and orange vegetables. Dried beans and peas can count as
  vegetables and as protein sources. The Dietary Guidelines are even more specific. They state that individuals on a 2,000-calorie diet need to eat three cups
  of dark-green vegetables, two cups of orange vegetables, and three cups of

TABLE 5.1. MAJOR CHANGES IN THE USDA FOOD GUIDE PYRAMID.

Previous Food Guide Pyramid (USDA, 1995)	Food Groups	MyPyramid (USDA, 2005) (based on a reference person who needs 2,000 calories daily)
6–11 servings daily Select a wide variety	Grain-based foods: breads, cereals, and pasta	6 ounces daily (1 oz. = 1 slice of bread, 1 cup ready-to-eat cereal, ½ cup cooked cereal, rice, or pasta) At least 3 whole-grain products daily
3–5 servings daily Select a wide variety	Vegetables	2½ cups daily Include more dark green vegetables, more orange vegetables, and include more cooked dry beans and peas
2–4 servings daily Select a wide variety	Fruits and juices	2 cups daily Choose a variety daily Limit juice to less than half of daily selections
2–3 servings daily	Dairy products	3 cups* of fat-free or low-fat milk (1%) or an equivalent daily (1 cup yogurt, 1.5 oz. natural cheese, 1 oz. processed cheese) *2 cups for children between 2 and 8 years
2–3 servings daily	Meat and meat substitutes	5½ ounces *lean* meat, poultry, or fish, or an equivalent (1 egg, ¼ cup dried beans or peas or nuts)
Use these items sparingly in daily meal plan	Foods to use sparingly (fats, oils, sugars, and alcohol)	Discretionary calories limited to 100–300 calories after above requirements have been met

Note: For more information or to determine your personal eating plan, go to www.mypyramid.gov.

dry beans and peas *each week*. Consumers need to be reassured that these choices do not have to be all fresh vegetables. Frozen or canned vegetables are also good sources of nutrients and fiber. This is also true of dried beans and peas.

- *Fruit group.* Individuals on a 2,000-calorie diet should eat two cups of fruit a day and should choose from a wide variety. The amount of fruit juice, however, should be limited to less than half of the total fruit intake. More fruit juice is not better because it adds more sugar. Again, canned, frozen, and dried fruits all can count toward meeting the fruit goals and will provide a variety of nutrients and fiber.

- *Dairy group.* The third tier of the previous pyramid was shared by the milk, yogurt, and cheese group and the meat, poultry, fish, dry beans, eggs, and nuts group. Now fat-free or low-fat (1 percent) dairy products are found on the fourth vertical tier. The new recommendation is to consume three cups of fat-free or low-fat milk or an equivalent amount of yogurt or cheese per day. Equivalent amounts for one cup of milk are one cup of yogurt, one and one-half ounces of natural cheese, or two ounces of processed cheese. The dairy group provides the nutrients needed for bone health and may be beneficial for maintaining a healthy weight. Children aged two to eight should have two cups of fat-free or low-fat milk or the equivalent. (Unless medically directed, children under age two should be given only whole milk after they have been weaned from breast milk or formula.) For individuals who can't or don't use dairy products, altered milk products such as Lactaid or a calcium- and vitamin-fortified soy milk are acceptable. However, consumers do need to be aware that rice milk is not an acceptable substitute for young children.

- *Meat, poultry, fish, dry beans, eggs, and nuts group.* These food products make up the fifth vertical tier, and the recommendation is to make choices that are very low in fat or lean. People who are consuming a 2,000-calorie daily diet need five and one-half ounce equivalents. An ounce equivalent in this group is the amount of food equal to one ounce of cooked meat, poultry, or fish. There should be an emphasis on selecting meat cuts that are at least 90 percent lean. Proper cooking techniques are also essential with foods in this group, and consumers need to be advised to try ways to cut fat, such as trimming excess fat before cooking, draining excess cooking fat, and cooking with as little fat as possible to start. One egg or a quarter-cup of dried beans or peas or nuts is a one-ounce equivalent for meat. However, nuts should be stressed as a snack or for inclusion in other foods, such as salads.

- *Discretionary calories.* New in MyPyramid and in the 2005 Dietary Guidelines are the discretionary calories, the calories remaining in a person's individual energy allowance after accounting for the number of calories needed to meet recommended nutrient intakes through consumption of foods that are low in fat or have no added sugar. For most Americans the number of allowed discretionary calories will be small—100 to 300 calories. This is where health care professionals will really have to work with consumers to help them understand using their choices wisely (Ferroli, 2005). Given the current discussion of saturated, polyunsaturated, and monounsaturated fats in the new Dietary Guidelines, it will be prudent for health care professionals to provide more explanation on the types of fats that consumers commonly use, as this subject can be very confusing. In addition, this is where discussion of limited use of sugar, salt, and alcohol is appropriate.

One key point for health care professionals to remember is that Americans are eating an ever increasing number of meals away from home, and no one seems to have any good ideas on how to reverse this trend. People can select healthful foods when they are away from home, but it takes planning and often requires making special requests, which many people are uncomfortable doing— requesting, for example, that a sandwich be made without mayonnaise or that salad dressing be on the side or that an entrée be broiled instead of sautéed. So the health care professional needs to help busy people eat defensively. It is possible to select healthy foods from restaurant and even some fast-food menus, but it takes a good eye and some initiative to avoid the high-calorie, high-fat, and high-sodium foods.

Realities of Effecting Positive Change in Eating Behavior

The promotion of changes in eating behavior can be daunting. For all the reasons discussed previously, consumers present to health care professionals with a variety of preexisting lifestyle practices that often do not promote healthy eating. Here are some general pointers that need to be incorporated into any educational plan.

- Although most people have some knowledge about nutrition and can usually list the foods that contribute to a healthy diet, they frequently cannot figure out a way to incorporate those foods into their daily lives. Nutrition education programs in many public schools have focused on the Food Guide Pyramid, and many American schoolchildren can recite the components of this pyramid, even though they may not incorporate this knowledge into what they routinely eat. For example, an informal survey of 200 adolescents at a popular shopping center in downtown Philadelphia found that at least 60 percent of them reported eating fast foods at least once a day. When questioned about what they thought a healthy diet should include, they tended to list the foods on the pyramid. When asked why they didn't eat more healthful foods, the most common answers were, "I don't like them," and, "I don't have time" (Matthews, 2004).

- The majority of people eat food—not just nutrients. When individuals are interested in improving their health status, they usually want to know which foods they should eat—not a specific level of nutrients. This is why calorie counting to specific levels often fails, and why many people would rather take a pill than try to select foods that are higher in specific nutrients.

- Humans eat for a number of reasons that have little to do with satisfying hunger. Personal preferences, habits, ethnic heritage or traditions, social pressures, positive associations, emotional needs, values, and beliefs are all factors that have little to do with hunger but a lot to do with what a person selects to eat. In almost all religions, food is a central focus during major holidays. Cultural background has a strong impact on what people decide to eat or not eat.

- Health care professionals sometimes forget that although it is their chosen work to spend all day thinking about health issues, these issues are usually not their clients' primary focus. Other people have careers and many issues to occupy their minds. Therefore most consumers need simple, concise directions that they can incorporate into their daily lives.

- Most adults prefer to have a role in the planning process to make changes in the way they eat. A person's personal and cultural preferences must be considered and valued. For a pregnant woman who either does not or cannot drink milk, a standardized diet sheet that recommends obtaining calcium from milk and mentions no other calcium sources will not meet with much success. A more successful approach would be to determine the foods she does eat, note which ones are good sources of calcium, and help her emphasize those foods in her diet. Some persons do not make the connection between milk and foods such as yogurt and cheese or between milk as a beverage and as a cooking ingredient in soups and puddings. In addition, dark-green, leafy vegetables, canned fish such as salmon and sardines, fortified soy products, and almonds are all reasonable sources of calcium. The health care professional must remember that people may be willing to try some new foods but they also want to see familiar ones.

- For successful long-term change the consumer must be satisfied that the proposed modifications can be incorporated into his or her existing lifestyle without major sacrifices. The first step in improving anyone's diet, no matter what his or her health status is, may be as simple as suggesting that an effort be made to eat at least five fruits and vegetables a day. If this is not a normal part of the person's current routine—and lots of studies indicate that it probably won't be—this small change will make a significant improvement in that person's diet. Eating more fruits and vegetables also may make some small differences in the way the person feels. If nothing else, a diet that includes more fruits and vegetables often improves regularity. McKinney, Ford, Riddell, and Lowe (2000) found that women who were helped to follow their normal diets with only minor changes and an emphasis on portion control that brought about decreases in calories were able to effect some weight loss. Because long-term positive changes are best accomplished in small increments that can be internalized, more changes can be added when a step such as this becomes a routine part of daily activity.

Health care professionals must be able to recognize severe nutrition problems and make a referral to an appropriate specialist. Dysfunctional eating is a relatively recent concept that incorporates abnormal and inappropriate eating behaviors. Berg (1996) calls it a disruption of normal eating, but it can also include restrained eating, disordered eating, and chronic dieting syndrome. It used to be most prevalent among middle- to upper-class white girls and women; however, dysfunctional eating can be seen across the spectrum today as cultural pressures to be thin continue (Berg, 1996). These individuals may need a specially trained team of professionals to help them.

Managing the Funding Problem

As federal and state governments tackle the issue of obesity, particularly in children, it is both interesting and frustrating to follow the proceedings. The U.S. Departments of Agriculture and Health and Human Services have begun to provide a wide variety of attractive educational materials, public service campaigns, and initiatives to improve American diets and increase physical activity (NHLBI, 2004; Institute of Medicine, 2004; USDHHS & USDA, 2005). State and local governments are grappling with issues of what children eat for school lunches, whether to mandate physical activity for schoolchildren, and whether to remove vending machines and other snacks from schools (American Dietetic Association, 2004).

In these days of limited health care dollars, however, health care professionals often find themselves frustrated by the lack of funding for nutrition education programs that meet the needs of individuals and groups. For children and adults, in-depth nutrition counseling is not readily covered by commercial insurers until the patient has an identifiable condition such as hypertension, hypercholesterolemia, or hyperglycemia. Coverage under most state-run Medicaid programs is even more stringent (American Dietetic Association, 1999, 2005). Thus health care professionals must be very creative in planning how to effectively provide nutrition education to most clients with finite resources.

Developing a Dietary Intervention Model

The following description of a pilot pediatric obesity program in a public health clinic demonstrates some of the issues involved.

During 2003 and 2004, the Philadelphia Department of Public Health (PDPH) launched a multifaceted program to assess and address the problem of child obesity among patients in the city health care centers, which serve over 25,000 low-income children each year. An audit of patients aged three to seven showed a prevalence of 19 percent overweight at very young ages (less than five years old). In response, in 2004, PDPH established a pediatric obesity task force to look for solutions, and eventually set up two on-site programs for overweight and at-risk children. 215 GO! is a one-on-one clinic, with the patient and the parent or caregiver working with a pediatric nutrition specialist, a health educator, and a pediatrician. Within the 215 GO! program there are three areas of activity: individual evaluation and management of eating and exercise behavior with assessment of self-image and parenting, an after-school exercise group, and a parent support group. The initial appointment includes a detailed evaluation and is followed by monthly visits. Information obtained at the first visit includes weight history, family medical history, usual food and drink intake, individual and family eating behaviors, and food purchasing and preparation habits. Usual level of physical activity is assessed by means of a detailed daily activity history. Parental attitudes and beliefs toward their weight, their child's weight, and eating are evaluated. Self-image, parenting style, and family function are assessed by the health educator. With the findings from the evaluation, an individual food and exercise plan is designed. The patient establishes nutrition and exercise goals, and the parent sets parenting goals. A curriculum of culturally appropriate lessons, teaching materials, and homework has been designed, with one lesson provided at each program visit. Topics include reading food labels, counting calories in beverages, increasing physical activity, identifying stressors and eating triggers, and self-acceptance. Parenting challenges are also addressed.

The goals of the weekly exercise program, Kids in Control (KIC IT), are to provide a venue for the children to move, to demonstrate fun activities that can be done in the home, and to teach healthy exercise techniques. A specific lesson is designed for each session. The parent support group takes place while KIC IT is in session and allows parents to discuss the challenges of helping the overweight child and includes the same lesson the children are learning in the exercise group. Of the hundreds of families that have been referred to the clinic, a few present with fairly simple issues—decreasing juice and soda intake and selecting low-fat milk instead of whole milk. However, other families bring complicated social issues to the clinic that make food selection almost secondary. The family that lives in a homeless shelter has limited control over food selection and opportunities for physical activities. Children who have lost a parent and now live with a grand-parent or other relative are often grieving and show signs of serious depression and may eat for comfort. Children who live in violent or dysfunctional households may also turn to food for relief. Part of the treatment model has to be to help them improve or cope with their situation and to improve their health.

The clinic is currently being evaluated, using several levels of assessment. Ob-viously, weight is measured, as are key physical and biochemical markers such as blood pressure, serum cholesterol, and blood glucose levels. Other laboratory val-ues are diagnosis driven. For example, a child who is already exhibiting abnormal glucose values will have a hemoglobin A1c test as well. In addition, the following lifestyle changes and other issues are tracked:

- Reported changes in food selection, such as decreased soft drink and juice in-take and increased water intake
- Reported changes in amount of physical activity, such as increased walking or supervised play
- Reported changes in numbers of trips to fast-food restaurants or corner stores
- Reported changes in how the children feel about themselves—do they feel more in control of their lives?
- Whether the children are willing to return for follow-up visits

Parents' and childrens' satisfaction and evaluation of program effectiveness are also assessed. Parents are also asked about any lifestyle changes and how they feel about their children's progress and their own. An integral component of the clinic's philosophy is harm reduction. In view of work by O'Dea (2004), an im-portant message of the clinic is that although the staff care about weight loss, they are more concerned about improving overall health. Focusing solely on weight loss means that many children will fail. If a boy does not lose significant amounts of weight, but his blood pressure improves, he has improved his health and well-being. If the teenage girl does not lose a significant amount of weight but has de-creased her juice and soda intake and the family now eats at least one meal together, there has been an improvement in her health and well-being.

In the first ten months of clinic operation, over 600 children were referred, with about 50 percent returning on an ongoing basis. There have been some in-dividual successes and some failures, but according to preliminary findings, the overall impact has been positive.

Building in Safeguards

Building in safeguards for the client is also an important strategy. The client needs to know that anyone can have a bad day and that this does not negate the process and does not make him or her a bad person or a failure. Further, encouraging self-efficacy in clients is important to their movement toward achieving their goals. Particularly with support from the health care professional, clients stop what they are doing, take a quick look, make some course corrections, and proceed toward their goal. In most cases the health care professionals' best advice is to say, "Let's see if you can do better tomorrow." Although everyone, especially the client, is anxious for success, directing blame toward the client is not productive. In fact it can make the client react negatively, as it appears that he or she can't do anything right. This is especially true for children and adolescents and pertains to the harm reduction issue discussed earlier.

The health care professional must instill in the client the idea that if things go wrong, the client should just start over. Failure to provide this kind of support will damage the client's ability to internalize the agreed-on goals. Further, the client must be reassured that effecting changes in eating habits is a relatively long process. When a sixty-year-old woman returns to a health care professional with no change in her serum cholesterol, she may be disappointed even though her blood pressure is within normal range and she has lost two pounds. She believes she has done everything she was supposed to and is beginning to get discouraged. The health care professional should praise the woman and tell her that she has obviously been making an effort to change the way she and her family eat. She should be reminded that cholesterol levels often do not respond as quickly as some other factors, and told that she is definitely moving in the right direction. It is important to affirm the new changes so that the client does not backslide and so that these lifestyle changes can become internalized. Care of this client should also focus on her movement through the stages of change.

Efficacy of Nutrition Interventions

It is obvious that effecting change in eating patterns is a difficult process, particularly when the change requires restricting a food or foods previously eaten as desired. The numerous approaches referenced in this chapter show the difficulties faced by clients and health care professional alike. Nowhere is this more apparent than in the area of weight loss and control. Numerous studies have demonstrated that long-term weight loss after any type of intervention is limited to a small minority of obese persons (Foster et al., 2003). However, studies have also shown that even a small amount of weight loss, 5 to 10 percent of body weight, can have positive effects on blood pressure, blood glucose levels, and cholesterol. Based on working with clients of all ages over a span of three decades, it is this author's opinion that the best focus for changing most persons' eating habits is to emphasize improved overall health. Demonstrating practical ways to eat a healthy diet that meets a person's lifestyle requirements and encouraging increased physical activity, however small the increase may be, are more frequently embraced by most clients than are other approaches.

In some cases it is more effective in the long run to downplay the emphasis on weight loss until the client is able to master the basics of dietary and life changes. A model such as the transtheoretical, or stages of change, may be a beneficial framework to enrich the health care professionals' understanding of change.

For evaluating outcomes, clearly measurable goals must be in place; otherwise both the client and the health care professional are setting themselves up for failure. As previously stated, it is usually better to have several small goals than one or two large ones. It is usually not productive to say, "Patient will lose 50 pounds over the next six months." However, it is reasonable to have written goals that say, "(1) Patient will increase intake of fruits and vegetables to at least 5 small servings daily; (2) patient will drink at least 4 cups of water daily; (3) patient will begin walking daily and, using a pedometer, will walk at least 5,000 steps daily by the end of three months; (4) patient will lose at least 1 to 2 pounds per month over the next six months." These are small steps that the patient can accomplish, and they can be measured. In addition, there may be laboratory values that can be measured to get a better view of health improvement.

Summary

Effecting change in human behavior of any kind is difficult. Helping someone to change lifelong habits is sometimes one of the most challenging tasks faced by health care professionals. Yet clients do willingly make changes if they perceive a need and if there is a practical, relatively simple way to do it. Health care professionals will be more successful in bringing about positive changes in behavior if they can adapt a health promotion model that meets the needs of their clients. The health care professional must alternatively function as a teacher, cheerleader, and partner in the process; however, the primary goal should be to give the client the tools he or she needs to succeed. (Exhibit 5.1 on page 188 lists some helpful resources.)

References

American Dietetic Association. (1999). *The three C's of MNT: Coverage, codes, and compensation.* Retrieved November 2005 from http://www.eatright.org/cps/rde/xchg/SID-5303 FFEA-OFAFF50B/ada/hs.xsl/nutrition_34

American Dietetic Association. (2004). Dietary guidance for healthy children aged 2 to 11 years. *Journal of the American Dietetics Association, 104,* 660–677.

American Dietetic Association. (2005). Position paper of the American Dietetic Association: Nutrition across the spectrum of aging. *Journal of the American Dietetic Association, 105,* 616–633.

Ball, S., Keller, K., Moyer-Mileur, L., Ding, Y., Donaldson, D., & Jackson, W. D. (2003). Prolongation of satiety after low versus moderately high glycemic index meals in obese adolescents. *Pediatrics, 111,* 488–494.

Baranowski, T., Perry, C., & Parcel, G. (2002). How individuals, environments, and health behavior interact: Social cognitive theory. In K. Glanz, B. K. Rimer, & F. M. Lewis (Eds.), *Health behavior and health education: Theory, research, and practice* (3rd ed., pp. 225–241). San Francisco: Jossey-Bass.

Barlow, S., Dietz, W., Klish, W., & Trowbridge, F. (2002). Treatment of overweight children and adolescents: A needs assessment of health practitioners. *Pediatrics, 110* (Suppl.), 205–238.

Berg, F. (1996). Afraid to eat. *Health at Any Size, 10*(2), 2–3.

Binns, H. J., & Ariza, A. J. (2004). Guidelines help clinicians identify risk factors for overweight in children. *Pediatric Annals, 33*(1), 19–22.

Brown, J. E. (2002). *Nutrition through the life cycle.* Belmont, CA: Wadsworth/Thomson Learning.

Callahan, M. (2004). Outrageous portions. *Networking News* (American Dietetic Association), *26,* 3.

Cartright, Y. (2004). Battling excess postpartum weight retention. *Journal of the American Dietetic Association, 104,* 1108–1109.

Centers for Disease Control and Prevention. (2000). Folate status in women of childbearing age—United States, 1999. *Morbidity and Mortality Weekly Report, 49*(42), 962–965.

Centers for Disease Control and Prevention. (2002). *Safer—healthier—people.* Retrieved January 15, 2005, from www.cdc.gov/nchs/data/hus/tables

Chernoff, R. (1999). *Geriatric nutrition: The health professional's handbook* (2nd ed.). Gaithersburg, MD: Aspen.

Edge, M. S. (2004). Promoting healthful diets from a public perspective. *Journal of the American Dietetic Association, 104,* 827–831.

Ferroli, C. (2005, Spring). The new food guidance system: An opportunity for RD's to step forward and make a difference. *The Digest* (American Dietetic Association), pp. 2–6.

Finkelstein, E. A., Fiebelkorn, I. C., & Wang, G. (2003, May 14). National medical spending attributable to overweight and obesity: How much and who's paying? *Health Affairs,* pp. 219–226.

Foster, G. D., Wadden, T. A., Makris, A., Davidson, D., Sanderson, R. S., Allison, D. B., et al. (2003). Primary care physicians' attitudes about obesity and its treatment. *Obesity Research, 11,* 1168–1177.

Hu, F. B., Stampfer, M. J., Manson, J. E., Ascherio, A., Colditz, G. A., Speizer, F. E., et al. (1999). Dietary saturated fats and their food sources in relation to the risk of coronary heart disease in women. *American Journal of Clinical Nutrition, 16,* 530–534.

Institute of Medicine. (2004). *Preventing childhood obesity: Health in the balance.* Washington, DC: National Academies Press.

International Food Information Counsel. (2003). *The road to enhancing the food supply: Consumer survey indicates USDA research on target.* Retrieved November 2005 from http://www.ific.org/foodinsight/1998/mj/enhancefi398.cfm

Janz, N., Champion, V., & Strecher, V. (2002). The health belief model. In K. Glanz, B. K. Rimer, & F. M. Lewis (Eds.), *Health behavior and health education: Theory, research, and practice* (3rd ed., pp. 45–65). San Francisco: Jossey-Bass.

Krummel, D., Semmens, E., Boury, J., Gordan, P., & Larkin, T. (2004). Stages of change for weight management in postpartum women. *Journal of the American Dietetic Association, 104,* 1102–1108.

Matthews, L. (2004). *Adolescent consumer survey: Title V needs assessment survey* (unpublished data). Philadelphia: Philadelphia Department of Public Health.

McGinnis, J. M., & Foege, W. H. (1993). Actual causes of death in the United States. *JAMA, 270,* 2207–2212.

McKenzie, J., & Smeltzer, J. L. (2001). *Planning, implementing and evaluating health promotion programs: A primer* (3rd ed.). Needham Heights, MA: Allyn & Bacon.

McKinney, S., Ford, E. G., Riddell, L. J., & Lowe, M. R. (2000). Assessment of nutrition education in leading cognitive behavioral therapy weight management programs. *Obesity Research, 8,* 88–91.

National Heart, Lung, and Blood Institute & North American Association for the Study of Obesity. (2000). *The practical guide: Identification, evaluation, and treatment of overweight and obesity in adults* (NIH Publication No. 00-4084). Washington, DC: National Institutes of Health.

National Heart, Lung, and Blood Institute. (2004). *Obesity education initiative.* Bethesda, MD: National Heart, Lung, and Blood Institute.

Nestle, M. (2003). *Food politics: How the food industry influences nutrition and health.* Los Angeles: University of California Press.

Nigg, C. R., Burbank, P. M., Padula, C., Dufresne, R., Rossi, J. S., Velicer, W. F., et al. (1999). Stages of change across ten health risk behaviors for older adults. *Gerontologist, 39,* 473–482.

O'Dea, J. (2004). Prevention of child obesity: "First do no harm." *Health Education Research Theory and Practice, 20*(2), 259–265.

Opoku-Boateng, A. (2004). *215 GO! A healthy lifestyle clinic for low-income adolescents and their families.* Unpublished thesis, Drexel University, Philadelphia.

Ornish, D. (1994). Dietary treatment of hyperlipidemia. *Journal of Cardiovascular Risk, 1,* 283–286.

Ornish, D. (2004). Was Dr. Atkins right? *Journal of the American Dietetic Association, 104,* 537–541.

Pennsylvania Advocates for Nutrition and Activity. (2003). Home page. Retrieved November 2005 from www.panaonline.org

Public Health Institute. (2004, Spring). Food advertising and marketing to children and youth. *The Digest* (American Dietetic Association), pp. 14–15.

Rosenstock, I. M. (1966). Why people use health services. *Milbank Quarterly, 44,* 99–124.

U.S. Department of Agriculture. (1992). *The Food Guide Pyramid* (Home and Garden Bulletin No. 249). Washington, DC: U.S. Government Printing Office.

U.S. Department of Agriculture. (2005). *MyPyramid: Steps to a healthier you.* Retrieved November 2005 from www.mypyramid.gov

U.S. Department of Agriculture & U.S. Department of Health and Human Services. (1995). *Nutrition and your health: Dietary guidelines for Americans* (4th ed.) (Home and Garden Bulletin No. 232). Washington, DC: U.S. Government Printing Office.

U.S. Department of Health and Human Services. (2001). *The surgeon general's call to action to prevent and decrease overweight and obesity.* Washington, DC: U.S. Government Printing Office.

U.S. Department of Health and Human Services. (2004). MCHB Women's Health Grant Programs.

U.S. Department of Health and Human Services & U.S. Department of Agriculture. (2005). *Dietary guidelines for Americans* (6th ed.) (Home and Garden Bulletin No. 232). Washington, DC: U.S. Government Printing Office.

Willet, W. C. (2003). *Eat, drink and be healthy: The Harvard Medical School guide to healthy eating.* Cambridge, MA: Harvard University Press.

EXHIBIT 5.1. HELPFUL RESOURCES.

Client Education Materials

The American Heart Association, 7272 Greenville Ave., Dallas, TX 75231-4596; Phone: (800) 242-8721; Web site: http://www.americanheart.org; offers many diet-related brochures and also downloadable materials. For example:

Controlando su peso [in Spanish]. Available from http://www.americanheart.org/presenter.jhtml?identifier=9267

Diet and nutrition. Available from http://www.americanheart.org/presenter.jhtml?identifier=1200010

An eating plan for healthy Americans: Our American Heart Association diet (Brochure No. 50-1481). Available from http://www.americanheart.org/presenter.jhtml?identifier=3007654

Eating plan: Fruits and vegetables. Available from http://www.americanheart.org/presenter.jhtml?identifier=108

A guide to losing weight (Brochure No. 50-1035, in English and Spanish).

How do I read food labels? Available from http://www.americanheart.org/presenter.jhtml?identifier=3007450

How to lose weight and keep it off. Available from http://www.americanheart.org/presenter.jhtml?identifier=506

Managing your weight: A guide to help you reach and maintain your ideal weight. Available from http://www.americanheart.org/presenter.jhtml?identifier=3007650

Reading food labels. Available from http://www.americanheart.org/presenter.jhtml?identifier=334

Taking it off (Brochure No. 50-079A).

Some useful National Institutes of Health materials are the following:

Eat more fruits and vegetables: 5 a day for better health (NIH Publication No. 92-3248). Washington, DC: U.S. Government Printing Office.

Diet, nutrition and cancer prevention (NIH Publication No. 87-2878). Washington, DC: U.S. Government Printing Office.

EXHIBIT 5.1. HELPFUL RESOURCES, Cont'd.

The National Diabetes Information Clearinghouse, 1 Information Way, Bethesda, MD 20892-3560; Phone: (301) 468-2162, (800) 860-8747; provides materials such as these:

Insulin-dependent diabetes (NIH Booklet No. 94-2098).

Non-insulin dependent diabetes (NIH Booklet No. 92-241).

Diabetes: Taking charge of your diabetes (Brochure No. 1530).

Diabetes and your body: How to take care of your eyes and feet (Brochure No. 1553).

Download the following client education materials through links on the Nutrition Information and Resource Center Web site: http://nirc.cas.psu.edu/online.cfm?area=440

Diabetes awareness and management. (2000). Kansas State University, Agricultural Experiment Station and Cooperative Extension. Provides information on risk factors for diabetes, symptoms, treatment, and resources.

Diet and diabetes. (2000). Colorado State University, Cooperative Extension. This four-page publication provides information on goals of diabetic management, type 1 and type 2 diabetes, major nutrient recommendations, methods for planning diets, and using nutritional labeling.

Keep your diabetes under control. (2000). National Institute for Diabetes & Digestive & Kidney Diseases, National Institutes of Health. This eighteen-page booklet provides information about blood sugar management and includes a chart to record blood sugars, meals, and medicines.

Keep your eyes healthy. (2000). National Institute of Diabetes & Digestive & Kidney Diseases, National Institutes of Health. This fourteen-page booklet provides information on how to prevent or delay eye damage caused by diabetes.

Keep your feet and skin healthy. (2000). National Institute of Diabetes & Digestive & Kidney Diseases, National Institutes of Health. This seventeen-page booklet provides information on feet and skin problems that can result from diabetes and how people with diabetes can prevent these problems from occurring.

Keep your nervous system healthy. (2000). National Institute of Diabetes & Digestive & Kidney Diseases, National Institutes of Health. Provided in this twenty-one-page booklet are detailed illustrations of the nervous system, and how uncontrolled diabetes can cause damage, including how to prevent and treat these problems.

Keep your teeth and gums healthy. (2000). National Institute of Diabetes & Digestive & Kidney Diseases, National Institutes of Health. Provided in this thirteen-page booklet is information on damage to the teeth and gums that can occur as the result of diabetes as well as how to prevent it.

Know your blood sugar numbers. (2000). National Diabetes Education Program, National Institutes of Health. This brochure explains how to measure blood sugar levels with a finger-stick test and hemoglobin A1c.

The power to control diabetes is in your hands. (2001). National Diabetes Education Program, National Institutes of Health. Provided in this twelve-page brochure is information on the importance of self-monitoring blood glucose levels.

EXHIBIT 5.1. HELPFUL RESOURCES, Cont'd.

What I need to know about eating and diabetes. (2003). National Institute of Diabetes &
Digestive & Kidney Diseases, National Institutes of Health. This forty-eight-page publication reviews nutrition and diabetes, including what, when, and how much a person with
diabetes should eat. Also provided is information on medications, exercise, and the food
guide pyramid.

Heart Health Action Windsor-Essex and the Windsor-Essex County Health Unit offer the following detailed weight loss brochure:

Working toward wellness: Live better, live longer. Available from http://www.wechealthunit.
org/Content/Resources/Healthy_Weights_Brochure_Winter2004_February2004.pdf

Additional Organizations

American Academy of Family Physicians
P.O. Box 11210
Shawnee Mission, KS 66207-1210
Phone: (913) 906-6000; (800) 274-2237
Web site: http://www.aafp.org/index.xml

American Dietetic Association
120 South Riverside Plaza, Suite 2000
Chicago, IL 60606-6995
Phone: (800) 877-1600
Web site: www.eatright.org

National Center for Nutrition and Dietetics of the American Dietetic Association
Phone: (800) 877-1600

Resources for Health Care Professionals

American Academy of Pediatrics. (2004). *Pediatric nutrition handbook* (5th ed.). Elk Grove,
IL: Author. Available from http://www.aap.org/bst/showdetl.cfm?&DID=15&Product_
ID=760

American Diabetes Association. (2005). *American Diabetes Association Complete guide to diabetes* (4th ed.). Available from http://store.diabetes.org/products/product_details.jsp?

*Bright Futures: Guidelines for health supervision of infants, children and adolescents; Bright
Futures pocket guide; Bright Futures anticipatory guidance cards.* Available from the National
Center for Education in Maternal and Child Health, 2000 15th Street North, Suite 701,
Arlington, VA 22201-2617; (703) 524-7802; http://www.brightfutures.org

Hamill, P.V.V., Drizd, T. A., Johnson, C .L., Reed, R. B., Roche, A. F., & Moore, W. M. (1979).
Physical growth: National Center for Health Statistics percentiles. *American Journal of Clinical Nutrition, 32,* 607–629. (Available as weight and length charts for boys and girls, ages
0–36 months, from Ross Products Division of Abbott Laboratories, Columbus, Ohio.)

EXHIBIT 5.1. HELPFUL RESOURCES, Cont'd.

Joint National Committee on Detection, Evaluation and Treatment of High Blood Pressure. (1993). The fifth report of the Joint National Committee on Detection, Evaluation and Treatment of High Blood Pressure (JNCV). *Archives of Internal Medicine, 153,* 154–183. Available from http://www.findarticles.com/p/articles/mi_m3225/is_n2_v47/ai_13432802

National Cholesterol Education Program. (1993). *Second report of the expert panel on detection, evaluation and treatment of high blood cholesterol of adults (Adult Treatment Panel II).* (NIH Publication No. 93-3095). Bethesda, MD: National Heart, Lung, and Blood Institute. See also http://www8.utsouthwestern.edu/utsw/cda/dept27717/files/97623.html

National Research Council, Food and Nutrition Board. (1989). *Recommended dietary allowances* (10th ed.). Washington, DC: National Academies Press. Available from http://www.nap.edu/catalog/1349.html; see also http://ods.od.nih.gov/index.aspx

Shils, M., Shike, M., Caballero, B., & Cousins, R. (2005). *Modern nutrition in health and disease* (10th ed.). Baltimore: Williams & Wilkins. Available from http://www.lww.com/product/?0-7817-4133-5

U.S. Department of Health and Human Services. (1994). *Clinician's handbook of preventive services* (See the height and weight tables for adults age 25 and over). Washington, DC: Author. Available from http://www.ahrq.gov/ppip/handbkup.htm For additional growth charts, contact Mead Johnson Nutritional Division (for the name and telephone number of an area representative) (812) 429-5000; or Ross Laboratories, Dept L-1120, Columbus, OH 43260; (800) 227-5767.

U.S. Department of Health and Human Services & U.S. Department of Agriculture. (2005). *Dietary guidelines for Americans.* Washington, DC: U.S. Government Printing Office. Available from http://www.healthierus.gov/dietaryguidelines

Web Sites

American Diabetes Association, http://www.diabetes.org

Arbor Nutrition Guide, www.arborcom.com

Ask the Dietitian, http://www.dietitian.com

diabetes.com, http://www.diabetes.com

National Council Against Health Fraud, http://www.ncahf.org

National Institute of Diabetes & Digestive & Kidney Diseases, http://www.niddk.nih.gov

Tufts University Nutrition Navigator, http://navigator.tufts.edu

CHAPTER SIX

PHYSICAL ACTIVITY

Karen J. Calfas
Athena S. Hagler

I t is well-known that regular physical activity works to maintain psychological and physical well-being and prevents chronic diseases and premature death (U.S. Department of Health and Human Services [USDHHS], 1996). Despite the numerous benefits of leading a physically active lifestyle, many Americans are sedentary.

Health care professionals can have a meaningful impact on their clients' level of physical activity and as a result improve clients' quality of life. Leading professional health care organizations specifically recommend physical activity counseling in the primary care setting (USDHHS, 1996, 2000).

This chapter will specifically address physical activity counseling in the primary care setting, broadly defined as any clinical setting where clients are being seen for preventive health care. The counseling may be delivered by nurses, nurse practitioners, physicians, or health educators, among others. The chapter is organized into six major sections. The first deals with the specific health benefits of physical activity. The second describes theoretical models used to understand physical activity behavior. The third section examines provider barriers to counseling and reviews studies of the different counseling approaches used in primary care

The authors wish to acknowledge the team of PACE researchers: Kevin Patrick, James F. Sallis, Gregory Norman, Marion Zabinski, Barbara J. Long, and Wilma J. Wooten.

and their efficacy. The fourth section discusses how to use Project PACE (Patient-Centered Assessment and Counseling for Exercise) protocols to counsel apparently healthy adults in an outpatient setting, and also offers examples of scripts. The fifth section provides an overview of physical activity counseling for children and older adults. The final section focuses on future directions for physical activity in health promotion.

Health Benefits and Epidemiology

This section considers the health benefits of physical activity, including the benefits for individuals with chronic disease and begins our examination of how much exercise people should get and how much they are currently getting.

Benefits for Those with Chronic Disease

Chronic diseases have had a profound impact on our nation. In fact, seven out of every ten deaths in the United States are attributable to chronic disease (USDHHS, 2004). Coronary heart disease (CHD) is the leading cause of death and disability in the United States (USDHHS, 2000). Physical inactivity is more prevalent than other risk factors for CHD, such as high blood pressure, high blood cholesterol, and cigarette smoking. Physically inactive Americans are almost twice as likely to develop CHD than are those who engage in regular physical activity. These findings are consistent with previous research indicating an inverse relationship between physical activity and CHD (Havranek, 1999; USDHHS, 1996).

Regular physical activity can also decrease an individual's risk of developing other chronic diseases, including obesity, certain types of cancer, and diabetes, and of experiencing such other health problems as a heart attack or hypertension (USDHHS, 2004). Regular physical activity can prevent and reduce obesity by increasing lean muscle mass and energy expenditure and decreasing body fat (Blair & Holder, 2002). Physical activity is a critical factor in weight loss maintenance (Brownell, 1995; Klem, Wing, McGuire, Seagle, & Hill, 1997; USDHHS, 2004). The American College of Sports Medicine (ACSM) has reported that regular physical activity, including appropriate endurance and resistance training, is therapeutic for type 2 diabetes because it lowers glucose levels and improves insulin sensitivity (ACSM, 2000). Studies of intensive behavioral interventions, including physical activity and diet modifications, have demonstrated dramatic improvements in health-related outcomes among persons at risk for type 2 diabetes and significantly reduced the incidence of diabetes (Knowler et al., 2002; Tuomilehto et al., 2001). Physical activities that promote endurance can not only prevent the development of hypertension but can also lower blood pressure in hypertensive and nonhypertensive adults (ACSM, 2004; Chodzko-Zajko, 1998).

Other Benefits of Physical Activity

Many other benefits are associated with an active lifestyle (USDHHS, 2000). First, physical activity increases muscle and bone strength. Weight-bearing exercises facilitate normal skeletal development in children and adolescents and help young adults reach and maintain their peak bone mass. Second, physical activity has various mental health benefits, such as reduced anxiety and stress levels and improved mood (Task Force on Community Preventive Services, 2002; USDHHS, 1996, 2000). Additionally, physical activity may protect against the development of depression in the future (Paffenbarger, Lee, & Leung, 1994; Van Gool et al., 2003). In depressed populations two meta-analyses reported mean effect sizes ranging from –.72 (Craft & Landers, 1998) to –1.1 (Lawlor & Hopker, 2001) for reducing symptoms of depression, relative to no-treatment control groups.

How Much Physical Activity Is Enough?

Regular, moderate-intensity physical activity, done at once or broken up into two or three shorter bouts of activity during the course of the day, is associated with lower death rates and other general health benefits (Altena, Michaelson, Ball, & Thomas, 2004; USDHHS, 1996, 2000). Therefore, a new guideline for moderate-intensity physical activity was developed in 1995. This guideline states that "every US adult should accumulate 30 minutes or more of moderate-intensity physical activity on most, preferably all, days of the week" (Pate et al., 1995). Moderate-intensity physical activities include walking, gardening, vacuuming, or social dancing. Additional health benefits are gained by those who also perform vigorous-intensity physical activity three or more times per week for at least twenty minutes each time (USDHHS, 2000). Vigorous physical activities, such as swimming and jogging, require more energy exertion than moderate activities and therefore noticeably increase the heart rate. In addition to cardiovascular-based recommendations for physical activity, the USDHHS also recommends adults engage in physical activities that enhance and maintain muscular strength, endurance, and flexibility (USDHHS, 2000).

Experts agree that expending 700 to 2,000 extra calories per week (approximately 100 to 285 calories per day) via physical activity can provide many health benefits including increased longevity ("Exercise Your Right to Health," 2004). Examples of activities that burn calories within this range include walking two miles in thirty minutes to burn 150 calories, heavy cleaning for forty-five minutes to burn 250 calories, and an hour of singles tennis to burn 300 calories. These activities may be completed in two to three shorter bouts, but must accumulate to at least thirty minutes per day (on at least five days a week) to meet the minimum guidelines for improved health (USDHHS, 2000).

From a behavioral point of view, research identifying the benefits of moderate-intensity physical activity is good news. Moderate-intensity physical activity may be more acceptable and achievable than vigorous activity for Americans who are currently inactive. For example, walking or gardening is often very acceptable to those not interested in "exercise."

How Active Are Americans?

Despite the known benefits of physical activity, only 15 percent of adults engage in the recommended amount (USDHHS, 2000). In fact, 40 percent of adults engaged in no physical activity during their leisure time in 1997. There are disparities in the amount of physical activity done by various persons. For example, physical activity decreases with age. Women and those with lower incomes and less education are less active than men and those with higher incomes and education (Dowda, Ainsworth, Addy, Saunders, & Riner, 2003; Van Mechelen, Twisk, Post, Snel, & Kemper, 2000; USDHHS, 2000). In addition, African Americans and Hispanics are generally less physically active than are whites, and adults in the northeastern and southern states are typically less active than adults in the north-central and western states (USDHHS, 2000). According to estimates published in 2000, approximately 23 percent of adults engage in vigorous activity on a regular basis (twenty minutes, three times a week), and 15 percent of U.S. adults met the moderate physical activity guideline (thirty minutes of moderate activity most days of the week). In addition, merely 18 percent did physical activities that promoted flexibility, and only 30 percent did activities that promoted strength and endurance (USDHHS, 2000).

Healthy People 2010

Healthy People 2010 objectives aim to increase the proportion of Americans who engage in moderate-intensity physical activity, from 15 percent in 1997 to 30 percent (USDHHS, 2000). Healthy People 2010 also contains two separate goals (objectives 3–10h and 1–3a) focused on increasing the proportion of primary care providers who conduct physical activity counseling. Approximately 22 percent of physicians counseled their at-risk patients about physical activity in 1995; a decrease of 8 percent from 1988 (USDHHS, 2000). A survey of physicians' physical activity counseling practices in North Dakota found that only 9 percent "always" or "most times" provided their patients with written materials on physical activity, and 91 percent reported that they "sometimes" or "never" provided these materials (North Dakota Department of Health, 2000). These estimates say nothing of the quality of the counseling or written materials.

Physicians' beliefs about health habits influence their counseling practices. For example, physicians who currently practice a healthy lifestyle themselves or are in the process of improving their own lifestyles are more likely to counsel clients about health habits (Abramson, Stein, Schaufele, Frates, & Rogan, 2000; Frank & Kunovich-Frieze, 1995; Toyry et al., 2000). Physicians can optimize their counseling efforts by incorporating methods already known to promote health behavior change (Elder, Ayala, & Harris, 1999), though there are few theoretical models for understanding physician counseling practices (Honda & Sheinfeld Gorin, 2006). Efficacious methods of counseling are derived from various theoretical models.

Theoretical Models for Understanding Physical Activity

There are many theories about how people change health behaviors. Increasing people's knowledge about the risks or benefits of a health behavior is generally considered to be necessary but insufficient to change behavior. This section will focus on three theoretical models of health behavior change, which address factors known to influence health behaviors, and apply them to physical activity counseling.

Determinants of Physical Activity

Sedentary clients present a long list of barriers to participation in physical activity, including lack of time, poor motivation, lack of support from family and friends, bad weather, and displeasure with physical activity. In fact, competing demands are among the most common reasons people are not physically active (USDHHS, 1996; Calfas, Sallis, Lovato, & Campbell, 1994). Additionally, few things in our modern society promote physical activity. Electric garage door openers, escalators, televisions (including their remote controls), all such things encourage inactivity; therefore the environment can also be a barrier to an active lifestyle. Because so many factors influence participation in physical activity, it is a difficult behavior to change. Successful attempts to change activity patterns require modification of personal, social, and environmental factors. To maximize its effect, an intervention must have a theoretical foundation, target known mediators of the behavior, and apply the most effective intervention approaches.

Behavioral theories have been applied to the study of physical activity determinants (or correlates). Modifiable correlates of physical activity have been reviewed (USDHHS, 1996; Sallis, Prochaska, Taylor, Hill, & Geraci, 1999; Marcus, Nigg, Riebe, & Forsyth, 2000). These theories, or models, have been used to generate hypotheses about how best to help someone adopt (or maintain) physical activity. Two theories will be discussed here: social cognitive theory and the transtheoretical model.

Social Cognitive Theory

Social cognitive theory states that personal factors and the environment interact to determine behavior and that all three can influence each other (Bandura, 1986). This theory takes into account the complexity of behaviors like participation in physical activity. A key component of social cognitive theory is self-efficacy. *Self-efficacy* is the belief in one's ability to competently perform a behavior. To determine a client's self-efficacy the health care professional could ask, "How confident do you feel about meeting this exercise goal over the next two weeks?" If the client is highly confident, then he or she is experiencing high self-efficacy, and research suggests that those who experience high self-efficacy are more likely to be physically active (Rovniak, Anderson, Winett, & Stephens, 2002; Sallis et al., 1989).

Other determinants of physical activity include social support, perceived barriers and benefits, and enjoyment. Research indicates that social support (for example, exercising with a friend, praising a friend for being active, or doing a chore for a family member so he or she has time to be active) is consistently associated with increased physical activity (Dowda et al., 2003; Giles-Corti & Donovan, 2002; Sallis et al., 1999). Perceiving benefits from physical activity (for example, endorsing statements such as, "I know if I exercise this morning, I'll feel good all day") has been consistently and positively associated with participation in physical activity (Ali & Twibell, 1995; Marcus et al., 2000). Similarly, perceiving barriers to activity is negatively associated with physical activity (Dishman & Steinhardt, 1990). Finally, enjoyment is consistently positively associated with physical activity (Courneya & McAuley, 1994). These predictors of physical activity are modifiable and should be targeted during an intervention aimed at improving adherence to an activity program (Baranowski, Lin, Wetter, Resnicow, & Hearn, 1997).

Transtheoretical Model

In the transtheoretical model, developed by Prochaska and DiClemente (1982), behavioral change is conceptualized as progressing through five *stages of change*. With respect to physical activity the five stages are described as follows: (1) *precontemplation,* when one is not engaging in physical activity and is not interested in doing so in the near future; (2) *contemplation,* when one is not engaging in activity (or is irregularly active) but is interested in becoming more active; (3) *preparation,* when one is making small changes in physical activity or is ready to begin activity soon; (4) *action,* when one is beginning a new activity program; and (5) *maintenance,* when one has been regularly active for more than six months (Marcus, Rakowski, & Rossi, 1992; Prochaska & Marcus, 1994). Persons may progress through these stages out of order and may revert back to earlier stages from later stages. An important implication of the stages of change model is that clients need different intervention messages, depending on their current stage of change, or *readiness to change.* By assessing a client's stage of change, the health care professional will be able to identify the client's current behavioral patterns, supports and barriers to change, interest in changing these patterns, and likelihood of actually changing these patterns.

Some methods of supporting behavioral change are more effective than others. Many health education approaches focus on giving information to clients. This is certainly necessary and appropriate, but it is usually insufficient to change behavior, and changing behavior is required to obtain the desired outcome. Interventions that target improved behavioral skills are more likely to lead to behavioral change. For example, helping a client increase his or her social support (by identifying a friend or family member who will encourage the client, for example) and increase his or her self-efficacy (by setting realistic and measurable goals, for example) will do more to increase physical activity than just telling someone to be more active. In fact, a review of the literature compared didactic, knowledge-based interventions to behavioral, skill-based interventions and showed that the latter were more than twice as likely to lead to behavioral change (Mazzuca, 1982). More specifically, research shows a positive prospective relationship between social support, self-efficacy, and physical activity (Rovniak et al., 2002; Giovannucci et al., 1998; Sallis et al., 1999).

The PACE program (described in detail later in this chapter) uses the stages of change model to identify where clients are on the continuum of readiness to change and specifically targets known determinants of physical activity for each stage, using concepts from social cognitive theory.

Health Care Professional Physical Activity Counseling

Patients report that they value their physician's advice and want to receive counseling about physical activity (Godin & Shephard, 1990). Recent data indicate that only 22 to 28 percent of patients receive provider administered physical activity *counseling* (Glasgow, Eakin, Fisher, Bacak, & Brownson, 2001; Podl, Goodwin, Kikano, & Stange, 1999), although approximately 54 percent of patients were at least *questioned* about exercise (Nawaz, Adams, & Katz, 2000). On average, about .78 of a minute was spent in physical activity counseling (Podl et al., 1999). In addition, provider administered exercise counseling appears to occur more frequently with patients who are older and have a chronic illness (Glasgow et al., 2001; Podl et al., 1999).

Provider Barriers to Counseling

Several barriers exist that discourage or limit physical activity counseling by health care professionals. Time constraints and lack of reimbursement for services rendered are among the most frequently cited barriers (Estabrooks, Glasgow, & Dzewaltowski, 2003; Wee, 2001). Certainly, as constraints from managed care and other measures of efficiency are introduced into more medical settings, spending even five minutes on this topic during a fifteen-minute patient encounter may be unrealistic, especially if it is nonreimbursable time. Health care professionals are often unaware of what physical activity to recommend (that is, what frequency and intensity level). Health care professionals may also perceive that their advice will not be followed. An example from the obesity literature indicates that although half of providers felt they were competent in prescribing weight loss (a large component of which is administering a physical activity prescription [USDHHS, 2004], only 14 percent believed that they were typically successful in helping their obese patients lose weight (Foster et al., 2003). Other data indicate that providers may be unsure how to appropriately tailor their counseling to an individual's readiness for change, gender, socioeconomic status, race or ethnicity, or level of education (ACSM, 2004).

Efficacy of Current Physical Activity Counseling Approaches

The average American makes approximately 2.7 doctor visits annually (USDHHS, 1999), so the opportunity for physical activity counseling clearly exists. But does the counseling work? Results from reviews of the literature indicate mixed results. Although some reports conclude that physician-administered physical activity counseling generally results in moderate increases in physical activity levels (Eakin, Glasgow, & Riley, 2000; Pinto, Goldstein, & Marcus, 1998; Simons-Morton, Calfas, Oldenburg, & Burton, 1998), others find that the accumulated evidence is insufficient to conclude whether or not this type of counseling is generally effective (Eden, Orleans, Mulrow, Pender, & Teutsch, 2002).

The Activity Counseling Trial (ACT) was a five-year, randomized clinical trial aimed at promoting exercise via physician counseling (Writing Group for the

Activity Counseling Trial, 2001). A total of 874 sedentary men and women (aged thirty-five to seventy-five years) were randomized to (1) standard care (that is, given physician advice to exercise for at least thirty minutes daily and given written materials), (2) assistance (physician advice plus interactive mail and behavioral counseling), or (3) counseling (physician advice, interactive mail, and behavioral counseling, plus telephone counseling and behavioral classes). Providers were trained to deliver three to four minutes of physical activity advice. After two years, the women in both the assistance and counseling group improved their cardiorespiratory fitness significantly more (5 percent) than women in the advice only group did ($p = .02$ and $.046$, respectively). There were no significant group differences in cardiorespiratory fitness among men. Also, the addition of the physical activity counseling did not disrupt the routine primary care visits. In fact, 83 percent of the providers spent less than five to six minutes counseling, and 46 percent spent three to four minutes. Sixty-three percent of the providers reported that the advice added little or no length to the visit. Although the advice-only group did not yield significant results among women or men, the positive results seen with both the assistance and counseling groups among women provides promising preliminary evidence for physical activity counseling in the primary care setting.

Another approach to physical activity counseling in primary care was developed and implemented by Project PACE (Patient-Centered Assessment and Counseling for Exercise). Various studies have been conducted to date on this intervention. The first found the PACE intervention to be acceptable and usable by providers, office staff, and patients in four parts of the United States (Long et al., 1996). Specifically, the PACE materials were rated highly acceptable, usable, and readily understandable to providers and patients. Seventy-five percent of providers reported that they would recommend PACE to other primary care providers, 80 percent said that their patients were "receptive" or "very receptive" to counseling, and most stated that the counseling was easy to do and improved their ability to do physical activity counseling. Patient assessment of the PACE process was uniformly positive, with 80 percent of patients reporting that the forms were "easy" or "very easy" to understand, and 72 percent reporting that the counseling was helpful. However, only 35 percent of providers reported that office staff were able to adopt PACE with minimal difficulty. Similarly, over one-third of office staff reported difficulty with paperwork or procedures related to PACE (Long et al., 1996). The PACE materials were acceptable and usable, but the process is heavily dependent on the office staff, and subsequent studies of PACE have included more specific procedures and training for office staff.

The second PACE study was designed to determine its efficacy, or effect, on the client's physical activity level when the intervention was delivered as written

(Calfas et al., 1996). In this quasi-experimental study, 212 sedentary, apparently healthy clients received either the PACE counseling or standard care (no physical activity counseling) during a scheduled *well visit*. Clients were assessed before and four to six weeks after their scheduled appointment with a PACE-trained provider. Compared to control patients, those who received PACE counseling increased their use of cognitive and behavioral strategies to increase physical activity; behavioral methods and improved self-efficacy were associated with an increase in physical activity (Calfas, Sallis, Oldenburg, & Ffrench, 1997). Also, patients who received the PACE intervention reported more minutes of walking for exercise compared to those who did not receive the counseling (75.4 versus 42.2 minutes per week; $p < .05$). Although all patients were in the contemplation stage of change at baseline, more participants in the intervention group moved into the action stage of change compared to controls (52 percent versus 12 percent; $p < .001$).

The PACE paper-based materials were later modified to be completed by using a computer kiosk in the physician's waiting room. They were further modified to include nutrition goals (reduced dietary fat and increased fruit and vegetable intake). Clients completed the assessment and goal setting on the computer, and a tailored counseling protocol was printed for use by the physician during a previously scheduled visit. Two additional pilot studies evaluated this newer version of the PACE intervention among adolescents (Patrick et al., 2001) and adults (Calfas et al., 2002). In both studies, participants completed a computerized assessment (Prochaska, Zabinski, Calfas, Sallis, & Patrick, 2000), chose one physical activity and one nutrition goal to *target* (that is, work on), and then discussed the plan with their physician (Calfas et al., 2002; Patrick, Sallis, et al., 2001). Subsequently, patients were randomly assigned to one of four groups: (1) no further contact (control), (2) mail only, (3) infrequent telephone and mail, or (4) frequent telephone and mail. Behavioral targets included moderate- and vigorous-intensity physical activity and dietary fat and fruit and vegetable intake. Both studies found that participants who targeted a particular behavior to change were more successful than those who did not target a specific behavior. Although participants' behaviors in all conditions improved, those in the extended intervention did not have better outcomes than those who received the computer and provider counseling components only. Overall, both studies supported the feasibility of the PACE interactive computer program and physician counseling components of PACE.

Although many professional medical organizations recommend some type of physical activity counseling in the primary care setting (American Academy of Pediatrics, 2001; American College of Obstetrics and Gynecology, 2000; ACSM, 1998; American Heart Association, 2003), the U.S. Preventive Services Task Force (USPSTF), in a review of the evidence, concluded that the existing evidence is insufficient to recommend for or against physical activity counseling in primary care settings (Eden et al., 2002; USPSTF, 2002). This does not mean that counseling is unimportant and should not be conducted. Rather, it indicates that more effective methods are necessary. Generally, studies with shorter-term follow-up assessments and studies that used behavioral theories to inform the intervention had better physical activity outcomes than did those without these components (Simons-Morton et al., 1998).

In summary, the data regarding the efficacy of physical activity counseling in primary care settings are inconsistent. The promising results of many studies and the importance of physical activity for ameliorating the recent increase in obesity make further research in this field a priority.

The next section describes the PACE paper-based counseling approach in detail.

PACE Counseling Approach

PACE counseling was developed in the early 1990s in response to the health objective for the year 2000 that calls for a greater proportion of physicians to counsel their patients about physical activity. Those goals have been carried over into the year 2010 health objectives (USDHHS, 2000). The focus of PACE is to alter known determinants of physical activity, using a simplified version of the stages of change approach to categorize patients into one of three stages of readiness for change (precontemplators, contemplators, and actives). A specific counseling approach has been developed for clients in each of the three stages, and each approach corresponds to one of the three counseling protocols. A *one-page assessment tool* is used to identify the client's stage of change. The back of the assessment page contains the Physical Activity Readiness Questionnaire (PAR-Q) (Chisholm, Collis, Kulak, Davenport, & Gruber, 1975), which screens for contraindications to exercise and is meant to be a risk assessment for the health care professional to use in addition to the medical record.

PACE was developed for primary care providers to use with their apparently healthy, adult patients in the outpatient setting. Although the original purpose of the PACE project was to develop tools for physicians to use, it is appropriate for nurses, health educators, and other members of the primary care team to conduct this counseling. The PACE approach has been adapted for use in many other medical settings, including diabetes management and physical therapy settings. The goal of PACE is to promote modest increases in physical activity; therefore health care professionals often recommend that clients begin a program of moderate physical activity. For clients already doing moderate or vigorous physical activity, recommendations that include vigorous activity may be made, as appropriate.

The PACE Process

Clients are given the one-page PACE assessment tool (a measure of interest and their current level of physical activity) (see Figure 6.1) when they arrive for their nonacute visit. The front of the page contains stage-relevant questions about physical activity, which the client is asked to complete and return to the receptionist. The receptionist then notes the client's stage of change and gives the client the appropriate one-page counseling protocol. The back of the protocol contains stage-relevant information for the client's use at home.

After the client completes the first half of the protocol in the waiting room and returns it to the receptionist, it is placed in the chart for the health care professional to review before entering the examination room. The counseling takes two to five minutes, depending on the protocol. During the counseling, the health care professional discusses stage-tailored content with the client, and they come to an agreement about a physical activity goal, if one is to be set.

General Principles for PACE Counseling

PACE was developed to address the many barriers that affect physician counseling for behavioral change. There was little researchers could do about the reimbursement issue. However, researchers could develop standardized counseling protocols and good training and could minimize the time required to conduct the counseling.

The first general principle for PACE counseling is *time efficiency*. The challenge with any type of health behavior counseling in primary care is that it needs to be brief enough for health care professionals to actually do it, yet it also needs to have enough substance to change patient behavior. Imbalance in either direction will produce little or no change in physical activity. Primary care providers want to do the best thing for their clients, and if they believe that it is important for a specific client to increase his or her physical activity and that spending a few minutes will result in increased activity, they are usually willing to try it. The PACE protocols are based on theories of behavioral change known to affect physical activity, and they can be delivered in two to five minutes.

Another general principle is that counseling must be a *team effort*. If office staff are not fully aware of and willing to distribute and collect the assessment and counseling forms, the process will not work. Likewise, different health care professionals in the same office may deliver different parts of the message. Generally, there are two parts of the PACE message—the advice, or recommendation, to be active and the counseling about how to be or stay active. In some settings the physician may give the recommendation, and a nurse or health educator may do

FIGURE 6.1. PACE ASSESSMENT TOOL.

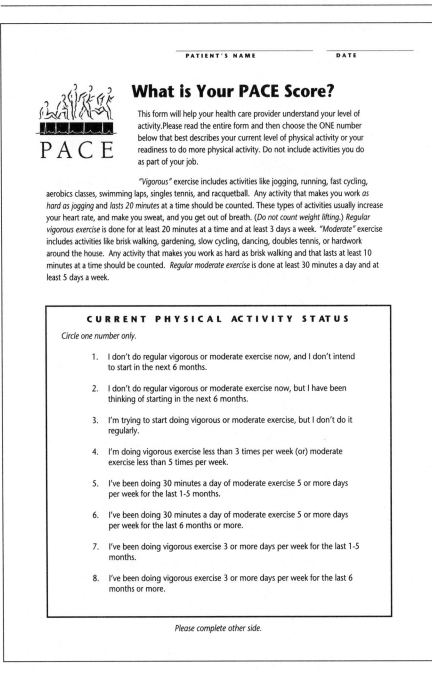

PATIENT'S NAME   **DATE**

What is Your PACE Score?

This form will help your health care provider understand your level of activity. Please read the entire form and then choose the ONE number below that best describes your current level of physical activity or your readiness to do more physical activity. Do not include activities you do as part of your job.

"Vigorous" exercise includes activities like jogging, running, fast cycling, aerobics classes, swimming laps, singles tennis, and racquetball. Any activity that makes you work *as hard as jogging* and *lasts 20 minutes* at a time should be counted. These types of activities usually increase your heart rate, and make you sweat, and you get out of breath. (*Do not count weight lifting.*) *Regular vigorous exercise* is done for at least 20 minutes at a time and at least 3 days a week. *"Moderate"* exercise includes activities like brisk walking, gardening, slow cycling, dancing, doubles tennis, or hardwork around the house. Any activity that makes you work as hard as brisk walking and that lasts at least 10 minutes at a time should be counted. *Regular moderate exercise* is done at least 30 minutes a day and at least 5 days a week.

CURRENT PHYSICAL ACTIVITY STATUS

Circle one number only.

1. I don't do regular vigorous or moderate exercise now, and I don't intend to start in the next 6 months.

2. I don't do regular vigorous or moderate exercise now, but I have been thinking of starting in the next 6 months.

3. I'm trying to start doing vigorous or moderate exercise, but I don't do it regularly.

4. I'm doing vigorous exercise less than 3 times per week (or) moderate exercise less than 5 times per week.

5. I've been doing 30 minutes a day of moderate exercise 5 or more days per week for the last 1-5 months.

6. I've been doing 30 minutes a day of moderate exercise 5 or more days per week for the last 6 months or more.

7. I've been doing vigorous exercise 3 or more days per week for the last 1-5 months.

8. I've been doing vigorous exercise 3 or more days per week for the last 6 months or more.

Please complete other side.

FIGURE 6.1. PACE ASSESSMENT TOOL, Cont'd.

PHYSICAL ACTIVITY READINESS QUESTIONNAIRE (PAR-Q)*

A SELF-ADMINISTERED QUESTIONNAIRE FOR ADULTS

PAR-Q is designed to help you help yourself. Many health benefits are associated with regular exercise, and the completion of PAR-Q is a sensible first step to take if you are planning to increase the amount of physical activity in your life.

For most people, physical activity should not pose any problem or hazard. PAR-Q has been designed to identify the small number of adults for whom physical activity might be inappropriate or those who should have medical advice concerning the type of activity most suitable for them.

Common sense is your best guide in answering these questions. Please read them carefully and check YES or NO opposite the question as it applies to you.

YES   NO

○   ○   1.   Has your doctor ever said that you have a heart condition and that you should only do physical activity recommended by a doctor?

○   ○   2.   Do you feel pain in your chest when you do physical activity?

○   ○   3.   In the past month, have you had chest pain when you were not doing physical activity?

○   ○   4.   Do you lose your balance because of dizziness or do you ever lose consciousness?

○   ○   5.   Do you have a bone or joint problem that could be made worse by a change in your physical activity?

○   ○   6.   Is your doctor currently prescribing drugs (for example, water pills) for your blood pressure or heart condition?

○   ○   7.   Do you know of any other reason why you should not do physical activity?

Note: If you have a temporary illness, such as a common cold, or are not feeling well at this time—Postpone.

*Adapted from the 1994 revised version of the Physical Activity Readiness Questionnaire PAR-Q and YOU. The PAR-Q and YOU is a copyrighted pre-exercise screen owned by the Canadian Society for Exercise Physiology.

Copyright © 1999 by San Diego State University Foundation and San Diego Center for Health Interventions, LLC.

The San Diego Center for Health Interventions and San Diego State University Foundation give permission to the Mass. Dept. of Public Health, Women's Health Network to duplicate these materials for **provider use only**, effective January 1, 2002 thru December 31, 2004. This contract expires January 1, 2005.

the rest of the counseling. In other settings the nurse or physician delivers all the counseling, and that is how the process will be described here. The point is that this counseling is delivered in the *primary care setting* and that the health care professional should use whatever resources are available to deliver the counseling in whatever manner makes the most sense for that setting. The PACE materials were designed to accommodate different settings and have been used by a variety of providers, including physicians, nurse practitioners, nurses, health educators, and physical therapists.

A third principle is to *get the right message to the right person.* In almost every encounter, time is at a premium. Health care professionals do not have time to waste giving detailed advice to patients who are not interested, but that is what many do. They do not take into account how *ready* the client is to deal with a particular clinical issue. Similarly, they should not spend time extolling the benefits of physical activity to someone who is already active (that is, they should not "preach to the choir"). The PACE approach allows the health care professional to target his or her message to meet a client's unique needs.

The PACE materials use a modified version of the stages of change theory to place each client into one of three groups: (1) *precontemplators,* those not presently active and not interested in becoming active; (2) *contemplators,* those not presently active or irregularly active but interested in beginning an activity program; and (3) *actives,* those already active. As previously stated, a different message has been specifically designed to be relevant to clients in each stage. The stages were collapsed from five to three because the intervention messages were not significantly different for those in preparation and those in contemplation or for those in action and those in maintenance, and three protocols (messages) were more practical than five for use in a medical setting. See Table 6.1 for a summary of PACE counseling by stage.

The value of identifying each client's group is that the health care professional can then spend the most time with the middle group, the contemplators. They are the most ready for change and the most likely to actually adopt an activity program based on their health care professional's recommendation. Also, patients moving from mostly sedentary to moderately active lifestyles are the ones who will derive the most benefit from behavioral change (Blair et al., 1995). Using this tailoring approach allows health care professionals to be more efficient with their time because they do not waste time outlining an exercise program for a precontemplator nor do they waste time by espousing the benefits of activity to someone in the active stage.

The final general principle is to *involve the client.* Clients are more likely to meet goals when they are able to participate in setting those goals. PACE counseling uses an interactive approach in which the health care professional and client agree on the physical activity goals, using recommendations from the health care

TABLE 6.1. SUMMARY OF PACE COUNSELING BY STAGE.

	Precontemplator	Contemplator	Active
Title of PACE protocol	"Getting Out of Your Chair"	"Planning the First Step"	"Keeping the PACE"
PACE Assessment Score	Score = 1	Score = 2–4	Score = 5–8
Goal for the patient	Think about the benefits of physical activity.	Set goal for a moderate physical activity program and identify roadblocks.	Maintain physical activity and avoid relapse.
Primary behavioral strategies to employ	Listening, identify benefits, problem solving.	Goal setting, self-efficacy, social support, praise.	Relapse prevention, goal setting, self-efficacy, praise.
Message and recommendation	Identify potential benefits of physical activity. Give a personalized message about considering beginning a program of moderate physical activity.	Praise patient for intending to begin a program. Recommend moderate physical activity program based on patient's interests. Together, agree on a realistic goal; identify who will help the client be active, reinforce benefits, and problem solve around anticipated barriers.	Recommend continued physical activity at the current level (or other suggestion you would give the client). Review current physical activity program and recommend changes if appropriate (encourage variety, enjoyment, and convenience). Identify potential sources of relapse, and problem solve around them. Advise about sport-related overuse injury prevention.
Action	No specific goal is set.	Provider records physical activity goal for a specified period of time at bottom of protocol; both sign.	Provider records physical activity goal (set for longer period of time).
Materials	Protocol only.	Protocol plus walking handout (or other).	Protocol and other handouts as appropriate.
Time	1–2 minutes.	5 minutes (or more if available).	2–4 minutes.

professional and information from the client about what would be most enjoyable and doable given the client's lifestyle. Involving the client in the decision-making process makes the client more accountable for the result and encourages him or her to take responsibility for his or her own health.

Scripts

This section presents specific recommendations for each of the three PACE protocols (summarized in Table 6.1).

Precontemplators. The protocol for precontemplators (PACE score = 1) is called "Getting Out of Your Chair," and applies to approximately 10 percent of clients. The goal for the precontemplator is not to set a physical activity goal but to *think* about the benefits of physical activity. These clients will appreciate not being pressured to begin an exercise program. They are asked to identify two potential benefits of being physically active, the reasons they are not currently active, and two ways to get around their roadblocks. If they can't think of how to get around roadblocks, examples are listed on the back of the protocol.

Primary care providers are encouraged to give precontemplator clients *personalized* advice to *think about beginning* a moderate-intensity program of physical activity. Health care professionals should use their clout and knowledge of the client's health status to give specific advice. For example, after reviewing a client's protocol a health care professional might say: "Mrs. Smith, I understand that you are not interested in starting a walking program now. However, since you are overweight and are on medication for high blood pressure, walking regularly (even just fifteen minutes per day to start) will help both of these conditions. You listed lack of time and interest as barriers to beginning a program. I'd like you to look over the potential ways to get around these barriers, on the back of this sheet, and think about starting a walking program. It is important for your health. If you decide you'd like to begin, come back and see me and I'll help you get started." This discussion will take only one to two minutes, and if the patient just thinks about it before his or her next visit, the primary care provider will have succeeded. The health care professional saves time with this group by not developing an exercise plan the client doesn't want to follow. Further, clients generally appreciate being *heard;* if the health care professional does not give advice about physical activity that the client is not interested in starting, the client may be more likely to listen to other advice that *is* given.

Contemplators. The protocol for contemplators is called "Planning the First Step" (PACE score = 2 to 4). Approximately 50 percent of the population is in this stage of change. Clients are asked to identify two benefits of physical activity and what type of program they would like to begin. They are asked to be fairly specific, identifying activities they enjoy, where they will be active, a realistic frequency of activity, the duration of activity, and who in their life can provide social support for their program. The health care professional should begin by praising the client for wanting to begin: "Mr. Jones, it is great that you are thinking about starting a walking program. You indicated on your form that you would like to have more energy, and being physically active will help you do that. I'd like to help you get started. Are there other things you would like to get out of being active? [*Client responds.*] In addition to having more energy, being active will help you control your weight, reduce the risk of cardiovascular disease, and even help you sleep better at night."

Next, the client and health care professional should review the proposed program together. Health care professionals should ask about enjoyment: "You need to choose an activity that you enjoy doing. What kind of activities have you done and enjoyed in the past?" Some clients will write a plan that is too ambitious or not challenging enough. Negotiate with the client: "I know you are anxious to get started and that's great, but why don't you start out with walking two to three days per week for fifteen to twenty minutes each time instead of every day. Once you've mastered that, you can gradually increase." A good way to assess self-efficacy is to ask the client, "How confident (sure) are you (on a scale from 0 percent [not confident at all] to 100 percent [totally confident]) that you can do this plan for the next two weeks?" If the client is less than 90 percent sure he or she can do it, adjust the goal to something easier to accomplish. It is very important for people to have a successful experience when they start out. Next, the health care professional assesses the client's social support: "Who will help you stick to your physical activity program? What kinds of things can they do that will be helpful to you? What kinds of things would you specifically not like them to do?"

The professional and client name barriers that might get in the way of meeting the goal. Planning in advance for these barriers is much more effective than waiting for them to happen. The professional might say: "You indicated that being too tired when you come home from work and being bored with exercise are barriers for you. You also said that you might try exercising in the morning. I think that's a great idea. You'll feel good all day knowing you have done something good for yourself. Another way people deal with this problem is to exercise before they go home at night. So take your walking shoes with you to work and walk there before you leave, or meet a friend at a park. Just avoid going home and sitting down in front of the television; because you're right, you might not leave to do your walk. The other thing you mentioned is that exercise can be boring. Try listening to music, vary what you do (walk one day, swim the next), or vary where you take your walk or do your activity with a friend. That will take the routine out of it."

Then the health care professional writes the agreed-upon plan in a box provided at the bottom of the protocol, indicating the frequency, intensity, type, and time (duration) of the physical activity. Both the health care professional and client sign the protocol, indicating a commitment by the client to meet this goal for a specified period. The back of the protocol contains suggestions for moderate and vigorous activities, suggestions about how to get around roadblocks, and an activity log. This protocol takes approximately five minutes to conduct. It allows health care professionals to invest their time wisely with a client who is ready—and therefore most likely—to change his or her lifestyle.

Actives. The protocol for actives is called "Keeping the PACE" (PACE score = 5 to 8). Approximately 40 percent of all clients will be in this category. The goal for this intervention is to review the client's current program, make suggestions for changes if appropriate, and discuss ways to avoid relapse. Clients are asked to document the type, intensity, frequency, and duration of their current activity program. They also document who supports them, any injuries they have had related to physical activity, what aspects of their program are most and least satisfying to them, and any changes they would like to make to their activity program to make it more convenient, enjoyable, or safe.

Health care professionals may recommend that clients continue with the *same* level of activity ("I see here that you are walking three times a week for half an hour. That's a good level for you. Keep up the good work.") or *increase* their current activity ("I see that you are riding your bike two times per week. Have you considered adding another exercise time to your schedule? Given your medical history and current physical condition, you can safely exercise three times per week and that is the recommended amount."), or even *decrease* their current activity ("I see that you run five miles six or seven days per week. That's a lot of exercise, and I'm concerned that you might get a sports-related injury. What is prompting you to exercise that much? Have you encountered any problems?").

Assess social support and potential relapse situations by asking, "Who can help you accomplish this goal?" and, "What is most likely to interfere with your activity program? What has caused you to stop exercising in the past? What can you do to avoid those barriers again? What did you do to get back on track last time you stopped exercising for a while?" The health care professional may refer to the back of the protocol to assist with making suggestions. Finally, assess the client's self-efficacy, "On a scale from 1 to 5, how confident are you that you can continue doing regular physical activity for the next three months?" Again, if the client is not highly confident, readjust the goal. The health care professional notes the agreed-upon program in the box at the bottom of the protocol and both sign.

This protocol will take two to four minutes, depending on whether or not the professional recommends changes to the program.

Having handouts ready to address patient questions you do not have time to answer fully is very helpful. Exhibit 6.2 on page 221 lists additional resources.

PACE Follow-Up

PACE counseling includes a brief follow-up, which may be done in person, by mail, or over the phone. If there is a reason for the client to return to the clinic, that is ideal, but not necessary. In the PACE efficacy study (Calfas et al., 1996), the follow-up was conducted during ten-minute phone interviews by a trained health educator two weeks after the office visit. Follow-up can be done by any trained health care professional. It does not have to be the same health care professional who conducted the original counseling. The purpose of the follow-up is to ask how a client is progressing with his or her physical activity goals, to identify problems and solutions, and to provide support. If formal follow-up is not possible, office staff may send a postcard follow-up. The health care professional should also be sure to ask about physical activity at the client's next office visit. Ideally, clients should complete a new PACE protocol at every well visit. This allows the health care professional to continue tailoring the exercise program to meet the client's changing needs. This may not be practical in some settings, but the health care professional should at least ask about physical activity at every nonacute visit.

Making PACE Part of the Clinical System

An effective protocol will not help if health care professionals do not use it. As medicine changes from a system where reimbursement occurs only when persons are sick to a capitated system in which a profit is made by keeping clients well, these protocols will be in more demand. If they are effective, health care professionals will eventually be reimbursed for conducting this counseling.

Additionally, the literature on exercise adoption and maintenance is relatively scant compared to that on smoking cessation and diet intervention. Physical activity was recognized as an independent risk factor for cardiovascular disease in 1992, much more recently than smoking or poor diet. It took many years for smoking cessation recommendations from physicians to become part of the "routine" primary care visit. We hope that physical activity recommendations will soon become routine.

There are six practical factors that can significantly increase the likelihood of PACE counseling occurring as planned. First, the office staff need to be included in PACE training and decision making about how the process will work in their particular clinical setting. If the office staff are not successful in having clients complete the forms, the health care professional cannot do the counseling. In our studies, office staff who were engaged in the process from the beginning were more enthusiastic about doing PACE in their offices than were others. Second, use chart stickers on medical records to identify clients who are being *paced*. This will alert any health care professional the client sees to ask about physical activity at every visit. Third, for counseling visits, put the completed protocol on (or in) the chart as a reminder to health care professionals to do the full PACE counseling. Fourth, the health care professional decides which clients will receive PACE counseling routinely in his or her clinic. Good candidates may be clients receiving annual pap smears, routine physical exams, or routine blood pressure checks for controlled hypertension. Fifth, the physical activity level (PACE score) should be included with the vital signs, similar to the way smoking status is recorded as a vital sign in many clinic settings today. Finally, no system can be designed to accommodate all possible settings, so the system can be changed as needed to work in a specific setting (for example, who does the counseling, how patients are identified, how records are kept, and how or if follow-up occurs might all be changed as needed).

Physical Activity Counseling for Children, Adolescents, and Older Adults

Some additional recommendations can be made for counseling children, adolescents, and older adults about physical activity.

Children and Adolescents

Researchers suggest that beginning physical activity programs early in life is the best way to prevent adolescent and later adult obesity. Current physical activity recommendations for adolescents include at least sixty minutes of moderate to vigorous physical activity daily (USDHHS, 2000; Biddle, Sallis, & Cavill, 1998; Cavill, Biddle, & Sallis, 2001). *Guidelines for Adolescent Preventive Services* (GAPS) (American Medical Association, 1992; Elster & Kuznets, 1994) recommends that adolescents (individuals aged eleven to twenty-one) receive annual preventive services visits that address both medical and behavioral aspects of health. With respect to physical activity, GAPS recommends that "all adolescents should receive health guidance annually about the benefits of exercise and should be encouraged to engage in safe exercise on a regular basis."

There are few physical activity interventions in primary care for adolescent clients. Walker et al. (2002) found that a larger proportion of those teens (fourteen- to fifteen-year-olds) who received physician advice regarding physical activity progressed on an exercise stage of change compared to teens who did not receive such advice; however, actual change in exercise behavior was not significant.

Based on results from the PACE pilot study with adolescents (described earlier), a new randomized controlled trial of the PACE intervention with adolescents is currently under way. The results from this study will be available soon. However, the manual *Bright Futures in Practice: Physical Activity* (Patrick, Spear, et al., 2001) describes approaches physicians can use with children and adolescents (from infancy through age twenty-one). General counseling recommendations include (1) assessing the child's level of physical activity at every visit; (2) recommending that children should be physically active every day or nearly every day, as part of play, games, physical education, planned physical activities, recreation, and sports, in the context of family, school, and community activities; (3) encouraging parents to be involved in physical activity with their child; and (4) encouraging older children to find physical activities that they enjoy and can continue into adulthood.

A recent review of physical activity interventions reported that school-based physical education interventions were effective in increasing levels of activity (Kahn et al., 2002). Kahn et al. also concluded that the existing evidence is insufficient to determine whether or not the following types of physical activity intervention are effective: classroom-based health education focused on information provision, classroom-based health education focused on reducing television viewing and video game playing, and college-based health education, among others. However, school-based programs that focus on skill building during physical education time are more promising. In SPARK-PE (Sports Play and Active Recreation for Kids), specialist-led or trained teacher–led physical education classes can increase the total number of minutes children spend in physical activity during recess as well as children's cardiovascular fitness (Sallis et al., 1997; McKenzie, Sallis, Kolody, & Faucette, 1997).

Older Adults

Counseling older adults about physical activity is similar to counseling younger adults, with a few exceptions. Older adults are more likely to require physician approval to begin a physical activity program. Once this permission is obtained, many seniors lead very active lifestyles. For this age group, emphasize the benefits of moderate physical activity. Brisk walking, gardening, and some forms of house-work can lead to health benefits. Living independently is very important to this age group. Strength training exercises can help older adults maintain independence by increasing their muscle strength and thus their ability to perform such activities of daily living as maintaining personal hygiene, maintaining a house-hold, and managing transportation. Health care professionals should encourage older clients to think of each physical challenge, like lifting groceries into the car or reaching for something on the top shelf, as an opportunity to maintain their muscle strength and independence. The American Association of Retired Persons and the Active for Life program have good client information and physical activity programs available for older adults (American Association of Retired Persons, n.d.; Active for Life, n.d.).

Future Directions for Health Promotion in Physical Activity

One of the most important goals for this field is to develop counseling protocols that work. A growing number of physical activity studies in primary care have been conducted with promising but inconsistent results (for reviews, see Simons-Morton et al., 1998; Eakin et al., 2000; Wee, 2001). Before we in the health promotion field can ask health care professionals to spend valuable time doing these kinds of interventions, we need to demonstrate more fully that these interventions work. Project PACE is evolving. Several new PACE studies are currently under way, including four randomized controlled trials focused on apparently healthy adolescents, overweight women, overweight men, and adolescents at risk of developing type 2 diabetes. The major changes being made in PACE counseling are (1) incorporating nutrition behavioral change goals, (2) tailoring to specific at-risk client populations, and (3) using computer technology to assist the health care professional in client assessment and delivery of the PACE intervention. Although these protocols are not yet available, the general counseling principles can be used with many health promotion topics and can be adapted for various populations and age groups.

An important clinical issue in preventive medicine is how to manage all the demands for preventive medicine counseling. Physical activity is only one of many important health topics. For this reason PACE researchers recently added nutrition as a health promotion behavioral change goal. Physical activity and nutrition are related health behaviors and both are important for weight management, an increasingly important health topic. Nine other personal health behaviors, or topics, are outlined in this volume, and each deserves special attention. How these topics will be addressed in the context of the primary care setting (for example, one at a time or multiple topics per visit) remains a valued area for future research.

Research suggests that computer technology is a promising medium to use for health behavior interventions, including weight loss (Tate, Wing, & Winett, 2001; Tate, Jackvony, & Wing, 2003), dietary improvements (Oenema, Brug, & Lechner, 2001), and eating disorder behaviors (Celio et al., 2000). Internet-based patient education systems have been found to be well accepted by patients in clinical settings (Helwig, Lovelle, Guse, & Gottlieb, 1999). The promise of Internet and cell phone technologies to support and enhance the efforts of health care professionals in counseling clients is a vast area for further research.

Summary

Physical activity is a major factor in risk reduction for cardiovascular disease, colon cancer, and non-insulin-dependent diabetes mellitus. It is a key element of weight control and maintenance of bone mass. Physical activity is related to reduced symptoms of depression and anxiety and overall psychological well-being (Task Force on Community Preventive Services, 2002; USDHHS, 1996). Yet more than 60 percent of all adults do not perform the recommended amount of physical activity (USDHHS, 2000). A common barrier to activity is competing time demands.

The transtheoretical model, which focuses on the stages of change through which a client moves in adopting physical activity, and social cognitive theory are the foundation of the PACE model described in this chapter. Several studies have demonstrated PACE's efficacy with adults and adolescents in outpatient settings. The client's stage of change, from precontemplation to contemplation to active, determines the counseling approach each health care professional adopts.

References

Abramson, S., Stein, J., Schaufele, M., Frates, E., & Rogan, S. (2000). Personal exercise habits and counseling practices of primary care physicians: A national survey. *Clinical Journal of Sports Medicine, 10*, 40–48.

Active for Life. (n.d.). *About the program.* Retrieved January 27, 2004, from http://www.activeforlife.info/about_the_program/active_living_network.htm

Ali, N. S., & Twibell, R. K. (1995). Health promotion and osteoporosis prevention among postmenopausal women. *Preventive Medicine, 24*, 528–534.

Altena, T. S., Michaelson, J., Ball, S. D., & Thomas, T. R. (2004). Single sessions of inter-
mittent and continuous exercise and postprandial lipemia. *Medicine and Science in Sports and
Exercise, 36,* 1364–1371.

American Academy of Pediatrics, Committee on Sports Medicine and Fitness, & Committee
on School Health. (2001). Policy statement: Organized sports for children and preadoles-
cents (RE0052). *Pediatrics, 107*(6), 1459–1462.

American Association of Retired Persons. (n.d.). *Step up to better health: The walking program that gets
everyone moving.* Retrieved January 27, 2004, from http://aarp.stepuptobetterhealth.com/
default.asp

American College of Obstetrics and Gynecology. (2000). *Primary and preventive care: Periodic assessments* (ACOG Committee Opinion 246). Washington, DC: Author.

American College of Sports Medicine. (1998). Exercise and physical activity for older adults
(Position Stand). *Medicine and Science in Sports and Exercise, 30*(6), 992–1008.

American College of Sports Medicine. (2000). Exercise and type 2 diabetes (Position Stand).
Medicine and Science in Sports and Exercise, 32(7), 1345–1360.

American College of Sports Medicine. (2004). Exercise and hypertension (Position Stand).
Medicine and Science in Sports and Exercise, 36(3), 533–553.

American Heart Association. (2003). Exercise and physical activity in the prevention and
treatment of atherosclerotic cardiovascular disease: A statement from the Council on
Clinical Cardiology and the Council on Nutrition, Physical Activity, and Metabolism
(Scientific Statement). *Circulation, 107,* 3109.

American Medical Association, Department of Adolescent Health. (1992). *Guidelines for
Adolescent Preventive Services.* Chicago: Author.

Bandura, A. (1986). *Social foundations of thought and action.* Upper Saddle River, NJ: Prentice
Hall.

Baranowski, T., Lin, L. S., Wetter, D. W., Resnicow, K., & Hearn, M. D. (1997). Theory as
mediating variables: Why aren't community interventions working as desired? *Annals of
Epidemiology, 7,* S89–S95.

Biddle, S., Sallis, J. F., & Cavill, N. (Eds.). (1998). *Young and active? Young people and health enhancing physical activity: Evidence and implications.* London: Health Education Authority.

Blair, S. N., & Holder, S. (2002). Exercise in the management of obesity. In C. G. Fairburn &
K. D. Brownell (Eds.), *Eating disorders and obesity: A comprehensive handbook* (2nd ed., pp. 518–
523). New York: Guilford Press.

Blair, S. N., Kohl, H. W., Barlow, C. E., Paffenbarger, R. S., Gibbons, L. W., & Macera, C. A.
(1995). Changes in physical fitness and all-cause mortality: A prospective study of healthy
and unhealthy men. *JAMA, 273,* 1093–1098.

Brownell, K. D. (1995). Exercise in the treatment of obesity. In K. D. Brownell & C. G. Fairburn
(Eds.), *Eating disorders and obesity: A comprehensive handbook* (pp. 473–478). New York: Guilford
Press.

Calfas, K. J., Long, B. J., Sallis, J. F., Wooten, W. J., Pratt, M., & Patrick, K. (1996). A controlled trial of physician counseling to promote the adoption of physical activity. *Preventive
Medicine, 25,* 225–233.

Calfas, K. J., Sallis, J. F., Lovato, C. Y., & Campbell, J. (1994). Physical activity and its determinants before and after college graduation. *Medicine Exercise Nutrition and Health, 3,* 323–334.

Calfas, K., Sallis, J., Oldenburg, B., & Ffrench, M. (1997). Mediators of change in physical
activity following an intervention in primary care: PACE. *Preventive Medicine, 26,* 297–304.

Calfas, K., Sallis, J., Zabinski, M., Wilfley, D., Rupp, J., Prochaska, J. J., et al. (2002). Preliminary evaluation of a multi-component program for nutrition and physical activity change in primary care: PACE+ for Adults. *Preventive Medicine, 34,* 153–161.

Cavill, N., Biddle, S., & Sallis, J. F. (2001). Health enhancing physical activity for young people: Statement of the United Kingdom expert consensus conference. *Pediatric Exercise Science, 13,* 12–25.

Celio, A. A., Winzelberg, A. J., Wilfley, D. E., Eppstein-Herald, D., Springer, E. A., Dev, P., et al. (2000). Reducing risk factors for eating disorders: Comparison of an Internet- and a classroom-delivered psychoeducational program. *Journal of Consulting and Clinical Psychology, 68*(4), 650–657.

Chisholm, D. M., Collis, M. L., Kulak, L. L., Davenport, W., & Gruber, N. (1975). Physical activity readiness. *British Columbia Medical Journal, 17,* 375–378.

Chodzko-Zajko, W. J. (1998). Physical activity and aging: Implications for health and quality of life in older persons. *President's Council on Physical Fitness and Sports Research Digest, 3*(4), 1–8.

Courneya, K. S., & McAuley, E. (1994). Are there different determinants of the frequency, intensity, and duration of physical activity? *Behavioral Medicine, 20,* 84–90.

Craft, L. L., & Landers, D. M. (1998). The effect of exercise on clinical depression and depression resulting from mental illness: A meta-analysis. *Journal of Sport and Exercise Psychology, 20,* 339–357.

Dishman, R. K., & Steinhardt, M. (1990). Health locus of control predicts free-living, but not supervised, physical activity: A test of exercise-specific control and outcome-expectancy hypotheses. *Research Quarterly for Exercise and Sport, 61,* 383–394.

Dowda, M., Ainsworth, B. E., Addy, C. L., Saunders, R., & Riner, W. (2003). Correlates of physical activity among U.S. adults, 18 to 30 years of age, from NHANES III. *Annals of Behavioral Medicine, 26*(1), 15–23.

Eakin, E. G., Glasgow, R. E., & Riley, K. M. (2000). Review of primary care-based physical activity intervention studies. *Journal of Family Practice, 49*(3), 158–168.

Eden, K. B., Orleans, T., Mulrow, C. D., Pender, N. J., & Teutsch, S. M. (2002). Does counseling by clinicians improve physical activity? *Annals of Internal Medicine, 137*(3), 208–215.

Elder, J. P., Ayala, G. X., & Harris, S. (1999). Theories and intervention approaches to health behavior change in primary care. *American Journal of Preventive Medicine, 17*(4), 275–284.

Elster, A. B., & Kuznets, N. J. (Eds.). (1994). *AMA guidelines for adolescent preventive services (GAPS): Recommendations and rationale.* Baltimore: Williams & Wilkins.

Estabrooks, P. A., Glasgow, R. E., & Dzewaltowski, D. A. (2003). Physical activity promotion through primary care. *JAMA, 289,* 2913–2916.

Exercise your right to health. (2004, July). *Harvard Heart Letter, 14*(11), 4–5.

Foster, G. D., Wadden, T. A., Makris, A. P., Davidson, D., Swain Sanderson, R., Allison, D. B., et al. (2003). Primary care physicians' attitudes about obesity and its treatment. *Obesity Research, 11,* 1168–1177.

Frank, E., & Kunovich-Frieze, T. (1995). Physicians' prevention counseling behaviors: Current status and future directions. *Preventive Medicine, 24,* 543–545.

Giles-Corti, B., & Donovan, R. J. (2002). The relative influence of individual, social and physical environment determinants of physical activity. *Social Sciences & Medicine, 54*(12), 1793–1812.

Giovannucci, E., Leitzmann, M., Spiegelman, D., Rimm, E. B., Colditz, G. A., Stampfer, M. J., et al. (1998). A prospective study of physical activity and prostate cancer in male health professionals. *Cancer Research, 58,* 5117–5122.

Glasgow, R. E., Eakin, E. G., Fisher, E. B., Bacak, S. J., & Brownson, R. C. (2001). Physician advice and support for physical activity: Results from a national survey. *American Journal of Preventive Medicine, 21*(3), 189–196.

Godin, G., & Shephard, R. (1990). An evaluation of the potential role of the physician in influencing community exercise behavior. *American Journal of Health Promotion, 4,* 225–229.

Havranek, E. P. (1999). Primary prevention of CHD: Nine ways to reduce risk. *American Family Physician, 59*(6), 1455–1465.

Helwig, A. L., Lovelle, A., Guse, C. E., & Gottlieb, M. S. (1999). An office-based Internet patient education system: A pilot study. *Journal of Family Practice, 48*(2), 123–127.

Honda, K., & Sheinfeld Gorin, S. (2006). A model of stage of change to recommend colonoscopy among urban primary care physicians. *Health Psychology, 25,* 65–73.

Kahn, E. B., Ramsey, L. T., Brownson, R. C., Heath, G. W., Howze, E. H., Powell, K. E., et al. (2002). The effectiveness of interventions to increase physical activity: A systematic review. *American Journal of Preventive Medicine, 22*(4 Suppl.), 73–107.

Klem, M. L., Wing, R. R., McGuire, M. T., Seagle, H. M., & Hill, J. O. (1997). A descriptive study of individuals successful at long-term maintenance of substantial weight loss. *American Journal of Clinical Nutrition, 66*(2), 239–246.

Knowler, W. C., Barrett-Connor, E., Fowler, S. E., Hamman, R. F., Lachin, J. M., Walker, E. A., et al. (2002). Reduction in the incidence of type 2 diabetes with lifestyle intervention or metformin. *New England Journal of Medicine, 346,* 393–403.

Lawlor, D. A., & Hopker, S. W. (2001). The effectiveness of exercise as an intervention in the management of depression: Systematic review and meta-regression analysis of randomised controlled trials. *British Medical Journal, 322,* 763–767.

Long, B. J., Calfas, K. J., Wooten, W., Sallis, J. F., Patrick, K., Goldstein, M., et al. (1996). A multisite field test of the acceptability of physical activity counseling in primary care: Project PACE. *American Journal of Preventive Medicine, 12*(2), 73–81.

Marcus, B. H., Nigg, C. R., Riebe, D., & Forsyth, L. H. (2000). Interactive communication strategies: Implications for population-based physical activity promotion. *American Journal of Preventive Medicine, 19*(2), 121–126.

Marcus, B. H., Rakowski, W., & Rossi, J. S. (1992). Assessing motivational readiness and decision making for exercise. *Health Psychology, 11,* 257–261.

Mazzuca, S. A. (1982). Does patient education in chronic disease have therapeutic value? *Journal of Chronic Diseases, 35,* 521–529.

McKenzie, T. L., Sallis, J. F., Kolody, B., & Faucette, F. N. (1997). Long-term effects of a physical education curriculum and staff development program: SPARK. *Research Quarterly for Exercise and Sport, 68*(4), 280–291.

Nawaz, H., Adams, M. L., & Katz, D. L. (2000). Physician-patient interactions regarding diet, exercise, and smoking. *Preventive Medicine, 31,* 652–657.

North Dakota Department of Health. (2000). *Physicians' physical activity assessment and counseling practices: A study of North Dakota primary-care practitioners.* Bismarck, ND: Author.

Oenema, A., Brug, J., & Lechner, L. (2001). Web-based tailored nutrition education: Results of a randomized control trial. *Health Education Research, 16*(6), 647–660.

Paffenbarger, R. S., Jr., Lee, I. M., & Leung, R. (1994). Physical activity and personal characteristics associated with depression and suicide in American college men. *Acta Psychiatrica Scandinavica, 377* (Suppl.), 16–22.

Pate, R. R., Pratt, M., Blair, S. N., Haskell, W. L., Macera, C. A., Bouchard, C., et al. (1995). Physical activity and public health: A recommendation from the Centers for Disease Control and Prevention and the American College of Sports Medicine. *JAMA, 273,* 402–407.

Patrick, K., Sallis, J. F., Prochaska, J. J., Lydston, D. D., Calfas, K. J., & Zabinski, M. F. (2001). A multicomponent program for nutrition and physical activity change in primary care: PACE+ for adolescents. *Archives of Pediatric Medicine, 155,* 940–946.

Patrick, K., Spear, B., Holt, K., & Sofka, D. (Eds.). (2001). *Bright futures in practice: Physical activity.* Arlington, VA: National Center for Education in Maternal and Child Health.

Pinto, B. M., Goldstein, M. G., & Marcus, B. H. (1998). Activity counseling by primary care physicians. *Preventive Medicine, 27*(4), 506–513.

Podl, T. R., Goodwin, M. A., Kikano, G. E., & Stange, K. C. (1999). Direct observation of exercise counseling in community family practice. *American Journal of Preventive Medicine, 17*(3), 207–210.

Prochaska, J. O., & DiClemente, C. C. (1982). Transtheoretical therapy: Toward a more integrative model of change. *Psychotherapy: Theory, Research and Practice, 20,* 161–173.

Prochaska, J. O., & Marcus, B. H. (1994). The transtheoretical model: Applications to exercise. In R. K. Dishman (Ed.), *Advances in exercise adherence* (pp. 161–180). Champaign, IL: Human Kinetics.

Prochaska, J. J., Zabinski, M. F., Calfas, K. J., Sallis, J. F., & Patrick, K. (2000). PACE+: Interactive communication technology for behavior change in clinical settings. *American Journal of Preventive Medicine, 19*(2), 127–131.

Rovniak, L. S., Anderson, E. S., Winett, R. A., & Stephens, R. S. (2002). Social cognitive determinants of physical activity in young adults: A prospective structural equation analysis. *Annals of Behavioral Medicine, 24*(2), 149–156.

Sallis, J. F., Hovell, M. F., Hoffstetter, C. R., Faucher, P., Elder, J. P., Blanchard, J., et al. (1989). A multivariate study of determinants of vigorous exercise in a community sample. *Preventive Medicine, 18,* 20–34.

Sallis, J. F., McKenzie, T. L., Alcaraz, J. E., Kolody, B., Faucette, N., & Hovell, M. F. (1997). The effects of a 2-year physical education program (SPARK) on physical activity and fitness in elementary school students: Sports, Play and Active Recreation for Kids. *American Journal of Public Health, 87*(8), 1328–1334.

Sallis, J. F., Prochaska, J. J., Taylor, W. C., Hill, J. O., & Geraci, J. C. (1999). Correlates of physical activity in a national sample of girls and boys in grades 4 through 12. *Health Psychology, 18*(4), 410–415.

Simons-Morton, D. G., Calfas, K. J., Oldenburg, B., & Burton, N. (1998). Effects of interventions in health care settings on physical activity or cardiorespiratory fitness. *American Journal of Preventive Medicine, 15*(4), 413–430.

Task Force on Community Preventive Services. (2002). Recommendations to increase physical activity in communities. *American Journal of Preventive Medicine, 22*(4 Suppl.), 67–72.

Tate, D. F., Jackvony, E. H., & Wing, R. R. (2003). Effects of Internet behavioral counseling on weight loss in adults at risk for type 2 diabetes. *JAMA, 289,* 1833–1836.

Tate, D. F., Wing, R. R., & Winett, R. A. (2001). Using Internet technology to deliver a behavioral weight loss program. *JAMA, 285,* 1172–1177.

Toyry, S., Rasanen, K., Kujala, S., Aarimaa, M., Juntunen, J., Kalimo, R., et al. (2000). Self-reported health, illness and self-care among Finnish physicians. *Archives of Family Medicine, 9,* 1079–1085.

Tuomilehto, J., Lindstrom, J., Erikkson, J. G., Valle, T. T., Hamalainen, H., Ilanne-Parikka, P., et al. (2001). Prevention of type 2 diabetes mellitus by changes in lifestyle among subjects with impaired glucose tolerance. *New England Journal of Medicine, 344,* 1343–1350.

U.S. Department of Health and Human Services. (1996). *Physical activity and health: A report of the surgeon general.* Atlanta, GA: U.S. Department of Health and Human Services, National Center for Chronic Disease Prevention and Health Promotion.

U.S. Department of Health and Human Services. (1999). *National Ambulatory Medical Care Survey: 1995–1996 Summary* (DHHS Publication No. [PHS] 2000-1713). Hyattsville, MD: Author.

U.S. Department of Health and Human Services. (2000). *Healthy people 2010: Understanding and improving health* (2nd ed.). Washington, DC: U.S. Government Printing Office.

U.S. Department of Health and Human Services. (2004). *Physical activity and good nutrition: Essential elements to prevent chronic diseases and obesity.* Atlanta, GA: U.S. Department of Health and Human Services, National Center for Chronic Disease Prevention and Health Promotion.

U.S. Preventive Services Task Force. (2002). *Guide to clinical preventive services* (3rd ed.). Retrieved February 1, 2005, from http://www.ahrq.gov/clinic/3rduspstf/preface.htm

Van Gool, C. H., Kempen, G. I., Penninx, B. W., Deeg, D. J., Beekman, A. T., & Van Ejik, J. T. (2003). Relationship between changes in depressive symptoms and unhealthy lifestyles in late middle aged and older persons: Results from the Longitudinal Aging Study Amsterdam. *Age & Ageing, 32*(1), 81–87.

Van Mechelen, W., Twisk, J. W., Post, B., Snel, J., & Kemper, H. C. (2000). Physical activity of young people: The Amsterdam Longitudinal Growth and Health Study. *Medicine and Science in Sports and Exercise, 32*(9), 1610–1616.

Walker, Z., Townsend, J., Oakley, L., Donovan, C., Smith, H., Hurst, Z., et al. (2002). Health promotion for adolescents in primary care: Randomised controlled trial. *British Medical Journal, 325,* 524–529.

Wee, C. C. (2001). Physical activity counseling in primary care: The challenge of effecting behavioral change. *JAMA, 286,* 717–719.

Writing Group for the Activity Counseling Trial. (2001). Effects of physical activity counseling in primary care: The Activity Counseling Trial: A randomized controlled trial. *JAMA, 286,* 677–687.

EXHIBIT 6.2. HELPFUL RESOURCES.

PACE: Physician's manual (2nd ed.). (1999). Available from San Diego State University, San Diego Center for Health Interventions, San Diego, CA 92182-4720; Phone: (619) 594-5949; Fax: (619) 594-3639; and can be ordered via a Web site: http://www. drjamessallis.sdsu.edu/paceform. This publication outlines the PACE process in more detail; patient materials available in English and Spanish.

Patrick, K., Spear, B., Holt, K., & Sofka, D. (Eds.). (2001). *Bright futures in practice: Physical activity.* Arlington, VA: National Center for Education in Maternal and Child Health. Provider materials for physical activity counseling with children and adolescents, including chapters on physical activity at different developmental stages, special issues for children and adolescents, and counseling tools.

SPARK PE: Sports Play and Active Recreation for Kids. Available from SPARK, Phone: (800) SPARK-PE; Web site: www.SPARKPE.org/index.jsp. SPARK is a physical activity training and curricula for elementary school teachers.

The Walking Kit. Available from the Stanford Center for Research and Disease Prevention; Web site: http://hprc.stanford.edu/pages/store/itemDetail.asp?23

Parlay International's one-page exercise handouts can be copied onto your letterhead and given to patients as appropriate. They cover multiple topics, such as how to take your pulse, dressing for exercise in warm or cold weather, buying good walking or running shoes, stretching, and injury prevention. Available (as a kit) from Parlay International; Phone: (800) 457-2752; Web site: http://www.parlay.com/aboutUs/index.html

National Organizations

American College of Sports Medicine; Phone: (317) 637-9200; Web site: www.ACSM.org

American Heart Association; Phone: (800) 787-8984; Web site: www.AmericanHeart.org

YMCA Program Store; Phone: (800) 872-9622; Web site: www.YMCA.net

American Alliance for Health, Physical Education, Recreation, and Dance (AAHPERD); Phone: 1-800-213-7193; Web site: http://www.aahperd.org

President's Council on Physical Fitness; Phone: (202) 690-9000; Web site: www.fitness.gov

CHAPTER SEVEN

SEXUAL HEALTH

Theo Sandfort

Very few people, if any, engage in sexual activity because of its health benefits. People have sex for a diversity of reasons. People have sex for pleasure;
to express affection, love, or dominance; to obtain money or other rewards; because it is expected from them; or, let us not forget, to procreate. Health rarely figures among these reasons.

Yet the term *sexual health* has found wide acceptance and figures dominantly
in the current discourse about sexuality. There are books about sexual health
(Miller & Green, 2002) and academic journals (for example, *Sexual Health* [http://
www.publish.csiro.au/nid/164.htm]), programs to enhance sexual health (for example, Agha & Van Rossem, 2004; DiClemente, 2001; *Promotion of Sexual Health,*
2000), Web sites devoted to sexual health (for example, www.sexualhealth.org),
and national and international sexual health policies (Adler, 2003; Giami, 2002;
Lottes, 2002; *Promotion of Sexual Health,* 2000). Even though the term *sexual health*
is regularly used as if its meaning were patently obvious, the concept behind it is
by no means uniformly understood and applied (Barrett, 1991; Coleman, 2002).

The preparation of this chapter was supported by NIMH center grant P30-MH43520 to the HIV Center for Clinical and Behavioral Studies (Anke A. Ehrhardt, principal investigator). The author would also
like to thank Sonya Romanoff and Jeffrey Weiss for their support in the preparation of this chapter.

What Is Sexual Health?

If people do not engage in sex for health reasons, how are sexuality and health related? It is important to first look at how both sexuality and health can be understood before addressing this question.

People experience their sexuality usually as a natural and personal affair. The private character of our sexuality makes it difficult for us to see how a range of factors that go far beyond the individual level affect of what we do and experience. However, when we look at differences between cultures or between time periods within a single culture, it becomes clear that sexuality is not as natural as it seems in our experience. For instance, although homosexuality was officially defined as a psychiatric disorder for a long time, only a few people now perceive it as such. Our sexuality is also affected by medical and technological developments. Viagra creates the possibility of prolonged sexual activity while the "natural" body refuses to work. The development of the Internet is radically changing how we find sexual partners and what we do with them. These examples illustrate that sexuality is, as Leonore Tiefer (2004) states, "not a natural act."

That sexuality is determined by a broad range of factors is clearly illustrated by the World Health Organization's definition of *sexuality:* "Sexuality is a central aspect of being human throughout life and encompasses sex, gender identities and roles, sexual orientation, eroticism, pleasure, intimacy and reproduction. Sexuality is experienced and expressed in thoughts, fantasies, desires, beliefs, attitudes, values, behaviours, practices, roles and relationships. While sexuality can include all of these dimensions, not all of them are always experienced or expressed. Sexuality is influenced by the interaction of biological, psychological, social, economic, political, cultural, ethical, legal, historical and religious and spiritual factors" (WHO, n.d.).

A definition of *health* is likewise less than self-evident. As discussed in Chapter One, a commonly accepted definition that health is the absence of disease suggests that health is an objective quality. History, however, shows that conceptions of health and disease, as well as ideas about the causes of diseases and how diseases can be treated, change over time. Turner (2000) describes, for instance, that in the premodern Western world illness was seen as resulting from nonnatural causes, such as divine punishment. Sickness was a moral category. The development of a scientific discourse has now replaced this religious framework. Within this scientific discourse illness is explained in natural terms and is understood as resulting from causal agents such as germs and viruses. This modern concept of health and disease is now dominant and coexists with various other belief systems.

Sexuality and Health: A Complex Relationship

The relationship between sexuality and health is complex. A review of the existing literature shows that the term *sexual health* covers a variety of phenomena. In the most common usage of sexual health, health—or better, ill health—refers to outcomes of sexual behavior, in particular negative outcomes such as sexually transmitted infections (STIs) or unwanted pregnancies. That is, there is nothing *unhealthy* about the sexual acts themselves or the desire to engage in such acts. Another understanding of sexual health refers to the working of the *sexual system* according to the wishes of the persons involved; this system is not working in the case of sexual disorders such as hyposexual desire and erectile dysfunctions. If sexual health is understood as a competency or a quality of a person, then avoiding sexual acts that potentially result in negative consequences might be seen as a sign of sexual health.

In a less orthodox approach, sexual health refers to the way sexual activities come about: those interactions that are not engaged in voluntarily or consensually are then understood as sexual health problems (Kalmuss, 2004). A lack of control might also imply an inability to protect oneself from undesirable outcomes, for instance by using condoms. Control might be lacking because a person is forced to engage in sexual activity by somebody else; it is also possible that an individual may not experience any control over his or her sexual behavior, as in what is labeled *sexual addiction* or *compulsivity.*

In an even broader understanding, sexual health refers to contexts in which sexuality is practiced. For instance, sexual health may be perceived as lacking in a system or culture that stigmatizes specific forms of sexual expression or that does not prepare people to engage in sexual interactions in a responsible manner.

Definitions of Sexual Health

The understandings of sexual health discussed so far imply absence of health. That a positive conception of sexual health is possible as well is clear from the definition established by the World Health Organization: "Sexual health is a state of physical, emotional, mental and social well-being related to sexuality; it is not merely the absence of disease, dysfunction or infirmity. Sexual health requires a positive and respectful approach to sexuality and sexual relationships, as well as the possibility of having pleasurable and safe sexual experiences, free of coercion, discrimination and violence. For sexual health to be attained and maintained, the sexual rights of all persons must be respected, protected and fulfilled" (WHO, n.d.).

This definition of sexual health has some useful, broadly encompassing features. The first of these is that sexual health not only has physical and mental aspects but also is defined within a social framework. Further, sexual health is defined in an affirmative way, stressing well-being and not just stating the absence of negative qualities.

This definition of sexual health is somewhat utopian, however. Who would be classified as sexually healthy according to this definition? Given the worldwide prevalence of sexual prejudice, most if not all sexual minorities would fail to meet the criteria. Phenomena such as sexual violence and sex trafficking, and also more generally the stereotyping of women as sexually passive, form serious limitations to the sexual health of women (Amaro, Raj, & Reed, 2001). Sexual health as defined by WHO seems more a worthwhile goal to aim for than a statement of what exists; it might guide us in our actions.

This and other definitions of sexual health can be easily criticized. They also elicit such questions (Edwards & Coleman, 2004; Sandfort & Ehrhardt, 2004) as these: Whose approach should be positive and respectful? Who is responsible for creating the possibility of "having pleasurable and safe sexual experiences, free of coercion, discrimination and violence" and for fulfilling the sexual rights of persons?

Sexual Health: A Contested Concept

Even though sexual health is now a well-accepted and commonly used concept, it is also extensively criticized. First, a strong stress on health might make us forget that sexuality is about lust, pleasure, and intimacy. Sexual health is not an ultimate but instrumental aim.

Another criticism is that health, first of all, is understood as a biomedical category. Consequently, adopting the concept of sexual health runs the danger of medicalizing sexuality and reinforcing an understanding of sexuality in terms of normal and abnormal (Bancroft, 2002; Easton, O'Sullivan, & Parker, 2002; Tiefer, 1996). A potential consequence of medicalization is that sexual problems and their solutions are conceived exclusively in biomedical terms, eclipsing the fact that sexuality is a social practice, occurring in specific sociohistorical contexts. Consider, however, that physical and mental health, its causes and treatment, are not exclusively understood from a biomedical perspective. Medical sociology, anthropology, history, and health psychology have substantially broadened our perspective on health and taken it far beyond a narrow medical focus (Armstrong, 2000; Parker & Ehrhardt, 2001; Turner, 2000).

The word *health* also suggests objective standards. However, any definition of sexual health implies psychological and societal norms about the expression of sexuality (cf. Schmidt, 1987). Norms are clearly related to values, and thus such definitions of sexual health evoke questions and concerns about whose values and beliefs are the determining ones and become the regulators. Historical examples show how *health* and *social hygiene* have been the pretexts for suppressing or regulating sexual practices in the past (Brandt, 1987; Hunt, 1999; Rubin, 1984; Vance, 1991), as in the pathologizing of masturbation and the battle against sexually transmitted diseases (STDs) and prostitution.

Involvement in sexual health always implies taking a normative stance. It requires an ongoing critical assessment of sexual values and norms, by health care practitioners as well as by policymakers, and assessment of the potential consequences of actions. Acknowledgment of the role of values and norms implies that sexual health promotion can never be based exclusively on empirical evidence. Research can help us to understand what causes a specific problem, and it can demonstrate what works and what doesn't when we want to solve a specific problem. Research cannot prescribe which problems should be solved and whether the methods used to solve problems are ethically acceptable.

In discussing the normative characteristics of sexual health promotion, it is important to understand that we are dealing with norms and values on various levels. There are norms dealing with concrete and specific sex acts or behaviors and norms dealing more generally with how people interact. Seidman (2001) calls the latter set of norms a "communicative sexual ethic" and contrasts it with a normalizing ethic that proclaims that sexual acts themselves have inherent moral meaning. In a communicative sexual ethic the focus of the normative evaluation shifts from the sex act to the social exchange. A way to appraise the normative aspect of sexual health interventions is to assess whether they prescribe how people should behave and regulate their behavior or whether they empower people by increasing their repertoire of strategies to manage sexual risks and opportunities.

Sexual Health and Sexual Rights

A helpful concept in evaluating the normative aspects of sexual health promotion activities and policies is that of sexual rights. The yardstick then is whether interventions restrict or promote such rights. In international declarations and treaties, the term *sexual rights* typically refers to reproductive self-determination (Cook, 1995) or to protection from sexual abuse and discrimination (Petchesky, 2000). Petchesky (2000) has developed a more affirmative vision of sexual rights, one containing a set of ethical principles as well as a range of enabling conditions (see also Miller, 2000). In this formulation, sexual rights include the principles of sexual diversity (a commitment to the principle that diversity of sexual expressions is beneficial to a society) and habitational diversity (recognition of a diversity of family arrangements). Other ethical principles that according to Petchesky are basic to sexual rights are the principle that people have the right to have a satisfying and safe sexual life, the principle of autonomy or personhood, which implies the right of people to make their own decisions in matters affecting their bodies and health, and finally, the principle of gender equality. Realization of these ethical principles requires the establishment of enabling conditions, which, according to Petchesky, includes providing access to information about sexuality and to preventive and caring services, as well as making broader societal changes in the way men and women and sexual minorities are envisioned.

WHO (n.d.) says that *sexual rights*

> embrace human rights that are already recognized in national laws, international human rights documents and other consensus documents. These include the right of all persons, free of coercion, discrimination and violence, to:
>
> - the highest attainable standard of health in relation to sexuality, including access to sexual and reproductive health care services;
> - seek, receive and impart information in relation to sexuality;
> - sexuality education;
> - respect for bodily integrity;
> - choice of partner;
> - decide to be sexually active or not;
> - consensual sexual relations;
> - consensual marriage;
> - decide whether or not, and when to have children; and
> - pursue a satisfying, safe and pleasurable sexual life.
>
> The responsible exercise of human rights requires that all persons respect the rights of others.

Sexual rights are important to sexual health. Having sexual rights may certainly be conducive to sexual health, as the lack or violation of such rights may seriously interfere with maintaining sexual health. Sexual rights do not, however, automatically bring about sexual health. Indeed, one may suggest that some aspect of sexual health is a prerequisite for a person to exert his or her sexual rights. The actual relationship between sexual rights and sexual health is, of course, an empirical question (cf. Burris, Lazzarini, & Loff, 2001).

The Need for Sexual Health Promotion

It may be clear from the preceding discussion that there is a need for sexual health promotion. That need becomes clear when we consider the people who try to find adequate sexual health care for a variety of issues. On a more general level, an extensive epidemiology of sexual health problems underscores this need.

Epidemiology of Sexual Health

STDs and HIV/AIDS are probably the best-documented sexual health problems. Chlamydia is the most commonly reported infectious disease in the United States. In 2003, over 850,000 infections were reported to the Centers for Disease Control and Prevention (CDC; 2004b). Because many cases of chlamydia are not reported or remain undiagnosed, the CDC estimates that there are about 2.8 million new cases of chlamydia per year. Gonorrhea is the second most commonly reported infectious disease in the United States. In 2003, more than 335,000 cases were reported; the CDC estimates the actual number of new infections per year at 718,000. While chlamydia infections seem to be rising, gonorrhea seems to be decreasing. The incidence of syphilis is rising dramatically, after having reached an all-time low in 2000.

Infections with the human papillomavirus (HPV) are not reportable to the CDC but are the most common sexually transmitted infection (STI) in the United States. Even though up to twenty million Americans are currently infected with sexually transmitted HPV, according to Planned Parenthood (n.d.) 70 percent of Americans have never heard of it. Overall it is estimated that more than one in five Americans is infected with a viral STI (other than HIV).

Probably publicly more acknowledged are the dramatic figures about HIV/AIDS. These figures show that this epidemic is ongoing and that goals to reduce new infections are not being met. Over twenty years into the epidemic, HIV/AIDS continues to be a major public health threat. Although the early 1990s showed a downward trend in estimated numbers of new HIV infections, the period from 1994 to 2000 showed a leveling off of this trend (CDC, 2002). Since 1999, the number of new HIV diagnoses per year has remained relatively stable, although it has started to increase again among men who have sex with men (MSM) (CDC, 2004a). Every year, 40,000 Americans newly test positive for HIV infection. This is the same number as a decade ago and double the annual goal of less than 20,000 new HIV cases per year that was laid out by the Centers for Disease Control and Prevention in 2001.

Another indicator of the need for sexual health promotion is the number of teenage pregnancies. In 2000, there were 83.6 pregnancies per 1,000 women aged fifteen to nineteen (Alan Guttmacher Institute, 2004). The good news is that this figure represents a fall of 28 percent since the number peaked in 1990. Still, in 2000, one-third of the pregnancies among fifteen- to nineteen-year-olds ended in abortion. Teen pregnancy rates vary widely by race and ethnicity and by state.

The prevalence of sexual dysfunctions is more difficult to assess and will depend to a large extent on how it is measured. For the United States the most reliable data probably come from a study that Laumann, Paik, and Rosen (1999) did in 1992 in a demographically representative cohort of 1,410 male and 1,749 female adults (aged eighteen to fifty-nine). They concluded that 43 percent of the women and 31 percent of the men had had at least one sexual problem in the preceding year. These problems are most prevalent in persons with poor physical and emotional health and are closely associated with negative experiences in sexual relationships and in overall well-being.

Sexual health problems rarely exist independently. For instance, sexual dysfunctions can result from sexual violence or abuse, which constitutes another major sexual health problem. The U.S. Department of Health and Human Services (2000a) estimated in 2000 that there are about 104,000 child victims of sexual abuse every year. The CDC reports in a fact sheet that approximately 9 percent of high school students have been forced to have sexual intercourse against their will at some point in their lifetimes, with female students (11.9 percent) being more likely than male students (6.1 percent) to report having been sexually assaulted (CDC, 2005). One in six women and one in thirty-three men in the United States have experienced an attempted or completed rape at least once during their lives.

Sexual abuse and violence are part of a cultural system of sexism and homophobia, which, in itself as well as in its consequences, makes up another sexual health issue. The stigma of being nonheterosexual is experienced by people in various ways, ranging from subtle forms of intolerance to overt forms of discrimination and actual violence. Actual figures about the occurrence of these phenomena are hard to get. Figures from surveys among gay and lesbian people show that such experiences are widespread (see, for instance, Herek, Gillis, & Cogan, 1999) and also occur in health care settings.

The various sexual health problems discussed here cause a lot of short- and long-term distress and misery for the people involved. Although that should be sufficient reason to prevent them, these problems also have economic consequences. Holtgrave and Pinkerton (2003) assessed the economic implications of the CDC failure to reduce the incidence of HIV infections by 50 percent by 2005 in the United States and calculated that the cost of the consequences exceeds $18 billion (see also Ebrahim, McKenna, & Marks, 2005).

Diversity of Sexual Health Needs and Specific Target Groups

Although sexually active people face several common sexual health threats, such as STDs, some needs may be more specific to some people than to others. Age, gender, sexual orientation, and ethnic background may diversely affect sexual health needs, and intersections between these factors contribute further to the diversity of needs. Not only do the sexual health needs of men and women vary, but young men and older men will have different needs, and ethnic background adds yet another layer of differences (Davidson, Fenton, & Mahtani, 2002). Numerous other factors, beyond gender and age also affect people's sexual health needs. Examples of such factors are being homeless (Rew, Fouladi, & Yockey, 2002), having been sexually abused (Loeb et al., 2002), and having specific diseases (Keller & Buchannan, 1993).

Furthermore, even though people may face common sexual health threats, the way these threats can be most effectively addressed requires understanding and acknowledgment of people's specific backgrounds. For instance, gender affects whether people will take the initiative in addressing their sex problems with physicians, men doing so less than women. Although this finding would warrant a more active response from physicians toward men, the practice seems to be opposite: physicians generally take less initiative in discussing sexual concerns with men than they do with women (Forrest, 2001; Metz & Seifert, 1993). Also, effective prevention of STIs among teenagers requires an approach that is different from STI prevention among gay men.

The differences in sexual health needs among specific categories of people can be variously understood. Sometimes the link between a category and needs is direct. For instance, aging affects people's capacity for sexual functioning, due to a greater likelihood of problems such as arthritis, diabetes, fatigue, fear of precipitating a heart attack, and side effects from prescription drugs (Miller, Zylstra, & Standridge, 2000; Vincent, 2002). Gender also affects functioning; a different physiology and differential roles in the reproductive process induce specific sexual health needs in men and women. Like age, however, gender also plays a more complicated role because it is also indicative of people's position in society. As Amaro and colleagues (2001) argue, women's sexual health is directly affected by their lower status in society. This lower status and relative lack of sexual autonomy increase their risk for sexual health problems. It also decreases women's ability to obtain treatment and support when a sexual health concern arises. Ethnicity affects sexual health needs and the way they are addressed because the levels of openness around sexuality differ among ethnic groups. Such openness, for instance, explained the higher prevalence of ever performing breast self-examination observed in Caucasian women compared to Asian women (Tang, Solomon, Yeh, & Worden, 1999).

On a more abstract level, sexual health needs, their perception, and the ways they are addressed are also affected by stereotypes about specific groups. For instance, the myth that physically disabled people have no sexuality prevents adequate treatment of their needs and might also be a self-fulfilling prophecy for the handicapped persons themselves (Milligan & Neufeldt, 2001). Older adults suffer from a comparable lack of recognition of their sexual desires (Calamidas, 1997). Sexuality is a fertile vehicle for stereotypes. These stereotypes can have detrimental consequences for the ways sexual health needs are perceived and addressed in various groups of people. Lewis and Kertzner (2004), for instance, convincingly argue that the sexual prowess attributed to black men results in a sexual health promotion approach focused on control instead of empowerment.

National Sexual Health Policies

The emergence of HIV/AIDS has contributed to renewed attention to sexual health and an acknowledgment of sexual health problems, not only by health professionals but also on the political level. In the United States, it has resulted in a call to action from the U.S. Surgeon General to promote sexual health and responsible sexual behavior (U.S. Department of Health and Human Services [USDHHS], 2001). In this document, sexual health issues are analyzed from a public health perspective and evidence-based intervention models are described. A strategy is presented that covers three fundamental areas: (1) increasing public awareness of issues relating to sexual health and responsible sexual behavior, (2) providing the health and social interventions necessary to promote and enhance sexual health and responsible sexual behavior, and (3) investing in research related to sexual health and disseminating findings widely. Similar plans have been developed in other countries, such as the United Kingdom (*The National Strategy for Sexual Health and HIV,* 2001), although the approaches taken differ (Giami, 2002; Wylie, 2001). *Healthy People 2010,* a report that articulates objectives for health in the United States in 2010, lists numerous objectives related to sexuality (USDHHS, 2000b).

Theoretical Foundations for Sexual Health Promotion

Sexual health promotion encompasses a broad field of activities. These activities can be distinguished by their overall aims, the contexts in which they take place, and the strategies that they apply. Sexual health promotion can be based on two kinds of theories, or theoretical frameworks. First, it may employ theories that focus on a specific object, and second, it may rely on theories that deal with how change can be accomplished. Both of these frameworks are needed for effective sexual health promotion. For instance, for effective HIV prevention we have to understand why people who could protect themselves by using condoms don't do so. However, even though understanding why these people don't use condoms is necessary, it does not tell us what we should do next. For this step we need theories that help us understand how we can produce change in their behavior.

Aims for Sexual Health Promotion

One of the first aims that comes to mind when looking at sexual health promotion is the prevention of harm. Preventive action aims not only at preventing the first occurrences of negative events or outcomes, such as unwanted pregnancies, STIs, and sexual violence. Preventive action can also be aimed at the avoidable reoccurrence of negative events, such as consequent infections of other people; screening can be a relevant tool for such preventive action. Instead of focusing on prevention, sexual health promotion can also aim at enhancing positive health, which would mean increasing people's capacity to achieve sexual intimacy and have a joyful sexual life.

Health promotion is usually thought about in terms of people who have to change their behavior if they are to have better health or social outcomes: for example, they need to learn how to use condoms, learn how to do breast self-examination, or develop more positive attitudes about sexual diversity. Although the focus is usually on learning new skills and behaviors, there is a growing awareness that newly acquired behaviors are not necessarily automatically retained and that maintenance of behavioral change is needed to prevent *relapse*. Relapse prevention was originally developed in the context of alcohol abuse and has seemed useful in the treatment of sex offenders. It may also be relevant for other health behaviors, such as condom use, where the people who need to perform the behavior perceive its associated costs as higher than its benefits.

Sexual health promotion can be aimed at specific goals, such as the prevention of HIV transmission. Specific goals can also be embedded in more global strategies. Technological arguments usually favor working with specific goals: for prevention to be effective you need to understand the factors that determine the behaviors that cause the problem. Preventive action should then focus on the identified determinants. Others argue that to be effective, one should connect with the needs of a specific population, which are usually broader than the needs identified by an outsider. For instance, in the case of young people the reasoning is that they are less likely to have unprotected sexual intercourse if they have acquired a variety of social skills relevant to dealing with romantic and sexual relationships. Instead of a focus on condom use, a broader sex education approach is expected to be more effective (Schaalma, Abraham, Gillmore, & Kok, 2004). However broad, in order for preventive action to be effective, it should address needs that are experienced as such by the target population. Several studies have been done to map out the needs of various groups of people, such as young people (Forrest, Strange, & Oakley, 2004), transgendered people (Bockting, Robinson, & Rosser, 1998), and patients with prostate cancer (Lintz et al., 2003).

Sexual health promotion cannot be limited to people's behavior and the factors affecting that behavior. Effective health promotion also includes and sometimes gives primary attention to various structural components. Examples of such components are specific resources, such as the availability of condoms; promoting skills to use condoms is senseless if condoms are hard or impossible to come by. The availability of condoms in public places where people have sex, such as specific bathhouses, can also support and foster behavioral change. Other examples of structural components are social environments that support behavioral change among people for whom such change is relevant. Policies and regulations are examples of structural components on a more general level that might contribute to sexual health promotion. Promoting access to sexual health care for specific groups, such as young people or gay and lesbian people, usually requires structural changes (Brotman, Ryan, Jalbert, & Rowe, 2002).

Levels of Intervention in Various Contexts

Sexual health promotion can be delivered at various levels and in various contexts. On the most general level, sexual health has been promoted via mass media campaigns. Such campaigns have, for instance, been used to promote responsible sexual behavior (Keller & Brown, 2002). A widely accessible and rapidly growing venue for sexual health promotion is the Internet, which has been used to reach general populations (see, for example, Barak & Fisher, 2003) and specific groups such as the elderly (Harris, Dersch, Kimball, Marshall, & Negretti, 1999), teenagers (Keller, Labelle, Karimi, & Gupta, 2002), and gay men (Bolding, Davis, Sherr, Hart, & Elford, 2004; Klausner, Levine, & Kent, 2004). Even though the Internet offers promising possibilities for sexual health promotion, it also functions as a source of sexual pleasure and as a threat to sexual health (Carnes, 2003).

The targets of sexual health promotion vary from individuals, families, and groups to communities. Individuals are the target of health promotion in a variety of settings, including health care interactions. Sometimes parents are targeted to promote positive parenting and effective parent-child communication about sexuality and sexual risk reduction, with the ultimate goal being to reduce sexual risk behavior among adolescents (Ball, Pelton, Forehand, Long, & Wallace, 2004; Dittus, Miller, Kotchick, & Forehand, 2004). Sexual health interventions sometimes involve schools or broader communities (see, for example, Paine-Andrews et al., 2000). One remarkable community prevention program used peer outreach, peer-led small groups, a publicity campaign, and a young men's center to promote safer sex among young gay men (Hays, Rebochook, & Kegeles, 2003).

Understanding Sexual Health Problems

All effective sexual health promotion activities require an in-depth understanding of the problem being addressed. The better a sexual health problem is understood, the more likely it is that an effective intervention can be developed. Sexual health problems have been conceptualized and studied from diverse and overlapping theoretical perspectives. Most of these theories—such as the health belief model, the theory of reasoned action, and the information-motivation-behavioral skills model—are general and can be applied to various health issues. Other theories, such as the AIDS risk reduction model, are topic specific. Most of these perspectives include a set of common psychosocial variables. How these variables are related depends upon the specific sexual health issue under consideration and the population of interest. Other perspectives on sexual health issues are broader and include interactional and cultural factors.

Information. Regardless of the sexual health issue, both information and misinformation are of crucial importance. There is a lot to know about sexuality that can protect a person from sexual problems or promote one's sexual well-being. To give a few examples, knowing the workings of effective contraception is a prerequisite for the prevention of unwanted pregnancies. Understanding how STIs are transmitted will help people protect themselves. Knowing the symptoms of major STIs will help people who contract them to seek early treatment. Understanding the side effects of various drugs on a person's sexual life will help prepare people to adapt to such changes. Understanding gender differences in sexual functioning will improve adjustment in heterosexual couples.

Whereas being sufficiently informed about sexuality might prevent sexual health problems, being misinformed is likely to cause or perpetuate such problems. Moreover, the consequences of misinformation usually go beyond the immediate health issue. For instance, the misconception that HIV can be transmitted by simple bodily contact has unnecessarily dehumanized the treatment of people infected with HIV. Stereotypes about sexual minorities, which dehumanize interactions with members of such minorities, are another example. A national U.S. study among adolescents (Crosby & Yarber, 2001) shows how widespread misconceptions about condoms are.

A concept that stresses that it is not just bits of information but a coherent knowledge base that is needed for the attainment of sexual health is *health literacy.* More broadly, health literacy has been defined as "the evolving skills and competencies needed to find, comprehend, evaluate, and use health information and concepts to make educated choices, reduce health risks, and improve quality of life" (Zarcadoolas, Pleasant, & Greer, 2003, p. 119). Health literacy has not been conceptualized in the context of sexuality per se. If it were, it could be used as a framework to develop learning objectives for curricula in sexuality.

The relevance of information for specific health issues varies. For some issues, just having adequate information might be sufficient for people to avoid specific risks or to take relevant action. Quite often, though, information is not the factor that turns the balance. Even though having adequate information might be a prerequisite, it is in itself not always sufficient for healthy behaviors. So, although providing information might be helpful, it does not necessarily affect people's motivation to practice healthy behaviors. Other factors also influence why people do—or don't do—certain things.

Risk Perception. One of the reasons why having information is not always sufficient to induce healthy behaviors is that people do not necessarily apply the information to their own situation. This point is particularly relevant in relation to risk perception. People may know, for instance, how HIV is transmitted yet not necessarily consider themselves to be at risk when engaging in these behaviors, and as long as people do not consider themselves to be at risk they will not do anything to protect themselves. The example of risk perception makes it clear that we are not always dealing with factual knowledge. People may have specific reasons to believe they are not at risk even though they objectively are. One of these reasons is the optimistic bias that has been found to affect many health behaviors: when estimating the risk of a negative event, such as an HIV infection, people usually think that they themselves are less at risk than others.

Information about sexuality is now widely accessible via the Internet. Times have changed rapidly in that respect. The era when young people used to rely mostly on their peers for—not necessarily the most accurate—information about sexuality, seems about to disappear. A problem with the abundance of Internet resources is that their information about sexuality is usually not presented in a matter-of-fact way but is tainted by norms and values. Distinguishing fact from normative fiction is not always easy for somebody in search of information.

Attitudes. Other factors affecting people's sexual behavior can be grouped under the category of attitudes. Attitudes are usually understood as beliefs that people have and evaluations of those beliefs. A range of beliefs (or verbalized opinions) has been shown to be crucial to sexual health and relevant in understanding sexual health behaviors. An obvious example is beliefs about or attitudes toward condoms (Kelly, 1995). Attitudes are attached to all kinds of behaviors that are relevant to people's sexual health. People have attitudes about discussing sexuality, which might prevent them from talking to their partner or discussing sexual problems with their health care provider. Specific attitudes seldom stand on their own but are likely to be part of a larger system of attitudes or beliefs. Examples of such larger systems are ideologies about masculinity or femininity and religious convictions.

Skills and Self-Efficacy. People may have the right attitude toward a specific healthy behavior and also feel encouraged by others to engage in that behavior, but this is not sufficient if they do not have the skills to perform this behavior or do not feel convinced that they can perform it.

Social Norms. Some beliefs have to do with what one thinks other people think about specific activities or behaviors. Such beliefs may not directly affect one's behavior, however, because one may disagree with these perceived social norms. Thus in sexual health promotion it is also important to know whether people are willing to comply with the norms that they perceive.

Interpersonal Factors. Protecting oneself and others from sexual health risks and maximizing positive outcomes from sexual interactions require interpersonal skills. A lot of studies have been done about the negotiation of safer sex practices (see, for example, El-Bassel et al., 2001; Melendez, Hoffman, Exner, Leu, & Ehrhardt, 2003).

Cultural Influences and Structural Factors. There is a growing awareness that in order to understand sexual health we have to look beyond individual levels and look at cultural, structural, or contextual variables (see, for example, Parker, 2001). For instance, the way labor is organized in specific populations might affect the risk for HIV. If men are supposed to travel and be away from their homes in order to work and gain income, that will affect their pattern of sexual behavior and consequently the risk for their partners. The sexual risk attached to sex work—for the sex workers, the clients, and the partners of both—cannot be understood without knowledge of the factors that affect the existence and organization of the sex work. Legal regulation is another example of a structural factor.

Theories of Change

Once one gains an understanding of the individual and contextual factors that determine the sexual health problem to be addressed, one has to develop a plan for how these factors can be changed to either prevent or ameliorate the problem. Several empirically supported theories can be used when developing such a plan. These theories can be distinguished by the level at which they operate. Accordingly, Bartholomew, Parcel, Kok, and Gottlieb (2001) distinguish individual theories, interpersonal theories, organizational change models and theories, community organization models and theories, and societal and governmental theories. Depending on the problem one wants to address and the relevant determinants identified, elements of various theories can be used to complement one another in a combined approach.

Although there is a growing awareness of the relevance and feasibility of structural approaches, individual theories are the most developed. These individual theories include the various learning theories, such as classical and operant conditioning, which stress rewarding positive behaviors and punishing unhealthful behaviors. Other individual theories that Bartholomew and colleagues (2001) distinguish are the persuasion communication model, goal-setting theory, attribution theory, and self-regulatory theories, as discussed further in Chapters Two and Fourteen.

Another individual perspective is the stages of change model. This model acknowledges that with more complex behaviors—when just giving information does not solve the problem—people do not change completely in one instant; they do not, for instance, immediately become consistent condom users when they never before have considered using condoms. This model assumes that people start by thinking about a specific behavior or behavioral change; what has to be accomplished in this situation is that people must move from precontemplation to contemplation. Subsequently, people prepare for action, and then move from preparation to action. After people have performed a certain behavior, such as condom use, they will not automatically continue doing so. A strategy is needed to guarantee that action is maintained, and this can involve preparing people for potential lapses. This model makes clear that prevention strategies have to be tailored to the specific phase people are in and that dependent on the phase they are in, different activities might be needed.

In the category of interpersonal theories, Bartholomew and colleagues discuss social cognitive theory and social support (or network) theories. Both perspectives can be used when identifying ways to promote specific behaviors. Major constructs in social cognitive theory are outcome expectancies ("when I don't use condoms I will regret it") and self-efficacy ("I am confident that I am able to negotiate condom use with this partner"). These constructs can be affected by active learning, reinforcement, modeling, guided practice, and persuasion. Social support theories stress the role of the networks that people are part of in adopting new behaviors. Strategies using this perspective might, for instance, train individuals to mobilize and maintain their networks to support them in desired behavioral changes.

When interventions are needed on an external level, various methods and strategies are possible. One method is community organization, which includes strategies such as grassroots organizing, mounting demonstrations, and coalition building. Another method is advocacy, which includes strategies such as letter-writing campaigns, lobbying, and holding press conferences. In designing interventions, Bartholomew and colleagues stress the importance of identifying what it is that is intended to produce the desired change.

Sexual Health Interventions: Evidence of Effectiveness

Given the diverse and wide-ranging needs for sexual health promotion and the limited resources available, it is of crucial importance to know whether sexual health interventions are effective and, if so, why. And when interventions don't reach their desired outcomes, it is crucial to understand why they are not effective. *Effect evaluation* is applied to assess the outcomes of an intervention, and *process evaluation* aims at understanding why an intervention did or did not accomplish the desired goals.

Evaluating interventions is easier said than done (see Chapter Two). The evaluation of health interventions is an independent science and involves numerous practical and theoretical decisions (Stephenson, Imrie, & Bonell, 2003). A first question to answer is which effects should be assessed. Effect evaluations can focus on a specific behavior that an intervention intends to change, on the determinants of that behavior, or on the negative health consequences of the undesired behavior. Examples are, respectively, condom use, attitudes toward condoms, and actual STIs. A study might assess only the desired effects of an intervention, but it will be stronger if it also assesses adverse effects. The selection of effects to be evaluated should, of course, depend on what the intervention attempts to accomplish. If, according to the stages of change model, an intervention is meant to move people from contemplating condom use to preparing for condom use, actual use is not the right outcome to assess.

When should effects be assessed, and how long are effects supposed to last? Answers to these questions depend of course on the complexity of the sexual health issue one tries to address. Some effects might occur directly after the intervention but subsequently fade out. It is also possible that initial effects will be positive and long-term effects will be negative. If sexual health interventions do not include support for maintenance of accomplished behavioral change, it is likely that the effects of an intervention will disappear.

A final decision is what research design to adopt. It is generally understood that true experiments or random clinical trials are the most accurate at demonstrating the effectiveness of interventions. Adopting such designs is, however, sometimes infeasible or impractical—as in evaluations of community-based interventions—or undesirable (cf. Kippax, 2003).

Various evaluation studies of sexual health interventions have been done and are reported in the scientific literature. These studies vary in the activities or strategies evaluated—such as face-to-face counseling, peer education, leaflets, radio announcements, and Web sites—and in the populations studied—ranging from broad groups such as teenagers to more specific groups such as HIV-positive women with sexual abuse histories. More important, these studies vary in terms of the sexual health issues addressed. The following sections discuss evaluations of interventions for two sexual health issues: prevention of teen pregnancies and HIV prevention among men who have sex with men. Other studies have evaluated, for instance, the effects of programs to prevent recidivism among adolescent sex offenders (Seabloom, Seabloom, Seabloom, Barron, & Hendrickson, 2003) and of programs to reduce the acceptance of rape-myths in male college students (Flores & Hartlaub, 1998).

Prevention of Unwanted Teen Pregnancies

A wide variety of programs are aimed at preventing teenage pregnancies, which for a variety of reasons (see, for example, As-Sanie, Gantt, & Rosenthal, 2004) are generally considered to be unwanted. These programs vary in many ways, although current programs can be grouped into two major categories: abstinence-only and abstinence-plus programs. Whereas the aim of the former is to postpone sexual involvement, preferably until marriage, the latter encourages youths to be abstinent but also to use condoms and contraceptives if they do have sex. It will be obvious that intervention programs that can prevent pregnancy will also reduce the transmission of STIs. Although there are programs for teenagers that focus on pregnancy, STIs, and HIV, there are also programs that focus exclusively on STIs and HIV.

Kirby (2002) evaluated whether, as has been claimed by proponents of abstinence, abstinence-only programs indeed delay the initiation of sex among young people and reduce teen pregnancy. Ten programs were reviewed, and nine out of the ten failed to provide credible evidence, which leaves the question about their efficacy open. The tenth program's results suggested that a delay of initiation of sex occurred among youths fifteen years old and younger but not among older teenagers.

Support for positive effects of abstinence-plus programs is much more convincing. Kirby (2001) evaluated three kinds of programs: (1) programs that focus primarily on sexual antecedents; (2) programs that focus primarily on nonsexual antecedents; and (3) programs that focus on both; an example of the latter is the Children's Aid Society-Carrera Program (Philliber, Williams Kaye, Herrling, & West, 2002). Kirby identifies ten characteristics of effective programs. According to Kirby, effective programs are based on theoretical approaches that have been demonstrated to influence other behaviors that affect health, and they identify specific determinants that should be targeted to change behaviors. Effective programs also provide basic, accurate information, not only about the risk of sexual involvement but also about ways to avoid intercourse or to prevent pregnancy and STIs. Additionally, these programs provide examples of and practice with communication and negotiation and include activities that address social pressures that might influence sexual behavior. Effective programs also incorporate behavioral goals, teaching methods, and materials that are appropriate in terms of teenagers' age, level of sexual experience, and culture. Finally, effective programs last a sufficient length of time; a few hours is not enough (see Meschke, Bartholomae, & Zentall, 2002, for an overview and discussion of various sexual health programs aimed at teens).

HIV Prevention Among MSM

Johnson et al. (2002) did an extensive review of research on HIV prevention for men who have sex with men. They found the surprisingly low number of nine studies that met basic requirements for inclusion in their review. These studies evaluated a variety of prevention strategies, ranging from lectures on HIV risk and safer sex practices to community interventions. The focus of these interventions varied as well. Most focused on interpersonal skills, others also focused on personal skills, self-esteem, social acceptability, and responsibility.

Overall these studies showed that HIV interventions are capable of reducing risk among MSM. The summary effect calculated for these nine studies indicated that compared to other men in similar conditions, 26 percent fewer men reported unprotected anal sex after receiving an intervention. The few studies that measured outcomes at multiple endpoints showed that the intervention effects were stable across six-month intervals. Small-group interventions with longer duration appeared to be more effective. Risk reduction of such a magnitude can have important public health implications, especially if it is realized in settings with high prevalences of HIV and STI.

Although studies show that HIV prevention works, not only are rates of high-risk sexual behavior increasing among MSM but actual infections are increasing as well. How is that possible? Elford and Hart (2003) tried to answer this question. One reason could be that what was proven to be effective in ideal circumstances—in which experimental evaluations usually take place—does not necessarily have to work in a real-life setting. Furthermore, they argue, MSM face a risk environment today that is different from the one they faced in the 1980s and early 1990s. The availability of more effective HIV treatment may have decreased the sense of urgency for safe sex.

Sexual Health Promotion in Clinical Care

Clinical care offers important opportunities for sexual health promotion (Maurice, 1999; Nusbaum & Hamilton, 2002; Ross, Channon-Little, & Rosser, 2000). Health care providers are likely to be the first people with whom individuals bring up sexual health problems, and clients seeking care expect health care providers to be informed about sexual health issues. Sexuality may come up in relation to other problems a patient or client has. Current problems such as depression or anxiety might result from experiences with sexual abuse. Studies show that when practitioners take the initiative and address sexuality, more patients will report sexual problems (Nusbaum & Hamilton, 2002; van Lankveld & van Koeveringe, 2003).

Studies show that opportunities for sexual health promotion in clinical care are not always optimally used (Haley, Maheux, Rivard, & Gervais, 1999). There are various reasons why this is so. Maurice (1999) lists several of them. A major reason for not asking sexual health questions is that practitioners do not know what to do with the answers they get. Addressing sexuality is often seen as opening Pandora's box or "a can of worms" (Gott, Galena, Hinchliff, & Elford, 2004). Practitioners might also feel that the issue is too personal or that an obvious justification is lacking, and thus they avoid talking about sexuality because they don't want to offend clients. Some practitioners seem to fear a sexual misconduct charge. Sexual issues may be perceived as of dubious importance because patients have more pressing concerns; such a perception may not correspond with that of patients themselves, however. Sometimes practitioners experience barriers in discussing sexuality with specific patient groups, either because of a lack of information or a sense of discomfort. Talking might be difficult when the patient and the practitioner are of different genders, belong to different ethnic groups, or have different sexual orientations; age differences can also act as a barrier (Gott et al., 2004). Practitioners might also feel that it is not part of their job to get involved with their patients' sexual health.

There are also various structural reasons why health care providers do not address sexual health issues. One of them is the limited time practitioners have available. There are also factors that go beyond the individual practitioner. Morin et al. (2004), for instance, showed that when promoting safer sex is part of the mission of a health care institution, such promotion is practiced more frequently.

In this section I first present some general guidelines for discussing sexuality with patients. Subsequently, I describe a general model for proactive sexual health history taking (Nusbaum & Hamilton, 2002) and present a tested script for safer sex promotion, as an example of how sexual health promotion can be done.

General Guidelines

In principal, discussing sexual health in clinical care requires the same attitudes and skills as discussing other health issues. Because the way questions are asked might be more troubling to patients than the actual issue discussed, it is worthwhile to describe some general approaches that will facilitate addressing sexual issues (see Maurice, 1999; Nusbaum & Hamilton, 2002; Ross et al., 2000, for a more extensive discussion).

Because sexuality is usually experienced as private and sensitive, a practitioner might want to start with asking permission to address sexuality. By asking permission the practitioner shows respect for the feelings of the patient; the patient is in control, and the practitioner does not have to worry about being intrusive. Giving an explanation for addressing sexuality might make it more acceptable in the eyes of the patient. The practitioner's taking the initiative shows patients that discussing sexuality is legitimate. This might help a patient with volunteering information that he or she would not otherwise have shared.

The language that is used to discuss sexuality requires specific attention. Taking a matter-of-fact approach and avoiding euphemisms seem to be most productive. Practitioners should make sure that patients understand the terms they use and inquire when patients use words or expressions that the practitioner doesn't know. Discomfort or embarrassment might prevent the patient from asking for clarifications. Language problems are more likely when the patient and the practitioner belong to different groups in terms of ethnicity or sexual orientation. For example, by using the word *partner*, rather than *husband* or *wife*, practitioners avoid assumptions about patients' sexual orientation. Such assumptions are likely to discourage nonheterosexual people from disclosing sexual information.

Potential embarrassment in the patient might be overcome by giving factual information before asking specific questions. For instance, stating that some people have multiple sex partners and others live monogamously facilitates volunteering that one has multiple partners. Given the privacy around sexuality, people typically do not know how other people live their sexual lives, and might be anxious that their own fantasies or behaviors are abnormal. Disclosure will further be facilitated if patients are convinced that the information that they are sharing is dealt with confidentially. Confidentiality is of particular importance in contacts with adolescents and patients with multiple partners. In some specific cases a practitioner might expect that he or she might elicit information that according to criminal law has to be reported to the appropriate authorities. If so, it is advisable to warn the patient in advance about the limits of confidentiality.

Crucial to ongoing disclosure is a nonjudgmental attitude on the side of health practitioners. Judgmental attitudes can be expressed in various ways. Practitioners can convey what they consider to be socially desirable answers by the way they ask questions. Practitioners might also express a negative attitude toward a patient because of the group that patient belongs to and the associated lifestyle. Furthermore, practitioners might respond negatively to sexual information that a patient volunteers. Negative judgment can be expressed verbally but also physically, for instance by showing negative surprise or disgust.

Taking Sexual Histories

Nusbaum and Hamilton (2002) describe two approaches to the sexual health interview: a screening or abbreviated method (Figure 7.1) and an in-depth approach (Exhibit 7.1). They recommend the in-depth approach when the patient's sexual history seems to be directly related to the chief complaint. Both approaches can be followed by the preventive sexual health questions listed in Exhibit 7.2.

Nusbaum and Hamilton's (2002) approach is general and applicable in most situations. There are also models for history taking that focus on specific situations.

FIGURE 7.1. SCREENING FOR SEXUAL HEALTH HISTORY.

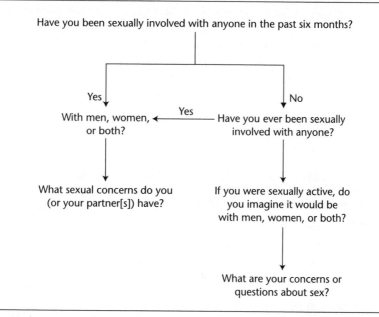

Source: Nusbaum & Hamilton, 2002.

EXHIBIT 7.1. QUESTIONS FOR A DETAILED SEXUAL HISTORY.

- Are you currently sexually active? Have you ever been?
- Are your partners men, women, or both?
- How many partners have you had in the past month? Six months? Lifetime?
- How satisfied with your (or your partner's) sexual functioning are you?
- Has there been any change in your (or your partner's) sexual desire or the frequency of sexual activity?
- Do you have, or have you ever had, any risk factors for HIV? (List blood transfusions, needlestick injuries, IV drug use, STDs, partners who may have placed you at risk.)
- Have you ever had any sexually related diseases?
- Have you ever been tested for HIV? Would you like to be?
- What do you do to protect yourself from contracting HIV?
- What method do you use for contraception?
- Are you trying to become pregnant (or father a child)?
- Do you participate in oral sex? Anal sex?
- Do you or your partner(s) use any particular devices or substances to enhance your sexual pleasure?
- Do you ever have pain with intercourse?
- Women: Do you have any difficulty achieving orgasm?
- Men: Do you have any difficulty obtaining and maintaining an erection? Difficulty with ejaculation?
- Do you have any questions or concerns about your sexual functioning?
- Is there anything about your (or your partner's) sexual activity (as individuals or as a couple) that you would like to change?

Note: HIV = human immunodeficiency virus; STDs = sexually transmitted diseases.

Source: Nusbaum & Hamilton, 2002.

EXHIBIT 7.2. PREVENTIVE SEXUAL HEALTH QUESTIONS.

- How do you protect yourself from HIV and other STDs?
- Have you ever been tested for HIV? Would you like to be?
- Do you use anything to prevent pregnancy? Are you satisfied with that method?
- Have you ever been immunized against hepatitis? Would you like to be?

Note: HIV = human immunodeficiency virus; STDs = sexually transmitted diseases.

Source: Nusbaum & Hamilton, 2002.

Ross and colleagues (2000) present sets of concrete questions to address topics such as menstruation, pregnancies, anorgasmia, sexual dysfunctions, STDs, and compulsive sexual behavior.

Sexual history taking can be an integral part of a broad screening strategy that includes other activities, such as serological tests and physical examinations. An extensive program for health care screening for men who have sex with men is described by Knight (2004).

A Strategy for Individual Safer Sex Promotion

Some people will profit from receiving support from a health care provider in acquiring or maintaining safer sex practices. One of the strategies for giving such support is motivational interviewing. Predominantly used to help people solve problems such as drinking and smoking, motivational interviewing is based on relationship-building principles of humanistic therapy and the more active cognitive-behavioral strategies. Taking into account stages of change, it makes use of the following four strategies: (1) expressing sympathy, (2) developing discrepancy between desired and actual behavior, (3) rolling with resistance, and (4) supporting self-efficacy (Burke, Arkowitz, & Menchola, 2003). Motivational interviewing has been administered in individual as well as group sessions, either as the only strategy or in combination with other approaches (cf. Harding, Dockrell, Dockrell, & Corrigan, 2001). Evidence for the effectiveness of this approach to address HIV risk behavior is mixed.

Motivational interviewing has been used to reduce risk in economically disadvantaged urban women (Carey et al., 1997) and in HIV-positive persons (Fisher et al., 2004). Harding et al. (2001) adopted motivational interviewing for reduction of HIV risk among gay men in commercial and public sex settings. Strategies developed in these studies can be easily adapted to specific situations. I summarize the approach of Harding and colleagues to give an impression of how motivational interviewing might work in safer sex promotion. Harding and colleagues wanted their approach to be appropriate for gay men in different stages of change. They also did not want to prescribe one form of safer sex behavior. The prevention had to be brief and had to provide participants with follow-up resources.

As an opening strategy, a peer educator asks a man some simple nonthreatening demographic questions. Subsequently, the man is asked to think about and identify all the places where he has had sexual contact in the preceding year. Then he is asked to indicate in what way he would like to practice safer sex. After having expressed empathy and permission by making clear that sometimes there are circumstances in which men ("we") are not always safe, the client is asked to express cognitions that he used to resolve the cognitive dissonance in situations in which he took a certain risk. Then the man is asked how many times in the past year he did not adhere to his personal safer sex strategy. The session ends with an open-ended conversation, in which the peer educator uses the elicited information and helps the man in looking at his risk taking and in identifying appropriate means for change.

Fisher and colleagues (2004), who used motivational interviewing in a clinical setting, added some components to this strategy. In their protocol the clinician also assesses the patient's readiness to change the behavior and the patient's confidence that he or she will be able to do so. To reinforce the behavioral change goal that the patient has identified, the clinician writes it down on a prescription pad and then hands it to the patient.

Summary

There is not only a great need for sexual health promotion; there are also diverse opportunities to promote sexual health effectively. In whatever way a person is involved in the promotion of sexual health, he or she always adopts a normative position. A sexual rights perspective might be helpful for staying on track. Substantial support exists for the effectiveness of sexual health interventions. New strategies are likely to be most effective when they build on existing evidence and acknowledge the needs of the people involved. Interventions can focus on individual people or groups or can be addressed to communities. They may also be structural. One of the most crucial barriers to sexual health will remain the fact people do not engage in sex for health reasons. Approaches that positively acknowledge pleasure, lust, and intimacy are consequently more likely to be effective than approaches that stress sickness and disease. (See Exhibit 7.3 on page 252 for helpful resources.)

References

Adler, M. (2003). Sexual health. *British Medical Journal, 327,* 62–63.

Agha, S., & Van Rossem, R. (2004). Impact of a school-based peer sexual health intervention on normative beliefs, risk perceptions, and sexual behavior of Zambian adolescents. *Journal of Adolescent Health, 34*(5), 441–452.

Alan Guttmacher Institute. (2004). *U.S. teenage pregnancy statistics: Overall trends: Trends by race and ethnicity and state-by-state information.* New York: Author.

Amaro, H., Raj, A., & Reed, E. (2001). Women's sexual health: The need for feminist analyses in public health in the decade of behavior. *Psychology of Women Quarterly, 25*(4), 324–334.

Armstrong, D. (2000). Social theorizing about health and illness. In G. L. Albrecht, R. Fitzpatrick, & A. C. Scrimshaw (Eds.), *Handbook of social studies in health and medicine* (pp. 24–35). Thousand Oaks, CA: Sage.

Arrington, R., Cofrancesco, J., & Wu, A. W. (2004). Questionnaires to measure sexual quality of life. *Quality of Life Research, 13*, 1643–1658.

As-Sanie, S., Gantt, A., & Rosenthal, M. S. (2004). Pregnancy prevention in adolescents. *American Family Physician, 70*(8), 1517–1524.

Ball, J., Pelton, J., Forehand, R., Long, N., & Wallace, S. A. (2004). Methodological overview of the Parents Matter! program. *Journal of Child and Family Studies, 13*(1), 21–34.

Bancroft, J. (2002). The medicalization of female sexual dysfunction: The need for caution. *Archives of Sexual Behavior, 31*(5), 451–455.

Barak, A., & Fisher, W. A. (2003). Experience with an Internet-based, theoretically grounded educational resource for the promotion of sexual and reproductive health. *Sexual and Relationship Therapy, 18*(3), 293–308.

Barrett, M. (1991). Sexual health education: Can a new vision avoid repetition of past errors? *SIECCAN Journal, 6*(4), 3–15.

Bartholomew, L. K., Parcel, G. S., Kok, G., & Gottlieb, N. H. (2001). *Intervention mapping. Designing theory- and evidence-based health promotion programs.* Mountain View, CA: Mayfield.

Bockting, W. O., Robinson, B. E., & Rosser, B. R. (1998). Transgender HIV prevention: A qualitative needs assessment. *AIDS Care, 10*(4), 505–525.

Bolding, G., Davis, M., Sherr, L., Hart, G., & Elford, J. (2004). Use of gay Internet sites and views about online health promotion among men who have sex with men. *AIDS Care, 16*(8), 993–1001.

Brandt, A. M. (1987). *No magic bullet: A social history of venereal disease in the United States since 1880* (Exp. ed.). New York: Oxford University Press.

Brotman, S., Ryan, B., Jalbert, Y., & Rowe, B. (2002). The impact of coming out on health and health care access: The experiences of gay, lesbian, bisexual and two-spirit people. *Journal of Health & Social Policy, 15*(1), 1–29.

Burke, B. L., Arkowitz, H., & Menchola, M. (2003). The efficacy of motivational interviewing: A meta-analysis of controlled clinical trials. *Journal of Consulting and Clinical Psychology, 71*(5), 843–861.

Burris, S., Lazzarini, Z., & Loff, B. (2001). Are human rights good for your health? *Lancet, 358*, 1901.

Calamidas, E. G. (1997). Promoting healthy sexuality among older adults: Educational challenges for health professionals. *Journal of Sex Education and Therapy, 22*(2), 45–49.

Carey, M. P., Maisto, S. A., Kalichman, S. C., Forsyth, A. D., Wright, E. M., & Johnson, B. T. (1997). Enhancing motivation to reduce the risk of HIV infection for economically disadvantaged urban women. *Journal of Consulting and Clinical Psychology, 65*(4), 531–541.

Carnes, P. (2003). The anatomy of arousal: Three Internet portals. *Sexual and Relationship Therapy, 18*(3), 309–328.

Centers for Disease Control and Prevention. (2002). Diagnosis and reporting of HIV and AIDS in states with HIV/AIDS surveillance—United States, 1994–2000. *Morbidity and Mortality Weekly Report, 51*, 595–598.

Centers for Disease Control and Prevention. (2004a). High-risk sexual behavior by HIV-positive men who have sex with men—16 sites, United States, 2000–2002. *Morbidity and Mortality Weekly Report, 53*(38), 891–894.

Centers for Disease Control and Prevention. (2004b). *Sexually transmitted disease surveillance, 2003.* Atlanta, GA: U.S. Department of Health and Human Services.

Centers for Disease Control and Prevention, National Center for Injury Prevention and Control. (2005). *Sexual violence: Fact sheet.* Retrieved September 2005 from www.cdc.gov/ncipc/factsheets/svfacts.htm

Coleman, E. (2002). Promoting sexual health and responsible sexual behavior: An introduction. *Journal of Sex Research, 39*(1), 3–6.

Cook, R. J. (1995). Human rights and reproductive self-determination. *American University Law Review, 44,* 975–1016.

Crosby, R. A., & Yarber, W. L. (2001). Perceived versus actual knowledge about correct condom use among U.S. adolescents: Results from a national study. *Journal of Adolescent Health, 28*(5), 415–420.

Davidson, O., Fenton, K. A., & Mahtani, A. (2002). Race and cultural issues in sexual health. In D. Miller & J. Green (Eds.), *The psychology of sexual health* (pp. 83–94). London: Blackwell Science.

Davis, C. M., Yarber, W. L., Bauserman, R., Schreer, G., & Davis, S. L. (Eds.). (1998). *Handbook of sexuality-related measures.* Thousand Oaks, CA: Sage.

Derogatis, L. R. (1998). The Derogatis Interview for Sexual Functioning. In C. M. Davis, W. L. Yarber, R. Bauserman, G. Schreer, & S. L. Davis (Eds.), *Handbook of sexuality-related measures* (pp. 267–269). Thousand Oaks, CA: Sage.

DiClemente, R. J. (2001). Development of programmes for enhancing sexual health. *Lancet, 358,* 1828–1829.

Dittus, P., Miller, K. S., Kotchick, B. A., & Forehand, R. (2004). Why Parents Matter! The conceptual basis for a community-based HIV prevention program for the parents of African American youth. *Journal of Child and Family Studies, 13*(1), 5–20.

Easton, D. E., O'Sullivan, L. F., & Parker, R. G. (2002). Sexualities and sexual health: Lessons from history. In D. Miller & J. Green (Eds.), *The psychology of sexual health* (pp. 53–67). London: Blackwell Science.

Ebrahim, S. H., McKenna, M. T., & Marks, J. S. (2005). Sexual behaviour: Related adverse health burden in the United States. *Sexually Transmitted Infections, 81,* 38–40.

Edwards, W. M., & Coleman, E. (2004). Defining sexual health: A descriptive overview. *Archives of Sexual Behavior, 33*(3), 189–195.

El-Bassel, N., Witte, S. S., Gilbert, L., Sormanti, M., Moreno, C., Pereira, L., et al. (2001). HIV prevention for intimate couples: A relationship-based model. *Families, Systems and Health, 19*(4), 379–395.

Elford, J., & Hart, G. (2003). If HIV prevention works, why are rates of high-risk sexual behavior increasing among MSM? *AIDS Education & Prevention, 15*(4), 294–308.

Fisher, J. D., Cornmand, D. H., Osborn, C. Y., Amico, K. R., Fisher, W. A., & Friedland, G. A. (2004). Clinician-initiated HIV risk reduction intervention for HIV-positive persons: Formative research, acceptability, and fidelity of the Options Project. *Journal of Acquired Immune Deficiency Syndromes, 37* (Suppl. 2), S78–S87.

Flores, S. A., & Hartlaub, M. G. (1998). Reducing rape-myth acceptance in male college students: A meta-analysis of intervention studies. *Journal of College Student Development, 39*(5), 438–448.

Forrest, K. A. (2001). Men's reproductive and sexual health. *Journal of American College Health, 49*(6), 253–266.

Forrest, S., Strange, V., & Oakley, A. (2004). What do young people want from sex education? The results of a needs assessment from a peer-led sex education programme. *Culture, Health & Sexuality, 6*(4), 337–354.

Giami, A. (2002). Sexual health: The emergence, development, and diversity of a concept. *Annual Review of Sex Research, 13,* 1–35.

Gott, M., Galena, E., Hinchliff, S., & Elford, H. (2004). "Opening a can of worms": GP and practice nurse barriers to talking about sexual health in primary care. *Family Practice, 21*(5), 528–536.

Haley, N., Maheux, B., Rivard, M., & Gervais, A. (1999). Sexual health risk assessment and counseling in primary care: How involved are general practitioners and obstetrician-gynecologists? *American Journal of Public Health, 89*(6), 899–902.

Harding, R., Dockrell, M.J.D., Dockrell, J., & Corrigan, N. (2001). Motivational interviewing for HIV risk reduction among gay men in commercial and public sex settings. *AIDS Care, 13*(4), 493–501.

Harris, S. M., Dersch, C. A., Kimball, T. G., Marshall, J. P., & Negretti, M. A. (1999). Internet resources for older adults with sexual concerns. *Journal of Sex Education and Therapy, 24*(3), 183–188.

Hays, R. B., Rebochook, G. M., & Kegeles, S. M. (2003). The Mpowerment Project: Community-building with young gay and bisexual men to prevent HIV1. *American Journal of Community Psychology, 31*(3–4), 301–312.

Herek, G. M., Gillis, J., & Cogan, J. C. (1999). Psychological sequelae of hate-crime victimization among lesbian, gay, and bisexual adults. *Journal of Consulting and Clinical Psychology, 67*(6), 945–951.

Holtgrave, D. R., & Pinkerton, S. D. (2003). Economic implications of the failure to reduce incident HIV infections by 50% by 2005 in the United States. *Journal of Acquired Immune Deficiency Syndromes, 33*, 171–174.

Hunt, A. (1999). *Governing morals: A social history of moral regulation.* New York: Cambridge University Press.

Johnson, W. D., Hedges, L. V., Ramirez, G., Semaan, S., Norman, L. R., Sogolow, E., et al. (2002). HIV prevention research for men who have sex with men: A systematic review and meta-analysis. *Journal of Acquired Immune Deficiency Syndromes, 30* (Suppl. 1), S118–S129.

Kalmuss, D. (2004). Nonvolitional sex and sexual health. *Archives of Sexual Behavior, 33*(3), 197–209.

Keller, S. N., & Brown, J. D. (2002). Media interventions to promote responsible sexual behavior. *Journal of Sex Research, 39*(1), 67–72.

Keller, S., & Buchannan, D. C. (1993). Sexuality and disability: An overview. In M. Nagler (Ed.), *Perspectives on disability: Text and readings on disability* (2nd ed., pp. 227–234). Palo Alto, CA: Health Markets Research.

Keller, S. N., Labelle, H., Karimi, N., & Gupta, S. (2002). STD/HIV prevention for teenagers: A look at the Internet universe. *Journal of Health Communication, 7*(4), 341–353.

Kelly, J. A. (1995). *Changing HIV risk behavior: Practical strategies.* New York: Guilford Press.

Kippax, S. (2003). Sexual health interventions are unsuitable for experimental evaluations. In J. M. Stephenson, J. Imrie, & C. Bonell (Eds.), *Effective sexual health interventions: Issues in experimental evaluations* (pp. 17–34). New York: Oxford University Press.

Kirby, D. (2001). *Emerging answers: Research findings on programs to reduce teen pregnancy.* Washington, DC: National Campaign to Prevent Teen Pregnancy.

Kirby, D. (2002). *Do abstinence-only programs delay the initiation of sex among young people and reduce teen pregnancy?* Washington, DC: National Campaign to Prevent Teen Pregnancy.

Klausner, J. D., Levine, D. K., & Kent, C. K. (2004). Internet-based site-specific interventions for syphilis prevention among gay and bisexual men. *AIDS Care, 16*(8), 964–970.

Knight, D. (2004). Health care screening for men who have sex with men. *American Family Physician, 69*(9), 2149–2156.

Laumann, E. O., Paik, A., & Rosen, R. C. (1999). Sexual dysfunction in the United States: Prevalence and predictors. *JAMA, 281*, 537–544.

Lewis, L. J., & Kertzner, R. (2004). Examining sexual health discourses in a racial/ethnic context. *Archives of Sexual Behavior, 33*(3), 223–234.

Lintz, K., Moynihan, C., Steginga, S., Norman, A., Eeles, R., Huddart, R., et al. (2003). Prostate cancer patients' support and psychological care needs: Survey from a non-surgical oncology clinic. *Psycho-Oncology, 12*(8), 769–783.

Loeb, T. B., Williams, J. K., Carmona, J. V., Rivkin, I., Wyatt, G. E., Chin, D., et al. (2002). Child sexual abuse: Associations with the sexual functioning of adolescents and adults. *Annual Review of Sex Research, 13*, 307–345.

Lottes, I. L. (2002). Sexual health policies in other industrialized countries: Are there lessons for the United States? *Journal of Sex Research, 39*(1), 79–83.

Maurice, W. L. (1999). *Sexual medicine in primary care.* St. Louis, MO: Mosby.

Melendez, R. M., Hoffman, S., Exner, T., Leu, C.-S., & Ehrhardt, A. A. (2003). Intimate partner violence and safer sex negotiation: Effects of a gender-specific intervention. *Archives of Sexual Behavior, 32*(6), 499–511.

Meschke, L. L., Bartholomae, S., & Zentall, S. R. (2002). Adolescent sexuality and parent-adolescent processes: Promoting healthy teen choices. *Journal of Adolescent Health, 31* (Suppl. 6), 264–279.

Metz, M. E., & Seifert, M. H. (1993). Differences in men's and women's sexual health needs and expectations of physicians. *Canadian Journal of Human Sexuality, 2*(2), 53–59.

Miller, A. M. (2000). Sexual but not reproductive: Exploring the junctions and disjunctions of sexual and reproductive rights. *Health and Human Rights, 4*, 68–109.

Miller, D., & Green, J. (Eds.). (2002). *The psychology of sexual health.* Oxford, England: Blackwell Science.

Miller, K. E., Zylstra, R. G., & Standridge, J. B. (2000). The geriatric patient: A systematic approach to maintaining health. *American Family Physician, 61*, 1089–1104.

Milligan, M. S., & Neufeldt, A. H. (2001). The myth of asexuality: A survey of social and empirical evidence. *Sexuality & Disability, 19*(2), 91–109.

Morin, S. F., Koester, K. A., Steward, W. T., Maiorana, A., McLaughlin, M., Myers, J. J., et al. (2004). Missed opportunities: Prevention with HIV-infected patients in clinical care settings. *Journal of Acquired Immune Deficiency Syndromes, 36*, 960–966.

The national strategy for sexual health and HIV. (2001). London: Department of Health.

Nusbaum, M.R.H., & Hamilton, C. D. (2002). The proactive sexual health history. *American Family Physician, 66*(9), 1705–1712.

Paine-Andrews, A., Fisher, J. L., Harris, K. J., Lewis, R. K., Williams, E. L., Vincent, M. L., et al. (2000). Some experiential lessons in supporting and evaluating community-based initiatives for preventing adolescent pregnancy. *Health Promotion Practices, 1*(1), 67–76.

Parker, R. (2001). Sexuality, culture, and power in HIV/AIDS research. *Annual Review of Anthropology, 30*, 163–179.

Parker, R., & Ehrhardt, A. A. (2001). Through an ethnographic lens: Ethnographic methods, comparative analysis, and HIV/AIDS research. *AIDS & Behavior, 5*, 105–114.

Petchesky, R. P. (2000). Sexual rights: Inventing a concept, mapping an international practice. In R. G. Parker, R. M. Barbosa, & P. Aggleton (Eds.), *Framing the sexual subject: The politics of gender, sexuality, and power* (pp. 81–103). Berkeley: University of California Press.

Philliber, S., Williams Kaye, J., Herrling, S., & West, E. (2002). Preventing pregnancy and improving health care access among teenagers: An evaluation of the Children's Aid Society-Carrera Program. *Perspectives on Sexual and Reproductive Health, 34*(5), 244–251.

Planned Parenthood. (n.d.). *HPV: The most common sexually transmitted virus.* Retrieved October 28, 2005, from http://www.plannedparenthood.org/pp2/portal/files/portal/medicalinfo/sti/fact-HPV-virus.xml

Promotion of sexual health: Recommendations for action. (2000). Proceedings of a Regional Consultation Convened by Pan American Health Organization and World Health Organization, Antigua Guatemala, Guatemala. Washington, DC: Pan American Health Organization.

Rew, L., Fouladi, R. T., & Yockey, R. D. (2002). Sexual health practices of homeless youth. *Journal of Nursing Scholarship, 34*(2), 139–145.

Ross, M. W., Channon-Little, L. D., & Rosser, B.R.S. (2000). *Sexual health concerns: Interviewing and history taking for health practitioners* (2nd ed.). Philadelphia: Davis.

Rubin, G. (1984). Thinking sex: Notes for a radical theory of the politics of sexuality. In C. Vance (Ed.), *Pleasure and danger: Exploring female sexuality* (pp. 267–319). New York: Routledge.

Sandfort, T.G.M., & Ehrhardt, A. A. (2004). Sexual health: A useful public health paradigm or a moral imperative? *Archives of Sexual Behavior, 33*(3), 181–187.

Schaalma, H. P., Abraham, C., Gillmore, M. R., & Kok, G. (2004). Sex education as health promotion: What does it take? *Archives of Sexual Behavior, 33*(3), 259–269.

Schmidt, G. (1987). *Sexual health within a societal context.* Working group on concepts of sexual health. Euro, 5–7 May, 1987. ICP/MCH 521–13, 9614F.

Seabloom, W., Seabloom, M. E., Seabloom, E., Barron, R., & Hendrickson, S. (2003). A 14- to 24-year longitudinal study of a comprehensive sexual health model treatment program for adolescent sex offenders: Predictors of successful completion and subsequent criminal recidivism. *International Journal of Offender Therapy and Comparative Criminology, 47*(4), 468–481.

Seidman, A. (2001). From identity to queer politics: Shifts in normative heterosexuality and the meaning of citizenship. *Citizenship Studies, 5,* 321–328.

Stephenson, J. M., Imrie, J., & Bonell, C. (Eds.). (2003). *Effective sexual health interventions: Issues in experimental evaluations.* New York: Oxford University Press.

Tang, T. S., Solomon, L. J., Yeh, C., & Worden, J. K. (1999). The role of cultural variables in breast self-examination and cervical cancer screening behavior in young Asian women living in the United States. *Journal of Behavioral Medicine, 22*(5), 419–436.

Tiefer, L. (1996). The medicalization of sexuality: Conceptual, normative, and professional issues. *Annual Review of Sex Research, 7,* 252–282.

Tiefer, L. (2004). *Sex is not a natural act and other essays.* Boulder, CO: Westview Press.

Turner, B. S. (2000). The history of the changing concepts of health and illness: Outline of a general model of illness categories. In G. L. Albrecht, R. Fitzpatrick, & S. C. Scrimshaw (Eds.), *Handbook of social studies in health and medicine* (pp. 9–23). Thousand Oaks, CA: Sage.

U.S. Department of Health and Human Services. (2000a). *Child maltreatment 1998: Reports from the states to the National Child Abuse and Neglect Data System.* Washington, DC: U.S. Government Printing Office.

U.S. Department of Health and Human Services. (2000b). *Healthy people 2010* (2nd ed.). Retrieved September 2005 from http://www.healthypeople.gov

U.S. Department of Health and Human Services. (2001). *The Surgeon General's call to action to promote sexual health and responsible sexual behavior.* Rockville, MD: Office of the Surgeon General.

van Lankveld, J. J., & van Koeveringe, G. A. (2003, April). Predictive validity of the Golombok Rust Inventory of Sexual Satisfaction (GRISS) for the presence of sexual dysfunctions within a Dutch urological population. *International Journal of Impotence Research, 15*(2), 110–116.

Vance, C. S. (1991). Anthropology rediscovers sexuality: A theoretical comment. *Social Science & Medicine, 33,* 875–884.

Vincent, C. (2002). Health challenges for older women: Some implications for sexual health. *Sexual and Relationship Therapy, 17*(3), 241–252.

World Health Organization. (n.d.). *Gender and reproductive rights.* Retrieved December 6, 2003, from http://www.who.int/reproductive-health/gender/sexual_health.html

Wylie, K. R. (2001). Is normal sexual function desirable when promoting sexual health? *Sexual and Relationship Therapy, 16*(4), 317–319.

Zarcadoolas, C., Pleasant, A., & Greer, D. S. (2003). Elaborating a definition of health literacy: A commentary. *Journal of Health Communication, 8* (Suppl. 1), 119–120.

EXHIBIT 7.3. HELPFUL RESOURCES.

Books

This chapter references a number of relevant books, reports, and articles. Two books deserve specific attention, because of their focus on health care interactions:

> Ross, M. W., Channon-Little, L. D., & Rosser, B.R.S. (2000). *Sexual health concerns: Interviewing and history taking for health practitioners* (2nd ed.). Philadelphia: Davis. This book informs about various sexual health issues, but also gives concrete and practical examples of which questions to ask in which situations.

> Maurice, W. L. (1999). *Sexual medicine in primary care.* St. Louis, MO: Mosby. This book is more extensive and also discusses treatment of various sexual health problems.

Assessment Tools

There are numerous questionnaires for assessing sexual functioning. Arrington, Cofrancesco, and Wu (2004) reviewed fifty-seven such measures to be used in clinical (and research) practice (see also Davis, Yarber, Bauserman, Schreer, & Davis, 1998). Forty-five of these questionnaires measured solely sexual functioning; the remaining twelve were more general. In reviewing the applicability, reliability, and validity of the various instruments, the authors concluded that most of these questionnaires assess such common dimensions as sexual interest, desire, excitement/arousal, frequency, performance, importance, and satisfaction. Furthermore, most of the questionnaires were gender specific and could be filled out only by heterosexual men or women. Questionnaires are also available for healthy or for chronically ill populations. Few scales are supported, however, by sufficient evidence about their reliability and validity.

One of the general measures positively reviewed by Arrington and colleagues (2004) is the Derogatis Interview for Sexual Functioning (Derogatis, 1998). This instrument is designed to provide an estimate of the quality of an individual's current sexual functioning. It consists of twenty-six questions and covers the following domains: (1) sexual cognition/fantasy, (2) sexual arousal, (3) sexual behavior/experience, (4) orgasm, and (5) sexual drive/relationship. It is available in distinct, gender-keyed versions for men and women. Outcomes can be assessed on three distinct levels: the discrete item itself, the general functional domains, and the global summary. The availability of gender-specific norms underscores the utility of this scale.

EXHIBIT 7.3. HELPFUL RESOURCES, Cont'd.

Web Sites

The following list contains the Web sites of a variety of organizations active in the field of sexual health promotion:

Alan Guttmacher Institute, http://www.agi-usa.org

American Association of Sex Educators, Counselors, and Therapists (AASECT), http://www.aasect.org

The Kinsey Institute, http://www.indiana.edu/~kinsey

Planned Parenthood, http://www.plannedparenthood.org

San Francisco State University, Program in Human Sexuality Studies, http://hmsx.sfsu.edu/index.html

Sexuality Information and Education Council of the United States, http://www.siecus.org

Society for the Scientific Study of Sexuality, http://www.sexscience.org

Humboldt-Universität zu Berlin, Magnus Hirschfeld Archive for Sexology, http://www2.hu-berlin.de/sexology

CHAPTER EIGHT

ORAL HEALTH

Joan I. Gluch
Susanne K. Giorgio
Barbara J. Steinberg

In 2000, *Oral Health in America,* the first report of the U.S. surgeon general on oral health, was released (U.S. Department of Health and Human Services [USDHHS], 2000b). The development and publication of this report marks a turning point; it acknowledges oral health as a key, interrelated component of general health care. The term *oral health* is used to indicate a broad view of health of the entire oral-facial complex, rather than only the health of the teeth. Health care professionals must realize the critical, interrelated role of oral health care within general health care and health promotion. For many clients, oral health issues often take a primary role in their perception of their quality of life and ideal health image. For example, oral health concerns (such as having a nice smile, physical attractiveness, the ability to eat and swallow, and freedom from mouth pain) are normally reflected in clients' discussions of their ideal health status, appearance, and function. Even when oral health concerns are not identified by clients as a separate issue, health care professionals can initiate these discussions by emphasizing the interrelationship of oral health and other healthy behaviors.

Understanding the connection between a client's oral health status and his or her perceived health status becomes even more important in light of the many health conditions that have manifestations in the mouth and face. The report of the surgeon general emphasizes the oral-facial area as a "mirror of health and disease" because many viral, bacterial, and fungal diseases frequently show lesions in and around the mouth and face (USDHHS, 2000b). The oral tissues also reflect immune status, and both HIV-infected individuals and patients whose immune systems are suppressed may show a number of variable oral lesions, depending on their level of immune function and severity of disease. Health care professionals should ask their patients about their history of oral lesions and any current lesions and should also complete a brief oral assessment for each patient in order to gain insight into a patient's health status. (The connections between health conditions and oral health are presented in more detail later in this chapter, in table format for ready reference.)

Recent research has uncovered early and intriguing associations between oral infections and diabetes, cardiovascular disease and stroke, and preterm delivery and low birth weight (USDHHS, 2000b). The link between diabetes and periodontal infections has received the most attention, and most studies report a greater prevalence and severity of periodontal infections with both type 1 and type 2 diabetes (Mattson & Cerutis, 2001; Ryan, Carnu, & Kamer, 2001). Although the research on the association between oral infections and both cardiovascular diseases (Lowe, 2004) and preterm delivery and low birth weight (Offenbacher, 2004) is in its early and evolving stages, health professionals should carefully monitor the oral health status of their patients with these conditions, with recommendations for frequent dental visits and optimum oral hygiene to promote oral health. Health care professionals should make oral health information an integral component of their health promotion advice to clients. For example, any discussion of medication compliance with clients should include the possible side effect of dry mouth and specific suggestions for optimizing health supportive patterns when little saliva is present in the client's mouth. Reducing the negative effects of the decreased salivary flow and related root decay often associated with dry mouth is a way to increase the client's comfort and overall health status.

Preventive oral health care represents a strong success story in health promotion activities (USDHHS, 2000b). Community water fluoridation and school-based oral health prevention programs, including dental sealant, topical fluoride, and oral hygiene programs have resulted in a general decline in the prevalence of dental decay. Oral health promotion is the connecting link between primary preventive regimens and their acceptance and use by the client, family, and community. The combined efforts of health care professionals and individual clients are needed to ensure that everyone has access to the information and services needed for appropriate oral health behaviors.

However, lack of access to oral health promotion strategies and dental treatment has become a major health issue for many individuals and is reflected in the uneven distribution of the prevalence of both caries and periodontal diseases. In 1997, 65.1 percent of individuals aged two years and older reported that they had visited a dentist within the past year (National Center for Health Statistics, 1996).

Data released by the National Center for Health Statistics (NCHS) in 1996 revealed that among individuals over the age of twenty-five, 64.3 percent of those at or above the poverty level reported dental visits, compared with 35.9 percent below the poverty level. The lower figure for those in poverty, however, is also confounded by issues of education and race or ethnicity. As reported by the 1996 NCHS data, 73.8 percent of those with thirteen or more years of education had visited the dentist in the past year, as compared with 38 percent of those with less than twelve years of education. In addition, this same data set revealed that among white, non-Hispanic individuals, 64 percent had visited a dentist in the past year, compared with 47.3 percent of black individuals and 46.2 percent of Hispanic individuals (NCHS, 1996).

An investigation into the reasons why individuals do not visit the dentist revealed that close to one-half (46.8 percent) report that they have no dental problems, and the next most common reason they cite is that they do not have any teeth (14.3 percent); 13.7 percent of individuals cited financial barriers to receiving dental care (Bloom, Gift, & Jack, 1992). In addition, individuals face many nonfinancial barriers to receiving dental care (Burt & Eklund, 2005). Fearful clients may postpone dental care, which inevitably complicates the care needed and increases the cost. Many individuals lack geographical access to a dentist or lack transportation to get to a dental office; for example, more than half of the homebound elderly have not seen a dentist for ten years (USDHHS, 2000b). In addition, many individuals do not visit a dentist because they do not perceive the need to receive routine preventive care to keep their mouths healthy (Strauss & Hunt, 1993). This is a special problem among older individuals who may not have experienced the benefits of modern preventive dentistry (Dolan & Atchison, 1993).

Negative attitudes and misinformation about oral health among both clients and some health care professionals can limit access to both preventive and restorative oral health care. The general perception of dental care as a discretionary, cosmetic service was reflected in the omission of oral health care as an essential primary care service in discussions regarding health care reform. In addition, a greater number of individuals lack dental insurance (approximately 150 million) than lack health insurance (37 million) (USDHHS, 2000b).

However, some current trends in health promotion have increased the scope of health care, so many policymakers and health care professionals have begun to include oral health as an integral part of general health care. The release of the surgeon general's report *Oral Health in America* in 2000 (USDHHS, 2000b) and of the surgeon general's *National Call to Action to Promote Oral Health* in 2003 (USDHHS, 2003) have helped to reposition oral health as an essential primary health service. In addition the latest edition of *Healthy People 2010* (USDHHS, 2000a) includes oral health as an essential component of the health protection objectives, with seventeen specific oral health objectives to guide and measure health promotion activities, as listed in Exhibit 8.1. Seven objectives focus efforts on the reduction of prevalence of gingivitis, periodontitis, dental caries, and oral cancer among specific population groups at risk; four objectives define risk reduction activities, including the use of community water fluoridation and sealants; and five objectives guide efforts in service provision, including examination utilization rates. These objectives provide guidance for this chapter.

Common Oral Health Issues and Clinical Interventions

The following sections examine the oral health issues of dental caries, periodontal diseases, oral trauma, common oral lesions, and oral cancers and also look at health conditions and medications that may be risk factors for oral disease.

Dental Caries

Although rates of dental caries (tooth decay) for both children and adults in the United States have been declining since 1940, dental caries remain a major persistent problem for many Americans. Dental decay is the most common childhood disease, five times more common than asthma and seven times more common than hay fever (USDHHS, 2000b). Dental caries experience increases as children age. Whereas about one-half (51.6 percent) of children aged five to nine have had dental caries, by age seventeen more than three-quarters (77.9 percent) have had dental caries (NCHS, 1996).

Greater dental decay is also concentrated among poor, minority children (USDHHS, 2000b). Of the youngsters who have experienced dental decay, non-Hispanic African American and Mexican American children and adolescents have higher percentages of decayed surfaces than non-Hispanic Caucasian youth do. Close examination of the data reveals that most of the decayed surfaces in the permanent teeth occur in a relatively small number of children (NCHS, 1996). One out of four children in America is born into poverty; children living below the poverty line (an annual income of $17,000 for a family of four) have more severe and untreated decay than higher-income children do (USDHHS, 2000b). Poverty-level African American and Mexican American children aged two to nine are the most likely to suffer with large amounts of untreated tooth decay (USDHHS, 2000b).

Dental decay continues to be a major oral health problem in adults (Burt & Eklund, 2005; USDHHS, 2000b). Root decay, which is more commonly seen in older adults, is strongly associated with age and the loss of periodontal (gum) attachment,

EXHIBIT 8.1. *HEALTHY PEOPLE 2010* (CHAPTER 21): SUMMARY OF OBJECTIVES FOR ORAL HEALTH.

Goal: Prevent and control oral and craniofacial diseases, conditions, and injuries and improve access to related services.

21-1. Reduce the proportion of children and adolescents who have dental caries experience in their primary or permanent teeth.

21-2. Reduce the proportion of children, adolescents, and adults with untreated dental decay.

21-3. Increase the proportion of adults who have never had a permanent tooth extracted because of dental caries or periodontal disease.

21-4. Reduce the proportion of older adults who have had all their natural teeth extracted.

21-5. Reduce periodontal disease.

21-6. Increase the proportion of oral and pharyngeal cancers detected at the earliest stage.

21-7. Increase the proportion of adults who, in the past 12 months, report having had an examination to detect oral and pharyngeal cancers.

21-8. Increase the proportion of children who have received dental sealants on their molar teeth.

21-9. Increase the proportion of the U.S. population served by community water systems with optimally fluoridated water.

21-10. Increase the proportion of children and adults who use the oral health care system each year.

21-11. Increase the proportion of long-term care residents who use the oral health care system each year.

21-12. Increase the proportion of low-income children and adolescents who received any preventive dental service during the past year.

21-13. Increase the proportion of school-based health centers with an oral health component.

21-14. Increase the proportion of local health departments and community-based health centers, including community, migrant, and homeless health centers, that have an oral health component.

21-15. Increase the number of States and the District of Columbia that have a system for recording and referring infants and children with cleft lips, cleft palates, and other craniofacial anomalies to craniofacial anomaly rehabilitative teams.

21-16. Increase the number of States and the District of Columbia that have an oral and craniofacial health surveillance system.

21-17. Increase the number of Tribal, State (including the District of Columbia), and local health agencies that serve jurisdictions of 250,000 or more persons that have in place an effective public dental health program directed by a dental professional with public health training.

Source: USDHHS, 2000a.

which accompanies periodontal diseases (Burt & Eklund, 2005; USDHHS, 2000b). The 2001 National Institutes of Health (NIH) Consensus Statement noted that 20 percent of the population has 60 percent of the caries (NIH, 2001).

Current research into the causes of dental decay reveals a complex, constant multifactorial process in which the tooth enamel is continuously in a state of losing minerals from the crystalline prisms (demineralization) and repairing the crystalline prisms (remineralization) (National Library of Medicine [NLM], 2001). The bacteria in the biofilm on the tooth metabolize available sugar and produce acids. These acids penetrate the microscopic channels inside the teeth and erode the space between the enamel prisms, driving calcium and phosphate out of the subsurface tissue, thereby demineralizing it (AHCPR). Although the surface of the tooth appears quite hard, these changes in the microscopic channels weaken the tooth. Demineralization occurs first below the surface of the enamel and cannot be detected until it becomes moderately advanced and a white chalky area appears on the tooth surface. At these early stages the decay process can be reversed by raising the low pH in the dental plaque, a step that helps to drive the salivary calcium and phosphate minerals back into the tooth, remineralizing it (Steinberg, 2004). Topical fluoride can also reverse the decay process by providing additional materials for remineralization (Centers for Disease Control and Prevention [CDC], 2001). It is only when the demineralization inside the tooth has advanced and the surface of the tooth has been undermined and broken that dental restorative care is needed to remove the decay and fill the tooth to restore it to function (Harris & Garcia-Godoy, 2004).

Although many patients may complain of having soft teeth and may see that as the cause of dental decay, the mineral content of mature enamel composes about 85 percent of the tooth by volume and 95 percent of the tooth by weight, and this does not vary greatly among individuals (Shore, Robinson, Kirkham, & Brookes, 1995). Shortly after the tooth erupts through the soft tissue into the mouth, minerals in the tooth begin a dynamic exchange of remineralization and demineralization with the surrounding fluids in the oral cavity.

Because of the complex nature of the dental decay process, there is no single preventive agent that will control dental caries (USDHHS, 2000b). Fluoride applied to the tooth, either topically or through systematic ingestion, will be a source of minerals to help reverse the decay process through remineralization (CDC, 2001). Fluoride has its greatest anticaries effect on the smooth surfaces of teeth. Dental sealants can be used to physically block the minute grooves from acid penetration but can be used only on the chewing (occlusal) surfaces of teeth. Current research has highlighted the critical and highly effective role both fluoride and sealants have in reducing decay. All clients with teeth should use at least one source of fluoride and should be evaluated for sealant placement on all unrestored teeth.

Dietary reductions in sugars and cooked starches can reduce the frequency and duration with which oral bacteria can form destructive acids; however, dietary changes are notoriously difficult to bring about, particularly in the present U.S. culture that enjoys sweetened products and where sugar consumption has continued to rise (Darby & Walsh, 2003; Harris & Garcia-Godoy, 2004). Although toothbrushing is often cited by most clients as the major method they use to prevent decay, toothbrushing alone is not effective in removing all microbial plaque, which may hide between the teeth and in small grooves and fissures. The major caries reduction benefit in toothbrushing involves the application of fluoridated toothpaste, which will increase remineralization of enamel prisms (Marinho, Higgins, Logan, & Sheiham, 2003).

Fluoride is essential in promoting remineralization of the subsurface tooth enamel that has been broken down by bacterial acids (CDC, 2001). Fluoridated toothpastes, mouth rinses, and professional gel treatments can provide this topical application of fluoride (Darby & Walsh, 2003; Harris & Garcia-Godoy, 2004). Table 8.1 summarizes the clinical guidelines for topical fluoride products that health care professionals can use to optimize oral health supportive activities. Daily use of sodium fluoride mouth rinses (0.05 percent concentration) can be helpful for clients who are at a moderate risk for dental decay. Clients with orthodontic appliances or who have experienced dental decay within the last year can use these fluoride rinses, which are readily available as over-the-counter products.

TABLE 8.1. FLUORIDE RECOMMENDATIONS FOR CLIENTS TO USE AT HOME TO PREVENT DENTAL DECAY.

Client	Recommendation
All clients	Fluoride toothpaste twice per day
Children aged 6 months to 16 years who do not drink fluoridated water	Sodium fluoride liquid drops or tablet supplementation at 0.25, 0.5, or 1.0 mg concentration per day, based on child's age and amount of fluoride in water system
Children older than 6 years and adults at moderate risk for dental decay	0.05% sodium fluoride mouth rinse once per day
Adults at high risk for dental decay	0.4% stannous fluoride gel or 1.1% sodium fluoride gel used once or twice daily

Source: CDC, 2001.

For individuals at high risk for dental decay, oral health professionals can prescribe home gel treatments, which provide intensive levels of fluoride to remineralize teeth. Both 1.1 percent neutral or 0.4 percent stannous fluoride can be prescribed to reduce the risk of caries development (CDC, 2001). Two types of patients at high risk for decay are those who develop dry mouth because of medications and those who have completed radiation therapy to the head and neck region. Impaired salivary gland function, with little or no saliva produced, increases the risk for decay. The best treatment in these situations is a twice daily application of 1.1 percent sodium fluoride gel, placed in a custom-fitted tray to ensure that an intensive amount of fluoride reaches all surfaces of the teeth without salivary dilution (Harris & Garcia-Godoy, 2004). The area known as the cervical portion, or neck, of the tooth, has a thin layer of enamel covering the underlying dentinal portion of the root and is more readily demineralized than other parts of the tooth. Without the buffering and cleansing effects of saliva, decay can proceed rapidly.

Fluoride treatments can also be provided by oral health care professionals, and these treatments include both 2.0 percent sodium and 1.23 percent acidulated phosphate fluoride, used either as a foam, a gel, or a varnish, placed in a tray or painted directly onto the teeth for one to four minutes (Darby & Walsh, 2003; Harris & Garcia-Godoy, 2004). These professional fluoride treatments are popular among oral health care professionals and provide high amounts of fluoride on a low-frequency basis, especially if given every six months to one year at the dental recall visit. However, the most effective regimens for increasing remineralization and preventing decay include the low-dosage products (toothpastes and mouth rinses) used on a high-frequency basis, at least once daily (CDC, 2001).

Although topical application of fluoride through a variety of fluoride-containing products provides a direct source for remineralization, this action depends on the patient's cooperation in purchasing and using the product. The most cost-effective and simple method to ensure that individuals use fluoride is to fluoridate community water supplies. Two of the *Healthy People 2010* objectives describe goals for fluoride usage to prevent decay. One objective sets a goal of having fluoride in community water systems for at least 75 percent of the nation's population, and the other objective identifies the need to increase the use of professionally and self-administered fluoride products so they are used by at least 85 percent of the individuals who are not drinking optimally fluoridated water.

Since 1945, fluoride has been added to many community water supplies at very low levels (one part per million) to increase access to this proven preventive measure for all children, despite economic and nonfinancial barriers to oral health care. Early studies, completed in the 1950s, documented that children who drank

fluoridated water experienced a reduction in dental decay, with reductions ranging from 30 percent to 60 percent. More recent studies, which take into account
the widespread distribution of fluoride toothpastes and other products, indicate
decay reductions from 20 percent to 40 percent for children and 15 percent to 35
percent for adolescents (Burt & Eklund, 2005; CDC, 2001). Adults who have been
lifelong residents of communities with fluoridated water supplies show a reduction in dental decay of as much as 35 percent (Burt & Eklund, 2005).

Unfortunately, the fluoridation of community water supplies has often created
political controversy, which has limited the number of community water systems
that are optimally fluoridated. In 2002, 67.3 percent of the United States population served by public water systems received fluoridated water (CDC, 2002). Since
1945, when Grand Rapids, Michigan, was the first city to fluoridate its water supply, the political controversy has centered around several key arguments. Claims of
forced mass medication usage, ineffective preventive activity against dental decay,
carcinogenic effects, chemical safety issues in storing and adding the fluoride product to the water, and other toxic effects have been argued by antifluoridationists,
often in an emotional context that is quite compelling to legislators and consumers
unfamiliar with scientific principles and practices (Burt & Eklund, 2005). Multiple
studies have documented the safety and effectiveness of fluoride as a caries-
preventive agent, and a summary report from the U.S. Public Health Service has
confirmed both human safety issues and caries reduction when fluoride is added
to public water supplies (Burt & Eklund, 2005).

Health care professionals should be prepared for the few clients who may state
objections to fluoride recommendations because of concerns related to safety and
effectiveness. A list of helpful resources for oral health promotion resources appears at the end of this chapter (Exhibit 8.2) to provide clients with accurate information from credible, reliable sources on such matters as the safety and efficacy
of water fluoridation in reducing dental decay. In areas of unfluoridated community water supplies, health care professionals should recommend and prescribe
fluoride supplementation for children between the ages of six months and sixteen
years. This systemic fluoride supplementation, either in the form of liquid drops
(sometimes combined with other vitamin supplementation) or tablets, provides a
source of fluoride for the developing permanent teeth (Burt & Eklund, 2005;
Harris & Garcia-Godoy, 2004).

The increased consumption of bottled water in the United States has created
a new challenge in caries risk reduction strategies. Most bottled waters do not contain fluoride, and when they do contain fluoride, there is no consistent information
required or contained on the labels. In the past the majority of water consumed by
Americans came from their home faucets. Consumption now has shifted from the
home faucet to bottled water. Consumers using solely bottled water for con-

sumption and cooking purposes need bottle-labeling information so they can identify the brands that contain an optimal fluoride concentration (CDC, 2001). Health care professionals should ask about the type of water consumed and advise parents to investigate their choice of bottled water further in order to properly assess, plan, and implement a comprehensive fluoride regimen (Levy, Kairitsy, & Warren, 1995; Harris & Garcia-Godoy, 2004). Health care professionals can also recommend that families use the charcoal-based filters found on water pitchers and units that attach to the home water faucet. These charcoal-based systems do not remove fluoride from the water, and often provide consumers with water that has a more acceptable taste and smell.

In addition to fluoride, dental sealants have been documented as a highly effective means of preventing decay by blocking the penetration of demineralizing acids into the enamel grooves of the teeth (CDC, 2001; Darby & Walsh, 2003). The molar and premolar teeth in the posterior region of the mouth contain narrow and uneven grooves and fissures on the occlusal (chewing) surfaces so that these teeth can chew and grind food properly. However, the grooves are often smaller than a single toothbrush bristle, and they frequently trap small pieces of food and retain acids from bacteria, which produce decay. The application of the dental sealant, a plastic resin material that is bonded to the enamel, seals and blocks the grooves so that food particles can be easily brushed from the tooth. Dental sealants have been shown to reduce virtually all decay when the sealant is retained in the occlusal surface of the tooth (Harris & Garcia-Godoy, 2004).

One of the objectives in *Healthy People 2010* is to increase to at least 50 percent the proportion of children who have received dental sealants, which is quite a large increase from the current 11 percent who have received them. Current recommendations are for all children to have their first and second permanent molars sealed as soon as the teeth erupt (Harris & Garcia-Godoy, 2004). The first permanent molars erupt between the ages of five and seven years (and therefore are often called six-year molars, because of the average age at which they erupt into the mouth); the second permanent molars (often called the twelve-year molars) erupt between the ages of eleven and fourteen years. Sealants may be placed only on the chewing surfaces of teeth not previously restored with a filling material, so it is important to seal the teeth as soon as they erupt to prevent decay. Adults should consult with their dentist to determine the appropriateness of sealing their unfilled teeth, depending on their risk for dental decay. Clients who are taking medications that produce dry mouth, who have experienced decay in the past, and who have difficulty in adequately performing their own oral hygiene should be evaluated carefully for sealant placement (Harris & Garcia-Godoy, 2004; Steinberg, 2004).

Nutritional counseling is important to limit the frequency and duration of individuals' consumption of fermentable carbohydrates and to avoid the constant use of mints, gum, candy, or high-sugar drinks. Corn chips, crackers, and pancakes need to be recognized as caries-risky foods along with those "sticky" fermentable carbohydrates (such as caramel and taffy candies) that are retained on tooth surfaces (Harris & Garcia-Godoy, 2004). The best time to eat fermentable carbohydrates is during a meal, when the salivary flow volume is the greatest and can wash the food from the mouth quickly and buffer any acids produced. Foods that have been found to promote less decay include cheese, nuts, popcorn, and sugarless chewing gum. Sugarless chewing gum, particularly gum containing xylitol (a five-carbon sugar alcohol that cannot be metabolized by Streptococcus mutans), has the added benefit of increasing saliva, which in turn can serve as an additional source of remineralization (Hayes, 2001; Harris & Garcia-Godoy, 2004).

Although traditional efforts to prevent dental decay have focused on reducing the consumption of sweets and other fermentable carbohydrates and removing plaque thoroughly through brushing and flossing, current research is showing that these efforts are less effective than traditionally believed (Burt & Eklund, 2005). Combining the use of water fluoridation, fluoride products, dental sealants, and prompt professional care to reduce the risk of decay and reverse early areas of decay inside the tooth is an effective method for reducing dental decay (Harris & Garcia-Godoy, 2004).

Periodontal Diseases

Like dental decay, periodontal diseases will affect most adults at some time in their lives, and the consequences, including pain, dysfunction, tooth loss, and treatment costs, can be high (USDHHS, 2000b; NIH, 2001). *Healthy People 2010* notes that approximately 48 percent of adults have gingivitis, which is the mildest form of periodontal disease. The most severe forms of destructive periodontal diseases are seen in 22 percent of the population (USDHHS, 2000b; Brown, Brunelle, & Kingman, 1996). Periodontal diseases are largely preventable (Harris & Garcia-Godoy, 2004).

Periodontal disease is any disease or disease process that affects the gum (gingiva) or the supporting bone structure of the teeth (periodontium) (USDHHS, 2000b; Page & Kornman, 1997). Periodontal diseases are predominantly caused by a collection of bacteria, commonly referred to as a *bacterial plaque biofilm.* However, even though these diseases are bacterial plaque associated, their occurrence and progression may be modified by risk factors. Effective preventive activities need to include the recognition, identification, and elimination or minimalization of both the etiologic factors and the risk factors associated with the diseases (Armitage, 2003). Bacterial biofilm is a soft deposit consisting of a salivary glycoprotein matrix to which colonies of bacteria and food debris adhere. Bacterial biofilm is found on surfaces of the teeth and gingival tissues and in the space between the gum and the tooth, which is called the *gingival sulcus,* or *gingival crevice* (Sbordone & Bortolaia, 2003). The epithelial tissue lining this gingival crevice gives bacteria and their waste products (endotoxins) easy access to connective tissues and blood vessels. This systemic assault has the potential to affect tissues and organs at distant sites (Page, 1998). The disease site also serves as a reservoir of proinflammatory mediators (molecules that enhance the inflammatory response), which can also induce or perpetuate systemic effects by entering the systemic circulation (Page, 1998). Mineralization of undisturbed or inadequately removed plaque biofilm results in hard deposits known as tartar (calculus). These deposits make thorough cleaning more difficult because their rough surfaces trap more bacteria, and the result is that more plaque biofilm will accumulate.

Two of the most common periodontal diseases are gingivitis and periodontitis. Gingivitis is inflammation of the gingival tissues, resulting in an increase in redness, swelling, and bleeding. The most common sign of gingivitis is bleeding, although many clients instead perceive overzealous brushing as the cause of the blood they see on their toothbrush or after rinsing (Darby & Walsh, 2003). Health care professionals should explain to clients that healthy gum tissue does not bleed and that any bleeding, even if minor, should be investigated during an examination visit with an oral health care professional. There is usually no pain involved with gingivitis except in severe acute conditions. Gingivitis can be found in children from the time teeth erupt, and can continue throughout a person's life (Darby & Walsh, 2003).

As the gingival tissue becomes more inflamed and swollen the accumulation of plaque biofilm increases. As the tissues swell the gingival sulcus or crevice deepens and the bacteria in the biofilm in this space under the gum shift to gram-negative anaerobic bacteria. These microorganisms are mediated by host factors and become destructive, causing recession of soft tissue and loss of bone support around the tooth. The tooth becomes mobile and eventually is lost. This destructive periodontal disease is periodontitis. A number of studies have shown that although periodontitis is preceded by gingivitis, not all sites with gingivitis progress in a predictable manner to periodontitis (Brown et al., 1996; Greene, Louie, & Wycoff, 1990).

The challenge for the client comes in keeping the teeth biofilm-free, because this demands time, good dexterity, and motivation to brush thoroughly and clean between the teeth with dental floss. Health care professionals can emphasize to clients the positive benefits of a clean, healthy mouth. Clinical studies have shown power toothbrushes do better than manual toothbrushes at effectively removing plaque biofilm and improving gingival health (Heanue et al., 2003; Haffajee, Thompson, Torresyap, Guerrero, & Socransky, 2001). To clean the difficult areas in between the teeth (*interproximal* areas), dental floss, interproximal brushes, or appropriately shaped wooden picks are necessary. Twice per day rinsing with approved antimicrobial rinses will also aid in the reduction of plaque and gingivitis

(Bauroth et al., 2003). The thoroughness of biofilm control is more important than the frequency of cleaning. Biofilm should be disrupted thoroughly at least once a day, preferably at night and more often if possible (Harris & Garcia-Godoy, 2004; Greene et al., 1990). Interrupting the destruction caused in periodontitis requires professional scaling and root planing by oral health care professionals to remove calcified deposits and to control the subgingival bacteria in order to minimize both the etiologic factors and the risk factors associated with the disease (Harris & Garcia-Godoy, 2004).

Oral Trauma

Traumatic injuries that cause damage to the face and teeth can create long-term dilemmas in clinical diagnosis and treatment in oral health. After an injury clients will need assistance in reevaluating oral health in relation to their current status. Traumatic injuries manifest in many ways but most commonly involve fractures of the maxilla or mandible or damage to the temporomandibular joint. Teeth may also be fractured, knocked out of alignment (occlusion), or lost. Repairs to injuries to teeth heal more slowly than repairs in other areas in the body. For example, it may take up to five years to determine whether a treated tooth will survive an injury (Kaste, Gift, Bhat, & Swango, 1996; Greene et al., 1990).

The prevention of trauma to the face and teeth is addressed in *Healthy People 2010* and is underscored in two objectives: one dealing with unintentional injury and the other with oral health. These objectives call for extending requirements for the use of oral-facial protective devices (head, face, eye, and mouth protection) in sporting and recreation events that present risks of injury. Clients seeking school or sports physicals may need guidance in determining ways to keep their face and mouth intact and not altered by injury. Health care professionals can counsel clients in the use of mouthguards, helmets, face shields, and seat belts. Baseball players do not look on their sport as a high-risk activity with heavy contact, yet a high percentage of baseball injuries (41 percent) are to the head, face, mouth, and eyes (Nowjack-Raymer & Gift, 1996).

The National Collegiate Athletic Association (NCAA) implemented mandatory mouth protector wear for its players in 1974 (Greene et al., 1990). It has been estimated that up to 200,000 injuries to the mouth from football contact are prevented annually through the use of mouthguards (Kumamoto & Maeda, 2004). Other athletic associations involved in contact sports have followed the NCAA's direction, thus the number of dental injuries from sports is decreasing. However, injury prevention depends on consistent use of protective devices, and not all sport associations, especially those involving children and youths, enforce these regulations consistently.

Clients and their families should be directed to obtain one of the following three types of mouthguards readily available today: the ready-made or the mouth-formed appliances, which can be purchased at any athletic store and are often available through a coach or school administration, or the custom-fitted athletic mouthguard, which can be fabricated by an oral health care professional for the athlete. The custom-fitted mouthguard is recommended for athletes participating in high-contact sports and those athletes unable to use the other types of mouthguards.

The facial region is the most commonly injured body area in automobile accidents (Cox et al., 2004). Encouraging seat belt usage will greatly reduce these injuries. Two investigations reported decreases in facial injuries of 50 percent and 72 percent after the implementation of seat belt laws (Cox et al., 2004; Huelke & Compton, 1983).

Health care professionals can promote clients' use of helmets when biking, skateboarding, snowboarding, or skiing by conducting helmet decorating contests and bicycle and skateboarding rodeos in elementary schools and recreation centers. These activities can extend to families and to advocacy at the community and public policy level. Head injuries have decreased in states that have implemented mandatory helmet use for bicyclers of certain ages, although specific policies vary by state (Kumamoto & Maeda, 2004; Greene et al., 1990).

Common Oral Lesions

Two of the most common disorders of the mouth, causing discomfort and annoyance to millions of people, are fever blisters (herpes simplex and herpes labialis) and canker sores (aphthous stomatitis) (Siegel, Silverman, & Sollecito, 2001). Fever blisters, seen most frequently around the lips, are highly contagious and frequently spread by direct contact, most commonly kissing. Most persons who experience fever blisters of the type I herpes simplex virus were infected with the virus by ten years of age. Health care professionals can counsel their clients who have fever blisters not to kiss or have direct contact when blisters are present. Reactivation of this latent virus can be triggered by the following factors: fever, stress, exposure to sunlight, trauma, and hormonal alterations (Siegel et al., 2001). Recommending that clients be placed on an antiviral medication aids in decreasing the duration of the lesion. Visualizing a face free of fever blisters could be one way of encouraging a client to use lip sunscreen.

Aphthous ulcers, or canker sores, are not contagious and are an altered immune response to certain precipitating factors, including stress, trauma, allergies, and endocrine alterations; some acidic foods and juices; and foods that contain gluten. In addition, individuals who are anemic, have diabetes mellitus or inflammatory bowel disease, or are immunocompromised may also report frequent aphthous ulcers (Neville, Damm, Allen, & Bouquot, 2000). Health care professionals should counsel these clients not to eat abrasive foods, which could traumatize the mouth; to use care when cleaning the mouth to prevent trauma; and to avoid acidic and spicy foods.

Dry mouth (xerostomia) and yeast infections (candidiasis) are two common oral conditions that often lead to clients' complaints of burning mouth syndrome. Dry mouth is most commonly induced by the anticholinergic properties of most medications and by some medical treatments and is also seen in a number of autoimmune disorders, particularly among women. Oral candidiasis is associated with immunocompromised status and is commonly seen in older clients because of prolonged wearing of dentures. Oral candidiasis is best treated with a wide range of antifungal medications; however, there is no clear-cut treatment for dry mouth, with symptom relief forming the basis for recommendations for clients (Siegel et al., 2001). Dry mouth can cause difficulties in swallowing, tasting, chewing, and speaking; it places the client at increased risk for tooth decay and other infections. Xerostomia can be an indication of certain conditions or diseases. Health care professionals should encourage clients to sip water frequently to keep the mouth moist and to use artificial saliva, which is sold as an over-the-counter gel or liquid. Clients can also stimulate their salivary glands by sucking on sugarless lemon drops or mints. Avoidance of products that cause drying, such as caffeine, alcohol, and tobacco, is recommended (Siegel et al., 2001). Additional supportive patterns include keeping the lips moisturized and using a dehumidifier in the sleeping area to decrease skin and lip chapping and to promote hydration in the oral-facial region (Siegel et al., 2001).

Oral Cancers

Healthy People 2010 identifies the reduction of deaths resulting from cancer of the oral cavity and pharynx as a priority objective in oral health care. Oral-facial cancers make up approximately 3 to 4 percent of total cancers; however, the morbidity and mortality rates are high (Swango, 1996). In 2004, approximately 29,370 new cases (19,100 men and 10,270 women) of oral and pharyngeal cancer were diagnosed in the United States (American Cancer Society, 2005). One *Healthy People 2010* objective is to increase early detection to reduce deaths from oral and pharyngeal cancers. In 2004, there were approximately 7,320 deaths (4,910 males and 2,410 females) due to oral and pharyngeal cancers (American Cancer Society, 2005).

The tragedy of oral and pharyngeal cancers is that 75 percent of the cases are preventable and up to 90 percent are treatable if detected early (USDHHS, 2000b). Health care professionals should encourage their clients to complete a variety of health promotional activities to prevent oral cancers (Horowitz, Goodman, Yellowitz, & Nourjah, 1996). Tobacco cessation is an important, life-saving intervention that health care professionals can complete with their clients. The use of smokeless, or spit, tobacco has especially severe negative effects in the oral-facial complex and is a habit often overlooked by health care professionals. Limiting exposure to the sun, always wearing sunscreen and lip protection, and limiting alcohol ingestion are also specific behaviors that decrease the risk of oral and pharyngeal cancers.

Early detection of any cancerous lesions is critical to ensure prompt care, and clients can be taught to examine their face, mouth, and neck for common signs of early oral lesions. Any growth or swelling that is tender and firmly bound to the head or neck should be investigated. Any mixed red and white lesion in the mouth that does not heal within a week should be examined by a dentist, especially when the lesion is located on the lips, in the floor of the mouth, or on the posterior lateral border of the tongue—common sites for oral cancer. Clients who are at risk for oral cancer include men older than forty-five years and men and women who smoke or use smokeless tobacco or who drink alcohol. All adults, especially those at high risk for oral cancer, should visit a dental office at least once a year for head and neck examinations.

Health Conditions as Oral Disease Risk Factors

Many health conditions, including diabetes and HIV/AIDS, affect oral health, and in turn, poor oral health often affects and exacerbates these conditions. Health care professionals need to monitor the oral health of patients with these conditions and recommend appropriate health promotion strategies and dental care. Table 8.2 summarizes some of these health conditions and the relevant health promotion strategies.

Effects of Medications on Oral Health

In addition to the health conditions that are risk factors for oral diseases, many medications that clients take for these conditions pose challenges to maintaining optimal oral health. The following sections explain the interrelationship between selected medications and oral health status.

Drugs Causing Gingival Overgrowth. Three drugs that exhibit gingival overgrowth are phenytoin, cyclosporine, and calcium channel blockers. Clients using these medications should be encouraged to complete thorough daily oral hygiene and self-care. In addition, these clients should visit a dental professional on a regular basis, because the research has shown that meticulous plaque control combined with professional care will prevent or significantly decrease the severity of the hyperplasia.

TABLE 8.2. ORAL HEALTH PROMOTION
FOR CLIENTS WITH HEALTH RISK FACTORS.

Health Risk Factor	Oral Implications	Health Promotion
Diabetes	Increased incidence and severity of periodontal diseases. Poor healing and slow response to care.	Encourage thorough daily oral hygiene. Encourage more frequent dental care. Complete dietary counseling to reduce dental decay-promoting patterns.
Cardiovascular disease	Potential for endocarditis with valvular diseases. Risk of transient bacteremia. Potential association with periodontal diseases.	Encourage thorough daily oral hygiene. Encourage compliance with antibiotic premedication prior to dental care. Refer for frequent dental evaluation and care.
Organ transplant	Oral infection may be life threatening. Immunosuppressant medications may cause gingival enlargement and can mask signs of oral infection.	Refer for dental treatment before transplant when possible. Encourage frequent dental care. Encourage thorough daily oral hygiene.
Acute leukemia	Gingival hemorrhage. Oral discomfort and pain. Loss of appetite.	Encourage gentle, thorough daily oral hygiene. Recommend use of chlorhexidine rinse. Refer for emergency dental care only during acute phase. Refer to dental care during remission.
Thrombocytopenia	Purpura. Gingival hemorrhage.	Refer for dental consultation. Recommend oxidizing mouth rinses. Encourage thorough, gentle oral hygiene.
Hemophilia	Spontaneous gingival hemorrhage. Hemarthrosis.	Encourage thorough, gentle oral hygiene.
HIV infection and AIDS	Oral candidiasis. Oral hairy leukoplakia. Kaposi's sarcoma. Gingivitis and periodontitis.	Refer for dental evaluation and care. Refer for early treatment with antifungal medications. Recommend chlorhexidine rinses. Encourage thorough daily oral hygiene.
Chemotherapeutic agents	Mucositis. Oral ulcerations.	Encourage only minimal dental care during oral chemotherapy. Use therapeutic mouth rinse as needed. Encourage dental care after active chemotherapy.

Gingival overgrowth occurs in about one half of individuals who ingest phenytoin as their sole antiepileptic medication on a long-term basis. However, the prevalence of gingival overgrowth is much higher when phenytoin is taken in combination with other antiepileptic agents. Gingival overgrowth often becomes clinically apparent during the first six to nine months of therapy and has a clinically similar appearance to the tissue enlargement seen with the antirejection medication cyclosporine, which is used with transplant clients, and the cardiac drugs classified as calcium channel blockers (Patton & Glick, 2001).

Chemotherapeutic Agents. Health care professionals should strongly recommend a referral to a dentist before the onset of chemotherapy so that all oral sources of infection (for example, periodontal disease and infected teeth) can be eliminated. Only minimal necessary dental intervention should be provided to control acute oral problems that occur during the active phases of myelosuppression secondary to chemotherapy. After chemotherapy is completed, comprehensive dental care may be provided for the client after consultation with the oncologist.

Frequent recall examinations, symptomatic support (for mucositis or ulcerations), and aggressive preventive intervention should be part of the medical and dental care of clients receiving chemotherapy. A 0.12 percent chlorhexidine gluconate mouth rinse (Peridex or PerioGard) to reduce fungal and bacterial overgrowth and assist in oral hygiene care is strongly recommended. Topical analgesia in an oral suspension may be prescribed to provide relief from painful mucositis or ulceration (Siegel et al., 2001).

Oral Health Promotion Throughout the Life Span

In addition to specific service objectives, *Healthy People 2010* emphasizes specific health concerns for each stage of the life span. Like all other health promotion activities, oral health promotion activities should be targeted according to the specific at-risk factors for each age group. The following sections discuss oral health promotion activities for four age groups: infants and children, adolescents, adults, and older adults (summarized in Table 8.3). A final section underlines the importance of providing targeted oral health promotion activities to meet the special oral health needs of women.

Infants and Children

Currently, there is much interest in dental decay seen in children younger than three years. The traditional term for this is *baby bottle tooth decay* (BBTD); however, many oral health researchers are now using the term *early childhood caries* (ECC) to

TABLE 8.3. ORAL HEALTH ISSUES THROUGHOUT THE LIFE SPAN.

Age Group	Specific Oral Health Concern	Oral Health Promotion
Infants and children	Early childhood caries (ECC) Dental decay Eruption of primary teeth	Evaluate teeth as soon as they erupt. Teach parents and child oral care and offer nutritional counseling. Encourage cessation of bottle feeding by age 1. Refer for dental care at age 1. Recommend fluoride supplements at 6 months if drinking water is not fluoridated.
Adolescents	Dental decay Tobacco use Periodontal diseases Oral-facial injury	Refer to dental visits, including fluoride and sealants. Recommend fluoride supplements if drinking water is not fluoridated. Encourage thorough daily oral hygiene, use of fluoride, and proper nutrition. Encourage use of protective devices, such as mouthguards and helmets. Discourage tobacco use.
Adults	Dental decay Dry mouth Periodontal diseases Tobacco use Oral facial injury Specific conditions, based on health risk factors	Encourage thorough daily oral hygiene, use of fluoride, and proper nutrition. Encourage use of protective devices, such as mouthguards and helmets. Discourage tobacco use. Refer for dental evaluation and care. Recommend salivary substitutes.
Older adults	Dental decay Root decay Periodontal diseases Candidiasis	Encourage thorough daily oral hygiene, use of fluoride, and proper nutrition for self and caretakers. Discourage tobacco use. Refer for dental evaluation and care. Recommend salivary substitutes. Teach denture care.

more accurately describe this type of decay (Harris & Garcia-Godoy, 2004). ECC is characterized by multiple areas of dental decay on the primary teeth, generally affecting the anterior teeth but also sometimes the posterior teeth. Research has shown that the bacteria that cause ECC come primarily from mothers or caregivers who have active untreated decay in their mouths. Through salivary contact via kissing or food sharing, the bacteria are passed from mother to child and serve to initiate decay. When the bacteria remain on the teeth and are not brushed away, they can combine with sugars to begin the decay process.

The traditional causal explanation for such decay, as the term *baby bottle tooth decay* suggests, focuses on children's habit of falling asleep with a bottle in their mouth, so that the bottle liquid—formula, milk, juice, or sweetened drink—when allowed prolonged contact with the primary teeth (most often the maxillary anterior teeth), causes dental decay (Harris & Garcia-Godoy, 2004). Health care professionals should discourage these night bottle-feeding practices and also encourage thorough bacterial removal and frequent dental visits both for parents or caretakers and for infants to reduce the risk for ECC.

Health care professionals should also examine all infants for evidence of early decay and teach parents proper appraisal of their child's oral health. White spot lesions on the surface of the tooth are the earliest signs of decay; these progress to small, white and brown or gray depressions in the tooth, which then continue to enlarge until portions of the tooth are lost because of fracture. Parents should be taught to cleanse the child's teeth as soon as the first tooth erupts, usually between six and eight months of age. Teeth can be cleaned with a washcloth or cloth wipe, and a small toothbrush can be used when comfortable for the child. A small smear of toothpaste should be used during infancy, with no more than a pea-sized amount of toothpaste placed on the brush for children up to six years of age.

Health care professionals should also teach parents to discontinue bottle feeding at one year of age and to promote mealtime drinking from a trainer cup until the child can master drinking from a glass. If parents allow the child to continue sleeping with a bottle, it should contain only water. Many parents and caregivers have only a poor understanding of the health-depleting aspects of bottle feeding on erupting teeth. Health care professionals can use resource information from the American Dental Hygienists' Association and the American Dental Association to illustrate to parents the critical importance of fostering oral health (DeBiase, 1991).

The American Academy of Pediatric Dentistry recommends that all children visit the dentist by one year of age. Parents should take the time to speak with oral health care professionals about appropriate care for children's teeth and should be encouraged to use fluoride tablet supplementation with their children if the community drinking water does not contain fluoride (CDC, 2001; Harris & Garcia-Godoy, 2004).

Adolescents

Because adolescents are in one of the highest risk groups for dental decay, special efforts should be made to ensure that all adolescents visit a dental office at least once a year (Harris & Garcia-Godoy, 2004). All adolescents should use fluoride toothpaste, and fluoride rinses either at home or school are recommended if even one area of decay has been noted recently. Supplemental fluoride tablets should be continued to at least age sixteen if the drinking water is not fluoridated. All adolescents should have dental sealants placed on their first and second molars, and these sealants should be evaluated each year and reapplied if necessary. Other preventive measures, such as proper toothbrushing and dietary counseling, should be provided as appropriate.

It is often during adolescence that sports injuries occur, so the health care professional should provide education and referral to a dental office to ensure that proper protection is available for the oral-facial region. Unfortunately, many coaches and other individuals are unaware of the need for mouthguards and eye protection, and injuries may occur that need prompt treatment (Kumamoto & Maeda, 2004). When teeth are avulsed from the mouth, it may be possible to successfully replant them, depending on the type of injury. Replanting must be done within twelve hours. Parents should be taught to bring the teeth with the child to the dental office or emergency room and to preserve the teeth in milk or saliva, without cleaning or brushing the avulsed teeth in any way. When some fibers or cells are retained on the teeth, they can be replanted more successfully.

Adults

Many adults are at risk of dental decay because of the common medications they take for a variety of health conditions (Dolan & Atchison, 1993). Many medications have anticholinergic properties that produce xerostomia. When saliva is reduced or absent, its protective buffering properties are also decreased, food is retained longer in the mouth, and bacteria can more readily produce acid, which increases the demineralization process (Harris & Garcia-Godoy, 2004). In addition, dental decay can proceed more quickly, especially around the gum line and between teeth. Health care professionals should warn their clients about these dangerous effects and should recommend that these clients drink more water to lubricate the mouth. Artificial saliva products (for example, Optimoist) provide temporary relief for many clients and contain fluoride to promote remineralization. Unfortunately, many clients keep sugar-containing hard candy or gum in their mouths to increase saliva and provide a fresh taste to their breath. The use of sugar mints or candy only increases the risk for decay by providing more nutrients for oral bacteria, which can then produce additional acid for demineralization.

Bad breath, or halitosis, affects most adults and many children during their lifetimes. Halitosis can occur occasionally, regularly, or chronically and at specific times of the day or month. Breath freshness is a major cause of concern for most adolescents and adults, especially in social situations. Oral malodor can be caused by certain medications; dry mouth; respiratory infections; and certain foods, such as garlic, onions, or spicy foods. At times certain diseases, such as tumors of the upper respiratory and gastrointestinal track or liver or kidney failure, can cause halitosis, which usually occurs late in the disease process, with rapid onset and progressive intensity (Richter, 1996).

Volatile sulfur compounds have been suggested to be the cause of halitosis in the absence of any of the previously mentioned factors. Volatile sulfur compounds are formed from anaerobic bacterial activity on sulfur-containing amino acids derived from degraded proteins present in the saliva. These compounds can be removed by thorough oral hygiene, particularly tongue brushing and scraping, and use of antimicrobial and oxidizing mouth rinses (Richter, 1996).

Health care professionals can recommend that clients decrease their ingestion of culprit foods, use salivary substitutes and other products to hydrate the mouth, and complete thorough daily oral hygiene to prevent halitosis. Thorough brushing of all mouth structures, including the cheeks and tongue—especially the posterior portion—helps to remove any food particles and microorganisms that may be causing the offending odor. All clients should receive a dental referral to rule out existing dental disease or other infections.

It is often during the adult years that periodontal diseases are initiated and progress in their destructive pattern (Harris & Garcia-Godoy, 2004). Although the major etiologic factor for periodontal diseases is microbial plaque, many health conditions present risk factors that complicate oral hygiene and exacerbate the inflammatory patterns of periodontal diseases (Tyler, Lozada Nur, & Glick, 2001).

Older Adults

The expanding population of older individuals has begun to provide oral health care professionals with many challenges and opportunities. Although one in eight Americans is currently older than sixty-five years, the most recent projections from the U.S. Census Bureau predict significant increases by the year 2020 and beyond. In 2020, one in six Americans, approximately fifty-three million individuals, will be older than sixty-five, and by the year 2050, the overall population of older individuals will reach eighty million, or one of every five Americans. These demographic projections should be a message to all health care professionals to increase their knowledge and develop their skills to provide appropriate and sensitive care to older adults (Darby & Walsh, 2003).

In addition to living longer, healthier lives, older individuals are keeping their teeth longer, and they need specialized dental care to continue in optimal oral health. As documented in progress reports on the oral health objectives set in *Healthy People 2010,* complete tooth loss has continued to be limited to approximately one-third of older adults (USDHHS, 2000b). However, root caries and periodontal diseases are still proportionately higher in older individuals (Burt & Eklund, 2005). Because this age cohort has not had long experience of the benefits of modern dental care or preventive dentistry, health care professionals face many challenges in persuading older adults to engage in frequent dental care and activities that promote oral health.

Older individuals experience a significantly higher rate of root caries, primarily seen in the exposed root areas, because of the loss of tissue and bone attachment associated with periodontal diseases, which also increase with age. Root caries can be prevented with thorough daily oral hygiene and the use of intensive, topical home fluoride gels (Darby & Walsh, 2003). Root caries should be treated early because these lesions are more difficult to treat as they progressively enlarge. Dry mouth associated with many medications increases the risk of root decay, so older clients, many of whom take medication, must use salivary substitutes. They should also receive dietary counseling, especially because many older clients may choose a relatively soft diet, one that is high in fermentable carbohydrates (Harris & Garcia-Godoy, 2004).

Health care professionals may recommend modifications in oral hygiene techniques for older clients with disabilities (Darby & Walsh, 2003). For example, powered toothbrushes are often easier than manual ones for a client with arthritis and can also prove easier for a caretaker who cleans the client's mouth. If the older client wears dentures, these should be cleaned thoroughly after eating; should always be soaked overnight, preferably in a commercially available cleansing solution; and should never be left in the mouth overnight. Older individuals should clean their mouth tissues with a soft toothbrush or washcloth and complete an oral-facial self-examination at least once a month to locate any suspicious lesions or sores (Harris & Garcia-Godoy, 2004).

Unfortunately, candidiasis is often a problem for clients when dentures are improperly cleaned or left in the mouth overnight, and it often manifests as a client's complaint of a *denture sore.* Denture sores should receive careful evaluation from an oral health care professional, who can determine whether the denture has been fractured or is ill fitting or whether a candida infection is present. Treatment with antifungal medications should also be applied to the denture to remove any residual sources of infection. In addition, the perception of a dry mouth will also affect the comfort of denture wear, so clients taking medications that produce dry mouth should be cautioned to sip water frequently and use a salivary substitute to reduce any denture discomfort (Siegel et al., 2001).

Women's Oral Health Issues

Women have special oral health needs and considerations that men do not have. Women often report aesthetic concerns, and motivational strategies are often effective when framed as supporting the transition to the client's idealized oral image. Also, hormonal fluctuations have a surprisingly strong influence on the oral cavity. Puberty, menses, pregnancy, and menopause all influence women's oral health and the way in which oral health care is provided (American Dental Association, 1995).

Puberty. During puberty the increased level of sex hormones, such as progesterone and possibly estrogen, in a young woman's maturing system causes increased blood circulation to the gingiva, which leads to a greater sensitivity and susceptibility for gingivitis. Localized enlargement of the gingival tissue is most commonly seen in young women, most often a result of the interaction of local irritants (microbial plaque and tartar) with fluctuating hormone levels. Health care professionals should alert girls and their parents to these phenomena and encourage self-examination of gingival tissues. Proper treatment involves both careful and thorough oral hygiene and professional scaling and root planing to remove all microbial biofilm. Continued attention to thorough brushing and flossing is necessary, or the swelling will return (American Dental Association, 1995).

Menses. Gingivitis is also prevalent during menstruation because of the combination of increased levels of progesterone with microbial plaque. Menstruation gingivitis usually occurs right before a woman's period and clears up once menses has started. As always, good home oral hygiene care, including brushing and flossing, is important to maintain oral health, especially during hormonal fluctuations. In addition, more frequent dental visits for cleanings may be indicated, and an antimicrobial mouth rinse may need to be prescribed for more thorough plaque removal. Occasionally during menses some women may experience aphthous ulcers in the mouth or herpetic lesions on the lips. They may appear three or four days before menses begins and heal after menstruation. Palliative treatment, such as topical anesthetic agents or systemic analgesics, may be necessary for the discomfort associated with aphthous ulceration and herpetic lesions. Topical corticosteroids may also be indicated for severe aphthous ulcers (American Dental Association, 1995).

Pregnancy. Recent studies have implicated a variety of infections, including periodontal disease, as a risk factor for adverse pregnancy outcomes such as prematurity and low birth weight (Offenbacher, 2004; Jeffcoat et al., 2001). Although there appears to be an association between periodontal disease and preterm low birth weight, it is not yet clear that periodontal disease plays a causal role in adverse pregnancy outcomes (Scannapieco, Bush, & Paju, 2003). Preliminary evidence to date suggests that periodontal intervention may reduce adverse pregnancy outcomes (Jeffcoat et al., 2003). Additional large-scale, longitudinal epidemiologic and interventional studies are ongoing to investigate further the association and determine whether it is causal. In light of these early and intriguing studies, health care providers should emphasize the importance of oral health to general health and recommend dental evaluation early in pregnancy (Offenbacher, 2004).

During pregnancy many women experience increased gingivitis, beginning in the second or third month, increasing in severity through the eighth month, and beginning to decrease in the ninth month. This condition, called *pregnancy gingivitis,* is marked by an increased amount of swelling, bleeding, and redness in the gum tissue in response to a very small amount of plaque or calculus and is caused by an increased level of progesterone that occurs during pregnancy (Laine, 2002). If the gingival tissues are in a state of good health before pregnancy occurs, a woman is less likely to have any gum problems during her pregnancy. Pregnancy gingivitis usually affects areas of previous inflammation—not healthy gum tissue. If a woman experiences some swelling and bleeding of the gums before pregnancy, she might be at increased risk for pregnancy gingivitis. Just like any other type of gingivitis, if left untreated, pregnancy gingivitis can have damaging effects on the gums and bone surrounding the teeth, resulting in tissue (bone and gum) loss. Occasionally, the inflamed gum tissue will form an enlarged growth, called a *pregnancy granuloma* or *epulis,* as an extreme inflammatory response to any local irritation. These areas of enlargement vary in size and usually appear by the third month of pregnancy but may occur at any time during the pregnancy. A pregnancy epulis is usually painless; however, it can become painful if it interferes with chewing or becomes further inflamed by local irritants.

Health care professionals should encourage their pregnant clients to seek professional dental care when signs of either pregnancy gingivitis or epulis occur. Dental care usually involves conservative periodontal therapy and oral hygiene instructions, with further treatment or removal generally delayed until after delivery. Pregnancy gingivitis and pregnancy epulis usually diminish after pregnancy, but they may not go away completely. Because of this, it is of utmost importance that after the completion of the pregnancy, a dental examination be performed to assess periodontal health. Any treatment that might be needed can be determined at this time (Darby & Walsh, 2003).

Any woman contemplating pregnancy should see her dentist to make sure her mouth is in an optimal state of health and that any source of infection is eliminated before pregnancy. During pregnancy it is important that she seeks more frequent professional cleanings for the removal of irritants, and maintains a diligent daily home oral care routine, including brushing and flossing. If tender, swollen, and bleeding gums, or any other dental problems, occur at any time during the pregnancy, a dentist must be contacted immediately. The pregnant client can be treated safely as long as the dentist is aware that the client is pregnant so that modifications can be made in the proposed treatment if necessary. It may be necessary for the dentist to communicate with the health care practitioner prior to treating the pregnant patient in certain situations (American Dental Association, 1995).

Oral Contraceptives. Women taking oral contraceptives may be susceptible to the same oral health conditions that affect pregnant women, as a result of the documented effects of progesterone on the gingival tissues. Treatment of gum inflammation exaggerated by oral contraceptives should include establishing an excellent oral hygiene home care program and ongoing dental examinations and cleanings to eliminate all predisposing factors. More definitive periodontal therapy may also be indicated. Antimicrobial mouth rinses may also be prescribed as part of the home care regimen (Darby & Walsh, 2003).

Menopause. For the most part menopause does not directly cause any oral problems. Estrogen supplements have little effect on oral health status; however, progesterone supplements may increase the gingival response to local irritants, causing redness, bleeding, and swelling of the tissues. On rare occasions a woman may experience a condition called menopausal gingivostomatitis. This condition is marked by gingival tissues that are dry and shiny, bleed easily, and range in color from abnormally pale to deep red (American Dental Association, 1995).

Additional oral symptoms that women may experience during menopause include a dry or burning sensation in the mouth and abnormal taste sensations, especially salty, peppery, or sour tastes. In some women, oral symptoms and complaints respond favorably to estrogen supplement therapy. Professional scaling and root planing in combination with thorough daily oral hygiene care can relieve symptoms by controlling the inflammatory response and any enlargement of the gingival tissues. In addition, there is some empirical evidence to show that nutritional supplements in the form of vitamin B complexes and vitamin C are somewhat successful. Saliva substitutes and use of sugarless candy and mints may also be prescribed to reduce mouth dryness (Tyler et al., 2001).

Oral Care

Numerous clinical trials have shown that effective oral self-care can control plaque and gingivitis in most individuals (Burt & Eklund, 2005; Harris & Garcia-Godoy, 2004). Other studies have shown, however, that proper client teaching and reinforcement of oral hygiene care is critical to ensure adherence to recommended oral hygiene practices (Darby & Walsh, 2003). Health care professionals can initiate activities that promote oral health by encouraging clients to visualize clean and healthy teeth, fresh breath, and the ideal appearance of their smile. Health care professionals should encourage frequent visits to a dental office for oral prophylaxis, oral hygiene instructions, and examinations. Health care professionals can recommend one or more of the oral hygiene techniques described in the following sections as ways to optimize the client's current oral health supportive techniques.

Brushing

Soft toothbrushes are recommended because they help avoid damage to gum tissue and enamel. Powered toothbrushes, clinically proven superior to manual toothbrushes, provide additional assistance to clients with physical or other disabilities that limit the effectiveness of their brushing technique (Haffajee et al., 2001). If the cost of a powered brush is a deterring factor, a variety of hand grips can be improvised to help the client brush; these include a rubber ball with the toothbrush inserted in the center, a large wad of tin foil wrapped around the handle of the toothbrush, or a rubber bicycle grip with the toothbrush inserted into the end.

Although oral health care professionals recommend at least a three-minute period for thorough toothbrushing, most individuals brush for thirty seconds or less—an inadequate amount of time to ensure thorough cleansing. Reminders, such as using an egg timer or brushing for the length of one radio song, can encourage clients, especially children, to spend more time brushing. The following two brushing techniques are most commonly recommended and are often combined to most thoroughly clean the mouth:

Rolling stroke brushing method. Place the bristles of the brush at a 45-degree angle to the gum line. Sweep the brush away from the gum toward the chewing surface of the tooth. Continue throughout the mouth, covering each tooth. Brush the chewing surfaces of the teeth next by holding the brush flat on the chewing surface and gently scrubbing. With paste still on the brush, gently sweep the brush with several strokes along the tongue from the back of the throat to the front. After brushing the tongue, gently sweep the brush along the inside of the cheeks (Harris & Garcia-Godoy, 2004).

Bass (sulcular) brushing method. Place the thoroughly rinsed brush at a 45-degree angle to the gum line. Direct the bristles of the brush under the margin of the gum so that a slight pressure is felt. Vibrate the brush and slightly rotate in small circles under the gum line to clean the sulcular space between the gum and the tooth. As each area is cleaned, withdraw the brush from under the gum and reposition the brush to the next tooth under the gum (Harris & Garcia-Godoy, 2004).

In young children or older adults with dexterity problems, a circular or scrub brushing technique is considered an acceptable alternative to these two traditional brushing techniques. However, older adults should be cautioned to use a gentle stroke and an extra soft toothbrush to avoid excessive abrasion, especially around exposed root surfaces (Harris & Garcia-Godoy, 2004).

Interproximal Cleansing

The anatomy of the teeth makes it very difficult for toothbrushing alone to be sufficient for cleansing the entire tooth surface. Additional products, such as dental floss, small tapered brushes, and wooden picks, are necessary to maneuver between the teeth to disrupt the bacterial plaque. Although there are a number of acceptable techniques for using dental floss, the following procedures are most commonly recommended:

Pull about eighteen inches of floss from the dispenser and wrap the ends around the middle fingers; hold the floss firmly, using the fingers to gently guide the floss between two teeth; curve the floss snugly around the sides of one tooth, and gently slide the floss under the gum until a slight pressure is felt; keeping the floss adapted around the tooth, scrape the floss several times on the tooth surface to remove the bacterial plaque; after cleansing that tooth, slide the floss up to the tight contact area and adapt the floss to the sides of the other tooth; repeat the flossing procedure on each tooth, upper and lower, using a clean segment of the floss on each area (Harris & Garcia-Godoy, 2004).

Antimicrobial Rinses and Toothpastes

Many clients will report using mouth rinses for fresh breath and clean teeth. Although most over-the-counter mouth rinses provide a temporary fresh taste, only two products (essential oils and 0.12 percent chlorhexidine gluconate) are accepted for the control of gingivitis; neither of these products has been shown to reduce periodontitis.

The essential oil rinse (sold as Listerine and as generic equivalents) has a potent antimicrobial effect and has been shown to reduce plaque, gingivitis, and bleeding (Bauroth et al., 2003). However, ethyl alcohol is used to increase the solubility of the essential oils (eucalyptus oils, oil of wintergreen) in the mouth rinse. The concentration of alcohol may be as much as 21 to 28 percent, which could create problems for clients taking certain medications or clients recovering from alcohol abuse (Harris & Garcia-Godoy, 2004).

The 0.12 percent chlorhexidine gluconate mouth rinse is the most effective antiplaque and antigingivitis mouth rinse currently available. A 0.12 percent chlorhexidine gluconate mouth rinse has been used in many randomized, controlled studies since the mid-1960s, and there is strong evidence to support its use to prevent gingivitis (Harris & Garcia-Godoy, 2004). However, because clients commonly report uncomfortable side effects, such as alterations in taste perception, unpleasant taste, tooth staining, and tartar formation, this rinse is recommended for a limited time period for a targeted use, such as managing acute gingivitis, controlling periodontal involvement in immunocompromised clients, and promoting healing after periodontal treatment. Most oral health care professionals recommend that 0.12 percent chlorhexidine gluconate be prescribed in a limited, conservative manner, rather than for routine use for either symptom relief or simplified oral hygiene, because of its ability to mask existing periodontal conditions (Harris & Garcia-Godoy, 2004).

One antimicrobial agent, triclosan, has been shown to control plaque biofilm, gingivitis, and bleeding when formulated in a toothpaste with a stabilizing copolymer (Harris & Garcia-Godoy, 2004). An antimicrobial toothpaste is often easier for client compliance, especially for those clients who cannot tolerate a mouth rinse with alcohol due to discomfort or recovery from alcohol abuse.

Professional Care

Professional dental care is necessary to control subgingival bacteria, remove calcified deposits, and reinforce personal oral hygiene techniques. Neither supragingival plaque control alone nor professional care alone will effectively limit the progression of periodontitis or maintain periodontal health, but the combination of the two is effective for the majority of clients (Darby & Walsh, 2003). The appropriate frequency for professional therapy depends on the client's medical history, medical status, age, and risk factors and the state of his or her dentition. Most oral health care professionals recommend that periodontal and high-risk clients be evaluated every three months and nonperiodontally involved clients every six months to one year.

Health care professionals need to be aware of clients who are at high risk for periodontal diseases. High-risk clients include immunocompromised individuals; diabetic patients; longtime users of antiepileptic drugs; pregnant women; alcoholics; tobacco users; individuals receiving radiation therapy; and individuals with certain blood dyscrasias, Down syndrome, or Sjögren's syndrome (Tyler et al., 2001). Health care professionals counseling these individuals should promote effective oral health interventions to reduce their risks. (Table 8.2, shown earlier in this chapter, provides a summary of some health risk factors that affect oral health care.)

Summary

Oral health is essential to ensure optimal general health. The oral health educational information and activities presented in this chapter allow the health care professional to explore different methods of encouraging the client to identify and incorporate oral health promotion and disease prevention and dental care as an integral part of his or her health behaviors. All of us, professionals and clients, need continuous reinforcement to meet the challenges of staying healthy and to integrate oral health care to reach an optimal level of wellness. (See Exhibit 8.2 on page 286 for a list of additional helpful resources.)

References

American Cancer Society. (2005). *Cancer facts and figures 2005.* Atlanta, GA: Author.

American Dental Association, Council on Access, Prevention, and Interprofessional Relations. (1995). *Women's oral health issues.* Chicago: Author.

Armitage, G. C. (2003). Diagnosis of periodontal diseases. *Journal of Periodontology, 74,* 1237–1247.

Bauroth, K., Charles, C. H., Mankodi, S. M., Simmons, K., Zhao, Q., & Kumar, L. D. (2003). The efficacy of an essential oil antiseptic mouthrinse versus dental floss in controlling interproximal gingivitis. *Journal of the American Dental Association, 134,* 359–365.

Bloom, B., Gift, H. C., & Jack, S. S. (1992). Dental services and oral health: United States, 1989. *Vital Health Statistics, 10*(183), 1–95.

Brown, L. J., Brunelle, J. A., & Kingman, A. (1996, February). Periodontal status in the United States, 1988–1991: Prevalence, extent, and demographic variation. *Journal of Dental Research, 75* (Special issue), 672–683.

Burt, B. A., & Eklund, S. A. (2005). *Dentistry, dental practice and the community* (6th ed.). Philadelphia: Saunders.

Centers for Disease Control and Prevention. (2001). Recommendations for using fluoride to prevent and control dental caries in the United States. *Morbidity and Mortality Weekly Report, 50,* 1–42. Retrieved November 2005 from http://www.cdc.gov/mmwr/preview/mmwrhtml/rr5014a1.htm

Centers for Disease Control and Prevention, National Oral Health Surveillance System. (2002). *Fluoridation status.* Retrieved November 2005 from http://www2.cdc.gov/nohss/FluoridationV.asp

Cox, D., Vincent, D. G., McGwin, M., MacLennan, P. A., Holmes, J. D., & Ruo, L. W. (2004). The effect of restraint systems on maxillofacial injury in frontal motor vehicle collisions. *Journal of Oral and Maxillofacial Surgery, 62*(5), 571–575.

Darby, M. L., & Walsh, M. M. (2003). *Dental hygiene theory and practice* (2nd ed.). Philadelphia: Saunders.

DeBiase, C. B. (1991). *Dental health education.* Philadelphia: Lea & Febiger.

Dolan, T. A., & Atchison, K. A. (1993). Implications of access, utilization and need for oral health care by the non-institutionalized and institutionalized elderly on the dental delivery system. *Journal of Dental Education, 57*(16), 876–887.

Greene, J. C., Louie, R., & Wycoff, S. (1990). Preventive dentistry: II. Periodontal disease, malocclusion, trauma, and oral cancer. *JAMA, 263,* 421–425.

Haffajee, A. D., Thompson, M., Torresyap, G., Guerrero, D., & Socransky, S. S. (2001). Efficacy of manual and powered toothbrushes: 1. The effect on clinical parameters. *Journal of Clinical Periodontology, 28,* 937–946.

Harris, N. O., & Garcia-Godoy, F. (2004). *Primary preventive dentistry* (6th ed.). Upper Saddle River, NJ: Pearson Prentice Hall.

Hayes, C. (2001). The effect of non-cariogenic sweeteners on the prevention of dental caries: A review of the evidence. *Journal of Dental Education, 65,* 1106–1109.

Heanue, M., Deacon, S. A., Deery, C., Robinson, P. G., Walmsley, A. D., Worthington, H. V., et al. (2003). Manual versus powered toothbrushing for oral health (Cochrane Review). *Cochrane Library, 1.*

Horowitz, A. M., Goodman, H. S., Yellowitz, J. A., & Nourjah, P. A. (1996). The need for health promotion in oral cancer prevention and early detection. *Journal of Public Health Dentistry, 56*(6), 319–330.

Huelke, D. F., & Compton, C. P. (1983). Facial injuries in automobile crashes. *Journal of Oral and Maxillofacial Surgery, 41*(4), 241–244.

Jeffcoat, M. K., Geurs, N. C., Reddy, M. S., Cliver, S. P., Goldenberg, R. L., & Hauth, J. C. (2001). Periodontal infection and preterm birth: Results of a prospective study. *Journal of the American Dental Association, 132,* 875–880.

Jeffcoat, M. K., Hauth, J. C., Geurs, N. C., Reddy, M. S., Cliver, S. P., Hodgkins, P. M., et al. (2003). Periodontal disease and preterm birth: Results of a pilot intervention study. *Journal of Periodontology, 74,* 1214–1218.

Kaste, L. M., Gift, H., Bhat, M., & Swango, P. A. (1996, February). Prevalence of incisor trauma in persons 6 to 50 years of age: United States, 1988–1991. *Journal of Dental Research, 75* (Special issue), 696–705.

Kumamoto, D. P., & Maeda, Y. (2004). A literature review of sports-related orofacial trauma. *General Dentistry, 52*(3), 270–280.

Laine, M. A. (2002). Effect of pregnancy on periodontal and dental health. *Acta Odontologica Scandinavica, 20,* 257–264.

Levy, S. M., Kairitsy, M. C., & Warren, J. J. (1995). Sources of fluoride intake in children. *Journal of Public Health Dentistry, 55*(1), 39–52.

Lowe, G. D. (2004). Dental disease, coronary heart disease and stroke, and inflammatory markers. *Circulation, 109,* 1076–1078.

Marinho, V.C.C., Higgins, J.P.T., Logan, S., & Sheiham, A. (2003). Fluoride toothpastes for preventing dental caries in children and adults (Cochrane Review). *Cochrane Library, 4.*

Mattson, J. S., & Cerutis, D. R. (2001). Diabetes mellitus: A review of the literature and dental implications. *Compendium of Continuing Education in Dentistry, 22,* 757–760.

National Center for Health Statistics. (1996). *Third National Health and Nutrition Examination Survey (NHANES III): Reference manuals and reports.* Hyattsville, MD: Author.

National Institutes of Health. (2001). *Diagnosis and management of dental caries throughout life* (NIH Consensus Statement). Retrieved November 2005 from http://consensus.nih.gov/2001/2001DentalCaries115html.htm

National Library of Medicine. (2001, February). *Current bibliographies in medicine 2001: Diagnosis and management of dental caries.* Retrieved November 2005 from http://www.nlm.nih.gov/pubs/cbm/dental_caries.html

Neville, B. W., Damm, D. D., Allen, C. M., & Bouquot, J. E. (2000). *Oral and maxillofacial pathology* (2nd ed.). Philadelphia: Saunders.

Nowjack-Raymer, R. E., & Gift, H. (1996). Use of mouthguards and head gear in organized sports by school-aged children. *Public Health Reports, 3*(1), 82–86.

Offenbacher, S. (2004). Maternal periodontal infections, prematurity, and growth restriction. *Clinical Obstetrics and Gynecology, 47*(4), 808–821.

Page, R. C. (1998). The pathobiology of periodontal diseases may affect systemic diseases: Inversion of a paradigm. *Annals of Periodontology, 3,* 108–120.

Page, R. C., & Kornman, K. S. (1997). The pathogenesis of human periodontitis: An introduction. *Periodontology 2000, 14,* 9–11.

Patton, L. L., & Glick, M. (2001). *Clinician's guide to treatment of HIV-infected patients* (2nd ed.). Chicago: American Academy of Oral Medicine.

Richter, J. (1996, April). Diagnosis and treatment of halitosis. *Compendium of Continuing Education in Dentistry, 17*(4), 370–386.

Ryan, M. E., Carnu, A., & Kamer, A. (2001). The influence of diabetes on the periodontal tissues. *Journal of the American Dental Association, 134,* 3345–3405.

Sbordone, L., & Bortolaia, C. (2003). Oral microbial biofilms and plaque related disease: Microbial communities and their role in the shift from oral health to disease. *Clinical Oral Investigations, 7,* 181–188.

Scannapieco, F. A., Bush, R. B., & Paju, S. (2003). Periodontal disease as a risk factor for adverse pregnancy outcomes: A systematic review. *Annals of Periodontology, 8,* 70–78.

Shore, R. C., Robinson, C., Kirkham, J., & Brookes, S. J. (1995). *Structure of mature enamel in dental enamel: Formation to destruction.* Boca Raton, FL: CRC Press.

Siegel, M. A., Silverman, S., & Sollecito, T. P. (2001). *Clinician's guide to treatment of common oral conditions* (5th ed.). Chicago: American Academy of Oral Medicine.

Steinberg, A. (2004). Paradigm shift for caries diagnosis and treatment: Part I. Diagnosis. *Practical Dental Hygiene, 13,* 27–30.

Strauss, R. P., & Hunt, R. J. (1993, January). Understanding the value of teeth to older adults: Influences on the quality of life. *Journal of the American Dental Association, 124,* 105–110.

Swango, P. A. (1996). Cancers of the oral cavity and pharynx in the United States: An epidemiologic overview. *Journal of Public Health Dentistry, 56*(6).

Tyler, M. T., Lozada Nur, F., & Glick, M. (2001). *Clinician's guide to treatment of medically complex dental patients.* Chicago: American Academy of Oral Medicine.

U.S. Department of Health and Human Services. (1991). *Review of fluoride benefits and risks.* Washington, DC: U.S. Government Printing Office.

U.S. Department of Health and Human Services. (2000a). *Healthy people 2010: Understanding and improving health* (2nd ed.). Washington, DC: U.S. Government Printing Office.

U.S. Department of Health and Human Services. (2000b). *Oral health in America: A report of the surgeon general.* Rockville, MD: Author.

U.S. Department of Health and Human Services. (2003). *National call to action to promote oral health* (NIH Publication No. 03-5303). Rockville, MD: Author.

EXHIBIT 8.2. HELPFUL RESOURCES.

Associations

American Dental Hygienists' Association
444 N. Michigan Ave.
Chicago, IL 60611
Phone: (800) 243-ADHA
Web site: http://www.adha.org

American Dental Association
Order Department, Ste. 1430
211 E. Chicago Ave.
Chicago, IL 60611
Phone: (800) 621-8099
Web site: http://www.ada.org

American Academy of Periodontology
211 E. Chicago Ave., Ste. 800
Chicago, IL 60611
Phone: (312) 787-5518
Web site: http://www.perio.org

American Society of Dentistry for Children
211 E. Chicago Avenue
Chicago, IL 60611
Phone: (800) 637-ASDC
Web site: http://www.asdc.org

Companies

Sunstar Butler
Phone: (800) JBUTLER
Web site: http://www.jbutler.com

Colgate-Palmolive Company
Colgate Oral Pharmaceuticals
One Canton Way
Canton, MA
Phone: (800) 2-COLGATE
Web site: http://www.colgatebsbf.com

Health Edco, Inc.
P.O. Box 21270
Waco, TX 76702
Phone: (800) 299-3366
Web site: http//www.healthedco.com

Oral B
600 Clipper Dr.
Belmont, CA 94002
Phone: (800) 446-7252
Web site: http://www.oralb.com

Procter & Gamble
One Procter & Gamble Plaza
Cincinnati, OH 45202
Phone: (800) 543-2577
Web site: http://www.dentalcare.com

Practicon
102 Station Court, Ste. D
Greenville, NC 27934
Phone: (800) 334-0956

CHAPTER NINE

SMOKING CESSATION

Sherri Sheinfeld Gorin
Robert A. Schnoll

Cigarette smoking is the most important single preventable cause of death in human society. Despite decades of research and major treatment advances, the U.S. adult rate of tobacco use has decreased only modestly, from 22.8 percent in 2001 to 22.1 percent in 2003 (Centers for Disease Control and Prevention [CDC], 2004a, 2004f). Today, about forty-six million Americans, or close to one-quarter of the U.S. population, are smokers (CDC, 2004a, 2004f). Given these facts, the national objective set by *Healthy People 2010* of reducing the population prevalence of smoking to less than 12 percent by 2010 will not be attained.

According to the World Health Organization and the World Bank, tobacco kills eight people every minute or more than four million people per year. If current trends continue, the global tobacco death toll will grow to ten million annually by the year 2030, with about one-half of these deaths in people aged thirty-five to sixty-nine years. By 2030, people from developing countries will account for 70 percent of all tobacco deaths (World Bank Group, 2001; American Society of Clinical Oncology, 2003). Tobacco use among youths is an expanding public health problem globally (Yang et al., 2004).

The nicotine contained in tobacco is highly addictive, making it very difficult for people to quit smoking. Of the fifty million Americans who smoke, thirty-five million would like to quit, and twenty million try each year. Only one million smokers annually are successful in their attempts to quit. Research on new cessation approaches is critical if this success rate is to be improved (American Society of Clinical Oncology, 2003).

It is to be hoped that recent advancements in research and policy—such as the spread of municipal bans on smoking in public places, the use of tobacco quit lines, the release of the surgeon general's report *The Health Consequences of Smoking* (U.S. Department of Health and Human Services [USDHHS], 2004), and the *national action plans* for nicotine addiction treatment (Fiore et al., 2004)—will translate into substantial reductions in the prevalence of smoking in the coming years.

Epidemiology of Smoking

As research and public policy move forward, initiatives should be guided by data on the epidemiology of tobacco use.

Gender

More men smoke than women (25.2 percent versus 20 percent). At the same time, the rate of tobacco use among men has decreased by 50 percent since 1960, and the rate among women has decreased by only 25 percent (Giovino, 2002), a trend largely attributed to aggressive tobacco industry marketing aimed at women in the past several decades and the use of tobacco by women for weight control. As expected, then, lung cancer morbidity and mortality rates among women have been increasing relative to the rates among men (Patel, Bach, & Kris, 2004). Even when controlling for smoking history and other key risk factors, women appear more susceptible than men to developing lung cancer, perhaps because of unique molecular changes that occur more frequently in women, such as *P53* mutations, or because of estrogen signaling in tumorigenesis (Patel et al., 2004). The risks for women from tobacco use are also elevated because certain cancers linked to smoking are exclusive to women, such as cervical cancer (Boyle, Leon, Maisonneuve, & Autier, 2003) and because women who smoke are at risk of experiencing adverse effects during pregnancy if they continue to smoke while pregnant (Oncken & Kranzler, 2003). Concerning the latter issue, although overall tobacco use among pregnant women has decreased over the past decade, such gains have not been dramatic among younger pregnant women. Whereas tobacco use fell from 18.4 percent to 11.4 percent among pregnant women of all ages from 1990 to 2002, the rates among pregnant women aged fifteen to nineteen fell from 20.3 percent to 17.1 percent (CDC, 2004e).

Age

The prevalence of tobacco use is highest among younger adults, with a linear decrease in the proportion of tobacco use as age increases. For instance, although 28.5 percent of adults aged eighteen to twenty-four are smokers, this rate drops to 22.7 percent for adults aged forty-five to sixty-four and to 9.3 percent for adults aged sixty-five and over (CDC, 2004a). The latest Youth Risk Behavior Survey (YRBS) (CDC, 2004g) results indicate that the prevalence of current cigarette use among high school students has decreased from 27.5 percent in 1991 to 21.9 percent in 2003. (The Youth Risk Behavior Surveillance System conducts a national, anonymous school-based survey of all students in grades nine to twelve in every odd-numbered year to examine the major risk factors that threaten the health and safety of young people.) Data from middle school students indicates that recently the decrease in tobacco use has slowed, however, and is not matching the benefits seen for high school students. The National Youth Tobacco Survey indicated that smoking among middle school students decreased from 11 percent in 2000 to 10.1 percent in 2002, a nonsignificant change (CDC, 2003). Male and white middle school and high school students remain high-risk groups for tobacco use (CDC, 2003). Further, tobacco may serve as a "gateway drug" to other licit (e.g., alcohol) or illicit substances (e.g., marijuana) (Kandel & Davies, 1996; see Chapter Ten). Finally, with slightly over 9 percent of U.S. adults over age sixty-five as current smokers, the overall aging of the U.S. population, the increased risk with age for tobacco-related illnesses, and the specific barriers to cessation exhibited by this population (for example, level of addiction, feelings of invulnerability to the adverse health impact of smoking), older smokers should not be neglected for targeted cessation treatments (Appel & Aldrich, 2003).

Education and Income Levels

The rate of tobacco use is inversely related to levels of education and income. Current smoking prevalence among adults with a GED is 42.5 percent, versus 12.1 percent for those with a BA degree and 7.2 percent for those with a graduate degree (CDC, 2004a). Since 1983, smoking prevalence has been higher among both men and women with lower levels of education (CDC, 2004a). Interestingly, the current rates of tobacco use among women with either a BA or a graduate degree and among men with a graduate degree are lower than the 12 percent goal set by *Healthy People 2010* (CDC, 2004a). It is important to note that the decrease in tobacco use between 1983 and 2002 has been 9 to 10 percent for those with a BA or a graduate degree, whereas it has been only 5 to 6.6 percent for those with a high school diploma or less (CDC, 2004a). This means the actual difference in tobacco use rates between college graduates and those with less than a high school education has actually widened since 1983 (CDC, 2004a). Likewise, whereas one-third of U.S. adults who live below the poverty line are current smokers, 22.2 percent of those who live at or above the poverty line are current smokers (CDC, 2004a). Like the difference in prevalence rates across education groups, the difference in the rates of smoking of those below the poverty line and those at or above the poverty line has actually increased from 1983 to 2002, from 8.7 percent to 10.7 percent (CDC, 2004a). Thus, overall, the socioeconomic status of U.S. adults is a strong correlate of tobacco use and the gap in smoking prevalence rates across education and income levels has widened in the past two decades.

Race and Ethnicity

There is substantial variability across racial and ethnic groups in terms of the prevalence of tobacco use. The rates of tobacco use are highest among American Indians and Alaska Natives (40 percent); Caucasians and African Americans rank second and third at 23 percent and 22 percent, respectively (CDC, 2004f). A close look at the trend in tobacco use prevalence rates across ethnic groups over the past decade underscores the need for targeted tobacco cessation programs for African Americans in particular. Comparisons among the prevalence rates of tobacco use among high school students across different ethnic and racial groups from 1991 to 2003 show that, although the rates for Caucasians and Hispanics have decreased substantially (30.9 percent to 24.9 percent for Caucasians and 25.3 percent to 18.4 percent for Hispanics), the rate for African Americans has actually increased, from 12.6 percent to 15.1 percent (CDC, 2004b). African American men, in particular, are likely to show a substantial increase in the prevalence of tobacco use in the coming years, because trend data indicate that although the rate of tobacco use among Caucasian and Hispanic male adolescents has significantly decreased from 1991 to 2003, the rate of tobacco use among African American male adolescents has increased over this period, from 14.1 percent to 19.3 percent (CDC, 2004b).

Additional Vulnerable Populations

Two additional populations are worthy of specific mention, considering their high rates of tobacco use or unique susceptibility to the adverse health consequences of smoking. First, about one-third of cancer patients who were smokers before their diagnoses continue to smoke during treatment, and many who do quit return to smoking posttreatment (Browning & Wewers, 2003; McBride & Ostroff,

2003; Schnoll & Lerman, 2003). Continued patient smoking reduces survival duration; heightens risk of disease recurrence and a second primary tumor; reduces treatment efficacy; and causes pulmonary embolisms, venous thrombosis, and mucositis (Schnoll & Lerman, 2003). Therefore the development and assessment of smoking cessation treatments in the oncologic setting is an important priority. In addition, there is well-documented evidence that an exceedingly high rate of tobacco use exists among those with psychiatric disorders (Lasser et al., 2000). For instance, the results of a national epidemiologic study showed that the rates of nicotine addiction for those with an alcohol disorder were 34.5 percent, a drug disorder 52.4 percent, a mood disorder 29.2 percent, an anxiety disorder 25.3 percent, and a personality disorder 27.3 percent (Grant, Hasin, Chou, Stinson, & Dawson, 2004). Rates of nicotine dependence were particularly high among those with major depression (30 percent), manic disorder (35.3 percent), panic disorder with agoraphobia (39.8 percent), and dependent (44 percent) or antisocial (42.7 percent) personality disorder (Grant et al., 2004). Further, additional studies have reported extremely high rates of tobacco use among schizophrenic patients, ranging from 65 to 76 percent of samples (de Leon, Tracy, McCann, McGrory, & Diaz, 2002; McCreadie, 2002; Patkar et al., 2002). The paucity of treatment trials with these vulnerable populations indicates the need for future research to develop specific interventions tailored to the particular needs of these groups of smokers.

Other Forms of Tobacco

No form of tobacco is safe. It is therefore important that patients not transfer from smoking cigarettes to the use of other tobacco products. Public education campaigns should also focus on the specific health care dangers inherent in noncigarette tobacco products, particularly in cultures where their use is more accepted (American Society of Clinical Oncology, 2003).

Smokeless Tobacco. Chewing tobacco, loose leaf, and snuff tobacco pose increased risks of oral cancers, gum disease, and dental problems, particularly for those who keep the tobacco in their mouths for long periods of time (USDHHS, 1986). The widespread use of variations of these products (for example, pan, which is a mixture of tobacco and other substances wrapped in a vegetable leaf) in Southeast Asia and India make oral cancer the most common type of cancer in these areas. The amount of nicotine absorbed from these products is two to three times greater than that delivered by a cigarette (USDHHS, 1986, 1998a). Because smokeless tobacco use is common among athletes and many young people emulate sports figures, these products are of particular concern (American Society of Clinical Oncology, 2003).

Cigars are associated with lung, oral, laryngeal, esophageal, and pancreatic cancers. For those who inhale or smoke several cigars a day, there is also increased risk of coronary heart and chronic obstructive lung diseases (Iribarren, Tekawa, Sidney, & Friedman, 1999; USDHHS, 1986, 1998a; CDC, 1997). Because cigars have more tobacco per unit, they generally take longer to smoke and generate more smoke and carbon monoxide. The NCI has concluded that "cigar smoke is as, or more, toxic and carcinogenic than cigarette smoke" (USDHHS, 1998a, p. 3). Of particular note is that cigars are not under the same federal oversight and control as other tobacco products (USDHHS, Office of Inspector General, 1999). Studies have demonstrated that cigar use in the United States increased during the 1990s among adults and teens (CDC, 1997). Pipe smoking is associated with oral, laryngeal, esophageal, and lung cancers, as well as chronic obstructive pulmonary disease (Nelson, Davis, Chrismon, & Giovino, 1996).

Exposure to Environmental Tobacco Smoke

The causal links between exposure to environmental tobacco smoke (ETS) and serious illnesses and diseases such as cancer (Sasco, Secretan, & Straif, 2004), heart disease (Leone, Giannini, Bellotto, & Balbarini, 2004), and asthma and acute and lower and upper respiratory illnesses (such as bronchitis and pneumonia) (U.S. Environmental Protection Agency, 1997) are well documented. Particularly vulnerable to these health consequences of ETS are children and adolescents and employees at worksites without bans on public smoking (for example, blue-collar and service workers). About 50 percent of all U.S. children may be exposed to ETS (Gehrman & Hovell, 2003), and many industries, such as restaurants, bars, and casinos, still permit smoking. Serum cotinine can be detected among children exposed to parental smoking (Klerman, 2004), and tobacco-specific lung carcinogens (for example, NNK, NNAL) are detectable among casino patrons (Anderson et al., 2003).

The Tobacco Industry and Tobacco Control

The tobacco industry, through its enormous economic power, influences the promotion and sale of cigarettes worldwide. Although the major tobacco companies have diversified and also produce food items, soft drinks, beer, and other commodities, cigarettes are among their most profitable products. Tobacco companies are the largest national advertisers in print media. Seeking to sell tobacco with the least hindrance, they have had considerable influence on state legislatures across the United States, using lobbying, the media, public relations, front groups, industry allies, and contributions to legislators (Givel & Glantz, 2001).

Cigarettes are produced, promoted, and sold everywhere in the world. Although cigarette consumption is highest in developed countries, it is beginning to decline. As a result, tobacco companies are aggressively promoting their products in developing countries and in selected developed countries, such as Japan (with a 2002 volume of seventy-eight billion cigarettes, or 61 percent of the total U.S. cigarette exports). The results of tobacco promotion have been disastrous, with 82 percent or 950 million of the world's smokers living in developing countries (American Society of Clinical Oncology, 2003).

Smoking in the Movies. The tobacco industry has a unique influence on smoking through the movies. About 85 percent of all movies that appear on U.S. screens show a smoker, smoking, or cigarettes; many of these films are rated as acceptable for children (Stanton Glantz, personal communication, March 15, 2005), despite the tobacco industry's voluntary restrictions on such practices. Movies have considerable power to promote the *social acceptability* and desirability of tobacco use, notably among youths (Makemson & Glantz, 2002). Because of the top role of movies in the entertainment industry, reducing smoking in films would influence television and other media, enhancing tobacco control among youth.

Federal and State Government Involvement. With the recent passage of the Fair and Equitable Tobacco Reform Act (FETRA) on October 22, 2004 (7 U.S.C. 518), tobacco is no longer grown under a federal price support and production control program that was initiated during the Great Depression. In that former program, farmers agreed to limit production in return for a guaranteed buyer and a minimum price. The price of tobacco was therefore kept at an artificially high level. Of late, as imported tobacco has supplanted domestic product for use by U.S. cigarette manufacturers, many tobacco farmers, especially small ones, have fallen on hard times, and domestic tobacco production is on the wane (Schroeder, 2004).

The federal government, all fifty states, the District of Columbia, and several hundred local governments tax cigarettes. Taxes increase prices, and increased prices, in turn, reduce purchases of cigarettes. Increases in the price of cigarettes may significantly affect children's likelihood to smoke (Chaloupka, 1999). Some research suggests that for every 10-cent price increase, 4 percent fewer persons will purchase cigarettes (Warner, 1981). A subcommittee of the USDHHS Interagency Committee on Smoking and Health released a report in February 2003 recommending a $2 increase in the federal excise tax on cigarettes and other tobacco products. To reduce the possibility of substituting one tobacco product for another, these taxes should be applied equally to all tobacco products by federal, state, and local governments.

Transnational Approaches

Worldwide, the World Health Organization (WHO) has encouraged tobacco control through the development of national programs, support of advocacy, and information dissemination (Chollat-Traquet, 1992). Importantly, member states of the World Health Organization have recently produced the impressive Framework Convention on Tobacco Control (WHO, 2004), which was adopted during the 56th World Assembly, May 28, 2003, in Geneva, Switzerland. This important international document is the first that contains a comprehensive ban on tobacco advertising, promotion, and sponsorship (WHO, 2004). The United States, although a signatory, has not yet ratified the document.

The television advertising ban in this document seems key to its effectiveness for transnational cessation efforts. According to recently released internal tobacco company documents, advertising (including sponsorships and promotions) plays a pivotal role in opening new markets, notably by encouraging brand switching, attracting younger smokers, and creating aspirational heroes who smoke (Lambert, Sargent, Glantz, & Ling, 2004).

U.S. Policy Approaches to Tobacco Control

In the United States, policy approaches including the Master Settlement Agreement, other legislation, and large, community-based antitobacco programs have had considerable impact on smoking cessation. The Supreme Court has ruled that the Federal Drug Administration (FDA) does not have the authority to regulate tobacco as an addictive drug, however, thus restricting national legislation to limit cigarette sales to minors, in particular (*FDA* vs. *Brown & Williamson Tobacco Corp.*, 98-1152 [2000]).

The Master Settlement Agreement. The Master Settlement Agreement (MSA) is a landmark agreement, signed November 23, 1998, between states' attorneys general; other representatives of forty-six states, Puerto Rico, the U.S. Virgin Islands, American Samoa, the Northern Mariana Islands, Guam, and the District of Columbia; and the five largest tobacco manufacturers at that time (Brown & Williamson Tobacco Corporation, Lorillard Tobacco Company, Philip Morris Incorporated, R. J. Reynolds Tobacco Company, and Liggett & Myers). It settles a variety of claims against the tobacco companies for relief from the costs resulting from consumers' use of tobacco products. It establishes a $206 billion settlement to be paid over the next twenty-five years to the states, including provisions for a $250 million national foundation (The American Legacy Foundation) and a $1.45 billion public education fund for tobacco control.

The provisions of the MSA prohibit advertising, marketing, and promotions that target youths (including a ban on using cartoon characters in advertising), restrict brand-name sponsorship of events with significant youth audiences, ban outdoor tobacco advertising, ban youth access to free samples, and set the minimum cigarette package size at twenty. The tobacco companies are required to make a commitment to reducing youth access and consumption (by implementing changes in their own corporate cultures), disbanding tobacco trade associations, restricting industry lobbying, and opening industry records and research to the public. The MSA provides for enforcement of these commitments by the court and establishes a state enforcement fund ($50 million in a one-time payment) (National Association of Attorneys General, 1998).

Despite the enormous promise of this settlement, with few exceptions states have used the funds for nearly all budgetary needs except tobacco control (American Heart Association, 2002; Givel & Glantz, 2002, 2004; Gross, Soffer, Bach, Rajkumar, & Forman, 2002). A report released by a number of public health organizations reveals that states have enacted spending cuts ($86.2 million, or 11 percent) in tobacco prevention and cessation programs in 2003, despite record-high revenues from tobacco sources ($20.3 billion) (Campaign for Tobacco-Free Kids, American Lung Association, American Cancer Society, American Heart Association, & SmokeLess States National Tobacco Policy Initiative, 2003).

Youth Access Laws. Among the most widespread and popular approaches to reducing tobacco use have been *youth access* laws, which make it illegal to sell cigarettes to anyone under twenty-one years of age. By August 2001, all fifty states and 1,139 local governments had passed youth access laws (American Nonsmokers' Rights Foundation, 2005). These programs have made it more difficult for teens to purchase cigarettes. A recent study using the Youth Risk Behavior Survey found that, in addition to purchasing cigarettes from stores, students give others money to buy cigarettes, borrow cigarettes from others, and sometimes steal cigarettes or use vending machines. These findings suggest that the effectiveness of youth access laws is undermined by these alternative sources of cigarettes (Jones, Sharp, Husten, & Crossett, 2002; Ling, Landman, & Glantz, 2002; Ling et al., 2002).

Comprehensive Bans on Public Smoking. Reducing or eliminating ETS exposure requires the establishment of comprehensive bans on public smoking (Fichtenberg & Glantz, 2002). Bans may yield a 10 percent reduction in the prevalence of smoking (Levy & Friend, 2003), and a recent study showed that the levels of respirable suspended particles (RSPs), a marker for ETS exposure, can be reduced by 84 percent by a ban on smoking in indoor workplaces (CDC, 2004d). A revealing study by Sargent, Shepard, and Glantz (2004) illustrated the health benefits of public smoking bans. Rates of hospital admissions for myocardial infarction (MI) in Helena, Montana, were tracked during a comprehensive ban on public smoking and then again after the ban was lifted. The analyses showed that the rates of MI admissions shifted significantly in Helena, from an average of forty admissions per year in years when the ban was not in place to twenty-four per year during the ban. There was no change in MI admission rates in areas outside Helena, where such a ban was not enacted, illustrating that bans on indoor public tobacco use can translate into measurable health benefits. Further, several studies have shown that the implementation of clean indoor air legislation does not diminish revenues in restaurants and bars (CDC, 2004c) or in recreational venues, such as bingo halls or other charity-run gaming facilities (Glantz & Wilson-Loots, 2003), despite what the tobacco industry and other detractors of public smoking bans would have people believe (Barnoya & Glantz, 2003; Bialous & Glantz, 2002).

Because the primary source of ETS exposure among children is parental tobacco use, and because many workers in workplaces without bans are smokers, formal smoking cessation interventions must also be provided to address ETS. In a recent review of interventions to reduce child ETS exposure, Klerman (2004) concluded that interventions directed to assist parents to quit smoking have been effective, even when they involve interventions of minimal intensity. Eight of twelve randomized controlled trials in this area have yielded significant reductions in child ETS exposure (see Gehrman & Hovell, 2003).

Community-Based Approaches

Community-based programs use multiple channels to provide reinforcement, support, and norms for cessation (Secker-Walker, Gnich, Platt, & Lancaster, 2005). The earliest of the community-based approaches in the United States was COM-MIT (Community Intervention Trial for Smoking Cessation), which included public education, work with health care professionals, worksite presentations, and the provision of other cessation resources within eleven intervention communities (compared with eleven controls) across North America (COMMIT Research Group, 1995a, 1995b). COMMIT had a significant effect on quitting among light-to-moderate smokers (fewer than twenty-five cigarettes per day); if that rate were achieved nationally, it would translate into 1.2 million additional adults quitting. The importance of the nicotine patch as an aid to quitting was also validated in COMMIT, with patch users more than twice as likely to succeed in quitting than those who did not use patches (Cummings, Hyland, Ockene, Hymowitz, &

Manley, 1997). More addicted, heavy smokers, however, were not affected by the COMMIT programs (COMMIT Research Group, 1995a, 1995b).

COMMIT formed the basis for ASSIST (American Stop-Smoking Intervention Study), begun in 1991 to implement policy, media, and program services through five channels: community environments, worksites, schools, health care settings, and community groups. In 1999, after a one-year extension, the ASSIST program was transferred from the National Cancer Institute (NCI) to the Office of Smoking and Health within the Centers for Disease Control and Prevention and merged with the IMPACT (Initiatives to Mobilize for the Prevention and Control of Tobacco Use) program to become a new nationwide program, titled the National Tobacco Control Program. The National Tobacco Control Program funded all fifty states with about $1 million per state as a core public health service, rather than using the research model of ASSIST. An interim analysis of the results, comparing seventeen ASSIST states with thirty-two others, revealed decreases in tobacco consumption (Manley et al., 1997).

Multilevel Approaches

Over time other policy initiatives, provided at multiple levels, such as smoke-free workplaces and homes (Biglan & Glasgow, 1991; Wakefield et al., 2000), cigarette taxes (Chaloupka & Wechsler, 1997; Grossman & Chaloupka, 1997; Wasserman, Manning, Newhouse, & Winkler, 1991; USDHHS, 2000b), media campaigns (Bauer & Johnson, 2000), and anti-secondhand-smoke messages (Glantz & Jamieson, 2000) have developed strong evidence for the benefits of tobacco control.

California Tobacco Control Program. The largest of the recent multilevel tobacco control initiatives is the California Tobacco Control Program, begun in 1988 under Proposition 99, which increased the tax on cigarettes by $0.25 per package and allocated $0.05 of that amount for an antitobacco educational campaign. The program combined the effects of the tax increase with an aggressive media campaign that attacked the tobacco industry and stressed clean indoor air and also community-based programs promoting clean indoor air and policies designed to foster a smoke-free society (Glantz & Balbach, 2000; Goldman & Glantz, 1998; Bal, Kizer, Felten, Mozar, & Niemeyer, 1990; Tobacco Control Section, 1998). Several well-designed longitudinal evaluations of the impact of the California Tobacco Control Program have demonstrated that it accelerated a decline in the number of cigarettes smoked and in the prevalence of smoking (Glantz, 1993; Pierce, Gilpin, Emery, Farkas, et al., 1998; Pierce, Gilpin, Emery, White, et al., 1998; Lightwood & Glantz, 1997; Siegel et al., 2000; National Cancer Policy Board, 2000). Similar declines in the number of cigarettes smoked and in the prevalence of smoking have been found in other large, statewide programs in Florida (Bauer & Johnson, 2000), Massachusetts (CDC, 1996; Biener, Harris, & Hamilton, 2000), and Oregon (CDC, 1999). In a striking set of recent findings, Fichtenberg and Glantz (2000) compared per capita cigarette consumption and age-adjusted rates of death from heart disease in California to those for the rest of the United States and found an accelerated decline in the rates of mortality from heart disease with the program-related declines in cigarette consumption. The incidence of lung cancer fell significantly below that predicted; with a three-year lag the incidence of bladder cancer (associated with the tar in cigarettes) fell. There were no associations of the program with the incidence of either prostate or brain cancer (Barnoya & Glantz, 2004), as predicted. These consistent and highly influential findings strongly suggest that advocacy for large, multilevel tobacco control programs, directed at adults as well as children and youths, is critical to accelerating the current declines in smoking prevalence.

Importance of Multilevel Approaches

Tobacco interventions are both clinically effective and cost effective relative to other medical and disease prevention interventions. Cessation services have the potential to pay for themselves over the course of a decade through savings of direct and indirect tobacco-related medical expenses (Campaign for Tobacco-Free Kids, 2002). Thus health care delivery systems (including insurers, administrators, and purchasers) should institutionalize the consistent identification, documentation, and treatment of every tobacco user seen in a health care setting. Tobacco counseling and pharmacotherapeutic treatments that have demonstrated effectiveness should be reimbursed; similarly, clinicians should be reimbursed for providing tobacco dependence treatment, just as they are reimbursed for treating other chronic conditions (Fiore et al., 2000a). Generally, influencing social norms and other social processes at the organizational, community, or even societal level may be a more effective approach than approaches directed at individuals and will certainly reach more smokers (Lichtenstein & Glasgow, 1992; Biglan & Glasgow, 1991).

Smoking Initiation, Maintenance, and Relapse

Because nearly all smokers begin to use tobacco when they are under age eighteen, age may be the most significant risk factor for tobacco use initiation. Understanding the factors related to initiation of tobacco use by adolescents can help explain the etiology of nicotine addiction. A recent review outlines the multidimensional framework for smoking initiation among adolescents, highlighting the following as risk factors: low socioeconomic status (SES), weight concern (among girls), conduct disorder (among boys), tolerance for nicotine, attention deficits, depression, peer influence, parental exposure, tobacco advertising, low cost for cigarettes, and genetic polymorphisms (Turner, Mermelstein, & Flay, 2004). Specific factors play greater roles at specific times in the trajectory from experimentation to regular use. Experimentation is more likely when the child is exposed to peer encouragement, has poor parental monitoring or lack of parental disapproval for tobacco use, is exposed to commercial advertising for tobacco use, and exhibits curiosity about the consequences of tobacco use. In contrast, a high tolerance for nicotine or genetic polymorphisms that lower endogenous dopamine concentrations may play a greater role in determining progression from experimentation to regular use (Lerman et al., 2003).

The extreme variability in people's susceptibility to tobacco initiation suggests that genetic factors may play a role in nicotine addiction. Although psychological and social factors are critical, genetic polymorphisms, individually or in combination, may explain 50 percent of the variability in smoking initiation (Li, 2003; Munafo, Clark, Johnstone, Murphy, & Walton, 2004). Several genetic pathways have been proposed to explain the possible genetic influence on smoking behavior, including genes responsible for metabolizing nicotine (for example, CYP2A6) and for regulating physiological reward (such as dopaminergic and serotonergic genes) (Munafo et al., 2004). Researchers have assessed polymorphisms on dopamine *receptor* genes DRD2, dopamine *transporter* gene (DAT VNTR), serotonin *transporter* gene (5HTT LPR), and cytochrome P450 2A6 gene.

Understanding the genetic basis of nicotine addiction is a complex process, which poses unique conceptual and methodological challenges (Schnoll & Lerman, 2003). This literature is dominated by case-control studies, has rarely considered gene-gene or gene-environment (for example, personality or depression) interactions, and has been limited by methodological shortcomings such as low statistical power and population stratification bias (owing to the examination of genetic predispositions in population subgroups). As studies in this pioneering area of research move forward, there is a growing promise that understanding the genetic correlates of nicotine addiction can pave the way for innovative personalized methods for preventing the development of nicotine addiction (Lerman, Patterson, & Berrettini, 2005; Swan, 1999).

Predicting Treatment Effectiveness

Perhaps the strongest predictors of responsiveness to treatments for nicotine addiction are the level of pretreatment nicotine addiction and the level of tobacco use. Smokers who exhibit lower pretreatment nicotine dependence are more likely to achieve cessation following treatment with nicotine replacement therapy (NRT) (Lerman et al., 2004), behavioral smoking cessation counseling (Ferguson et al., 2003), and bupropion (Harris et al., 2004; Swan et al., 2003). Likewise, smokers who report greater levels of pretreatment tobacco use exhibit poorer response to physician-based smoking cessation counseling (Vanasse, Niyonsenga, & Courteau, 2004) and to bupropion (Harris et al., 2004). Given these findings, an important direction for current research is to examine the effectiveness of more intensive cessation treatments, including the efficacy of combined NRTs, with smokers who exhibit such smoking-related characteristics.

Pharmacogenetics

One of the most significant advancements in the field of nicotine addiction treatment is the emergence of pharmacogenetic studies. These studies focus on the examination of inherited variability in genes that relate to responsiveness to nicotine addiction treatment (Lerman et al., 2005). In the context of bupropion, Lerman and colleagues have examined several possible genetic variants that may influence response to treatment. In one study the CYP2B6 gene, which influences the rate of nicotine metabolism, was shown to interact with gender and bupropion to affect quit rates (Lerman et al., 2002). In particular, women who were *slow metabolizers* showed higher quit rates when provided with bupropion than *rapid metabolizers* did.

In the context of NRT, Johnstone et al. (2004) examined the moderating effects of alleles on the DRD2 gene on responsiveness to treatment with the transdermal patch. Although there was no long-term effect of the DRD2 A1 versus A2 allele on quit rates, the presence of both the A1 allele of DRD2 and the dopamine hydroxylase A allele, which enhance levels of dopamine, enhanced the likelihood for cessation following patch treatment. These findings were maintained, among women only, up to twelve months after the quit date.

Lastly, in a recent study, Lerman et al. (2004) examined the role of the mu-opioid receptor gene in modulating response to the transdermal patch and the nicotine nasal spray. Smokers in this trial with the OPRM1 Asp40 variant of this gene, which enhances binding affinity of beta-endorphin, were significantly more likely than smokers without this genetic variant to quit smoking if given the transdermal patch. Despite these interesting and encouraging results, pooled analyses indicate that polymorphisms in the DRD2 and DAT VNTR genes are not associated with the ability to quit smoking, but effects have been detected for polymorphisms in 5HTT LPR and in CYP2A6 genes (Munafo et al., 2004). Undoubtedly, future studies in this area are needed, but the implications for the tailoring of cessation treatments based on the smoker's genetic profile are potentially extremely useful for the enhancement of the efficacy of existing cessation treatments.

Relapse Prevention

Relapses are common in smoking treatment. An average of two to three relapses is common among successful abstainers (Fisher, Haire-Joshu, Morgan, Rehberg, & Rost, 1990; Fisher, Lichtenstein, Haire-Joshu, Morgan, & Rehberg, 1993). Freestanding *relapse-prevention* interventions have been suggested to assist individuals to remain smoke-free, even though the evidence is strongest for supporting initial cessation attempts (Hajek, Stead, West, Jarvis, & Lancaster, 2005). A recent study has suggested that a series of relapse-prevention booklets mailed to recent quitters may significantly reduce smoking relapse (Brandon, Herzog, & Webb, 2003).

Smoking and Body Weight

The belief that cigarette smoking reduces body weight and that cessation produces a marked weight gain is an incentive for clients, particularly women, to both continue to smoke and to relapse (Klesges, Meyers, Klesges, & La Vasque, 1989; Gritz et al., 1992; Klesges & Klesges, 1988; Pirie, Murray, & Leupker, 1991). A 1990 U.S. surgeon general's report stated that smoking cessation could be followed by a mean weight gain of five pounds (two to three kilograms); smoking seems to lower an individual's body weight *set point,* and cessation raises the set point (Perkins, 1993). More positively, however, even with weight gain, the pattern of fat deposition (for example, waist-to-hip ratio) improves after cessation (Shimokata, Muller, & Andres, 1989). Further, levels of high-density lipoproteins increase with no change in total cholesterol of low-density lipoprotein levels after an individual quits (Gerace, Hollis, Ockene, & Svendsen, 1991). Therefore cessation approaches, particularly with women, involve strategies for healthy eating and physical activity while quitting.

Intervention Approaches for Smoking Cessation

Quitting smoking is not usually an event, it is a process. Many individuals must try several times before they succeed. The influential *Treating Tobacco Use and Dependence* (Fiore et al., 2000a) suggests that cessation requires repeated interventions and may differ according to the client's gender, age, pretreatment level of addiction, and stage of quitting (see Exhibit 9.2, which offers an example of the 5 A's approach).

Many smokers give up smoking on their own, but printed or electronic materials giving advice and information may help them and increase their numbers. A recent systematic review of fifty-one rigorous studies found that compared to standard materials or none at all, materials tailored to the individual smoker may increase cessation (Lancaster & Stead, 2002).

Three types of counseling and behavioral therapies have been found especially effective and should be used with all patients who are attempting to quit: (1) provision of practical counseling (problem-solving or skills training), (2) provision of social support intratreatment (for example, from other smokers who are trying to quit), and (3) assistance with extratreatment social support (for example, from a spouse or other family members). Pharmacotherapies for smoking cessation are important to the quit effort. Except in the presence of contraindications, they should be used with all patients who are attempting to quit. Five first-line therapies have reliably increased long-term cessation rates: bupropion SR, nicotine gum, nicotine inhaler, nicotine nasal spray, and the nicotine patch. Two second-line therapies, clonidine and nortriptyline, have been found efficacious and should be implemented if the first-line therapies fail. Because smoking is both an addiction and a learned, or habitual, behavior, behavioral approaches are designed to disrupt long-established patterns associated with smoking.

There is a strong dose-response relationship between the intensity of tobacco dependence counseling and its effectiveness. Treatments involving individual, group, or proactive telephone counseling (for example, on smoking quit lines) are effective, and their effectiveness increases with intensity (for example, minutes of contact).

Primary Care Approaches

Visits with a health care provider offer an important opportunity for a *teachable moment* in which to discuss quitting smoking. Therefore all smokers who are willing to stop should be offered a treatment at each visit. The basic components of effective, brief primary care interventions include the five A's: (1) *ask* all patients about their smoking status; (2) *advise* smokers, clearly, to stop smoking; (3) *assess* the client's willingness to quit; (4) *assist* the client's efforts with self-help materials, a quit date, and possibly nicotine gum or the transdermal patch, particularly with smokers who are not yet ready to quit; and (5) *arrange* follow-up support (Exhibit 9.1). A sixth step has been added for children and adolescents: *anticipate* guiding smoking cessation with each client (Glynn & Manley, 1991; Manley, Epp, Husten, Glynn, & Shopland, 1991). For those smokers who are unwilling to quit, the five R's should be added at every visit: *relevance, risk, rewards, roadblocks,* and *repetition* (Exhibit 9.2). For more intensive cessation efforts, health care providers should refer the client to a local cessation therapist, group, or clinic or one of the few inpatient cessation programs.

Physicians' and Other Health Care Professionals' Support. As 70 percent of Americans visit a health care professional every year (Schubiner, Herrold, & Hurt, 1998), physicians, nurses, and dentists have much potential for contact with U.S.

EXHIBIT 9.1. A BASIC COMPONENT OF
EFFECTIVE, BRIEF INTERVENTIONS: THE 5 A'S.

ASK: **inquire about smoking status routinely**

- Gather some specific information, such as:
  - How much? How often? When? Where?
  - Do your parents smoke?
  - Do your parents know that you smoke?
  - Any connection b/w presenting issues and smoking?
- Follow with:
  - Have you ever thought about quitting?
  - Ever tried to quit?

ADVISE: **urge the client to quit**

- Message should be CLEAR, STRONG, and PERSONALIZED
- Offer of assistance from self and/or staff is key

ASSESS: **assess the client's willingness to quit**

- If client would like to make a quit attempt, move on to ASSIST
- If the client wavers or is unwilling
  - Determine reasons why
  - Address concerns
  - Provide support and assurance of help
  - If necessary, provide a motivational intervention
    - Offer possible connections b/w smoking and other problems
    - Consider providing motivational statements that relate to health, social life, money, self-esteem
- If client unwilling at this time, return to topic again at a later contact

ASSIST: **aid the client in quitting**

- Can make quitting part of the client's individualized clinical plan
- A variety of interventions are possible

Set a quit date	Make a plan to tell others, enlist support
Teach to monitor smoking behavior	Help anticipate challenges
Teach problem-solving skills	Teach adaptive coping skills
Review past quit attempts	Help make changes to the environment
Provide positive reinforcement	Help the client develop a reward system
Refer the client to other means of support	

EXHIBIT 9.1. A BASIC COMPONENT OF
EFFECTIVE, BRIEF INTERVENTIONS: THE 5 A'S, Cont'd.

ARRANGE: follow up on progress
- Problem solve and elicit recommitment when there are setbacks

WITH PARENTS:
- After ASK, cautiously pursue further 5A steps if the parent responds in a resistant manner
- If receptive, can refer to primary care physician and provide list of additional resources

Source: Fiore et al., 2000b.

EXHIBIT 9.2. A BRIEF STRATEGY FOR
ENHANCING MOTIVATION TO QUIT TOBACCO: THE 5 R'S.

Relevance	Encourage the patient to indicate why quitting is personally relevant, being as specific as possible. Motivational information has the greatest impact if it is relevant to a patient's disease status or risk, family or social situation (for example, having children in the home), health concerns, age, gender, and other important patient characteristics (for example, prior quitting experience, personal barriers to cessation).
Risks	The clinician should ask the patient to identify potential negative consequences of tobacco use. The clinician may suggest and highlight those that seem most relevant to the patient. The clinician should emphasize that smoking low-tar or low-nicotine cigarettes or using other forms of tobacco (for example, smokeless tobacco, cigars, and pipes) will not eliminate these risks. Examples of risks are:

- *Acute risks*: Shortness of breath, exacerbation of asthma, harm to pregnancy, impotence, infertility, increased serum carbon monoxide.

- *Long-term risks*: Heart attacks and strokes, lung and other cancers (larynx, oral cavity, pharynx, esophagus, pancreas, bladder, cervix), chronic obstructive pulmonary diseases (chronic bronchitis and emphysema), long-term disability and need for extended care.

- *Environmental risks*: Increased risk of lung cancer and heart disease in spouses; higher rates of smoking in children of tobacco users; increased risk for low birth weight, SIDS, asthma, middle ear disease, and respiratory infections in children of smokers.

Rewards	The clinician should ask the patient to identify potential benefits of stopping tobacco use. The clinician may suggest and highlight those that seem most relevant to the patient. Examples of rewards follow:

- Improved health.
- Food will taste better.

EXHIBIT 9.2. A BRIEF STRATEGY FOR
ENHANCING MOTIVATION TO QUIT TOBACCO: THE 5 R'S, Cont'd.

- Improved sense of smell.
- Save money.
- Feel better about yourself.
- Home, car, clothing, breath will smell better.
- Can stop worrying about quitting.
- Set a good example for children.
- Have healthier babies and children.
- Not worry about exposing others to smoke.
- Feel better physically.
- Perform better in physical activities.
- Reduced wrinkling and aging of skin.

Roadblocks	The clinician should ask the patient to identify barriers or impediments to quitting, and should note elements of treatment (problem solving, pharmacotherapy) that could address barriers. Typical barriers might include the following: • Withdrawal symptoms. • Fear of failure. • Weight gain. • Lack of support. • Depression. • Enjoyment of tobacco.
Repetition	The motivational intervention should be repeated every time an unmotivated patient visits the clinic setting. Tobacco users who have failed in previous quit attempts should be told that most people make repeated quit attempts before they are successful.

Source: Fiore et al., 2000a.

smokers. Currently, about 70 percent of physicians report advising their patients to stop smoking (Lindsay et al., 1994). Although few U.S. physicians smoke, smoking prevalence among these health care providers remains relatively high in developing countries of the world, such as Guatemala (Barnoya & Glantz, 2002). Given the proportion of U.S. adults who smoke, even if health professionals have only a small impact on quit rates, the public health impact of this change could potentially be enormous.

Anywhere from 34 to 74 percent (Eckert & Junker, 2001; Rogers, Johnson, Young, & Graney, 1997; CDC, 1993) of patients have reported receiving cessation advice from their providers. A recent survey of 1,400 smokers found that over one-half welcomed physician advice and stated that it would have a strong influence on their decision to quit (Ossip-Klein et al., 2000).

Depending on the setting, 45 to 81 percent of physicians (Easton, Husten, Elon, Pederson, & Frank, 2001; O'Loughlin et al., 2001; Gottlieb, Guo, Blozis, & Huang, 2001), 36 to 71 percent of nurses (Sarna et al., 2000; McEwen & West, 2001), and 51 to 61 percent of dentists (Lodi et al., 1997; John, Yudkin, Murphy, Ziebland, & Fowler, 1997) report having advised patients to quit, although fewer report assisting patients in cessation or arranging follow-up (Goldstein et al., 1998; Grimley, Bellis, Raczynski, & Henning, 2001).

Counseling practices vary by several patient factors, including age, race or ethnicity, and gender. Counseling is most likely when the patient is young, Caucasian, male, and relatively healthy. It is more likely when the patient has insurance. It also varies by the physician's specialty; primary care physicians and obstetricians and gynecologists report higher rates of counseling than do pediatricians (Easton et al., 2001; Doescher & Saver, 2000; Borum, 2000; McIlvain, Crabtree, Backer, & Turner, 2000; Kviz et al., 1995; Secker-Walker, Solomon, Flynn, & Dana, 1994). Research has found that counseling is done most often during new patient visits, and is most thorough (that is, follows all of the 5 A's through follow-up) among physicians who are practicing in solo, private offices rather than group, HMO, or other settings (Fiore et al., 2000a; Goldstein et al., 1998). Among pediatricians, counseling varies by the age of the child or youth and by the topic, as well as by the amount of time spent on the visit (Galuska et al., 2002).

Surveys of medical professionals have evaluated their receptivity to providing tobacco cessation counseling. One recent report found that two-thirds of nurses believe that it is their obligation to provide cessation advice (McCarty, Hennrikus, Lando, & Vessey, 2001); surveys of dentists have found similar results (Fried & Cohen, 1992; Allard, 2000). Some of the common barriers cited by health care professionals are time (Pollak et al., 2001), perceived complexity of a smoking cessation protocol (Bolman, de Vries, & Mesters, 2002), and insufficient confidence in ability to counsel in this area (Sheinfeld Gorin, 2001). Other factors related to the provision of counseling include educational level (for example, year of residency) (Gottlieb et al., 2001), having received training in cessation counseling (Hepburn, Johnson, Ward, & Longfield, 2000), whether the provider smokes (Sheinfeld Gorin, 2001), the provider's race or ethnicity (Sheinfeld Gorin, 2001), and the strength of the provider-patient relationship (Coleman, Murphy, & Cheater, 2000). A recent report suggested that providing feedback to physicians improves their motivation to counsel patients in cessation (Andrews, Tingen, Waller, & Harper, 2001).

Training programs have been designed to improve medical professionals' skills and self-efficacy in this area. In the short term these programs have been effective in improving providers', particularly physicians', confidence and perceived effectiveness and increasing their rates of asking, advising, and providing cessation counseling and self-help materials (Cornuz et al., 1997). Openness to providing counseling can be influenced by the provider's own smoking status, and if the provider does smoke, by his or her desire to quit (Kawakami, Nakamura, Fumimoto, Takizawa, & Baba, 1997).

Several meta-analyses and literature reviews have assessed the efficacy of smoking cessation advice from varied health care professionals. Studies have found that brief physician advice can increase one-year smoking abstinence rates among adults by more than 20 percent compared with controls (American Cancer Society, 1990; Montner, Bennett, & Brown, 1994). Even minimal contact of adults with physicians (three minutes or less) increases the efficacy of the intervention, although effectiveness increases with both increased intensity and duration of contact and with the addition of nicotine replacement therapies, such as the patch (Kottke, Battista, DeFriese, & Brekke, 1988; Ockene & Zapka, 1997; Fiore et al., 2000a). The findings from a recent meta-analysis revealed that receiving advice from any health care professional—physician, nurse, dentist, or team of providers—produced a small increase in quit rates (Sheinfeld Gorin & Heck, 2004). Physicians have been found more effective in tobacco cessation than any other professional group alone (Fiore et al., 2000a). Two clinicians (that is, a team) are the most effective, however (Fiore et al., 2000a).

Sustaining quit attempts over time is difficult, particularly without additional prompts and reinforcement. Continued provider prompts to smokers to quit, through chart reminders and computerized office-based systems, for example, are important to sustained cessation. Over time these contacts may be particularly effective means for encouraging longer-term abstinence.

The results of these studies support the efficacy of cessation counseling by all health care professionals but particularly by teams and physicians. There is promise for counseling by community pharmacists (Sinclair, Bond, & Stead, 2004) and dentists, and a need for increased training of nurses in smoking cessation counseling, particularly among African American clients (Ellerbeck, Ahluwalia, Jolicoeur, Gladden, & Mosier, 2001).

Health Care Professional Counseling with Youths. Even though more than one in three adolescents smokes, and the great majority of adult smokers began smoking prior to the age of eighteen, there have been few studies on brief interventions for adolescent smoking in health care settings. From 60 to 70 percent of adolescents visit their pediatricians on an annual basis (Gans, McManus, & Newacheck, 1991); three visits per year is the average (Pamuck, Makuc, Heck, Reuben, & Lochner, 1998). Further, children and adolescents perceive physicians to be credible health experts and may heed their advice more than that of parents or other adults (Perry & Silvis, 1987; Gans, McManus, & Newchuck, 1991; Thorndike, Ferris, Stafford, & Rigotti, 1999). Nonetheless, two recent population-based and large HMO surveys of physicians who treat adolescents continued to document the gap between the need for tobacco cessation among adolescents and the primary care provider's response (Klein, Levine, & Allan, 2001; Thorndike et al., 1999; Ellen, Franzgote, Irwin, & Millstein, 1998; Franzgrote, Ellen, Millstein, & Irwin, 1997; Gregorio, 1994; Zapka et al., 1999). In a telephone survey of 7,960 adolescents, only 25 percent reported that a health care provider had said something to them about cigarette smoking in the last year (Baker, 1995).

Health care professionals can be trained to increase their skills in screening and counseling adolescents in tobacco cessation, as they do with adults, within the confines of a routine outpatient visit (Klein et al., 2001). Although the rigorous evidence for the effectiveness of tobacco control with youth by health care professionals is not yet available, given that nicotine dependence develops quickly in adolescents, methods of smoking cessation intervention used for adults have been recommended for adolescents (Sussman, Lichtman, Ritt, & Pallonen, 1999; Schubiner et al., 1998; Fiore et al., 2000a). It is suggested that health care providers begin to ask about smoking when children reach the age of ten, teach parents to maintain smoke-free households, set nonsmoking expectations early on, and monitor adolescents for signs of smoking. Parents should limit exposure to adult media and use family television time to discuss the effects of seeing screen depictions of smoking on adolescent behavior. Adolescents who smoke should be assessed for signs of nicotine dependence and counseled about quitting (Sargent & DiFranza, 2003) (see Table 9.1 on page 311).

Pharmacological Interventions

The main effect of nicotine replacement therapies (NRTs)—including nicotine gum (nicotine polacrilex), the nicotine patch (transdermal nicotine), and nicotine nasal spray, inhalers, and tablets—is the relief of nicotine withdrawal symptoms and the prevention of short-term relapse. A systematic review of these varied NRT approaches found that all forms increase the odds of quitting from 1.5- to 2-fold, regardless of setting, duration of therapy, or the intensity of the additional support provided. In comparing the varied forms of NRT, the nasal spray was most effective in cessation, followed by inhaled nicotine, nicotine sublingual tablets or lozenges, the nicotine patch, and nicotine gum. In highly dependent smokers, there is a significant benefit from higher doses (for example, 4 mg gum versus 2 mg gum). Higher doses of the nicotine patch may also produce small increases in quit rates. Combinations of NRT do not seem to increase cessation. There is some evidence that quit rates with bupropion are higher than rates with the nicotine patch (Silagy, Lancaster, Stead, Mant, & Fowler, 2004).

Acupuncture and Hypnosis

Acupuncture, acupressure, laser therapy, and electrostimulation may help smokers deal with the addictive component of smoking by focusing attention on and appearing to treat the problem, but they do not increase cessation. A recent systematic review confirmed that acupuncture seems to have a placebo effect similar to that of pills containing sugar but no medication (White, Rampes, & Ernst, 2002). Although individuals may undergo hypnosis to help them to stop smoking, there is no evidence for its effectiveness (Abbot, Stead, White, Barnes, & Ernst, 2000).

Aversive Conditioning

Aversive conditioning approaches that pair the pleasurable stimulus of smoking a cigarette with some unpleasant stimulus may diminish the attractiveness of smoking or may result in the cigarette itself becoming aversive. One such approach is rapid smoking, in which a client puffs a cigarette every 6 to 8 seconds until the client senses that he or she will become nauseated. This is repeated several times in sessions that accompany quit dates and that are continued until urges to smoke are reduced (Lichtenstein, Harris, Birchler, Wahl, & Schmahl, 1973; Danaher, Jeffery, Zimmerman, & Nelson, 1980). Despite its early demonstration of effectiveness in conjunction with cessation counseling and abstinence rates of 50 percent (Glasgow, Lichtenstein, Beaver, & O'Neill, 1981), more recent reviews have been inconclusive (Hajek & Stead, 2004). Further, acceptance of this approach is limited. Components of aversive conditioning, such as a butt jar, are often used in conjunction with other approaches.

Intensive Cessation Clinics

Often clients need more intensive treatment to quit, such as an intensive cessation clinic. A state-of-the-art clinic for smoking cessation tends to use approaches that include (1) setting a quit date, (2) interrupting conditioned responses that support smoking, (3) identifying and preparing plans for coping with temptations after cessation, (4) attending to relapse episodes and encouraging the continuation of cessation, and (5) providing follow-up contact and social support for quitting and abstinence (Lowe, Green, Kurtz, Ashenberg, & Fisher, 1980; Lando, 1977; Lichtenstein, 1982; Hall, Rugg, Tunstall, & Jones, 1984). The American Lung Association (ALA), for example, offers Freedom from Smoking clinics that have demonstrated a long-term abstinence rate of 29 percent (Rosenbaum & O'Shea, 1992). These clinics, which can be located through the ALA, hospitals, health maintenance organizations (HMOs), and other centers, serve a small percentage of all quitters. The health care professional's support is critical to clinic clients' follow-through.

Interventions in Particular Settings

Particular settings, such as hospitals, substance abuse treatment or cancer treatment facilities, or worksites or schools, may offer unique opportunities for intervention (see Table 9.2 on page 313).

Summary

Interventions, whether brief exchanges or oriented toward intensive clinical work, rely on several features of the dynamics of smoking. The decision to smoke is determined by many factors, from the economics of cigarette marketing and prices to the physiology of nicotine addiction. Addiction and conditioning enrich each other; smoking thus becomes connected with numerous cues of daily life. This sets the stage for equally numerous cues to relapse.

Clinically, the health care professional should ask about smoking, offer brief counseling using the 5 A's (ask, advise, assess, assist, and arrange) and the 5 R's to motivate quitting, provide a prescription or recommendation for over-the-counter NRT, and provide a referral for more intensive counseling. Counseling and ongoing support for the client and also encouragement of quitting by health care professionals and others in the client's support network will enhance the client's likelihood of stopping.

As advocates for smoke-free environments, health care professionals can have an impact not only on an individual's successful cessation but also on the creation of a healthier society. Health care professionals have the power to help clients live longer and healthier lives through smoking cessation. (Also see the list of helpful online resources in Exhibit 9.3 on page 327.)

TABLE 9.1. INTERVENTION APPROACHES PARTICULAR TO SELECTED GROUPS BY GENDER, AGE, AND STATUS.

	Primary Smoking Issues	Specific Cessation Approaches
Women	Targeted marketing efforts	Emphasize self-control, illogic in advertisements and smoking in the movies; develop counteradvertising
	Less education, lower socioeconomic class	Target interventions to high-risk groups
	Weight gain	Vigorous physical activity (Marcus et al., 1999)
		Advocate for changed legislation, policies for tobacco control
Pregnant women	Smoking by others in the home (environmental tobacco smoke [ETS])	Develop plan to reduce smoking in various settings
Infants	Smoking by mother during pregnancy or while nursing	Emphasize effects on child from mother's smoke (for example, by measuring cotinine in breast milk)
Children	Smoking by others in the home (modeling and ETS)	Develop "no smoking" times, days at home
	Peer group influence	Cessation as an affirmative response
Adolescents	Process of separation and individuation	Not smoking is one's own decision; challenge them to stop
	Peer group influence	Peer pressure as self-pressure; cessation as an affirmative response
	Egocentricity and increased self-concern	Emphasize effects on appearance (for example, smelly hair, yellow teeth)
	Feelings of invulnerability	Focus on relevant effects (for example, shortness of breath)
	Present-orientation	Emphasize short-term effects (for example, cost, bad breath)
	Smoking by others in the home	Explore smoking as a family problem
Adolescent women	Targeted marketing efforts	Analyze smoking in the movies and advertisements for illogic; develop counteradvertising
Adolescent men	Interest in portraying a "macho" image	Portray smokers as weak and babyish

**TABLE 9.1. INTERVENTION APPROACHES PARTICULAR TO
SELECTED GROUPS BY GENDER, AGE, AND STATUS, Cont'd.**

	Primary Smoking Issues	Specific Cessation Approaches
	Marketing of smokeless tobacco	Analyze smoking in the movies and advertisements for illogic; encourage client to make his own choice
Elderly	Exacerbates conditions more common among elderly, such as heart disease, high blood pressure, circulatory and vascular conditions, duodenal ulcers, reductions in smell and taste, osteoporosis, diabetes	Emphasize short-term health benefits of stopping
	Drug dose alterations	Highlight increased efficacy of medications
Vulnerable populations	Divorced or separated men; those with lower levels or education and income	Target interventions efforts to these high-risk groups
Minorities	Higher prevalence among African Americans	Use culturally sensitive messages and community leaders (for example, church leaders)
	Hispanic males have higher prevalence, women have lower rates	Use culturally sensitive messages; emphasize the impact on the family
	American Indians have higher rates of smokeless tobacco use	Use culturally sensitive messages; work with Indian Health Service or spiritual healers or both
		Advocate for changes in advertising, promotion practices targeted to high-risk groups
Persons experiencing psychological distress	Depression and anxiety are risk factors	Focus on link between symptoms and smoking
	Psychiatric inpatients have higher rates	Make nicotine addiction part of treatment process
Cancer survivors	Second primary tumor often fatal	Focus on alternative stress reduction approaches (other than smoking)
	Risk persists for up to twenty years	

TABLE 9.1. INTERVENTION APPROACHES PARTICULAR TO SELECTED GROUPS BY GENDER, AGE, AND STATUS, Cont'd.

Primary Smoking Issues	Specific Cessation Approaches
Long-term survivors of childhood cancers at particular risk (American Society for Clinical Oncology, 2003)	Peer counseling doubles smoking cessation among childhood cancer survivors (Emmons et al., 2005)

TABLE 9.2. SMOKING CESSATION IN SPECIFIC ORGANIZATIONAL SETTINGS.

Setting	Intervention Components
General hospital	• Brief, multicomponent bedside treatment can produce 20–25% long-term quit rates (Orleans, Kristeller, & Gritz, 1993). • 5 A's and 5 R's to increase motivation. • In-hospital contact ≥ 20 minutes. • Extended postdischarge contact (≥ 1 month; Rigotti, Munafo, Murphy, & Stead, 2003). • ≥ 5 contacts. • ≥ 3 months. • Include NRT except if contraindicated. • Supported by hospital systems (for example, chart reminders or stamps) (Wolfenden, Campbell, Walsh, & Wiggers, 2003) and hospital bans on smoking. • Computed tomography (CT) screening for those at high risk for lung cancer may increase cessation opportunities (Henschke et al., 1999; Mulshine & Henschke, 2000).
Prenatal clinics	• Multicomponent program integrated with other healthcare. • 5 A's and 5 R's to increase motivation. • Share risks of smoking on preterm births and low weight infants; risks of smoking for infant during breast feeding and early infancy and childhood. • Give suggestions for problem-solving approaches for coping with multiple stresses of early mothering. • Use of motivational interviewing (nonjudgmental approach focused on resolving ambivalence about behavioral change) is effective. • Follow-up telephone booster sessions (Gehrman & Hovell, 2003).

TABLE 9.2. SMOKING CESSATION
IN SPECIFIC ORGANIZATIONAL SETTINGS, Cont'd.

Setting	Intervention Components
	• Maximize unique social supports, such as spousal (Orleans, 1985; Coppotelli & Orleans, 1985).
	• Provide cessation manuals (for example, those published by the American Cancer Society (see the Helpful Resources section in Exhibit 9.3, and Windsor, 1986).
	• Relapse prevention programs generally ineffective (Lumley, Oliver, Chamberlain, & Oakley, 2004).
Substance abuse treatment facilities	• Determine stage of readiness to quit.
	• Stage-based counseling (McIlvain & Bobo, 1999).
	• Cessation counseling may be more effective one year after alcoholic has become sober (Bobo, 1992).
Dental Offices	• Oral examination and feedback about tobacco-induced mucosal changes decrease use of smokeless tobacco (see Chapter Eight; Ebbert et al., 2004; Gordon & Severson, 2001; Newton & Palmer, 1997).
	• Dental team effective in cessation (Sheinfeld Gorin & Heck, 2004).
Worksites	• Formal behavioral counseling or NRT, or both (Moher, Hey, & Lancaster, 2003).
	• Provision of personalized risk assessment feedback to smokers (Schnoll et al., 2005).
	• Smoke-free worksite policies (Glasgow, Cummings, & Hyland, 1997).
Schools	• Increase skills for identifying social influences to smoke (for example, tobacco advertising, movies, and marketing strategies) and peer influence.
	• Increase skills for resisting influences to smoke (for example, advertising analysis and resistance skills).
	• Increase information for correcting erroneous normative perceptions regarding smoking (for example, "everyone smokes") and for promoting tobacco-free social norms.
	• Involve teachers in cessation curriculum development, review, training, program implementation (Connell, Turner, & Mason, 1985; Gold et al., 1991).
	• Supplement with peer leaders to model social skills, lead role rehearsals (Perry, Telch, Killen, Burke, & Maccoby, 1983; Clarke, MacPherson, Holmes, & Jones, 1986).

TABLE 9.2. SMOKING CESSATION
IN SPECIFIC ORGANIZATIONAL SETTINGS, Cont'd.

Setting	Intervention Components
	• Parents may further enhance the influence of school efforts through program development, reinforcement at home, assessment of program effectiveness (Perry, Pirie, Holder, Halper, & Dudovitz, 1990).
	• Educate students about the short- and long-term negative consequences of tobacco use, the social influences on smoking, peer norms regarding smoking, and communication and refusal skills (CDC, 1994).
	• Emphasize age-appropriate topics.
	• *Evidence-based approach* suggests that school-based programs emphasize teaching youths a broad array of life skills training (Botvin, Baker, Dusenbury, Botvin, & Diaz, 1995).
	• Combining school-based components with community-based elements, such as mass media, may be considered.
	• Smoke-free school policies have some effects on reducing smoking among students (Pentz et al., 1989).
	• School-based social influences approach using best practices does not produce long-term deterrence of smoking among youth (Peterson, Kealey, Mann, Marek, & Sarason, 2000).

References

Abbott, N. C., Stead, L. F., White, A. R., Barnes, J., & Ernst, E. (2000). Hypnotherapy for smoking cessation (Cochrane Review). *Cochrane Library, 2.*

Allard, R. H. (2000). Tobacco and oral health: Attitudes and opinions of European dentists: A report of the EU Working Group on Tobacco and Oral Health. *International Dental Journal, 50,* 99–102.

American Cancer Society. (1990). 1989 survey of physicians' attitudes and practices in early cancer detection. *CA, 40,* 77–101.

American Heart Association. (2002). *State of tobacco control: 2002.* Retrieved June 2005 from http://www.lungusa.org/press/tobacco/tobacco_0010703.html

American Nonsmokers' Rights Foundation. (2005). *Tobacco-related disease research program.* Retrieved July 2005 from http://www.trdrp.org/research

American Society of Clinical Oncology. (2003). American Society of Clinical Oncology policy statement update: Tobacco control—Reducing cancer incidence and saving lives. *Journal of Clinical Oncology, 21,* 2777–2786.

Anderson, K. E., Kliris, J., Murphy, L., Carmella, S. G., Han, S., Link, C., et al. (2003). Metabolites of a tobacco-specific lung carcinogen in nonsmoking casino patrons. *Cancer Epidemiology, Biomarkers, & Prevention, 12*(12), 1544–1546.

Andrews, J. O., Tingen, M. S., Waller, J. L., & Harper, R. J. (2001). Provider feedback improves adherence with AHCPR Smoking Cessation Guideline. *Preventive Medicine, 33,* 415–421.

Appel, D. W., & Aldrich, T. K. (2003). Smoking cessation in the elderly. *Clinics in Geriatric Medicine, 19*(1), 77–100.

Associated Film Promotions. (1981). *Recall and recognition of commercial products in motion pictures: For Brown & Williamson Tobacco Company* (Bates No. 682158296-8307). Retrieved September 2005 from http://legacy.library.ucsf.edu/popular_documents_movies.html

Baker, L. (1995). Health care provider advice on tobacco use to persons aged 10–22 years— United States, 1993. *Morbidity and Mortality Weekly Report, 44,* 826–830.

Bal, D. G., Kizer, K. W., Felten, P. G., Mozar, H. N., & Niemeyer, D. (1990). Reducing tobacco consumption in California: Development of a statewide anti-tobacco use campaign. *JAMA, 264,* 1570–1574.

Barnoya, J., & Glantz, S. (2004). Association of the California Tobacco Control Program with declines in lung cancer incidence. *Cancer Causes and Control, 15,* 689–695.

Bauer, U., & Johnson, T. (2000). *Florida youth tobacco survey results* (Vol. 3, Report 1). Tallahassee: Florida Department of Health Survey Research Unit. Retrieved July 2005 from http://www.state.fl.us/tobacco

Bialous, S. A., & Glantz, S. A. (2002). ASHRAE Standard 62: Tobacco industry's influence over national ventilation standards. *Tobacco Control, 11,* 315–328.

Biener, L., Harris, J. E., & Hamilton, W. (2000). Impact of the Massachusetts Tobacco Control Program: Population-based trend analysis. *British Medical Journal, 321,* 351–354.

Biglan, A., & Glasgow, R. E. (1991). The social unit: An important facet in the design of cancer control research. *Preventive Medicine, 20,* 292–305.

Bobo, J. K. (1992). Nicotine dependence and alcoholism epidemiology and treatment. *Journal of Psychoactive Drugs, 24,* 123–129.

Bolman, C., de Vries, H., & Mesters, I. (2002). Factors determining cardiac nurses' intentions to continue using a smoking cessation protocol. *Heart & Lung, 31,* 15–24

Borum, M. L. (2000). A comparison of smoking cessation efforts in African Americans by resident physicians in a traditional and primary care internal medicine residency. *Journal of the National Medical Association, 92,* 131–135.

Botvin, G. J., Baker, E., Dusenbury, L., Botvin, E. M., & Diaz, T. (1995). Long-term follow-up results of a randomized drug abuse prevention trial in a white middle-class population. *JAMA, 273,* 1106–1112.

Boyle, P., Leon, M. E., Maisonneuve, P., & Autier, P. (2003). Cancer control in women: Update 2003. *International Journal of Gynaecology and Obstetrics, 83* (Suppl. 1), 179–202.

Brandon, T. H., Herzog, T. A., & Webb, M. S. (2003). It ain't over till it's over: The case for offering relapse-prevention interventions to former smokers. *American Journal of the Medical Sciences, 326,* 197–200.

Browning, K. K., & Wewers, M. E. (2003). Smoking cessation and cancer. *Seminars in Oncology Nursing, 19*(4), 268–275.

Campaign for Tobacco-Free Kids. (2002). *Medicaid and Medicare costs & savings from covering tobacco cessation.* Retrieved July 2005 from http://tobaccofreekids.org/research/factsheets/pdf/0192.pdf

Campaign for Tobacco-Free Kids, American Lung Association, American Cancer Society, American Heart Association, & SmokeLess States National Tobacco Policy Initiative. (2003, January 23). *Show us the money: A report on the states' allocation of the tobacco settlement dollars.* Retrieved July 2005 from http://www.tobaccofreekids.org/reports/settlements/2003/fullreport.pdf

Centers for Disease Control and Prevention. (1993). Physician and other health-care professional counseling of smokers to quit—United States, 1991. *Morbidity and Mortality Weekly Report, 42,* 854–857.

Centers for Disease Control and Prevention. (1994). Guidelines for School health programs to prevent tobacco use and addiction. *Morbidity and Mortality Weekly Report, 43,* 1–18.

Centers for Disease Control and Prevention. (1996). Cigarette smoking before and after an excise tax increase and an antismoking campaign—Massachusetts, 1990–1996. *Morbidity and Mortality Weekly Report, 45,* 966–970.

Centers for Disease Control and Prevention. (1997, May 23). *Facts about cigar smoking.* Retrieved August 2005 from http://www.cdc.gov/od/oc/media/factcigars.htm

Centers for Disease Control and Prevention. (1999). Decline in cigarette consumption following implementation of a comprehensive tobacco prevention and education program—Oregon, 1996–1998. *Morbidity and Mortality Weekly Report, 48,* 140–143.

Centers for Disease Control and Prevention. (2003). Tobacco use among middle and high school students—United States, 2002. *Morbidity and Mortality Weekly Report, 52,* 1096–1098.

Centers for Disease Control and Prevention. (2004a). Cigarette smoking among adults—United States, 2002. *Morbidity and Mortality Weekly Report, 53,* 427–431.

Centers for Disease Control and Prevention. (2004b). Cigarette use among high school students—United States, 1991–2003. *Morbidity and Mortality Weekly Report, 53,* 499–502.

Centers for Disease Control and Prevention. (2004c). Impact of a smoking ban on restaurant and bar revenues—El Paso, Texas, 2002. *Morbidity and Mortality Weekly Report, 53,* 150–152.

Centers for Disease Control and Prevention. (2004d). Indoor air quality in hospitality venues before and after implementation of a clean indoor air law. *Morbidity and Mortality Weekly Report, 53,* 1038–1041.

Centers for Disease Control and Prevention. (2004e). Smoking during pregnancy—United States, 1990–2002. *Morbidity and Mortality Weekly Report, 53,* 911–915.

Centers for Disease Control and Prevention. (2004f). State-specific prevalence of current cigarette smoking among adults—United States, 2002. *Morbidity and Mortality Weekly Report, 52,* 1277–1280.

Centers for Disease Control and Prevention. (2004g). Youth Risk Behavior Surveillance—United States, 2003. *Morbidity and Mortality Weekly Report Surveillance Summaries, 53*(2), 1–100.

Chaloupka, F. (1999). How effective are taxes in reducing tobacco consumption? In C. Jeanrenaud & N. Soguel (Eds.), *Valuing the costs of smoking: Assessment methods, risk perceptions and policy options: Studies in risk and uncertainty* (pp. 205–218). Boston, Kluwer.

Chaloupka, F., & Wechsler, H. (1997). Price, tobacco control policies, and smoking among young adults. *Journal of Health Economics, 16,* 359–373.

Chollat-Traquet, C. (1992). Tobacco or health: A WHO programme. *European Journal of Cancer, 28,* 311–315.

Clarke, J. H., MacPherson, B., Holmes, D. R., & Jones, R. (1986). Reducing adolescent smoking: A comparison of peer-led, teacher-led, and expert interventions. *Journal of School Health, 56,* 102–106.

Coleman, T., Murphy, E., & Cheater, F. (2000). Factors influencing discussion of smoking between general practitioners and patients who smoke: A qualitative study. *British Journal of General Practice, 50,* 207–210.

COMMIT Research Group. (1995a). Community Intervention Trial for Smoking Cessation (COMMIT): I. Cohort results from a four-year community intervention. *American Journal of Public Health, 85,* 183–192.

COMMIT Research Group. (1995b). Community Intervention Trial for Smoking Cessation (COMMIT): II. Changes in adult cigarette smoking prevalence. *American Journal of Public Health, 85,* 193–200.

Connell, D. B., Turner, R. R., & Mason, E. F. (1985). Summary of findings of the School Health Education Evaluation: Health promotion effectiveness, implementation, and costs. *Journal of School Health, 55,* 316–321.

Coppotelli, H. C., & Orleans, C. T. (1985). Partner support and other determinants of smoking cessation maintenance among women. *Journal of Consulting and Clinical Psychology, 53,* 455–460.

Cornuz, J., Zellweger, J. P., Mounoud, C., Decrey, H., Pecoud, A., & Burnand, B. (1997). Smoking cessation counseling by residents in an outpatient clinic. *Preventive Medicine, 26,* 292–296.

Cummings, K. M., Hyland, A., Ockene, J. K., Hymowitz, N., & Manley, M. (1997). Use of the nicotine skin patch by smokers in 20 communities in the United States, 1992–1993. *Tobacco Control, 6,* S63–S70.

Danaher, B. G., Jeffery, R. W., Zimmerman, R., & Nelson, E. (1980). Aversive smoking using printed instructions and audiotape adjuncts. *Addictive Behaviors, 5,* 353–358.

de Leon, J., Tracy, J., McCann, E., McGrory, A., & Diaz, F. J. (2002). Schizophrenia and tobacco smoking: A replication study in another US psychiatric hospital. *Schizophrenia Research, 56*(1–2), 55–65.

Doescher, M. P., & Saver, B. G. (2000). Physicians' advice to quit smoking: The glass remains half empty. *Journal of Family Practice, 49,* 543–547.

Easton, A., Husten, C., Elon, L., Pederson, L., & Frank, E. (2001). Non-primary care physicians and smoking cessation counseling: Women Physicians' Health Study. *Women & Health, 34,* 15–29

Ebbert, J. O., Rowland, L. C., Montori, V., Vickers, K. S., Erwin, P. C., Dale, L. C., et al. (2004). Interventions for smokeless tobacco use cessation (Cochrane Review). *Cochrane Library, 3.*

Eckert, T., & Junker, C. (2001). Motivation for smoking cessation: What role do doctors play? *Swiss Medical Weekly, 131,* 521–526.

Ellen, J. M., Franzgrote, M., Irwin, C. E., & Millstein, S. G. (1998). Primary care physicians' screening of adolescent patients: A survey of California physicians. *Journal of Adolescent Health, 22,* 433–438.

Ellerbeck, E. F., Ahluwalia, J. S., Jolicoeur, D. G., Gladden, J., & Mosier, M. C. (2001). Direct observation of smoking cessation activities in primary care practice. *Journal of Family Practice, 50,* 688–693.

Emmons, K. M., Puleo, E., Park, E., Gritz, E. R., Butterfield, R. M., Weeks, J. C., Mertens, A., & Li, F. P. (2005). Peer-delivered smoking counseling for childhood cancer survivors increases rate of cessation: The Partnership for Health study. *Journal of Clinical Oncology, 23,* 6516–6523.

Fair and Equitable Tobacco Reform Act, 7 U.S.C. § 518 (2004).

Ferguson, J. A., Patten, C. A., Schroeder, D. R., Offord, K. P., Eberman, K. M., & Hurt, R. D. (2003). Predictors of 6-month tobacco abstinence among 1224 cigarette smokers treated for nicotine dependence. *Addictive Behaviors, 28*(7), 1203–1218.

Fichtenberg, C. M., & Glantz, S. A. (2000). Association of the California Tobacco Control Program with declines in cigarette consumption and mortality from heart disease. *New England Journal of Medicine, 343,* 1772–1777.

Fichtenberg, C. M., & Glantz, S. A. (2002). Effect of smoke-free workplaces on smoking behaviour: Systematic review. *British Medical Journal, 325,* 188.

Fiore, M. C., Bailey, W. C., Cohen, S. J., Dorfman, S. F., Goldstein, M. G., Gritz, E. R., et al. (2000a). *Treating tobacco use and dependence* (Clinical Practice Guideline). Rockville, MD: U.S. Department of Health and Human Services, Public Health Service.

Fiore, M. C., Bailey, W. C., Cohen, S. J., Dorfman, S. F., Goldstein, M. G., Gritz, E. R., et al. (2000b). *Treating tobacco use and dependence* (Quick Reference Guide). Rockville, MD: U.S. Department of Health and Human Services, Public Health Service.

Fiore, M. C., Croyle, R. T., Curry, S. J., Cutler, C. M., Davis, R. M., Gordon, C., et al. (2004). Preventing 3 million premature deaths and helping 5 million smokers quit: A national action plan for tobacco cessation. *American Journal of Public Health, 94*(2), 205–210.

Fisher, E. B., Jr., Haire-Joshu, D., Morgan, G. D., Rehberg, H., & Rost, K. (1990). Smoking and smoking cessation. *American Review of Respiratory Disease, 142,* 702–720.

Fisher, E. B., Jr., Lichtenstein, E., Haire-Joshu, D., Morgan, G. D., & Rehberg, H. R. (1993). Methods, successes, and failures of smoking cessation programs. *Annual Review of Medicine, 44,* 481–513.

Franzgrote, M., Ellen, J., Millstein, S., & Irwin, C. (1997). Screening for adolescent smoking among primary care physicians in California. *American Journal of Public Health, 87,* 1341–1345.

Fried, J. L., & Cohen, L. A. (1992). Maryland dentists' attitudes regarding tobacco issues. *Clinical Preventive Dentistry, 14,* 10–16.

Galuska, D. A., Fulton, J. E., Powell, K. E., Burgeson, C. R., Pratt, M., Elster, A., et al. (2002). Pediatrician counseling about preventive health topics: Results from the Physicians' Practices Survey, 1998–1999. *Pediatrics, 109*(5), E83–E88.

Gans, G. E., McManus, M. A., & Newchuck, P. W. (1991). *Adolescent health care: Use, costs, and problems of access* (AMA Profiles of Adolescent Health, No. 6). Chicago: American Medical Association.

Gehrman, C. A., & Hovell, M. F. (2003). Protecting children from environmental tobacco smoke (ETS) exposure: A critical review. *Nicotine & Tobacco Research, 5*(3), 289–301.

Gerace, T. A., Hollis, J., Ockene, J. K., & Svendsen, K. (1991). Smoking cessation and change in diastolic blood pressure, body weight, and plasma lipids. *Preventive Medicine, 20,* 602–620.

Giovino, G. A. (2002). Epidemiology of tobacco use in the United States. *Oncogene, 21*(48), 7326–7340.

Givel, M., & Glantz, S. A. (2001). Tobacco lobby political influence on US state legislatures in the 1990s. *Tobacco Control, 10,* 124–134.

Givel, M., & Glantz, S. A. (2002). State tobacco settlement funds not being spent on vigorous tobacco control efforts. *Oncology, 16,* 152–157.

Givel, M., & Glantz, S. A. (2004). The "global settlement" with the tobacco industry: 6 years later. *American Journal of Public Health, 94,* 218–224.

Glantz, S. A. (1993). Changes in cigarette consumption, prices, and tobacco industry revenues associated with California's Proposition 99. *Tobacco Control, 2,* 311–314.

Glantz, S. A., & Balbach, E. D. (2000). Tobacco war: Inside the California battles. Berkeley: University of California Press.

Glantz, S. A., & Jamieson, P. (2000). Attitudes toward secondhand smoke, smoking, and quitting among young people. *Pediatrics, 106,* E82.

Glantz, S. A., & Wilson-Loots, R. (2003). No association of smoke-free ordinances with profits from bingo and charitable games in Massachusetts. *Tobacco Control, 12,* 411–413.

Glasgow, R. E., Cummings, K. M., & Hyland, A. (1997). Relationship of worksite smoking policies to changes in employee tobacco use: Findings from COMMIT. *Tobacco Control, 6,* S44–S48.

Glasgow, R. E., Lichtenstein, E., Beaver, C., & O'Neill, K. (1981). Subjective reactions to rapid and normal pace adversive smoking. *Addictive Behaviors, 6,* 53–59.

Glynn, T. J., & Manley, M. (1991). How to help your patients stop smoking: A National Cancer Institute manual for physicians (DHHS Publication No. 92-3064). Washington, DC: National Cancer Institute.

Gold, R. S., Parcel, G. S., Walberg, H. J., Luepker, R. V., Portnoy, B., & Stone, E. J. (1991). Summary and conclusions of the THTM evaluation: The expert work group perspective. *Journal of School Health, 61,* 39–42.

Goldman, L. K., & Glantz, S. A. (1998). Evaluation of antismoking advertising campaigns. *JAMA, 279,* 772–777.

Goldstein, M. G., DePue, J. D., Monroe, A. D., Lessne, C. W., Rakowski, W., Prokhorov, A., et al. (1998). A population-based survey of physician smoking cessation counseling practices. *Preventive Medicine, 27,* 720–729.

Gordon, J. S., & Severson, H. H. (2001). Tobacco cessation through dental office settings. *Journal of Dental Education, 65,* 354–363.

Gottlieb, N. H., Guo, J. L., Blozis, S. A., & Huang, P. P. (2001). Individual and contextual factors related to family practice residents' assessment and counseling for tobacco cessation. *Journal of the American Board of Family Medicine, 14,* 343–351.

Grant, B. F., Hasin, D. S., Chou, S. P., Stinson, F. S., & Dawson, D. A. (2004). Nicotine dependence and psychiatric disorders in the United States: Results from the national epidemiologic survey on alcohol and related conditions. *Archives of General Psychiatry, 61*(11), 1107–1115.

Gregorio, D. (1994). Counseling adolescents for smoking prevention: A survey of primary care physicians and dentists. *American Journal of Public Health, 84,* 1151–1153.

Grimley, D. M., Bellis, J. M., Raczynski, J. M., & Henning, K. (2001). Smoking cessation counseling practices: A survey of Alabama obstetrician-gynecologists. *Southern Medical Journal, 94,* 297–303.

Gritz, E. R., St. Jeor, S. T., Bennett, G., Biener, L., Blair, S. N., Bowen, D. J., et al. (1992). National working conference on smoking and body weight: Task Force 3: Implications with respect to intervention and prevention. *Health Psychology, 11,* 17–25.

Gross, C., Soffer, B., Bach, P., Rajkumar, R., & Forman, H. (2002). State expenditures for tobacco-control programs and the tobacco settlement. *New England Journal of Medicine, 347,* 1080–1086.

Grossman, M., & Chaloupka, F. J. (1997). Cigarette taxes: The straw to break the camel's back. *Public Health Reports, 112*(4), 290–297.

Hajek, P., & Stead, L. F. (2004). Aversive smoking for smoking cessation (Cochrane Review). *Cochrane Library, 3.*

Hajek, P., Stead, L. F., West, R., Jarvis, M., & Lancaster, T. (2005). Relapse prevention interventions for smoking cessation (Cochrane Review). *Cochrane Library, 1.*

Hall, S. M., Rugg, D., Tunstall, C., & Jones, R. T. (1984). Preventing relapse to cigarette smoking by behavioral skill training. *Journal of Consulting and Clinical Psychology, 52,* 372–382.

Harris, K. J., Okuyemi, K. S., Catley, D., Mayo, M. S., Ge, B., & Ahluwalia, J. S. (2004). Predictors of smoking cessation among African-Americans enrolled in a randomized controlled trial of bupropion. *Preventive Medicine, 38*(4), 498–502.

Henschke, C. I., McCauley, D. I., Yankelevitz, D. F., Naidich, D. P., McGuinness, G., Miettinen, O. S., et al. (1999). Early lung cancer action project: Overall design and findings from baseline screening. *Lancet, 354*, 99–105.

Hepburn, M. J., Johnson, J. M., Ward, J. A., & Longfield, J. N. (2000). A survey of smoking cessation knowledge, training, and practice among U.S. Army general medical officers. *American Journal of Preventive Medicine, 18*, 300–304.

Iribarren, C., Tekawa, I. S., Sidney, S., & Friedman, G. D. (1999). Effect of cigar smoking on the risk of cardiovascular disease: Chronic obstructive pulmonary disease, and cancer in men. *New England Journal of Medicine, 340*, 1773–1780.

John, J. H., Yudkin, P., Murphy, M., Ziebland, S., & Fowler, G. H. (1997). Smoking cessation interventions for dental patients: Attitudes and reported practices of dentists in the Oxford region. *British Dental Journal, 183*, 359–364.

Johnstone, E. C., Yudkin, P. L., Hey, K., Roberts, S. J., Welch, S. J., Murphy, M. F., et al. (2004). Genetic variation in dopaminergic pathways and short-term effectiveness of the nicotine patch. *Pharmacogenetics, 14*(2), 83–90.

Jones, S. E., Sharp, D. J., Husten, C. G., & Crossett, L. S. (2002). Cigarette acquisition and proof of age among US high school students who smoke. *Tobacco Control, 11*, 20–25.

Kandel, D. B., & Davies, M. (1996). High school students who use crack and other drugs. *Archives of General Psychiatry, 53*, 71–80.

Kawakami, M., Nakamura, S., Fumimoto, H., Takizawa, J., & Baba, M. (1997). Relation between smoking status of physicians and their enthusiasm to offer smoking cessation advice. *Internal Medicine, 36*, 162–165.

Klein, J. D., Levine, L. J., & Allan, M. J. (2001). Delivery of smoking prevention and cessation services to adolescents. *Archives of Pediatrics & Adolescent Medicine, 155*, 597–602.

Klerman, L. (2004). Protecting children: Reducing their environmental tobacco smoke exposure. *Nicotine & Tobacco Research, 6* (Suppl. 2), S239–S253.

Klesges, R. C., & Klesges, L. M. (1988). Cigarette smoking as a dieting strategy in a university population. *International Journal of Eating Disorders, 7*, 413–419.

Klesges, R. C., Meyers, A. W., Klesges, L. M., & La Vasque, M. E. (1989). Smoking, body weight, and their effects on smoking behavior: A comprehensive review of the literature. *Psychological Bulletin, 106*, 204–230.

Kottke, T. E., Battista, R. N., DeFriese, G. H., & Brekke, M. L. (1988). Attributes of successful smoking cessation interventions in medical practice: A meta-analysis of 39 controlled trials. *JAMA, 259*, 2883–2889.

Kviz, F. J., Clark, M. A., Prochaska, T. R., Slezak, J. A., Crittenden, K. S., Freels, S., et al. (1995). Attitudes and practices for smoking cessation counseling by provider type and patient age. *Preventive Medicine, 24*, 201–212.

Lambert, A., Sargent, J. D., Glantz, S. A., & Ling, P. M. (2004). How Philip Morris unlocked the Japanese cigarette market: Lessons for global tobacco control. *Tobacco Control, 13*, 379–387.

Lancaster, T., & Stead, L. F. (2002). Self-help interventions for smoking cessation (Cochrane Review). *Cochrane Library, 3*.

Lando, H. A. (1977). Successful treatment of smokers with a broad-spectrum behavioral approach. *Journal of Consulting and Clinical Psychology, 45*, 361–366.

Lasser, K., Boyd, J. W., Woolhandler, S., Himmelstein, D. U., McCormick, D., & Bor, D. H. (2000). Smoking and mental illness: A population-based prevalence study. *JAMA, 284,* 2606–2610.

Leone, A., Giannini, D., Bellotto, C., & Balbarini, A. (2004). Passive smoking and coronary heart disease. *Current Vascular Pharmacology, 2*(2), 175–182.

Lerman, C., Kaufmann, V., Rukstalis, M., Patterson, F., Perkins, K., Audrain-McGovern, J., et al. (2004). Individualizing nicotine replacement therapy for the treatment of tobacco dependence: A randomized trial. *Annals of Internal Medicine, 140*(6), 426–433.

Lerman, C., Patterson, F., & Berrettini, W. (2005). Treating tobacco dependence: State of the science and new directions. *Journal of Clinical Oncology, 23*(2), 311–323.

Lerman, C., Shields, P. G., Wileyto, E. P., Audrain, J., Hawk, L. H., Jr., Pinto, A., et al. (2003). Effects of dopamine transporter and receptor polymorphisms on smoking cessation in a bupropion clinical trial. *Health Psychology, 22*(5), 541–548.

Lerman, C., Shields, P. G., Wileyto, E. P., Audrain, J., Pinto, A., Hawk, L., et al. (2002). Pharmacogenetic investigation of smoking cessation treatment. *Pharmacogenetics, 12*(8), 627–634.

Levy, D. T., & Friend, K. B. (2003). The effects of clean indoor air laws: What do we know and what do we need to know? *Health Education Research, 18*(5), 592–609.

Li, M. D. (2003). The genetics of smoking related behavior: A brief review. *American Journal of the Medical Sciences, 326*(4), 168–173.

Lichtenstein, E. (1982). The smoking problem: A behavioral perspective. *Journal of Consulting and Clinical Psychology, 50,* 804–819.

Lichtenstein, E., Harris, D. E., Birchler, G. R., Wahl, J. M., & Schmahl, D. P. (1973). Comparison of rapid smoking, warm, smoky air, and attention placebo in the modification of smoking behavior. *Journal of Consulting and Clinical Psychology, 40,* 92–98.

Lightwood, J. M., & Glantz, S. A. (1997). Short-term economic and health benefits of smoking cessation: Myocardial infarction and stroke. *Circulation, 96,* 1089–1096.

Lindsay, E. A., Ockene, J. K., Hymowitz, N., Giffen, C., Berger, L., & Pomrehn, P. (1994). Physi cians and smoking cessation: A survey of office procedures and practices in the Community Intervention Trial for Smoking Cessation. *Archives of Family Medicine, 3,* 341–348.

Ling, P. M., Landman, A., & Glantz, S. A. (2002). It is time to abandon youth access tobacco programmes. *Tobacco Control, 11,* 3–6.

Lodi, G., Bez, C., Rimondini, L., Zuppiroli, A., Sardella, A., & Carrassi, A. (1997). Attitude towards smoking and oral cancer prevention among northern Italian dentists. *Oral Oncology, 33,* 100–104.

Lowe, M. R., Green, L., Kurtz, S. M., Ashenberg, Z. S., & Fisher, E. B., Jr. (1980). Self-initiated, cue extinction, and covert sensitization procedures in smoking cessation. *Journal of Behavioral Medicine, 3,* 357–372.

Lumley, J., Oliver, S. S., Chamberlain, C., & Oakley, L. (2004). Interventions for promoting smoking cessation during pregnancy (Cochrane Review). *Cochrane Library, 4.*

Makemson, C., & Glantz, S. A. (2002). How the tobacco industry built its relationship with Hollywood. *Tobacco Control, 11* (Suppl. 1), i81–i91.

Manley, M., Epp, R., Husten, C., Glynn, T., & Shopland, D. (1991). Clinical interventions in tobacco control: A National Cancer Institute training program for physicians. *JAMA, 266,* 172–173.

Manley, M. W., Pierce, J. P., Gilpin, E. A., Rosbrook, B., Berry, C., & Wun, L. M. (1997). Impact of the American Stop Smoking Intervention Study on cigarette consumption. *Tobacco Control, 6,* S12–S16.

Marcus, B. H., Albrecht, A. E., King, T. K., Parisi, A. F., Pinto, B. M., Roberts, M., et al. (1999). The efficacy of exercise as an aid for smoking cessation in women. *Archives of Internal Medicine, 159,* 1229–1234.

McBride, C. M., & Ostroff, J. S. (2003). Teachable moments for promoting smoking cessation: The context of cancer care and survivorship. *Cancer Control, 10*(4), 325–333.

McCarty, M. C., Hennrikus, D. J., Lando, H. A., & Vessey, J. T. (2001). Nurses' attitudes concerning the delivery of brief cessation advice to hospitalized smokers. *Preventive Medicine, 33,* 674–681.

McCreadie, R. G. (2002). Use of drugs, alcohol and tobacco by people with schizophrenia: Case-control study. *British Journal of Psychiatry, 181,* 321–325.

McEwen, A., & West, R. (2001). Smoking cessation activities by general practitioners and practice nurses. *Tobacco Control, 10,* 27–32.

McIlvain, H. E., & Bobo, J. K. (1999). Tobacco cessation with patients recovering from alcohol and other substance abuse. *Primary Care Clinics in Office Practice, 26,* 671–689.

McIlvain, H. E., Crabtree, B. F., Backer, E. L., & Turner, P. D. (2000). Use of office-based smoking cessation activities in family practices. *Journal of Family Practice, 49,* 1025–1029.

Moher, M., Hey, K., & Lancaster, T. (2003). Workplace interventions for smoking cessation (Cochrane Review). *Cochrane Library, 2.*

Montner, P., Bennett, G., & Brown, C. (1994). An evaluation of a smoking cessation training program for medical residents in an inner-city hospital. *Journal of the National Medical Association, 86,* 671–675.

Mulshine, J. L., & Henschke, C. I. (2000). Prospects for lung-cancer screening: Commentary. *Lancet, 355,* 592–593.

Munafo, M., Clark, T., Johnstone, E., Murphy, M., & Walton, R. (2004). The genetic basis for smoking behavior: A systematic review and meta-analysis. *Nicotine & Tobacco Research, 6*(4), 583–597.

National Association of Attorneys General. (1998). *NAAG projects: Tobacco: Master Settlement Agreement and Amendments.* Retrieved September 2005 from http://www.naag.org/issues/tobacco/index.php?sdpid=919

National Cancer Institute. (2003). *Questions and answers about smokeless tobacco and cancer.* Retrieved September 2005 from http://cis.nci.nih.gov/fact/10_15.htm

National Cancer Policy Board. (2000). *State programs can reduce tobacco use.* Washington, DC: National Academies Press.

Nelson, D. E., Davis, R. M., Chrismon, J. H., & Giovino, G. A. (1996). Pipe smoking in the United States, 1965–1991: Prevalence and attributable mortality. *Preventive Medicine, 25,* 91–99.

Newton, J. T., & Palmer, R. M. (1997). The role of the team in the promotion of smoking cessation. *British Dental Journal, 182,* 353–355.

Ockene, J. K., & Zapka, J. G. (1997). Physician-based smoking intervention: A rededication to a five-step strategy to smoking research. *Addictive Behaviors, 22,* 835–848.

O'Loughlin, J., Makni, H., Tremblay, M., Lacroix, C., Gervais, A., Dery, V., et al. (2001). Smoking cessation counseling practices of general practitioners in Montreal. *Preventive Medicine, 33,* 627–638.

Oncken, C. A., & Kranzler, H. R. (2003). Pharmacotherapies to enhance smoking cessation during pregnancy. *Drug and Alcohol Review, 22*(2), 191–202.

Orleans, C. T. (1985). Understanding and promoting smoking cessation: Overview and guidelines for physician intervention. *Annual Review of Medicine, 36,* 51–61.

Orleans, C. T., Kristeller, J. L., & Gritz, E. R. (1993). Helping hospitalized smokers quit: New directions for treatment and research. *Journal of Consulting and Clinical Psychology, 61,* 778–789.

Ossip-Klein, D. J., McIntosh, S., Utman, C., Burton, K., Spada, J., & Guido, J. (2000). Smokers ages 50+: Who gets physician advice to quit? *Preventive Medicine, 31,* 364–369.

Pamuck, E., Makuc, D., Heck, K., Reuben, C., & Lochner, K. (1998). *Socioeconomic status and health chartbook: Health, United States, 1998.* Hyattsville, MD: National Center for Health Statistics.

Patel, J. D., Bach, P. B., & Kris, M. G. (2004). Lung cancer in US women: A contemporary epidemic. *JAMA, 291,* 1763–1768.

Patkar, A. A., Gopalakrishnan, R., Lundy, A., Leone, F. T., Certa, K. M., & Weinstein, S. P. (2002). Relationship between tobacco smoking and positive and negative symptoms in schizophrenia. *Journal of Nervous and Mental Disease, 190*(9), 604–610.

Pentz, M., Brannon, B., Charlin, V., Barrett, E., MacKinnon, D., & Flay, B. (1989). The power of policy: The relationship of smoking policy to adolescent smoking. *American Journal of Public Health, 79*(7), 857–862.

Perkins, K. A. (1993). Weight gain following smoking cessation. *Journal of Consulting and Clinical Psychology, 61,* 768–777.

Perry, C., & Silvis, G. (1987). Smoking prevention: Behavioral prescription for the pediatrician. *Pediatrics, 79,* 790–799.

Perry, C. L., Pirie, P., Holder, W., Halper, A., & Dudovitz, B. (1990). Parent involvement in cigarette smoking prevention: Two pilot evaluations of the "Unpuffables Program." *Journal of School Health, 60,* 443–447.

Perry, C. L., Telch, M. J., Killen, J., Burke, A., & Maccoby, N. (1983). High school smoking prevention: The relative efficacy of varied treatments and instructors. *Adolescence, 18,* 561–566.

Peterson, A. V., Jr., Kealey, K. A., Mann, S. L., Marek, P. M., & Sarason, I. G. (2000). Hutchinson Smoking Prevention Project: Long-term randomized trial in school-based tobacco use prevention—Results on smoking. *Journal of the National Cancer Institute, 92,* 1979–1991.

Pierce, J. P., Gilpin, E. A., Emery, S. L., Farkas, A. J., Zhu, S. H., Choi, W. S., et al. (1998). *Tobacco control in California: Who's winning the war? An evaluation of the Tobacco Control Program 1989–1996.* LaJolla: University of California, San Diego.

Pierce, J. P., Gilpin, E. A., Emery, S. L., White, M. M., Rosbrook, B., & Berry, C. C., et al. (1998). Has the California Tobacco Control Program reduced smoking? *JAMA, 280,* 893–899.

Pirie, P. L., Murray, D. M., & Luepker, R. V. (1991). Gender differences in cigarette smoking and quitting in a cohort of young adults. *American Journal of Public Health, 81,* 324–327.

Pollak, K. I., Arredondo, E. M., Yarnall, K. S., Lipkus, I., Myers, E., McNeilly, M., et al. (2001). How do residents prioritize smoking cessation for young "high-risk" women? Factors associated with addressing smoking cessation. *Preventive Medicine, 33,* 292–299.

Rigotti, N. A., Munafo, M. R., Murphy, M. F., & Stead, L. F. (2003). Interventions for smoking cessation in hospitalised patients (update of 2001 Cochrane Review) (Cochrane Review). *Cochrane Library, 1.*

Rogers, L. Q., Johnson, K. C., Young, Z. M., & Graney, M. (1997). Demographic bias in physician smoking cessation counseling. *American Journal of the Medical Sciences, 313,* 153–158.

Rosenbaum, P., & O'Shea, R. (1992). Large-scale study of Freedom from Smoking clinics: Factors in quitting. *Public Health Reports, 107,* 150–155.

Sargent, J. D., & DiFranza, J. R. (2003). Tobacco control for clinicians who treat adolescents. *CA, 53,* 102–123.

Sargent, R. P., Shepard, R. M., & Glantz, S. A. (2004). Reduced incidence of admissions for myocardial infarction associated with public smoking ban: Before and after study. *British Medical Journal, 328,* 977–980.

Sarna, L. P., Brown, J. K., Lillington, L., Rose, M., Wewers, M. E., & Brecht, M. L. (2000). Tobacco interventions by oncology nurses in clinical practice: Report from a national survey. *Cancer, 89,* 881–889.

Sasco, A. J., Secretan, M. B., & Straif, K. (2004). Tobacco smoking and cancer: A brief review of recent epidemiological evidence. *Lung Cancer, 45* (Suppl. 2), S3–S9.

Schnoll, R. A., & Lerman, C. (2003). Smoking behavior and smoking cessation among head and neck cancer patients. In J. Ensley, J. Gutkind, J. Jacobs, & S. M. Lippman (Eds.), *Head and neck cancers* (pp. 185–200). San Diego, CA: Academic Press.

Schnoll, R. A., Rothman, R. L., Wielt, D. B., Lerman, C., Pedri, H., Wang, H., et. al. (2005). A randomized pilot study of cognitive-behavioral therapy versus basic health education for smoking cessation among cancer patients. *Annals of Behavioral Medicine, 30,* 1–11.

Schroeder, S. A. (2004). The tobacco buyout and the FDA. *New England Journal of Medicine, 351,* 1377–1380.

Schubiner, H., Herrold, A., & Hurt, R. (1998). Tobacco cessation and youth: The feasibility of brief office interventions for adolescents. *Preventive Medicine, 27,* A47–A54.

Secker-Walker, R. H., Solomon, L. J., Flynn, B. S., & Dana, G. S. (1994). Comparisons of the smoking cessation counseling activities of six types of health professionals. *Preventive Medicine, 23,* 800–808.

Secker-Walker, R. H., Gnich, W., Platt, S., & Lancaster, T. (2005). Community interventions for reducing smoking among adults. *The Cochrane Database of Systematic Reviews, 4,* 0 0075320–1 00000000–00976.

Sheinfeld Gorin, S. (2001). Predictors of tobacco control among student nurses. *Patient Education and Counseling, 44,* 251–262.

Sheinfeld Gorin, S., & Heck, J. E. (2004). Meta-analysis of the efficacy of tobacco counseling by health care providers. *Cancer Epidemiology, Biomarkers & Prevention, 13,* 2012–2022.

Shimokata, H., Muller, D. C., & Andres, R. (1989). Studies in the distribution of body fat: III. Effects of cigarette smoking. *JAMA, 261,* 1169–1173.

Siegel, M., Mowery, P. D., Pechacek, T. P., Strauss, W. J., Schooley, M. W., Merritt, R. K., et al. (2000). Trends in adult cigarette smoking in California compared with the rest of the United States, 1978–1994. *American Journal of Public Health, 90,* 372–379.

Silagy, C., Lancaster, T., Stead, L., Mant, D., & Fowler, G. (2004). Nicotine replacement therapy for smoking cessation (Cochrane Review). *Cochrane Library, 3.*

Sinclair, H. K., Bond, C. M., & Stead, L. F. (2004). Community pharmacy personnel interventions for smoking cessation (Cochrane Review). *Cochrane Library, 1.*

Sussman, S., Lichtman, K., Ritt, A., & Pallonen, U. E. (1999). Effects of thirty-four adolescent tobacco use cessation and prevention trials on regular users of tobacco products. *Substance Use and Misuse, 34,* 1469–1503.

Swan, G. E. (1999). Implications of genetic epidemiology for the prevention of tobacco use. *Nicotine & Tobacco Research, 1* (Suppl. 1), S49–S56.

Swan, G. E., Jack, L. M., Curry, S., Chorost, M., Javitz, H., McAfee, T., et al. (2003). Bupropion SR and counseling for smoking cessation in actual practice: Predictors of outcome. *Nicotine & Tobacco Research, 5*(6), 911–921.

Task Force on Community Preventive Services. (2001). Guide to community preventive services: Tobacco use prevention and control. *American Journal of Preventive Medicine, 20*(2, Suppl. 1), 1–87.

Thorndike, A. N., Ferris, T. G., Stafford, R. S., & Rigotti, N. A. (1999). Rates of US physicians counseling adolescents about smoking. *Journal of the National Cancer Institute, 91,* 1657–1662.

Tobacco Control Section. (1998). *A model for change: The California experience in tobacco control.* Sacramento: California Department of Health Services.

Turner, L., Mermelstein, R., & Flay, B. (2004). Individual and contextual influences on adolescent smoking. *Annals of the New York Academy of Sciences, 1021,* 175–197.

U.S. Department of Health and Human Services. (1980). *The health consequences of smoking for women: A report of the surgeon general.* Bethesda, MD: U.S. Department of Health and Human Services, Public Health Service.

U.S. Department of Health and Human Services. (1986). *The health consequences of using smokeless tobacco: A report of the advisory committee to the surgeon general* (NIH Publication No. 86-2874). Bethesda, MD: U.S. Department of Health and Human Services, Public Health Service.

U.S. Department of Health and Human Services. (1998a, February). *Cigars: Health effects and trends* (Smoking and Control Monograph 9). Bethesda, MD: U.S. Department of Health and Human Services, National Cancer Institute.

U.S. Department of Health and Human Services. (1998b). *Tobacco use among US racial/ethnic minority groups—African Americans, American Indians and Alaska Natives, Asian Americans and Pacific Islanders, and Hispanics: A report of the surgeon general.* Washington, DC: U.S. Government Printing Office.

U.S. Department of Health and Human Services. (2000a). *Healthy people 2010: Understanding and improving health* (2nd ed.). Washington, DC: U.S. Government Printing Office.

U.S. Department of Health and Human Services. (2000b). *Reducing tobacco use: A report of the surgeon general.* Rockville, MD: U.S. Department of Health and Human Services, Office of the Surgeon General.

U.S. Department of Health and Human Services. (2004). *The health consequences of smoking: A report of the surgeon general.* Atlanta, GA: U.S. Department of Health and Human Services, Office on Smoking and Health.

U.S. Department of Health and Human Services, Office of Inspector General (1999, February). *Youth use of cigars: Federal, state regulation and enforcement* (OEI-06-98-00020). Retrieved September 2005 from http://oig.hhs.gov/oei/reports/oei-06-98-00020.pdf

U.S. Environmental Protection Agency. (1997). Health effects of exposure to environmental tobacco smoke. *Tobacco Control, 6,* 346–353.

Vanasse, A., Niyonsenga, T., & Courteau, J. (2004). Smoking cessation within the context of family medicine: Which smokers take action? *Preventive Medicine, 38*(3), 330–337.

Wakefield, M., Chaloupka, F., Kaufman, N., Orleans, C. T., Barker, D. C., & Ruel, E. E. (2000). Effect of restrictions at home, at school, and in public places on teenage smoking: Cross sectional study. *British Medical Journal, 321,* 333–337.

Warner, K. E. (1981). Cigarette smoking in the 1970s: The impact of the antismoking campaign on consumption. *Science, 211,* 729–731.

Wasserman, J., Manning, W., Newhouse, J., & Winkler, J. D. (1991). The effects of excise taxes and regulations on cigarette smoking. *Journal of Health Economics, 10,* 43–64.

White, A. R., Rampes, H., & Ernst, E. (2002). Acupuncture for smoking cessation (Cochrane Review). *Cochrane Library, 2.*

Windsor, R. A. (1986). An application of the PRECEDE model for planning and evaluating health education methods for pregnant smokers. *Hygiene, 5,* 38–44.

Wolfenden, L., Campbell, E., Walsh, R., & Wiggers, J. (2003). Smoking cessation interventions for in-patients: A selective review with recommendations for hospital-based health professionals. *Drug and Alcohol Review, 22,* 437–452.

World Bank Group. (2001, March). *Tobacco at a glance.* Retrieved November 2005 from http://www1.worldbank.org/tobacco/tobacco.pdf

World Health Organization. (2004, May 21). WHO Framework Convention on Tobacco Control (Report No. WHA56,1). Retrieved June 2005 from www.who.int/gb/ebwha/pdf_files/WHA56/ea56r1.pdf

Yang, G. H., Ma, J. M., Chen, A. P., Brown, S., Taylor, C. E., & Samet, J. M. (2004). Smoking adolescents in China: 1998 survey findings. *International Journal of Epidemiology, 33,* 103–110.

Zapka, J. G., Fletcher, K., Pbert, L., Druker, S. K., Ockene, J. K., & Chen, L. (1999). The perceptions and practices of pediatricians. *Tobacco Intervention, 103,* 65.

EXHIBIT 9.3. HELPFUL RESOURCES.

Web Sites

Action on Smoking and Health, http://ash.org

This is an antismoking Web site that offers resources for activists.

The American Cancer Society, http://www.cancer.org

The ACS, a voluntary organization, offers programs and other resources, including a quit line, to help individuals quit smoking.

The American Heart Association, http://www.amhrt.org

The AHA home page contributes a directory of materials and programs for smoking cessation. It has developed a packet and runs programs for cessation titled Calling It Quits.

The American Lung Association, http://www.lungusa.org

This site contains several fact sheets, particularly one titled "Smoking and Teens Fact Sheet." The ALA also maintains the Freedom from Smoking online quit program.

Centers for Disease Control and Prevention, *Tobacco information and prevention source* (TIPS), http://www.cdc.gov/tobacco/index.htm

EXHIBIT 9.3. HELPFUL RESOURCES, Cont'd.

This CDC site offers the opportunity to download guidelines for tobacco control published by the CDC and other governmental agencies. It also offers a multitude of fact sheets on tobacco control.

National Cancer Institute, *Cancer topics,* http://www.nci.nih.gov/cancertopics/tobacco

The NCI's Cancer Topics home page provides links to a variety of resources for smoking cessation as well as other cancer prevention and control approaches. The NCI has a national quit line and a Web site (www.smokefree.gov) to help smokers stop. (See the following section on brochures and videotapes for more information on NCI materials.)

Brochures and Videotapes

National Cancer Institute, Office of Cancer Communications, Building 31, Room 10A16, 9000 Rockville Pike, Rockville, MD 20892; Phone: (800) 4-CANCER; offers the following client educational brochures and videotapes:

Clearing the air: Quit smoking today. Available from http://www.smokefree.gov/pubs/clearing_the_air.pdf

Dangerous game: The truth about spit tobacco. (Not yet available online.)

Good information for smokers. Available from http://www.surgeongeneral.gov/tobacco/lowlit.pdf

Guía para dejar de fumar: No lo deje para mañana, deje de fumar hoy (Guide to quitting smoking: Don't leave it for tomorrow, quit today). Available from http://cancercontrol.cancer.gov/tcrb/Spanish_Smoking_book.pdf

Quitting helps you heal faster. Available from http://www.surgeongeneral.gov/tobacco/hospital.pdf

Spit tobacco: A guide for quitting. Available from http://www.nidr.nih.gov/health/newsandhealth/spitTobacco

Treating tobacco use and dependence: Clinical practice guideline. Available from https://cissecure.nci.nih.gov/ncipubs/details.asp?pid=236

Usted puede dejar de fumar. Available from http://www.surgeongeneral.gov/tobacco/tearsheetspa.pdf

You can quit smoking: Support and advice from your clinician. Available from http://www.surgeongeneral.gov/tobacco/tearsheeteng.pdf

The American Cancer Society offers the following online brochures:

Set yourself free: A smoker's guide (English/Spanish) and *Living smoke free for you and your baby.* Both available from http://www.cancer.org/asp/freebrochures/fb_global.asp

CHAPTER TEN

SUBSTANCE SAFETY

Kristen Lawton Barry
Frederic C. Blow

Substance safety is a major public health concern. This public health concern, however, is complicated by the fact that social interaction in U.S. society is generally characterized by the use of some substance, such as alcohol. This chapter begins with a discussion of the differentiation of the classes of drugs, focusing specifically on alcohol and banned substances, and then outlines health promotion through substance safety for special populations. Specific criteria for recognizing levels of risk and problem use are identified, and effective brief interventions and brief therapies are discussed.

Classes of Substances

In dealing with health promotion related to substance use and abuse, the complexity of the issues is manifest in the different classes of drugs that are subsumed under the term *substances*.

Prescribed and Over-the-Counter Drugs and Medications

The purpose of prescribed and over-the-counter drugs is to foster health or to minimize symptoms of discomfort and ill health. The major health promotion issues concerning these drugs are related to prescribing practices and Food and

Drug Administration (FDA) monitoring of drugs sold over the counter. Health care professionals are often concerned about medication. Compliance (that is, the patient's following the instructions for the use of a particular medication) is an ambiguous issue because accurate follow-up to determine compliance is often difficult and the use of over-the-counter drugs, largely as self-medication, is widespread. Further, prescribing practices are influenced by variations in medical education, practice norms, and pharmaceutical marketing approaches.

Banned Substances

Banned substances are drugs that appear on Schedule I, defined under the Controlled Substances Act (1970). The medicinal value of these drugs is disputed, and these illegal substances are generally obtained for recreational usage. Banned substances include marijuana, cocaine, heroin, morphine, lysergic acid diethylamide (LSD), and phencyclidine (PCP). Issues inherent in the medical applications of marijuana for certain conditions notwithstanding, the use or abuse of banned substances is generally considered a risk to good health.

Social Drugs

Drugs such as caffeine, nicotine, and alcohol are often referred to as *social drugs*. These drugs are readily available—at least, by law, to adults—and are widely used. Caffeine, the most widely used psychoactive drug in the world, is considered a relatively mild stimulant (Greden & Walters, 1992). In recent decades people in the United States have been consuming caffeine more from soft drinks than from coffee. The amount of caffeine consumed in coffee, tea, and soft drinks produces relatively limited stimulant effects when compared with the effects of amphetamines. Evidence linking caffeine to benign breast disease and coronary disease is still unclear. Except for the occasional case of *caffeinism* and the mild discomfort of caffeine withdrawal, evidence for a linkage between poor health outcomes (such as diseases) and caffeine is limited, provided one consumes it moderately (Lamarine, 1994). There is, however, clear evidence of long-term consequences from nicotine use. Chapter Nine deals with health promotion through smoking cessation and, although persons may continue to choose to use nicotine, the relationship between nicotine and adverse health consequences has been clearly established for many decades. The first clear evidence of a relationship between smoking and lung cancer appeared in the 1955, and the first U.S. surgeon general's report that defined nicotine as a "health hazard" was issued decades ago (Ray & Ksir, 1996).

The use and abuse of alcoholic beverages is an area in which there is a good deal of information, and some work has been done on health promotion via prevention (Miller & Nirenberg, 1984; Gerstein, 1984; Morrissey, 1986; Nirenberg &

Gomberg, 1993; Fleming, Barry, Manwell, Johnson, & London, 1997; Barry, 1999; Whitlock et al., 2004). Because of the widespread use of alcohol and some of the consequences that follow, both for the individual user and for society, alcohol is treated separately in this chapter, as a specific challenge to health promotion.

Alternative Medicines

Alternative medicines include herbs and vitamins. Sales of "natural herbal remedies" have increased during the last decade. In 1993, the FDA issued a notice that regulation of these medicines was needed; this was followed by a well-organized program of letters to Congress, resulting in passage of the Dietary Supplement and Health Education Act of 1994. Herbal remedies were declared to be *supplements* and exempt from FDA investigatory rules before reaching the market. The FDA does, however, monitor dietary supplements for safety post-marketing. Whereas prescription and over-the-counter drugs must be proved effective and meet standards of safety both before and after they are marketed to the public, the plant products advertised to produce medicinal effects are generally exempt from these standards. Manufacturers have not been required by the FDA to test these products or to engage in quality control. It is expected that at some point the FDA will specify minimal quality controls, and the relationship of these alternative herbal remedies to health promotion will become better defined.

Alcohol and Health Promotion

Alcohol abuse is an issue for a far higher percentage of the U.S. population than is abuse of any other substances with the exception of nicotine. A summary of alcohol use in the lifetime, past year, and past month for individuals aged eighteen and older, by demographic characteristics, is presented in Table 10.1. Tables 10.2, 10.3, 10.4, with the most recent findings on Table 10.5, show the breakdown of that alcohol use for lifetime, past year, and past month, respectively, by year from 1994 to 2003 (National Institute of Alcohol Abuse and Alcoholism [NIAAA], 2004c; Substance Abuse and Mental Health Services Administration [SAMHSA], Office of Applied Studies, 2004). Additionally, as can be seen in Table 10.2, although not of legal drinking age, 43 percent of adolescents aged twelve to seventeen years report that they have consumed alcohol (SAMHSA, Office of Applied Studies, 2004).

Women report comparatively less alcohol use than men do. It should be noted that among women, the eighteen to twenty-five age group had the largest percentage of alcohol consumers in the past year and past month, and among men the twenty-six to thirty-four age group had the highest rate of drinkers. Generally, alcohol use is more common among men, whites, adults in age groups eighteen to

TABLE 10.1. ALCOHOL USE IN LIFETIME, PAST YEAR, AND PAST MONTH AMONG PERSONS AGED 18 OR OLDER, BY DEMOGRAPHIC CHARACTERISTICS: PERCENTAGES, 2002 AND 2003.

| Demographic Characteristic | Time Period | | | | | |
| | Lifetime | | Past Year | | Past Month | |
	2002	2003	2002	2003	2002	2003
Total	87.8	87.8	69.8[a]	68.6	54.9	53.9
Gender						
Male	91.8	91.9	75.4	74.3	62.4	62.4
Female	84.1	84.1	64.7	63.4	47.9[a]	46.0
Hispanic origin and race						
Not Hispanic or Latino	88.8	89.0	70.6	69.6	56.0	55.0
White	91.1	91.1	73.1	72.2	58.7	57.9
Black or African American	81.5	82.8	59.6	58.4	44.5	42.2
American Indian or Alaska Native	85.4	84.0	64.2	66.5	47.9	46.2
Native Hawaiian or other Pacific Islander	*	*	*	*	*	*
Asian	68.2	72.4	57.9	56.5	40.8	43.2
Two or more races	90.3	87.2	73.2	68.5	56.3	49.4
Hispanic or Latino	80.6	79.3	64.0	61.6	46.9	45.4
Education						
< High school	76.5	77.1	52.4	50.4	37.8	36.7
High school graduate	87.4	86.3	67.6[a]	65.6	51.5[a]	49.0
Some college	91.7	91.7	74.9	74.7	58.8	59.2
College graduate	92.4	93.4	80.1	79.1	67.4	66.5
Current employment						
Full-time	91.8	91.9	77.0	76.3	61.8	61.2
Part-time	89.2	87.9	73.3	72.4	58.6	55.9
Unemployed	87.5	88.9	75.0	73.4	57.9	57.0
Other[1]	79.3	79.6	53.3	51.1	39.0	37.9

*Low precision; no estimate reported.

[a]Difference between estimate and 2003 estimate is statistically significant at the 0.05 level.

[1]Retired person, disabled person, homemaker, student, or other person not in the labor force.

Source: Substance Abuse and Mental Health Services Administration, Office of Applied Studies, National Survey on Drug Use and Health, 2004.

TABLE 10.2. PERCENTAGE REPORTING ALCOHOL USE IN *LIFETIME,* BY AGE GROUP AND DEMOGRAPHIC CHARACTERISTICS: NSDUH (NHSDA), 1994–2002.

| Demographic Characteristic | Age Group (Years) | | | | Total |
	12–17	18–25	26–34	35+	
Total					
2002	43.4	86.7	90.2*	87.3*	83.1
2001	42.7	85.0	89.0*	85.7*	81.7
2000	41.7	84.0	89.2*	85.0*	81.0
1999	42.9	83.9	89.2*	85.3*	81.3
1998	37.3	83.2	88.2	86.6	81.3
1997	39.7	83.5	88.9	87.0	81.9
1996	38.8	83.8	90.3	87.8	82.6
1995	40.6	84.4	90.1	87.1	82.3
1994	41.7	86.3	91.8	89.0	84.2
Sex					
Male					
2002	43.4	88.0	93.1*	92.2*	86.4
2001	42.8	86.3	92.1*	91.3*	85.4
2000	41.9	85.6	92.1*	91.8*	85.3
1999	43.6	85.5	92.1*	90.5*	84.8
1998	36.6	87.2	90.9	92.2	85.2
1997	38.8	86.0	93.1	93.9	86.6
1996	38.3	86.3	93.8	93.9	86.6
1995	41.6	86.1	92.6	92.2	85.8
1994	42.9	87.9	94.6	95.4	88.4
Female					
2002	43.4	85.4	87.4*	82.9*	80.1
2001	43.0	83.7	86.1*	80.7*	78.3
2000	41.5	82.5	86.4*	79.0*	76.9
1999	42.2	82.3	86.5*	80.7*	78.1
1998	38.1	79.2	85.5	81.6	77.6
1997	40.7	81.0	84.7	80.9	77.5
1996	39.4	81.2	87.0	82.5	78.8
1995	39.5	82.7	87.6	82.6	79.2
1994	40.4	84.8	89.1	83.4	80.3

TABLE 10.2. PERCENTAGE REPORTING ALCOHOL USE IN *LIFETIME,* BY AGE GROUP AND DEMOGRAPHIC CHARACTERISTICS: NSDUH (NHSDA), 1994–2002, Cont'd.

Demographic Characteristic	Age Group (Years)				
	12–17	18–25	26–34	35+	Total
Race/ethnicity					
White non-Hispanic					
2002	45.8	90.1	94.5*	90.4*	86.8
2001	45.7	89.0	93.6*	89.6*	86.0
2000	44.3	88.2	93.9*	88.3*	84.9
1999	44.8	88.2	94.1*	88.3*	85.1
1998	40.4	87.9	92.8	89.4	85.2
1997	42.5	89.0	93.9	90.0	86.0
1996	40.7	88.9	94.7	90.4	86.2
1995	43.7	88.6	94.1	89.9	86.1
1994	45.3	91.6	95.5	91.1	87.6
Black non-Hispanic					
2002	35.9	81.2	87.3*	80.1*	75.3
2001	34.3	76.6	83.1*	77.3*	72.6
2000	32.1	76.2	80.9*	76.2*	71.5
1999	35.6	73.7	79.9*	76.2*	71.5
1998	26.7	74.2	81.9	78.6	71.7
1997	31.4	73.2	80.4	78.3	71.7
1996	32.2	73.5	83.8	79.3	72.8
1995	30.4	75.3	82.4	79.6	72.8
1994	32.9	74.8	83.0	80.8	73.9
Hispanic					
2002	44.7	81.2	81.9*	79.9*	75.7
2001	41.3	77.8	79.3*	73.3*	70.9
2000	41.8	76.7	80.2*	76.3*	71.9
1999	44.6	78.0	79.9*	78.9*	74.1
1998	36.4	74.4	78.3	76.2	70.8
1997	36.3	71.5	74.4	75.0	68.9
1996	40.3	73.9	80.6	76.1	71.7
1995	37.6	73.0	80.7	77.2	71.6
1994	39.1	76.7	83.4	84.2	76.2

Note: NSDUH = National Survey on Drug Use and Health; prior to 2002 it was called NHSDA = National Household Survey on Drug Abuse.

*Low precision; no estimate reported.

Source: NIAAA, 2004c.

TABLE 10.3. PERCENTAGE REPORTING ALCOHOL USE IN THE *PAST YEAR,* BY AGE GROUP AND DEMOGRAPHIC CHARACTERISTICS: NSDUH (NHSDA), 1994–2002.

Demographic Characteristic	Age Group (Years)				
	12–17	18–25	26–34	35+	Total
Total					
2002	34.6	77.9	77.7*	66.1*	66.1
2001	33.9	75.4	76.5*	63.1*	63.7
2000	33.0	74.5	75.1*	61.0*	61.9
1999	34.1	74.8	74.9*	61.3*	62.3
1998	31.8	74.2	74.5	64.6	64.0
1997	34.0	75.1	74.6	64.1	64.1
1996	32.7	75.3	77.2	64.9	64.9
1995	35.1	76.5	77.0	65.0	65.4
1994	36.2	78.5	78.8	66.2	66.9
Sex					
Male					
2002	33.3	80.1	83.0*	72.3*	70.7
2001	33.0	78.3	81.9*	68.3*	67.7
2000	32.1	77.2	80.2*	68.7*	67.2
1999	33.6	78.4	80.4*	66.1*	66.4
1998	31.0	79.3	77.7	70.2	68.3
1997	32.7	78.9	80.4	69.8	68.7
1996	32.0	78.6	81.5	72.0	70.0
1995	35.3	80.4	80.8	71.1	70.0
1994	36.2	82.3	83.7	72.5	71.8
Female					
2002	36.0	75.6	72.6*	60.5*	61.8
2001	34.9	72.6	71.4*	58.4*	59.9
2000	34.0	71.8	70.3*	54.2*	56.9
1999	34.7	71.3	69.7*	57.0*	58.5
1998	32.7	68.9	71.5	59.7	60.0
1997	35.3	71.2	69.0	59.0	59.8
1996	33.5	72.0	73.1	58.6	60.2
1995	34.8	72.7	73.3	59.6	61.1
1994	36.1	74.8	74.0	60.7	62.4

TABLE 10.3. PERCENTAGE REPORTING ALCOHOL USE IN THE *PAST YEAR,* BY AGE GROUP AND DEMOGRAPHIC CHARACTERISTICS: NSDUH (NHSDA), 1994–2002, Cont'd.

Demographic Characteristic	Age Group (Years)				Total
	12–17	18–25	26–34	35+	
Race/ethnicity					
White non-Hispanic					
2002	37.9	83.1	82.6*	69.3*	69.8
2001	37.3	80.8	81.5*	67.4*	68.1
2000	36.3	80.1	80.8*	64.7*	66.0
1999	36.7	80.3	80.4*	64.9*	66.2
1998	35.1	79.0	79.0	68.0	67.8
1997	36.0	81.0	80.2	67.2	67.8
1996	34.4	80.5	81.9	67.4	68.0
1995	38.1	81.4	81.3	67.9	68.8
1994	39.6	84.0	82.3	68.3	69.8
Black non-Hispanic					
2002	24.7	69.2	71.0*	53.6*	54.9
2001	22.9	63.9	65.9*	47.8*	49.9
2000	21.2	62.5	62.3*	46.6*	48.5
1999	23.8	62.7	62.5*	47.9*	49.6
1998	22.3	64.2	66.0	48.1	50.4
1997	27.3	62.9	64.0	52.2	52.7
1996	26.6	63.9	69.6	50.9	52.9
1995	25.8	65.0	67.4	53.0	53.8
1994	27.9	67.2	70.2	54.2	55.8
Hispanic					
2002	34.0	68.7	68.8*	60.1*	60.0
2001	32.2	65.0	66.9*	53.6*	55.2
2000	32.4	63.9	64.8*	55.1*	54.9
1999	35.2	65.3	66.3*	52.4*	54.9
1998	29.4	66.2	66.2	60.7	58.5
1997	32.5	63.2	63.0	56.2	55.6
1996	34.6	66.0	66.8	59.0	58.6
1995	32.2	64.4	68.5	58.1	57.9
1994	33.0	68.3	71.6	65.8	63.0

Note: NSDUH = National Survey on Drug Use and Health; prior to 2002 it was called NHSDA = National Household Survey on Drug Abuse.

*Low precision; no estimate reported.

Source: NIAAA, 2004c.

TABLE 10.4. PERCENTAGE REPORTING ALCOHOL USE
IN THE *PAST MONTH,* BY AGE GROUP AND DEMOGRAPHIC
CHARACTERISTICS: NSDUH (NHSDA), 1994–2002.

Demographic Characteristic	Age Group (Years)				Total
	12–17	18–25	26–34	35+	
Total					
2002	17.6	60.5	61.4*	52.1*	51.0
2001	17.3	58.8	59.9*	48.7*	48.3
2000	16.4	56.8	58.3*	46.8*	46.6
1999	16.5	57.2	57.4*	46.6*	46.4
1998	19.1	60.0	60.9	53.1	51.7
1997	20.5	58.4	60.2	52.8	51.4
1996	18.8	60.0	61.6	51.7	51.0
1995	21.1	61.3	63.0	52.6	52.2
1994	21.6	63.1	65.3	54.1	53.9
Sex					
Male					
2002	17.4	65.2	69.3*	60.0*	57.4
2001	17.2	64.7	68.6*	56.1*	54.8
2000	16.2	62.5	67.0*	55.3*	53.6
1999	16.7	63.9	67.0*	54.0*	53.2
1998	19.4	68.2	67.7	61.4	58.7
1997	21.0	65.9	67.9	60.6	58.2
1996	19.2	66.5	70.0	61.6	58.9
1995	22.5	68.2	70.3	62.4	60.1
1994	22.1	70.9	73.9	60.9	60.3
Female					
2002	17.9	55.7	53.6*	45.0*	44.9
2001	17.3	53.0	51.6*	42.0*	42.3
2000	16.5	51.3	50.1*	39.2*	40.2
1999	16.3	50.7	48.4*	40.0*	40.2
1998	18.7	51.7	54.2	45.8	45.1
1997	19.9	50.8	52.6	46.0	45.1
1996	18.3	53.5	53.7	43.0	43.6
1995	19.6	54.7	56.0	44.1	45.0
1994	21.1	55.3	57.1	48.1	47.9

TABLE 10.4. PERCENTAGE REPORTING ALCOHOL USE
IN THE *PAST MONTH,* BY AGE GROUP AND DEMOGRAPHIC
CHARACTERISTICS: NSDUH (NHSDA), 1994–2002, Cont'd.

Demographic Characteristic	Age Group (Years)				Total
	12–17	18–25	26–34	35+	
Race/ethnicity					
White non-Hispanic					
2002	20.1	66.8	66.7*	55.6*	55.0
2001	19.5	64.4	65.5*	52.7*	52.7
2000	18.4	63.3	63.7*	50.3*	50.7
1999	18.2	63.3	62.8*	49.9*	50.3
1998	20.9	65.0	65.2	56.2	55.3
1997	22.0	63.5	64.8	56.1	55.1
1996	20.4	65.5	66.0	54.3	54.2
1995	22.9	66.7	67.5	55.4	55.6
1994	23.9	68.2	68.6	56.2	56.7
Black non-Hispanic					
2002	10.9	48.3	56.0*	40.1*	39.9
2001	10.6	46.5	47.5*	34.3*	35.1
2000	8.8	43.9	47.8*	32.8*	33.7
1999	9.7	43.4	44.8*	34.5*	34.3
1998	13.1	50.3	54.8	38.3	39.8
1997	16.3	46.6	51.0	40.9	40.4
1996	14.7	49.6	55.7	42.0	41.9
1995	15.5	47.8	55.0	40.2	40.8
1994	18.2	51.5	59.2	42.4	43.8
Hispanic					
2002	16.6	49.8	51.2*	43.9*	42.8
2001	15.1	48.7	48.8*	39.4*	39.5
2000	16.8	44.7	47.7*	36.8*	39.8
1999	16.9	46.7	48.1*	38.2*	38.6
1998	18.9	50.8	53.1	47.7	45.4
1997	18.8	48.5	51.6	42.8	42.4
1996	19.9	49.8	50.6	44.0	43.1
1995	18.7	49.3	53.5	47.8	45.2
1994	18.3	53.6	56.6	50.0	47.7

Note: NSDUH = National Survey on Drug Use and Health; prior to 2002 it was called NHSDA = National Household Survey on Drug Abuse.

*Low precision; no estimate reported.

Source: NIAAA, 2004c.

TABLE 10.5. ALCOHOL USE IN LIFETIME, PAST YEAR, AND PAST MONTH AMONG PERSONS AGED 12 OR OLDER: NUMBERS IN THOUSANDS, 2002 AND 2003 (PERCENTAGES).

	Time Period					
	Lifetime		*Past Year*		*Past Month*	
Drug	**2002**	**2003**	**2002**	**2003**	**2002**	**2003**
Alcohol	195,452 (83.1%)	197,533 (83.1%)	155,476 (66.1%)	154,540 (65.0%)	119,820 (51.0%)	118,965 (50.1%)
Binge alcohol use[1]	—	—	—	—	53,787 (22.9%)	53,770 (22.6%)
Heavy alcohol use[1]	—	—	—	—	15,860 (6.7%)	16,144 (6.8%)

Note: — = Not available.

[1]*Binge alcohol use* is defined as drinking 5 or more drinks on the same occasion (that is, at the same time or within a couple of hours of each other) on at least 1 day in the past 30 days. Heavy alcohol use is defined as drinking 5 or more drinks on the same occasion on each of 5 or more days in the past 30 days; all heavy alcohol users are also binge alcohol users.

Source: SAMHSA, Office of Applied Studies, National Survey on Drug Use and Health, 2004.

twenty-five and twenty-six to thirty-four, college graduates, and those employed full time. As shown in Figure 10.1, heavy alcohol use is more common among young adults eighteen to twenty-nine years old; heavy and binge alcohol use are both most prevalent among young adults aged twenty-one to twenty-five. The gender gap in relation to alcohol use widens with increasing age.

Racial and ethnic comparisons show non-Hispanic whites reporting more lifetime, past-year, and current alcohol use than blacks or Hispanics do. The overall figures for Hispanics are most similar to those of blacks; however, older Hispanics (aged thirty-five and older) report higher recent rates of past-year and past-month alcohol consumption than do non-Hispanic blacks (see Tables 10.3 and 10.4). Adult white males (eighteen years and older) report greater current alcohol use than do females of the same age in any racial or ethnic group. Additionally, white adult females (eighteen years and older) report greater current alcohol use than do black or Hispanic females of the same age. Rates of past-year alcohol dependence show American Indian/Alaska Native populations with more than double the national percentage: 8.3 percent of the population indicated past-year alcohol dependence, compared to 3.2 percent of the national population

FIGURE 10.1. CURRENT, BINGE,
AND HEAVY ALCOHOL USE, BY AGE, 2003.

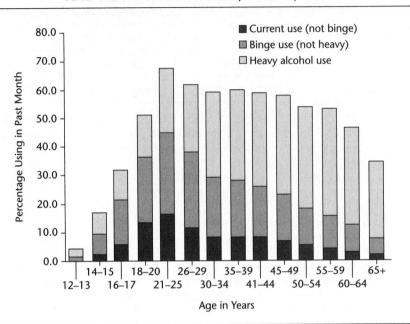

Source: SAMHSA, Office of Applied Studies, 2004.

(SAMHSA, Office of Applied Studies, 2004). Estimates of per capita alcohol consumption by state suggest that the District of Columbia and the following ten states have the heaviest consumption: Nevada, New Hampshire, Alaska, Wisconsin, Delaware, Arizona, Montana, Florida, Massachusetts, and Colorado (NIAAA, 2004d).

The latest figures available indicate that 38 percent of Americans totally abstain from alcohol; 30 percent of American male adults and 39 percent of American female adults abstain from alcohol consumption (NIAAA, 2004b).

Data from the Epidemiologic Catchment Area Study (Robins & Regier, 1991) showed, in general, a peak of alcohol abuse or dependence for both men and women in the age group eighteen to twenty-nine years old, followed by declines in the age groups thirty to forty-four, forty-five to sixty-five, and sixty-five and older. The epidemiologic data gathered from African American respondents showed a different age trajectory: there was a much smaller proportion of abuse or dependence diagnoses in the age group eighteen to twenty-nine years than in the same age group among whites, but starting with age thirty, the reported percentages of abuse or dependence were higher among African Americans than among whites; this was true for both men and women.

The epidemiologic literature provides targets for prevention and health promotion programs and details differences that exist between genders, age groupings, and ethnic or racial groupings in the U.S. population. As history demonstrates, Prohibition (the Eighteenth Amendment) was not successful in deterring Americans' use of alcoholic beverages. Recommending abstinence from alcohol is also not an effective or accurate health education strategy. Furthermore, some health benefits may apparently be gained from small or moderate amounts of alcohol.

The recent nutritional guidelines issued by the federal government list not only the medical and social consequences of drinking but also note that moderate drinking is associated with lower risk for coronary heart disease, mainly among men over age forty-five and women over age fifty-five (U.S. Department of Health and Human Services [USDHHS] & U.S. Department of Agriculture [USDA], 2000; Rimm, Klatsky, Grobbee, & Stampfer, 1996); and a good deal of medical evidence exists to support that association (Renaud & DeLorgeril, 1992; Grønbæk et al., 2000). Alcohol is a substance that when consumed in heavy amounts, however, produces a number of negative consequences and can lead to poor health outcomes.

Health care professionals need to recognize the relationship between heavy or problem drinking—the consumption of large quantities of alcohol that can produce health, social, and legal problems—and the diagnosable conditions of alcohol abuse and alcohol dependence. After an individual drinks one beer, glass of wine, or mixed drink (about half an ounce of alcohol), his or her blood alcohol concentration (BAC) is .02. With two and one-half beers, glasses of wine, or mixed drinks the BAC rises to .05, judgment is more impaired, and inhibitions can be decreased. The legal limit for blood alcohol concentration under *driving while intoxicated* (DWI) laws varies by state, from .08 to .10 grams per 100 milliliters. This amounts, respectively, to about four or five beers, glasses of wine, or mixed drinks (two and one-half ounces of alcohol). At ten beers, glasses of wine, or mixed drinks (five ounces of alcohol), the BAC is .20, and the individual experiences slowed reflexes. Fifteen beers, glasses of wine, or mixed drinks (seven and one-half ounces of alcohol) yield a BAC of .30, a stupor, complete loss of coordination, and little sensation. At twenty beers, glasses of wine, or mixed drinks (ten ounces of alcohol) (BAC of .40), the person may be comatose, and breathing may cease (Edlin & Golanty, 1992; Boston Women's Health Care Collective, 1992). The criteria for diagnoses are further described in the *Diagnostic and Statistical Manual of Mental Disorders* (*DSM-IV*) (American Psychiatric Association, 1994).

Risks for Substance Abuse

According to the traditional models of etiology and prevention, risk factors for alcohol or drug abuse among men and women include (1) alcoholism or drug abuse in a family member, (2) disruptive early family experiences, (3) membership in peer groups with heavy alcohol or drug use, (4) depression or antisocial personality factors, (5) life crises, (6) use of alcohol or drugs to relieve stress, (7) sociocultural factors (for example, neighborhood, community distribution of consumption), and (8) the degree of heavy drinking or drug use in the society. In addition, it is important to take into account what the individual *expects to happen* with the use of alcohol. A number of experimental studies of the concept of expectancy posit that the individual's view of the effect of the alcohol or drug when it is ingested is an important aspect of his or her attraction to it (see Blume, Lostutter, Schmaling, & Marlatt, 2003; Oei & Young, 1987; Jaffe & Lohse, 1991; Christiansen, Goldman, & Brown, 1985).

Lower-Risk Use

Does healthy behavior require total abstinence from alcohol and drugs? A distinction must be made among the different classes, or categories, of drugs. Prescribed and over-the-counter drugs that are taken for therapeutic purposes in prescribed amounts can be beneficial to general health. The safety of therapeutic drugs is monitored by the FDA and recommended dosages are well codified. However, it is important to note that these drugs may be misused. When persons are admitted to emergency departments and substance abuse treatment programs with drug-related diagnoses, the drugs at issue may be therapeutic medications (SAMHSA, Office of Applied Studies, 1996).

The use of banned substances, including cocaine, heroin, and marijuana, produces legal, medical, and psychological health consequences. Use of the social drugs caffeine and nicotine raises other questions. Nicotine remains a major health concern in the United States. Research on caffeine consumed in moderate amounts has not found it to be a major health hazard. As pointed out earlier, some writing documents a relationship between caffeine and benign breast disease and coronary disease, but the evidence is ambiguous and studies have found few negative effects from small to moderate amounts of caffeinated beverages (Lamarine, 1994). Some research has suggested that long-term caffeine consumption is associated with lower risk for type 2 diabetes (Salazar-Martinez et al., 2004).

The consumption of alcoholic beverages remains a controversial area of health promotion. Several population studies from different countries indicate a relationship between alcohol intake and mortality from all causes (Fuchs et al., 1995; Grønbæk et al., 1994, 2000; Farchi, Fidanza, Mariotti, & Menotti, 1992;

Klatsky, Armstrong, & Friedman, 1992; Yuan, Ross, Gao, Henderson, & Yu, 1997). For example, historically, cirrhosis death rates have been higher and cardiovascular disease death rates lower in countries with higher per capita alcohol consumption (World Health Organization [WHO], 1995; Embland, 1995; Renaud & DeLorgeril, 1992). Some studies have found an inverse relation between incidence rates of coronary heart disease and wine consumption, but a weak or nonexistent relation for the consumption of beer or spirits (Criqui & Rigel, 1994; Renaud & DeLorgeril, 1992). Different types of alcoholic beverages have different effects on mortality (Grønbæk et al., 2000; Hertog et al., 1995; Ruf, Berger, & Renaud, 1995; Frankel, Kanner, German, Parks, & Kinsella, 1993). Recommendations vary internationally regarding the benefits of moderate drinking (Shiflett, 1996; USDHHS & USDA, 2000). The view that small to moderate amounts of alcoholic beverages may have beneficial health effects appears in the most recent U.S. nutritional guidelines (USDHHS & USDA, 2000). This makes the question of whether substance safety means total abstinence from alcohol a difficult one.

Currently, it can be concluded that a consideration of substance safety in regard to alcohol points to the consequences of heavy consumption as a health risk. The problem that remains is how to define small, moderate, and heavy amounts of alcohol consumption. Based on current dietary guidelines, *moderate* drinking for women is defined as an average of one drink or less per day; moderate drinking for men is defined as an average of two drinks or less per day (USDHHS & USDA, 2000; NIAAA, 1995a). *Heavy* drinking is consuming alcohol in excess of one drink per day on average for women and greater than two drinks per day on average for men (NIAAA, 2004a). *Binge* drinking is generally defined as having five or more drinks on one occasion, meaning in a row or within a short period of time (Naimi et al., 2003). Among women, because of their smaller body size and hormonal and metabolic differences from men, binge drinking is often defined as having four or more drinks on one occasion (NIAAA, 2004a; Wechsler & Austin, 1998). Further, *excessive* drinking among men may be defined as more than four drinks per day, or an average of more than two drinks per day over a seven- or thirty-day period. Among women excessive drinking may be defined as more than three drinks per day, or an average of more than one drink per day over a seven- or thirty-day period (NIAAA, 2004a).

Current guidelines further specify that certain individuals should *not* drink at all (USDHHS & USDA, 2000). These include children and adolescents; individuals of any age who cannot restrict their drinking to moderate levels; women who may become pregnant or who are pregnant; individuals taking prescription or over-the-counter medications that can interact with alcohol; and individuals who plan to drive, operate machinery, or take part in other activities that require attention, skill, or coordination. Among these individuals *any* alcohol consumption may be too much. In addition, anyone who chooses to drink should be aware that individual reactions to alcohol can vary greatly. The recommended alcohol restrictions for women who are or may become pregnant is directed at least in part to the prevention of fetal alcohol syndrome, a confluence of clinical symptoms that includes growth retardation, central nervous system deficits, and altered facial features and that has been associated with moderate to heavy drinking by women during pregnancy (Centers for Disease Control and Prevention [CDC], 1997).

Minimizing Negative Health Consequences Related to Substance Use

Approaches to minimizing the negative health consequences of various classes of drugs will differ. When medication and over-the-counter drugs are being prescribed, the individual patient's understanding of the prescribed medications, ability and willingness to use the prescription as given, and the health care provider's training must be considered. Health care providers are trained to prescribe but not always adequately trained or reimbursed to counsel the patient. Both are important to client change.

The potential negative consequences of illegal substances are well documented. Some illegal substances create more negative health outcomes than others (for example, cocaine used regularly has swift and complex negative health effects) (Thompson, 2003; Bouknight & Bouknight, 1988; Woods, 1977; Billman, 1995; Thadani, 1995). Additionally, some individuals, due to their genetic predispositions or developmental stages, are more sensitive and susceptible than others to the effects of these drugs (Morse, Erwin, & Jones, 1995). Some of the banned substances do have medical uses (for example, the use of marijuana in glaucoma treatment or to alleviate chemotherapy responses); however, the foregoing discussion pertains to their recreational uses.

In terms of the legal drugs caffeine and alcohol, the key is moderation. The use of caffeinated or alcoholic beverages in modest amounts appears to do little harm to most adults, although there are persons who have genetic, familial, or personality vulnerability and probably should avoid such drugs (Simmons, 1996; Hinds, West, Knight, & Harland, 1996; USDHHS & USDA, 2000; Ozkaragoz, Satz, & Noble, 1997). *Moderation* is usually defined by the family, social groups, and community to which an individual belongs. Moderation may also be characterized as *low-risk drinking*, or alcohol use that does not lead to problems. Low-risk drinkers do not engage in binge drinking—more than two drinks per occasion for women or four for men—or in excessive regular drinking, more than seven drinks a week for women or fourteen for men (NIAAA, 1995a, 1995b, 2004a). With tobacco there is little ambiguity: the safest course is abstinence, and there is no substance safety in any tobacco alternative.

Substance-Related Health Promotion for Special Groups

Although the course and consequences of alcohol abuse and alcohol dependence may be about the same for all persons (Schuckit, 1991), the importance of tailoring health promotion scripts to specific populations cannot be overemphasized.

Gender. Research in the field of alcohol studies has clearly demonstrated that women are more vulnerable than men to some consequences of heavy use. They are, for example, more likely to develop medical problems related to heavy alcohol intake, particularly liver disorders. The enhanced vulnerability of women to developing alcohol-related diseases may be due to their higher blood alcohol levels after drinking, but the mechanism for this effect has been debated. The gender difference in alcohol levels is due mainly to a smaller gastric metabolism in females (Baraona et al., 2001). Alcohol use may have effects on sex steroid levels, partially contributing to increased cancer risk (Onland-Moret, Peeters, van der Schouw, Grobbee, & van Gils, 2004; Johnson & Williams, 1985). Women who are problem drinkers are at greater risk of alcoholic cardiomyopathy than are men who are problem drinkers (Urbano-Marquez et al., 1995). The prevalence of alcohol-dependent women with dilated cardiomyopathy has been shown to be similar to that among alcohol-dependent men, but women require a lower total lifetime dose of ethanol to develop the disease (Fernandez-Sola et al., 1997). There are also problems associated with drinking during pregnancy, as mentioned earlier, and issues regarding double-standard social attitudes toward heavy drinking and intoxication in men and women. Traditionally, from a societal standpoint, intoxication has been more stigmatizing for women than for men.

Minorities. Rates of alcohol use and misuse vary by race and ethnicity. Nationally representative samples of youths show different substance use patterns among adolescents from different ethnic groups (CDC, 2000). For the white population, the youthful years are the most risk laden; for African Americans and other minority groups the pattern is different. African American youths, for example, are less likely than white youths to be alcohol or drug users (Catalano et al., 1993; Ellickson, Collins, & Bell, 1999; Merrill, Kleber, Shwartz, Liu, & Lewis, 1999; Wallace, 1994). In 2003, whites were more likely than any other racial or ethnic group to report current use of alcohol, with an estimated 54.4 percent of whites reporting past-month use (SAMHSA, Office of Applied Studies, 2004). African Americans reported the lowest rates among all racial or ethnic groups of current past-month alcohol use, with 37.9 percent reporting such use. In the same study differences between whites and blacks narrowed with alcohol misuse patterns. The rate of binge alcohol use was 15.9 percent for whites and 14.5 percent for blacks; the rate of heavy alcohol use was 7.7 percent among whites and 4.5 percent among blacks (SAMHSA, Office of Applied Studies, 2004). In one study of elderly people who were alcohol dependent (Gomberg, 1995), African American men drank more heavily, manifested more negative health and community consequences, and were more likely than white men to use a variety of substances. All of these factors must be considered in prevention and health promotion strategies.

Age. It is obvious that alcohol and drug use patterns vary at different stages of the individual's life span. It is also clear that specific health promotion strategies need to be designed for youths and adolescents, for young adults, for the middle-aged, and for older adults. Health promotion strategies are not a case of one size fits all. Although numerous prevention programs have been developed and implemented for young persons and adolescents in the past two decades, many providers teach effective content but few use effective delivery techniques; the transfer to practice of research knowledge about school-based substance use prevention, including binge drinking, has been limited (Ennett et al., 2003). Health strategies for adults must address issues of marriage, occupation, and parenting. The middle-age and older years present some particular issues too; for example, for older persons the possibility of medication interactions and of alcohol and medication interactions is a major issue, and there are issues surrounding the life span of women (Blow, 1998a; Barry, Oslin, & Blow, 2001; Barry, Blow, & Oslin, 2002).

Older Adults. Older adults present special concerns when criteria for drinking and medication use are being set. Understanding alcohol use among older adults is important because what might be considered light or moderate drinking for younger individuals may have untoward health effects in an older person; compared to younger adults the elderly also have an increased sensitivity to over-the-counter and prescription medications (Blow, 1998a, 1998b; Finch & Barry, 1992; Barry, Oslin, & Blow, 2001; Barry, Blow, & Oslin, 2002). Older individuals experience an age-related decrease in lean body mass compared to total volume of fat, and the resultant reduction in total body volume increases the total distribution of alcohol and other mood-altering chemicals in the body. Central nervous system sensitivity increases, and liver enzymes that metabolize alcohol and certain other drugs are less efficient with age. Comparable amounts of alcohol produce higher blood alcohol levels in older adults than in younger persons and may exacerbate other health problems such as chronic illness, poor nutrition, and polypharmacy (Lucey, Hill, Young,

Demo-Dananberg, & Beresford, 1999; Vogel-Sprott & Barrett, 1984; Vestal et al., 1977). Symptoms of harmful drinking may be less visible among older adults because they may be masked by social, medical, or psychological conditions.

Heavy alcohol use is associated with a number of adverse health effects in the older population. These include greater risk for harmful drug interactions, injury, depression, memory problems, liver disease, cardiovascular disease, cognitive changes, deficits in physical functioning, pain, and sleep problems (Barry, 1997; Blow et al., 2000; Gambert & Katsoyannis, 1995; Liberto, Oslin, & Ruskin, 1992; Wetle, 1997).

The potential interaction of medication and alcohol is of great concern with this age group. For some clients, any alcohol use at all combined with the use of specific over-the-counter or prescription medications can result in problematic consequences. Therefore alcohol use recommendations are generally lower than those for adults aged sixty-five and younger and are usually made on a case-by-case basis. To determine the prescription and over-the-counter medication use of older clients, the health care professional can use the *brown bag* approach: ask clients to bring to their next office visit a brown paper bag that contains every medication they take. This will provide an opportunity to better determine potential medication problems.

Categories of Substance Use

Psychoactive drugs may be sanctioned medically to modify or control moods; however, any use of a psychoactive substance to change a person's state of mind that is harmful to that individual or others is considered abuse. The concepts of *abuse* and *dependence* pertain to both alcohol and drugs. Definitions for adults of low-risk, at-risk, and problem use focus primarily but not exclusively on alcohol (Barry, 1997). To determine whether a client could benefit from drinking less or needs to stop entirely, it is necessary to use operating definitions of varying levels of alcohol and drug use.

Low-risk drinking is alcohol use that does not lead to problems. Persons in this category can set reasonable limits on alcohol consumption and do not drink when pregnant or trying to conceive, driving a car or boat, operating heavy machinery, or using contraindicated medications. As stated earlier they do not engage in binge drinking—more than two drinks for women or four drinks for men per occasion—or in excessive regular drinking—more than seven drinks a week for women and fourteen drinks a week for men (NIAAA, 1995a). Low-risk use of medications or drugs would include having the individual use an antianxiety medication for an acute anxiety state according to the physician's prescription (Trachtenberg &

Fleming, 1994). Low-risk clients can benefit from prevention messages but do not need interventions. Prevention messages follow this format: "Our goal is to prevent future health problems. Your exercise program looks good and your weight has remained stable. Since you have no family history of alcohol or drug problems and are taking no medication to interfere with alcohol, not exceeding a glass of wine a few times a week should not cause any additional problems for you" (Barry, 1997, p. 354).

Alcohol consumption that increases the chances for a person to develop problems and complications is called *at-risk* drinking. Women who consume more than seven drinks per week, men who consume more than fourteen drinks per week, and persons who drink in risky situations are considered to be at-risk drinkers. Although these individuals may not currently have a health problem caused by alcohol, they may be experiencing family and social problems, and if this drinking pattern continues over time, health problems could result. In general, any illegal drug use is considered at-risk use, warranting further discussion.

Individuals who engage in *problem* drinking consume alcohol at a level that has already resulted in adverse medical, psychological, or social consequences. Potential consequences can include accidents and injuries, legal problems, sexual behavior that increases the risk of HIV infection, and family problems (Barry & Fleming, 1994). It is important to note that some persons who drink small amounts of alcohol, such as elderly individuals (see the "Older Adults" section) or persons with severe medical or psychiatric problems, may also experience alcohol-related problems. With special populations the presence of consequences, rather than quantity and frequency of alcohol use, should drive the need for intervention.

Alcohol or drug *dependence* refers to a medical disorder characterized by loss of control, preoccupation with alcohol or drugs, continued use despite adverse consequences, and physiological symptoms such as tolerance and withdrawal (American Psychiatric Association, 1994). A wide range of legal and illegal substances can be addictive. Motivational interviewing interventions can be especially helpful with this group of drinkers in defining the problem and assisting them to engage in more structured treatment as necessary (Miller & Rollnick, 1991).

Alcohol-Related Interventions

Alcohol interventions were developed based on principles originally used in the original smoking cessation studies. Scripts for reducing alcohol use thus have similarities to smoking cessation scripts. The main difference is the focus of the intervention. Smoking scripts are designed with the ultimate goal of smoking cessation; alcohol intervention scripts are based on motivational interviewing principles and are often designed to assist the at-risk or problem drinker in cutting down on alcohol use. If cutting down is ineffective, abstinence then becomes the goal.

All the alcohol-related brief interventions include the use of assessment and direct feedback, contracting and goal setting, behavioral modification techniques, and written materials such as self-help manuals. A number of trials have demonstrated the efficacy of brief advice in reducing alcohol use.

Kristenson, Ohlin, Hulten-Nosslin, Trell, and Hood (1983) reported the results of a trial conducted in Malmö, Sweden, in the late 1970s, in which the subjects were advised in a series of health education visits to reduce their alcohol use. They subsequently demonstrated significant reductions in gamma glutamyl transferase levels and in health care utilization up to five years after the brief interventions. Wallace, Cutler, and Haines (1988), in the Medical Research Council trial, conducted in forty-seven general practitioners' offices in Great Britain, found significant reductions in alcohol use by the intervention group as compared with the control group twelve months after the intervention. The World Health Organization trial, conducted in ten countries, found similar differences in alcohol use between the study and control groups (Babor & Grant, 1992). A recent review of the research indicates brief behavioral counseling interventions for risky or harmful alcohol use among adult primary care patients reduced consumption levels and improved drinking patterns over time and are an effective component of a public health approach to reducing risky or harmful alcohol use (Whitlock et al., 2004).

A brief, randomized controlled alcohol intervention trial was conducted in the United States, with sixty-seven community-based primary care physicians serving as intervenors. A total of 392 at-risk or problem drinkers aged sixty-five or younger received a physician-delivered brief advice protocol (the control group consisted of 382 individuals). The main outcome variables of this Trial for Early Alcohol Treatment (Project TrEAT) were decreased alcohol use, emergency department visits, and hospital days. At baseline the study and control groups were comparable on alcohol use, age, socioeconomic status, smoking status, rates of depression or anxiety, frequency of conduct disorders, lifetime drug use, and health care utilization. At the time of the twelve-month follow-up, compared with the control group, the experimental group showed a significant reduction in seven-day alcohol use ($t = 4.33$, $p < .001$), episodes of binge drinking ($t = 2.81$, $p < .001$), and frequency of excessive drinking ($t = 4.53$, $p < .001$). (A p value of <001 indicates a less than a 1 in 1,000 probability that this result would have occurred by chance alone.) Chi-square tests of independence revealed a significant relationship between group status and lengths of hospitalization over the study period for men ($p < .01$) although not for women. (A p value of $<.01$ indicates a less than a 1 in 100 probability that this result would have occurred by chance alone.)

Project TrEAT provided the first direct evidence that physician intervention with at-risk and problem drinkers decreases alcohol use and health resource utilization in a community-based U.S. health care system (Fleming et al., 1997). The basic design of most brief intervention studies is a randomized controlled trial of individuals with at-risk or problem-drinking patterns who are assigned either to an experimental condition, ranging from one to ten sessions, or to one or more control conditions (Kristenson et al. 1983; Chick, 1988; Heather, Campion, Neville, & MacCabe, 1987; Wallace et al., 1988; Persson & Magnusson, 1989; Harris & Miller, 1990; Anderson & Scott, 1992; Babor & Grant, 1992; Fleming et al., 1997). Overall, eight of the nine randomized controlled studies conducted have found significantly greater improvements in drinking outcomes for the brief intervention group compared with the control group.

Studies of Strategies to Change Drinking Behavior

Studies of brief interventions for alcohol problems have used various approaches to change drinking behaviors. Strategies have ranged from relatively unstructured counseling and feedback to more formal structured therapy and have relied heavily on concepts and techniques from the behavioral self-control training (BSCT) literature (Miller & Taylor, 1980; Miller & Hester, 1986; Miller & Munoz, 1976; Miller & Rollnick, 1991). Drinking goals of brief treatment interventions are flexible, allowing the individual to choose drinking in moderation or abstinence. The overall goal of brief counseling is to motivate the problem drinker to change his or her behavior, not to blame himself or herself or to assign blame.

Most studies of brief alcohol intervention have explicitly excluded dependent drinkers with significant withdrawal symptoms. The rationale for this has been that alcohol-dependent individuals, those affected most severely by alcohol, should be referred to formal specialized alcoholism treatment programs because their conditions are not likely to be amenable to a low-intensity intervention (Institute of Medicine, 1990; Babor, Ritson, & Hodgson, 1986). One study has addressed the validity of that assumption. Sanchez-Craig, Neumann, Souza-Formigoni, and Rieck (1991) found no significant differences in rates of abstinence or moderate drinking when comparing the treatment outcomes of severely alcohol-dependent men and non-alcohol-dependent men twelve months after they received brief treatment in Toronto and Brazil. Additionally, rates of spontaneous remission of alcoholism suggest that some members of the most severely alcoholic population will reduce their drinking or stop drinking without formal intervention (Institute of Medicine, 1990). The Project MATCH Research Group (1997) attempted to assess the benefits of matching alcohol-dependent clients to three different treatments (cognitive behavioral coping skills therapy, motivational enhancement therapy, or twelve-step facilitation therapy) with reference to a variety of client attributes. Results indicated little difference in outcomes by type of treatment, but client attributes of motivational readiness, network support for drinking, alcohol involvement, gender, psychiatric severity, and sociopathy were prognostic of drinking outcomes over time. The findings suggested that psychiatric severity should be considered when assigning clients to various forms of outpatient treatment.

Substance Safety Tools and Script

The following case example and script provide basic tools the health care professional can use to assess and intervene with an at-risk drinker. Other drug or medication use can be assessed using this same model. Following the script and adapting it to the individual's drinking level and gender, as in the case example, will provide the framework to assist clients in managing their alcohol intake. The recommendations for the client in the case example are based on the definitions described earlier in this chapter and the "health promotion matrix" described in Chapter Two (and see Sheinfeld Gorin & Arnold, 1998).

Case Example: Substance Safety

This case involves a thirty-four-year-old mother of two daughters, aged eight and ten. She is a secretary at a large marketing firm and was recently divorced. She shares child custody with her ex-husband. She has been experiencing stomach pain, difficulty in sleeping, mild hypertension, and stress at work and at home. She recently tripped and fell while getting out of the shower.

Goals for the Future

The health care professional works with the client to discuss her goals for herself in the next six months. The client's idealized picture of health may include the use of alcohol. In the case of the thirty-four-year-old woman, the image that she holds of herself with a drink in her hand is one of a relaxed and confident person. This influences her subsequent behavior in that she may see herself as healthier with than without the use of alcohol. The image the client holds in her mind that shows her healthier while drinking may be reinforced by the media, thus solidifying her idealized positive view of herself. To begin, the health care professional accepts the client's picture. As they work through health promotion activities, however, the health care professional collaborates with the client to modify the image and to make it more reflective of the positive and negative consequences of drinking and other risky substance use. The health care professional asks these questions:

Tell me what you see when you picture yourself as a healthy person.

What kinds of activities do you see yourself doing?

How would you feel physically? Emotionally?

Developing a Discrepancy

The health care provider works with the individual to develop a discrepancy between current circumstances and what the person desires for the future. This is done by asking screening questions and discussing current health status, the types of drinkers in the United States, and the person's reasons for drinking. The health care professional begins by asking a set of screening questions related to drinking patterns and other health habits (often including smoking and nutrition [see Chapters Five and Nine]). Questions about alcohol use are generally part of an overall health assessment. The responses to these queries enable the health care professional to determine whether the client is at risk and to customize the client feedback.

The health care professional then discusses the client's health status, including physical and emotional functioning. Some examples of problems resulting from risky drinking behaviors include difficulties with stress, sleep, family, stomach pains, depressed feelings, and accidents or injuries.

This element is followed by a discussion of the types of drinkers in the United States or elsewhere, as geographically appropriate. The health care professional places the individual's drinking pattern into the population norms for her age group. Using principles of motivational interviewing, the health care professional works to move the individual toward a commitment to change.

This section of the intervention ends with a discussion of the individual's reasons for drinking. This is particularly important because the health care professional needs to understand the role of alcohol in the life context. Here is an example:

Provider: From the screening questions you completed as part of your health assessment, you indicated that you walk three times a week for one-half to one hour. Do you have friends who walk with you? Where do you walk?

Client: I walk with another woman in my neighborhood.

Provider: That's great. I'm glad to hear that you are getting some good exercise. Your weight has stayed the same for quite a while now. You said that you stopped smoking four years ago. I know that was hard to do, but it's one of the best things you could do for your health.

On the screening, you indicated that, on average you drink alcohol six days a week and drink two to three drinks at a time. Tell me, how do you see your current health status? What kinds of issues are causing you the most stress at this time? How do you feel physically? Emotionally?

National guidelines recommend that women your age drink no more than seven drinks per week. Your pattern of alcohol use fits into the at-risk drinking category. You have also indicated that you have some sleep problems, stomach pains, and fell in the bathroom and that you feel a very real loneliness since your divorce.

Minimize Health-Depleting Patterns

At this point, the health care professional discusses the consequences of the individual's at-risk or heavy drinking pattern to encourage change. Often myriad physical, psychological, social, and economic aspects of the at-risk drinker's life have already been affected by drinking. These are addressed by the health care professional to move the person toward change.

Provider: You are drinking at a risky level at this time. I know that you have been experiencing a lot of stress. Sometimes people use alcohol to help in coping with stressful situations. I am concerned about some of the health problems you've had and your loneliness, and I think your alcohol use may be making these other problems even worse, rather than helping you cope with them.

Optimize Health-Supportive Patterns

The reasons to cut down or to quit drinking are emphasized at this point, and a drinking agreement or plan for change is negotiated and summarized. Maintaining good work and family relationships is often an important reason to control alcohol intake, and families can sometimes serve as primary supports for change.

During the discussion of the drinking agreement the client may negotiate for a higher level of drinking that is still within the national guidelines. Some at-risk drinkers are not willing to decrease consumption to the recommended levels of use. In this instance the health care professional should negotiate the lowest temporary limit possible and note that changing behavior is an ongoing process and that drinking limits, as well as other issues, can be discussed at subsequent visits.

Negotiated and written drinking agreements that are signed by the individual receiving the intervention and the health care professional are particularly effective in changing drinking patterns. It is important to summarize expectations and to set a follow-up appointment in one month.

Provider: Remember your drinking limit for the next month is [*specify the number*] beverages. [*State the agreement.*] Think of an activity you do frequently every day. Whenever you do that activity, think of your reasons to cut down on drinking. Every time you are tempted to drink more than allowed in the agreement and can resist, congratulate yourself on breaking an old habit and helping yourself. A follow-up visit is important to assess your progress and any problems that occur. I'll see you in one month on [*specify the date*].

Strategies That Promote Change

Strategies that are useful for cutting down or quitting include developing social opportunities that do not involve alcohol, getting reacquainted with hobbies and interests, and pursuing new activities unrelated to alcohol use.

The health care professional states his or her recognition of the effects of the at-risk drinker's social isolation, boredom, and negative family interactions (which can present special problems to those who drink) and works with the individual to develop strategies to deal with these issues. Role-playing specific situations can be helpful.

Any progress toward the goal needs to be rewarded. Risky situations need to be assessed to develop coping strategies. For example:

Provider: From your drinking diary cards, it looks like you did a very good job working toward your goal.

Provider: Congratulations! The only times you drank more than one drink a day were Sundays. What was happening on those days? Let's look at some ways to cope with days that are more stressful.

Summary

Potentially unsafe substances may be classified as prescribed and over-the-counter drugs; banned "street" drugs, such as marijuana, cocaine, and heroin; alternative medicines, such as herbs and vitamins; and social drugs, such as nicotine, caffeine, and alcohol. Alcohol is among the more widely used risky substances. Because the rates and effects of immoderate drinking differ by age, gender, and minority or racial status, strategies to promote moderate drinking should be customized. Each client should be screened by the health care professional for at-risk use of alcohol. A brief, focused script, designed for an adult outpatient population, may be effectively used to reduce drinking through direct feedback, a behavioral contract, goal setting, and social reinforcement. Clients may be encouraged to reduce their drinking, rather than eliminate it entirely. (See Exhibit 10.1 on page 360 for a list of helpful online resources.)

References

American Psychiatric Association. (1994). *Diagnostic and statistical manual of mental disorders* (4th ed.). Washington, DC: Author.

Anderson, P., & Scott, E. (1992). The effect of general practitioners' advice to heavy drinking men. *British Journal of Addiction, 87,* 891–900.

Babor, T. F., & Grant, M. (1992). *Project on identification and management of alcohol-related problems: Report on phase II: A randomized clinical trial of brief interventions in primary health care.* Geneva: World Health Organization.

Babor, T. F., Ritson, E. B., & Hodgson, R. J. (1986). Alcohol-related problems in the primary health care setting: A review of early intervention strategies. *British Journal of Addiction, 8*(1), 23–46.

Baraona, E., Abittan, C. S., Dohmen, K., Moretti, M., Pozzato, G., Chayes, Z. W., et al. (2001). Gender differences in pharmacokinetics of alcohol. *Alcoholism, Clinical and Experimental Research, 25*(4), 502–507.

Barry, K. (1997). Alcohol and drug abuse. In M. Mengel & W. Holleman (Eds.), *Fundamentals of clinical practice: A textbook on the patient, doctor, and society.* New York: Plenum.

Barry, K. L. (1999). *Treatment Improvement Protocol: Brief alcohol interventions and therapies in substance abuse treatment (TIP 34).* Rockville, MD: Center for Substance Abuse Treatment, Substance Abuse and Mental Health Services Administration.

Barry, K. L., Blow, F. C., & Oslin, D. (2002). Substance abuse in older adults: Review and recommendations for education and practice in medical settings (HRSA/AMERSA Monograph). *Substance Abuse, 23*(3), 105–131.

Barry, K. L., & Fleming, M. F. (1994). The family physician. *Alcohol Health and Research World, 18*(1), 105–109.

Barry, K. L., Oslin, D., & Blow, F. C. (2001). *Alcohol problems in older adults: Prevention and management.* New York: Springer.

Billman, G. E. (1995). Cocaine: A review of its toxic actions on cardiac function. *Critical Reviews in Toxicology, 25*(2), 113–132.

Blow, F. C. (1998a). Identification, screening, and assessment. In F. C. Blow, *Substance abuse among older adults* (pp. 47–64) (TIP 26, DHHS Publication No. [SMA] 98-3179). Rockville, MD: Center for Substance Abuse Treatment, Substance Abuse and Mental Health Services Administration.

Blow, F. C. (1998b). The spectrum of alcohol interventions for older adults. In E.S.L. Gomberg, A. M. Hegedus, & R. A. Zucker (Eds.), *Alcohol problems and aging* (pp. 373–396) (NIAAA Research Monograph 33, DHHS Publication No. 98-4163). Bethesda, MD: National Institute on Alcohol Abuse and Alcoholism.

Blow, F. C., Walton, M. A., Barry, K. L., Coyne, J. C., Mudd, S. A., & Copeland, L. A. (2000). The relationship between alcohol problems and health functioning of older adults in primary care settings. *Journal of the American Geriatrics Society, 48,* 769–774.

Blume, A. W., Lostutter, T. W., Schmaling, K. B., & Marlatt, G. A. (2003). Beliefs about drinking behavior predict drinking consequences. *Journal of Psychoactive Drugs, 35*(3), 395–399.

Boston Women's Health Care Collective. (1992). *Our bodies, ourselves.* New York: Simon & Schuster.

Bouknight, L. G., & Bouknight, R. R. (1988). Utilizing expectancies in alcoholism treatment. *Psychology of Addictive Behavior, 2*(2), 59–65.

Catalano, R. F., Hawkins, J. D., Krenz, C., Gillmore, M., Morrison, D., Wells, E., et al. (1993). Using research to guide culturally appropriate drug abuse prevention. *Journal of Consulting and Clinical Psychology, 61,* 804–811.

Centers for Disease Control and Prevention. (1997). Alcohol consumption among pregnant and childbearing aged women—United States, 1991 and 1995. *Morbidity and Mortality Weekly Report, 46*(16), 346–350.

Centers for Disease Control and Prevention. (2000). Youth risk behavior surveillance—United States, 1999. *Morbidity and Mortality Weekly Report Surveillance Summary, 49,* 1–96.

Chick, J. (1988). Early intervention for hazardous drinking in the general hospital setting. *Australian Drug and Alcohol Review, 7*(3), 339–343.

Christiansen, B. A., Goldman, M. S., & Brown, S. A. (1985). Differential development of adolescent alcohol expectancies may predict adult alcoholism. *Addictive Behaviors, 10*(3), 299–306.

Controlled Substances Act, 21 U.S.C. §§ 13-801 et seq. (1970).

Criqui, M. H., & Rigel, B. L. (1994). Does diet or alcohol explain the French paradox? *Lancet, 344,* 1719–1723.

Edlin, G., & Golanty, E. (1992). *Health and wellness.* Boston: Jones & Bartlett.

Ellickson, P. L., Collins, R. L., & Bell, R. M. (1999). Adolescent use of illicit drugs other than marijuana: How important is social bonding and for which ethic groups? *Substance Use and Misuse, 34,* 317–346.

Embland, H. (1995). What would happen in the world if sensible drinking was adopted as a reasonable concept and advertised universally? *Addiction, 90*(2), 169–171.

Ennett, S. T., Ringwalt, C. L., Thorne, J., Rohrbach, L. A., Vincus, A., Simons-Rudolph, A., et al. (2003). A comparison of current practice in school-based substance use prevention programs with meta-analysis findings. *Prevention Science, 4*(1), 1–14.

Farchi, G., Fidanza, F., Mariotti, S., & Menotti, A. (1992). Alcohol and mortality in the Italian rural cohorts of the Seven Countries Study. *International Journal of Epidemiology, 21,* 74–81.

Fernandez-Sola, J., Estruch, R., Nicolas, J. M., Pare, J. C., Sacanella, E., Antunez, E., et al. (1997). Comparison of alcoholic cardiomyopathy in women versus men. *American Journal of Cardiology, 80*(4), 481–485.

Finch, J., & Barry, K. (1992). Substance use in older adults. In M. Fleming & K. Barry (Eds.), *Addictive disorders: A practical guide to treatment.* St. Louis, MO: Mosby.

Fleming, M. F., Barry, K. L., Manwell, L. B., Johnson, K., & London, R. (1997). Brief physician advice for problem alcohol drinkers: A randomized controlled trial in community-based primary care practices. *JAMA, 117,* 1039–1045.

Frankel, E. N., Kanner, J., German, J. B., Parks, E., & Kinsella, J. E. (1993). Inhibition of oxidation of human low-density lipoprotein by phenolic substances in red wine. *Lancet, 341,* 454–457.

Fuchs, C. S., Stampfer, M. J., Colditz, G. A., Giovannucci, E. L., Manson, J. E., Kawachi, I., et al. (1995). Alcohol consumption and mortality among women. *New England Journal of Medicine, 332,* 1245–1250.

Gambert, S. R., & Katsoyannis, K. K. (1995). Alcohol-related medical disorders of older heavy drinkers. In T. Beresford & E. Gomberg (Eds.), *Alcohol and aging* (pp. 70–81). New York: Oxford University Press.

Gerstein, D. R. (1984). *Toward the prevention of alcohol problems: Government, business and community action.* Washington, DC: National Academies Press.

Gomberg, E. S. (1995). Older women and alcohol: Use and abuse. *Recent Developments in Alcoholism, 12,* 61–79.

Greden, J. F., & Walters, A. (1992). Caffeine. In J. L. Lowinson, P. Ruiz, R. B. Millman, & J. G. Langrod (Eds.), *Substance abuse* (2nd ed., pp. 357–369). Baltimore: Williams & Wilkins.

Grønbæk, M., Becker, U., Johansen, D., Gottschau, A., Schnohr, P., Hein, H. O., et al. (2000). Type of alcohol consumed and mortality from all causes, coronary heart disease, and cancer. *Annals of Internal Medicine, 133*(6), 411–419.

Grønbæk, M., Deis, A., Sørensen, T. I., Becker, U., Borch-Johnsen, K., Müller, P., et al. (1994). Influence of sex, age, body mass index, and smoking on alcohol and mortality. *British Medical Journal, 308,* 302–306.

Harris, K. R., & Miller, W. R. (1990). Behavioral self-control training for problem drinkers: Components of efficacy. *Psychology of Addictive Behaviors, 4*(2), 90–92.

Heather, N., Campion, P. D., Neville, R. G., & MacCabe, D. (1987). Evaluation of a controlled drinking minimal intervention for problem drinkers in general practice (the DRMS scheme). *Journal of the Royal College of General Practitioners, 27*(301), 358–363.

Hertog, M. G., Kromhout, D., Aravanis, C., Blackburn, H., Buzina, R., Fidanza, F., et al. (1995). Flavonoid intake and long-term risk of coronary heart disease and cancer in the Seven Countries Study. *Archives of Internal Medicine, 155*, 381–386.

Hinds, T. S., West, W. L., Knight, E. M., & Harland, B. F. (1996). The effect of caffeine on pregnancy outcome variables. *Nutrition Reviews, 54*(7), 203–207.

Institute of Medicine. (1990). *Broadening the base of treatment for alcohol problems.* Washington, DC: National Academies Press.

Jaffe, A., & Lohse, C. M. (1991). Expectations regarding cocaine use: Implications for prevention and treatment. *Addiction and Recovery, 11*(3), 9–12.

Johnson, R. D., & Williams, R. (1985). Genetic and environmental factors in the individual susceptibility to the development of alcoholic liver disease. *Alcohol and Alcoholism, 20*(2), 137–160.

Klatsky, A. L., Armstrong, M. A., & Friedman, G. D. (1992). Alcohol and mortality. *Annals of Internal Medicine, 117*, 646–654.

Kristenson, H., Ohlin, H., Hulten-Nosslin, M., Trell, E., & Hood, B. (1983). Identification and intervention of heavy drinking in middle-aged men: Results and follow up of 24–60 months of long-term study with randomized controls. *Alcoholism, Clinical and Experimental Research, 7*(2), 203–209.

Lamarine, R. J. (1994). Selected health and behavioral effects related to the use of caffeine. *Journal of Community Health, 19*(6), 49–466.

Liberto, J. G., Oslin, D. W., & Ruskin, P. E. (1992). Alcoholism in older persons: A review of the literature. *Hospital & Community Psychiatry, 43*, 975–984.

Lucey, M. R., Hill, E. M., Young, J. P., Demo-Dananberg, L., & Beresford, T. P. (1999). The influences of age and gender on blood ethanol concentrations in healthy humans. *Journal of Studies on Alcohol, 60*(1), 103–110.

Merrill, J. C., Kleber, H. D., Shwartz, M., Liu, H., & Lewis, S. R. (1999). Cigarettes, alcohol, marijuana, other risk behaviors and American youth. *Drug and Alcohol Dependence, 56*, 205–212.

Miller, P. M., & Nirenberg, T. D. (1984). *Prevention of alcohol abuse.* New York: Plenum.

Miller, P. M., Smith, G. T., & Goldman, M. S. (1990). Emergence of alcohol expectancies in childhood: A possible critical period. *Journal of Studies on Alcohol, 51*(4), 343–349.

Miller, W. R., & Hester, R. K. (1986). *Treating addictive behaviors: Processes of change.* New York: Plenum.

Miller, W. R., & Munoz, R. F. (1976). *How to control your drinking.* Upper Saddle River, NJ: Prentice Hall.

Miller, W. R., & Rollnick, S. (1991). *Motivational interviewing.* New York: Guilford Press.

Miller, W. R., & Tayor, C. A. (1980). Relative effectiveness of bibliotherapy, individual and group self-control training in the treatment of problem drinkers. *Addictive Behaviors, 5*, 13–24.

Morrissey, E. R. (1986). Of women, by women or for women? Selected issues in the primary prevention of drinking problems. In National Institute on Alcohol Abuse and Alcoholism (Ed.), *Women and alcohol: Health-related issues* (pp. 226–259) (Research Monograph No. 16,

DHHS Publication No. [ADM] 86-1139). Washington, DC: U.S. Government Printing Office.

Morse, A. C., Erwin, V. G., & Jones, B. C. (1995). Pharmacogenetics of cocaine: A critical review. *Pharmacogenetics, 5*(4), 183–192.

Naimi, T., Brewer, B., Mokdad, A., Serdula, M., Denny, C., & Marks, J. (2003). Binge drinking among U.S. adults. *JAMA, 289,* 70–75.

National Institute of Alcohol Abuse and Alcoholism. (1995a). Diagnostic criteria for alcohol abuse. *Alcohol Alert, 30,* 1–6.

National Institute of Alcohol Abuse and Alcoholism. (1995b). *The physicians' guide to helping patients with alcohol problems* (NIH Publication No. 95-3769). Bethesda, MD: National Institutes of Health.

National Institute of Alcohol Abuse and Alcoholism. (2004a). *Helping patients with alcohol problems: A health practitioners' guide.* Retrieved April 6, 2004, from http://www.niaaa.nih.gov/publications/Practitioner/HelpingPatients.htm#step1A

National Institute of Alcohol Abuse and Alcoholism. (2004b). *Percent who drink beverage alcohol, by gender, 1939–2003.* Retrieved December 21, 2004, from http://www.niaaa.nih.gov/database

National Institute of Alcohol Abuse and Alcoholism. (2004c). *Quick facts.* Retrieved December 10, 2004, from http://www.niaaa.nih.gov/databases/qf-text.htm

National Institute of Alcohol Abuse and Alcoholism. (2004d). *Total per capita alcohol consumption in gallons of ethanol by state—United States, 2000.* Retrieved December 20, 2004, from http://www.niaaa.nih.gov

Nirenberg, T. D., & Gomberg, E.S.L. (1993). Prevention of alcohol and drug problems among women. In E.S.L Gomberg & T. D. Nirenberg (Eds.), *Women and substance abuse* (pp. 339–359). Norwood, NJ: Ablex.

Oei, P. S., & Young, R. M. (1987). Roles of alcohol-related self-statements in social drinking. *International Journal of the Addictions, 11*(10), 905–915.

Onland-Moret, N. C., Peeters, P. H., van der Schouw, Y. T., Grobbee, D. E., & van Gils, C. H. (2004). Alcohol and endogenous sex steroid levels in postmenopausal women: A cross-sectional study. *Journal of Clinical Endocrinology and Metabolism* (Epub ahead of print; retrieved December 14, 2004).

Ozkaragoz, T., Satz, P., & Noble, E. P. (1997). Neuropsychological functioning in sons of active alcoholic, recovering alcoholic, and social drinking fathers. *Alcohol, 14*(1), 31–37.

Persson, J., & Magnusson, P. H. (1989). Early intervention in patients with excessive consumption of alcohol: A controlled study. *Alcohol, 6*(5), 403–408.

Project MATCH Research Group. (1997). Matching alcoholism treatments to client heterogeneity: Project MATCH posttreatment drinking outcomes. *Journal of Studies on Alcohol, 58*(1), 7–29.

Ray, O., & Ksir, C. (1996). *Drugs, society and human behavior.* St. Louis, MO: Mosby.

Renaud, S., & DeLorgeril, M. (1992). Wine, alcohol, platelets, and the French paradox for coronary heart disease. *Lancet, 229,* 1523–1526.

Rimm, E. B., Klatsky, A., Grobbee, D., & Stampfer, M. J. (1996). Review of moderate alcohol consumption and reduced risk of coronary heart disease: Is the effect due to beer, wine, or spirits? *British Medical Journal, 312,* 731–736.

Robins, L. N., & Regier, D. A. (1991). *Psychiatric disorders in America: The Epidemiologic Catchment Area Study.* New York: Free Press.

Ruf, J. C., Berger, J. L., & Renaud, S. (1995). Platelet rebound effect of alcohol withdrawal and wine drinking in rats: Relation to tannins and lipid peroxidation. *Arteriosclerosis, Thrombosis, and Vascular Biology, 15,* 140–144.

Salazar-Martinez, E., Willett, W. C., Ascherio, A., Manson, J. E., Leitzmann, M. F., Stampfer, M. J., et al. (2004). Coffee consumption and risk for type 2 diabetes mellitus. *Annals of Internal Medicine, 140*(1), 1–8.

Sanchez-Craig, M., Neumann, B., Souza-Formigoni, M., & Rieck, L. (1991). Brief treatment for alcohol treatment for alcohol dependence: Level of dependence and treatment outcome. *Alcohol and Alcoholism,* (Suppl. 1), 515–518.

Schuckit, M. A. (1991). Importance of subtypes in alcoholism. *Alcohol and Alcoholism,* (Suppl. 1), 511–514.

Sheinfeld Gorin, S., & Arnold, J. (Eds.). (1998). *Health promotion handbook.* St. Louis, MO: Mosby.

Shiflett, D. (1996, October). Here's to your health. *American Spectator,* pp. 26–30.

Simmons, D. H. (1996). Caffeine and its effect on persons with mental disorders. *Archives of Psychiatric Nursing, 10*(2), 116–122.

Substance Abuse and Mental Health Services Administration, Office of Applied Studies. (1996). *1996 DAWN (Drug Abuse Warning Network) survey.* Retrieved January 2005 from http://www.health.org/pubs/95dawn.

Substance Abuse and Mental Health Services Administration, Office of Applied Studies. (2004). *Results from the 2003 National Survey on Drug Use and Health: National findings* (NSDUH Series H–25, DHHS Publication No. SMA 04-3964). Retrieved December 20, 2004, from http://www.oas.samhsa.gov/NHSDA

Thadani, P. V. (1995). Biological mechanisms and perinatal exposure to abused drugs. *Synapse, 19*(3), 228–232.

Thompson, J. P. (2003). Acute effects of drugs of abuse. *Clinical Medicine, 3*(2), 123–126.

Trachtenberg, A., & Fleming, M. (1994, Summer). *Diagnosis and treatment of drug abuse in family practice* [monograph]. Leawood, KS: American Academy of Family Physicians.

Urbano-Marquez, A., Estruch, R., Fernandez-Sola, J., Nicolas, J. M., Pare, J. C., & Rubin, E. (1995). The greater risk of cardiomyopathy and myopathy in women compared with men. *JAMA, 274,* 149–154.

U.S. Department of Health and Human Services & U.S. Department of Agriculture. (2000). *Nutrition and your health: Dietary guidelines for Americans* (5th ed.) (Home and Gardening Bulletin No. 232). Washington, DC: Author.

Vestal, R. E., McGuire, E. A., Tobin, J. D., Andres, R., Norris, A. H., & Mezey, E. (1977). Aging and ethanol metabolism. *Clinical Pharmacology and Therapeutics, 21,* 343–354.

Vogel-Sprott, M., & Barrett, P. (1984). Age, drinking habits, and the effects of alcohol. *Journal of Studies on Alcohol, 45,* 517–521.

Wallace, J. (1994). Race differences in adolescent drug use. *African American Research Perspectives, 1*(1), 31–36.

Wallace, P., Cutler, S., & Haines, A. (1988). Randomized controlled trial of general practitioner intervention in patients with excessive alcohol consumption. *British Medical Journal, 197,* 663–668.

Wechsler, H., & Austin, S. B. (1998). Binge drinking: The five/four measure. *Journal of Studies on Alcohol, 59,* 122–124.

Wetle, T. (1997). Living longer, aging better: Aging research comes of age. *JAMA, 278,* 1376–1377.

Whitlock, E. P., Polen, M. R., Green, C. A., Orleans, T., & Klein, J.; U.S. Preventive Services Task Force. (2004). Behavioral counseling interventions in primary care to reduce risky/harmful alcohol use by adults: A summary of the evidence for the U.S. Preventive Services Task Force. *Annals of Internal Medicine, 140*(7), 557–568.

Woods, J. (1977). *Behavioral effects of cocaine in animals.* In R. C. Petersen & R. C. Stillman (Eds.), *Cocaine: 1977* (pp. 63–95) (NIDA Research Monograph No. 12). Washington, DC: U.S. Government Printing Office.

World Health Organization. (1995). *Alcohol: Less is better: European Action Plan* (WHO Regional Publications, European Series, 70). Geneva: Author.

Yuan, J. M., Ross, R. K., Gao, Y. T., Henderson, B. E., & Yu, M. C. (1997). Follow up study of moderate alcohol intake and mortality among middle aged men in Shanghai, China. *British Medical Journal, 314,* 18–23.

EXHIBIT 10.1. HELPFUL RESOURCES.

Al-Anon/Alateen, http://www.al-anon.alateen.org

This Web site describes the Twelve Steps, Twelve Traditions, and Twelve Concepts of Service adapted from AA for families and friends of alcoholics. It also lists local groups. Information is also available from Al-Anon Family Group Headquarters, Inc., 1600 Corporate Landing Pkwy., Virginia Beach, VA 23454-1655; phone: (757) 563-1600; fax: (757) 563-1655.

Alcoholics Anonymous (AA) World Services, Inc., http://www.alcoholics-anonymous.org

This Web site provides information and resources on AA programs in English, Spanish, and French.

National Clearinghouse for Alcohol and Drug Information, http://www.health.org/research/library.aspx

The PREVLINE, or Prevention Online, allows access to databases and substance abuse prevention materials that pertain to alcohol, tobacco, and illegal drugs.

Substance Abuse & Mental Health Services Administration, http://www.findtreatment.samhsa.gov

This site allows its users to search for local treatment programs by facility function (for example, substance abuse treatment, methadone treatment, detoxification), type of care (for example, inpatient or outpatient), subpopulation (for example, youths, dually diagnosed), special language services, and payment type (for example, Medicare, Medicaid).

National Institute on Alcohol Abuse and Alcoholism (NIAAA), http://www.niaaa.nih.gov

On this site the NIAAA, part of the U.S. Department of Health and Human Services, lists publications and databases that provide information on alcohol problems, as well as referrals and links to other organizations and associations.

CHAPTER ELEVEN

INJURY PREVENTION

David A. Sleet
Andrea Carlson Gielen

Injury is the third leading cause of death in the United States and is the lead-ing cause of death for children and young adults (Centers for Disease Control and Prevention [CDC], 2005a). Each year about 149,000 injury-related deaths result in 3.7 million potential years of life lost before the age of sixty-five. Every year nonfatal injuries account for 114 million visits to physicians' offices and more than one-quarter of the total visits to emergency departments. Injuries are the leading cause of hospital admissions for persons younger than forty-five years, and in 2005 alone, one in four Americans will suffer a potentially preventable injury serious enough to require medical attention.

In many respects injury is today's primary public health problem for Ameri-cans younger than forty-four years. Injuries among Americans of all ages could be dramatically reduced if health promotion approaches were used to prevent and control injuries.

Injury as a Public Health Problem

According to the National Academy of Sciences (1988), injury is probably the most underrecognized major public health problem facing the nation today. Each year injury is the number one cause of death among school-age children and youths, in virtually every country in the world. Yet until recently, injury prevention was not recognized as a public health issue.

Injury is now recognized as a health problem that can best be understood and controlled by using the same approaches used against other diseases. Injury results from interactions between persons (host factors), energy (agent and vehicle factors), and the environment (environmental factors) (Haddon, 1970). This epidemiologic approach to understanding injury is the foundation on which health promotion strategies to injury reduction are applied.

Injury can be controlled by reducing the number of times potentially injurious events occur and by reducing the severity when injury events do occur. In public health, injury is defined as "unintentional or intentional damage to the body resulting from acute exposure to thermal, mechanical, electrical, or chemical energy or from the absence of such essentials as heat or oxygen" (National Committee for Injury Prevention and Control, 1989). In the case of a sports injury, damage to the host (the person harmed) is brought about through a rapid transfer of kinetic energy. This exchange of energy can be modified in several ways—for instance, by making the host more resistant to it (by increasing injury tolerance) or by separating the host from the kinetic energy exchange (for example, interposing protective equipment between the host and the energy source) (Haddon, 1970).

Although injury is a public health problem, to solve it takes professionals from many disciplines, such as nurses, health educators, school teachers and officials, nursing home and hospital administrators, psychologists, social workers, police, product engineers, highway planners, criminologists, playground designers, sports physicians, coaches, and occupational safety managers. To be successful, injury prevention strategies require collaboration.

Injury or Accident?

Injury does not happen by accident. Accidents are not predictable or preventable. The *Oxford English Dictionary* defines the term *accident* as "an event without apparent cause . . . unexpected—happening by chance." The word *injury* has its root in the Latin term *injurius,* which means "unjust" or "not right." Funk and Wagnalls' *Standard College Dictionary* of 1966 defines injury as "harm, damage, or grievous distress inflicted or sustained." Because the term *accident* implies an unavoidable event, it should not be used when referring to injury, which is a predictable medical outcome. The science of injury prevention teaches that injuries are not accidental or random events—they are predictable, and many are preventable through changes in products, human behavior, and environments. Using terms such as *injury prevention* rather than *accident prevention* helps make clear the potential for preventing these adverse medical outcomes. Former U.S. surgeon general C. Everett Koop underscored this distinction in his preface to *Injury Prevention: Meeting the Challenge* (National Committee for Injury Prevention and Control, 1989) when he said: "We must accept that the injuries associated with motor vehicles are not 'accidents' and that much can be done to reduce them. We must realize that violence in the forms of abuse, assault or suicide is not only within the purview of the police and the criminal justice system but also the health system. An informed and aroused public can change the behavior of each of us, but more importantly, it must lead to community outrage and action in regard to unsafe playgrounds, automobiles, highways, work places, toys, homes and use of handguns" (p. ii).

Professionals in the injury prevention field should be encouraged by the findings that a majority among the public believe that accidents and injuries are preventable (Girasek, 1999). Focusing on prevention of both the injury event and its medical, social, and economic consequences may help us to reframe the issue of injury within a disease prevention and health promotion framework.

Causes of Injury

A specific cause of injury is the transfer of energy to a person at rates and in amounts more than the tolerance of human tissue (De Haven, 1942). The amount of the energy concentration that is outside the tolerance of tissue usually determines the severity of the injury. The terms *injury* and *trauma* are often used interchangeably.

Two generally recognized categories of injuries are *unintentional injuries* (caused by unintentional means: for example, falling; drowning; poisoning; or experiencing a motor vehicle, pedestrian, or motorcycle crash) and *injuries from violence* (intentionally inflicted: for example, homicide, assault, child maltreatment, elder abuse, or suicide). Domestic violence, particularly to children and youths, is one form of intentional injury in which the health care professional is generally legally obligated to intervene, and it is discussed in Chapter Twelve. Homicides and suicides are also explored in part in Chapter Twelve. We focus in this chapter principally on unintentional injuries.

Although there are many kinds and causes of injury, the following two main categories prevail:

1. *Acute exposure to energy:* refers to injuries resulting from falls, motor vehicle crashes, firearms, violence, and sports play (kinetic energy); fires and burns (thermal energy); poisonings (chemical energy); electrocution (electrical energy); and radiation (radiant energy)
2. *Absence of essentials:* includes lack of oxygen (for example, as occurs in asphyxiation, strangulation, or drowning) and lack of heat (for example, as occurs in hypothermia or frostbite)

Magnitude of the Injury Problem

Like diseases, injuries have geographic, socioeconomic, and seasonal variations. Injuries also vary according to characteristics of persons (for example, age, sex, income) and of persons' environments (for example, neighborhood, workplace, or home). Injury epidemiology has developed as a way to understand and explain these variations and as a way to target specific interventions to reduce injuries among persons in specific high-risk populations.

Table 11.1 shows the ten leading causes of death by age group in 2001. Injury (including unintentional injury, homicide, and suicide) is the leading cause of death for each age group category from ages one to forty-four years. Unintentional injuries dominate, with homicide and suicide occupying prominent places as major causes of death for those aged ten to thirty-four years.

Table 11.2 shows the number of deaths caused by each injury type and the rates per 100,000 population (including age-adjusted and crude rates) by gender in the United States in 2002. In sheer numbers in 2002, motor vehicle crashes were the leading cause of injury-related deaths, followed by suicide, homicide, falls, poisonings, drownings, and fires. Violence, when measured by the number of deaths resulting from both suicide and homicide, exceeds the combined total of both motor vehicle- and fall-related deaths. Among males, violent deaths exceeded the combined total of deaths resulting from motor vehicle crashes, falls, drownings, and fires.

Deaths are only a part of the devastating effects of injury on society. Each year about 1.5 million Americans sustain a traumatic brain injury (TBI). That's eight times the number of people diagnosed with breast cancer each year. Approximately one in four adults with TBI is unable to return to work one year after injury. It is estimated that 10,000 persons are hospitalized each year with a spinal cord injury, and about 200,000 persons live their entire lives with permanent effects from this type of injury (National Center for Injury Prevention and Control, 2001). Although motor vehicle crashes, firearms, falls, poisonings, fires and burns, and drownings account for 80 percent of deaths resulting from injury each year, they account for only about 36 percent of treated injuries not requiring hospitalization. (See Table 11.3.)

The costs of injury are enormous. In 2000, the United States spent $117 billion, or 10 percent of medical expenditures, on injury-related medical care (CDC, 2004).

The Epidemiology of Injury

The model developed to explain the epidemiology of infectious and chronic disease can be applied to injury (Gordon, 1949). This model considers the contribution of and interaction between the host (the person getting the disease), the agent (the specific disease-causing element) and vector (the carrier transmitting the agent to the host), and the environment (the physical and sociocultural factors influencing transmission and reception) (Haddon, 1980).

TABLE 11.1. TEN LEADING CAUSES OF DEATH BY AGE GROUP, 2001.

Age Groups

Rank	<1	1–4	5–9	10–14	15–24	25–34	35–44	45–54	55–64	65+	Total
1	Congenital Anomalies 5,513	Unintentional Injury 1,714	Unintentional Injury 1,283	Unintentional Injury 1,553	Unintentional Injury 14,411	Unintentional Injury 11,839	Malignant Neoplasms 16,569	Malignant Neoplasms 49,562	Malignant Neoplasms 90,223	Heart Disease 582,730	Heart Disease 700,142
2	Short Gestation 4,410	Congenital Anomalies 557	Malignant Neoplasms 493	Malignant Neoplasms 515	Homicide 5,297	Homicide 5,204	Unintentional Injury 15,945	Heart Disease 36,399	Heart Disease 62,486	Malignant Neoplasms 390,214	Malignant Neoplasms 553,768
3	SIDS 2,234	Malignant Neoplasms 420	Congenital Anomalies 182	Suicide 272	Suicide 3,971	Suicide 5,070	Heart Disease 13,326	Unintentional Injury 13,344	Chronic Low. Respiratory Disease 11,166	Cerebro-vascular 144,486	Cerebro-vascular 163,538
4	Maternal Pregnancy Comp. 1,499	Homicide 415	Homicide 137	Congenital Anomalies 194	Malignant Neoplasms 1,704	Malignant Neoplasms 3,994	Suicide 6,635	Liver Disease 7,259	Cerebro-vascular 9,608	Chronic Low. Respiratory Disease 106,904	Chronic Low. Respiratory Disease 123,013
5	Placenta Cord Membranes 1,018	Heart Disease 225	Heart Disease 98	Homicide 189	Heart Disease 999	Heart Disease 3,160	HIV 5,867	Suicide 5,942	Diabetes Mellitus 9,570	Influenza & Pneumonia 55,518	Unintentional Injury 101,537

TABLE 11.1. TEN LEADING CAUSES OF DEATH BY AGE GROUP, 2001, Cont'd.

Rank		<1	1-4	5-9	10-14	15-24	25-34	35-44	45-54	55-64	65+	Total
	Age Groups											
6		Respiratory Distress 1,011	Influenza & Pneumonia 112	Benign Neoplasms 52	Heart Disease 174	Congenital Anomalies 505	HIV 2,101	Homicide 4,268	Cerebro-vascular 5,910	Unintentional Injury 7,658	Diabetes Mellitus 53,707	Diabetes Mellitus 71,372
7		Unintentional Injury 976	Septicemia 108	Influenza & Pneumonia 46	Chronic Low. Respiratory Disease 62	HIV 225	Cerebro-vascular 601	Liver Disease 3,336	Diabetes Mellitus 5,343	Liver Disease 5,750	Alzheimer's Disease 53,245	Influenza & Pneumonia 62,034
8		Bacterial Sepsis 696	Perinatal Period 72	Chronic Low. Respiratory Disease 42	Benign Neoplasms 53	Cerebro-vascular 196	Diabetes Mellitus 595	Cerebro-vascular 2,491	HIV 4,120	Suicide 3,317	Nephritis 33,121	Alzheimer's Disease 53,852
9		Circulatory System Disease 622	Benign Neoplasms 58	Cerebro-vascular 38	Influenza & Pneumonia 46	Influenza & Pneumonia 181	Congenital Anomalies 458	Diabetes Mellitus 1,958	Chronic Low. Respiratory Disease 3,324	Nephritis 3,284	Unintentional Injury 32,694	Nephritis 39,480
10		Intrauterine Hypoxia 534	Cerebro-vascular 54	Septicemia 29	Cerebro-vascular 42	Chronic Low. Respiratory Disease 171	Liver Disease 387	Influenza & Pneumonia 983	Homicide 2,467	Septicemia 3,111	Septicemia 25,418	Septicemia 32,238

Note: Homicide and suicide counts include terrorism deaths associated with the events of September 11, 2001, that occurred in New York City, Pennsylvania, and Virginia. A total of 2,926 U.S. residents lost their lives in these acts of terrorism in 2001, of which 2,922 were classified as (transportation-related) homicides and 4 were classified as suicides.

Source: CDC, 2002. Thanks to Dionne D. White for providing these data.

TABLE 11.2. NUMBER OF DEATHS CAUSED BY INJURY AND RATES PER 100,000 UNITED STATES POPULATION—ALL AGES AND RACES, BY SEX, 2002.

Cause	Males		Females		Total		
	No.	Rate	No.	Rate	No.	Crude Rate	Age-Adjusted Rate*
Motor vehicle	29,989	21.2	14,076	9.6	44,065	15.3	15.2
Suicide	25,409	18.0	6,246	4.3	31,655	11.0	10.9
Homicide/legal intervention	14,009	9.9	4,013	2.7	18,022	6.3	6.2
Fall	8,463	6.0	7,794	5.3	16,257	5.7	5.6
Poisoning	12,059	8.5	5,491	3.8	17,550	6.1	6.1
Drowning/ submersion	2,761	2.0	686	0.5	3,447	1.2	1.2
Fire/flames	1,935	1.4	1,224	0.8	3,159	1.1	1.1
Other injury deaths	17,184	12.1	9,930	6.8	27,114	9.4	9.4
Total	111,809	79.0	49,460	33.8	161,269	56.0	55.7

Note: Standard population is 2000 United States all races and both genders. NCHS ICD-10 Preliminary Data are used for number of deaths; U.S. Census Populations with Bridged Race Categories provided by the National Center for Health Statistics (NCHS) are used for population numbers.

*Age-adjusted rate excludes those whose ages are unknown.

Source: CDC, 2005a. Thanks to Dionne D. White for providing these data.

Injury results from the interaction between injury-producing agents (for example, kinetic energy), the environment (for example, a playground), and a susceptible host (for example, a young and curious child). Injury can be controlled by preventing its occurrence or by minimizing its severity when it does occur. In the case of motor vehicle–related injury, damage to the host is caused by a rapid transfer of kinetic energy when the vehicle stops suddenly. Changing this pattern of energy transfer (either by making the host more resistant to it or by separating the host from the energy exchange) is part of the science of injury control.

When this model is applied to smoking it shows how host factors (amount smoked, depth of inhalation), agent factors (tar and ciliotoxins), and environmental factors (secondhand smoke, social pressure) each contribute to smoking-related morbidity and mortality. This model can be used similarly in injury control, showing, for example, the factors in injury morbidity and mortality resulting from traffic crashes (Figure 11.1). Host factors include age, inexperience at driving, and alcohol or drug use. Environmental factors include road surfaces, road signs, and

TABLE 11.3. NUMBER OF NONFATAL INJURIES AND RATES PER 100,000 UNITED STATES POPULATION—ALL AGES AND RACES, BY SEX, 2003.

Cause	Males		Females		Total		
	No.	Rate	No.	Rate	No.	Crude Rate	Age-Adjusted Rate*
Fall	3,626,985	2535.7	4,267,172	2887.6	7,895,385	2715.0	2720.9
Struck by/against	2,808,228	1963.3	1,613,498	1091.9	4,422,252	1520.7	1529.0
Overexertion	1,740,314	1216.7	1,583,722	1071.7	3,324,641	1143.2	1142.1
MV-occupant	1,363,684	953.4	1,662,341	1124.9	3,026,595	1040.7	1036.5
Cut/pierce	1,427,861	998.2	807,523	546.5	2,235,869	768.8	768.3
Assault/ legal intervention	1,039,396	726.7	659,554	446.3	1,699,142	584.3	583.8
Self-harm	178,568	124.8	232,439	157.3	411,128	141.4	141.2
Other nonfatal injuries	3,797,039	2654.6	2,424,647	1640.8	6,222,735	2139.8	2146.2
Total	15,982,075	11,173.4	13,250,896	8967.0	29,237,747	10,053.9	10,067.9

Note: Standard population is 2000 United States all races and both genders. The numbers of nonfatal injuries presented in WISQARS Nonfatal are national estimates based on weighted data from the U.S. Consumer Product Safety Commission's (CPSC) National Electronic Injury Surveillance System (NEISS). The Total No. column represents males, females, and unknown sex. NEISS-AIP data are used for number of nonfatal injuries; U.S. Census Populations with Bridged Race Categories provided by the National Center for Health Statistics (NCHS) are used for population numbers.

*Age-adjusted rate excludes those whose ages are unknown.

Source: CDC, 2005b. Thanks to Dionne D. White for providing these data.

traffic conditions. Vector and agent factors are those factors that affect (1) the amount of energy released, (2) the distribution of that energy, and (3) the transfer of the energy to the host. Examples of vector and agent factors that influence injury in a motor vehicle crash are size and weight of the vehicle, vehicle speed, force of impact, angle of crash, construction of the vehicle to absorb energy, and use of seat belts and air bags to reduce the energy transferred to the host in a crash. The combined use of safety belts (by the host), air bags and crumple zones (by vehicles), strengthened vehicle bodies (by the manufacturer), and dividing bar-

FIGURE 11.1. EPIDEMIOLOGY OF CIGARETTE-RELATED MORBIDITY AND MORTALITY AND EPIDEMIOLOGY OF TRAFFIC INJURY–RELATED MORBIDITY AND MORTALITY.

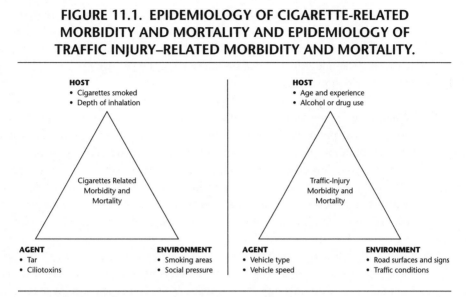

Source: Sleet & Gielen, 1998, Figs 10.1 and 10.2.

riers and guardrails on highways will limit the amount of kinetic energy transferred to the driver or passenger and can significantly reduce fatal injuries in vehicle crashes.

Axioms in Injury Prevention

The following injury prevention axioms can guide efforts to control injuries (Sleet & Rosenberg, 1997; Sleet, Egger, & Albany, 1991).

1. *Injury results from interactions between people and the environment.* The determinants of injury are both human and environmental. The agent of injury will cause relatively little damage if the amount of it reaching tissues is within the limits of human tolerance. For example, tap water can scald in seconds or not at all, depending on its temperature. Approaches that control the environment by reducing hot water temperatures at the tap and simultaneously targeting the parents of small children and the elderly with information about hot water scald risks (including the need for reduced tap water temperatures) recognize the importance of this interaction.

2. *Injury-producing interactions can be modified through changing behavior, products, or environments.* Injuries can be reduced by modifying the weakest or most adaptable link in the chain of causation. Unsanctioned swimming in a home swimming pool

is more easily reduced by placing an isolation fence or barrier between the child and the pool than by supervising the child's behavior at all times. During sanctioned swimming, while the child is in the pool, supervision is the most important strategy. Changing the environment, the laws, the person, or the product can all lead to reductions in injuries.

3. *Environmental changes have the potential to protect the greatest number of people.* Changes to the environment that automatically provide protection to every person have the potential to prevent the most injuries. Such automatic protection may be built into roads (as barriers, for example), into buildings (as fire sprinkler systems), into automobiles (as air bags), into homes (as fuses), and into products (as child-resistant packaging on medicines). Few "passive" interventions succeed without an active behavioral component (such as replacing the child-resistant lids on medicines), and so they perform better when the public is informed and convinced of their necessity and benefit.

4. *Effective injury prevention requires a mixture of strategies and methods.* Three primary strategies—education and behavioral change, legislation and enforcement, and technology and engineering—are widely recognized as effective in preventing injuries. Individual behavioral change, product engineering, public education, legal requirements, law enforcement, and changes in the physical and social environments work together to reduce injuries. The challenge in intervention planning is to select the most effective combination of strategies to produce the desired result.

5. *Public participation is essential for community action.* Effective public policy requires the support and participation of people. Local problems and resource availability often determine the direction of injury prevention programs. Factors influencing success in injury prevention are best identified by public participation in the process. Without public support, laws designed to protect the public (such as laws requiring the use of bicycle helmets) may be ignored, or worse, repealed.

6. *Intersectoral collaboration is necessary.* Injury prevention requires coordinated action by many groups. Participation by community leaders, in addition to health department and public health officials, is necessary in planning and implementing injury prevention programs. Different sectors can play different roles—ranging from identifying problems to mobilizing community action, evaluating intervention effectiveness, and advocating for change. Identifying and building a constituency and shifting or sharing resources requires collaboration across many different sectors.

Health Promotion and Injury Prevention

Although people must assume personal responsibility for maintaining their health, it is now widely recognized that environmental cues and reinforcers exert an important influence on behavioral choices and outcomes. Injury prevention behavior is shaped not only by individual choices and motivation, knowledge, skills, and attitudes but also by organizational, economic, environmental, and social factors (Ross, 1984). Approaches that attempt to bring about change in injury behaviors without consideration for these broader influences are likely to have limited or no success (Peden et al., 2004; Sleet, 1984). Approaches that combine education with other behavioral, environmental, policy, and organizational changes, elements central to health promotion, are likely to be the most effective (Howat, Sleet, Elder, & Maycock, 2004; World Health Organization [WHO], 1986).

Health promotion arose from the recognition of the complex determinants of health behavior and health status. One definition of health promotion is, "a combination of educational, organizational, economic and political actions designed with consumer participation, to enable individuals, groups and whole communities to increase control over, and to improve health through changes in knowledge, attitudes, behavior, policy, and social and environmental conditions" (Howat et al., 2003). This definition builds on and incorporates aspects of earlier definitions of health promotion (Green & Kreuter, 1999; Pan American Health Organization, 1996; WHO, 1984), which focus on building health public policy, creating supportive environments, strengthening community action and developing personal health skills. For example, a health promotion approach to the prevention of alcohol-related traffic injuries would incorporate a balance of strategies that focus on individual behavioral change and strategies that encourage supportive environments (Howat et al., 2004).

An example of applying this approach to the problem of injury is displayed in Figure 11.2. The figure presents a logic model and framework showing how the components of health promotion (economic actions, policy actions, organizational actions, and health education) can cumulatively contribute to the changes in knowledge, attitudes, behaviors, and policies and the social and environmental change necessary to reduce hazardous environments, products, and behaviors, which in turn reduce injury, ultimately leading to improved health status of individuals and communities.

We are reminded by Mason and Tolsma (1984) that "persons can hardly be expected to avoid the risks imposed by personal choices when they do not know or understand these risks, when they lack the knowledge or skills needed to choose a healthier lifestyle, or worst of all, when they seek guidance or support from their community and it is unavailable to them" (p. 772). Preventing injury is no exception. It too requires strong community support. Such support is not only necessary for legislative initiatives but is also critically important for shaping personal behavior and social norms (Gielen & Sleet, 2003).

Injury prevention has received less coverage than it deserves in the health promotion literature, perhaps because it does not fall within the traditional domain of preventive medicine and public health (Sleet & Rosenberg, 1997). This may

FIGURE 11.2. A HEALTH PROMOTION FRAMEWORK
FOR REDUCING ALCOHOL-RELATED TRAFFIC INJURY.

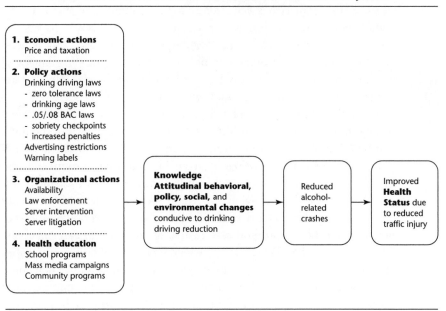

Source: Howat et al., 2004; reprinted by permission, Taylor and Francis Publishers.

have been partly due to the way *Healthy People* (U.S. Department of Health, Education and Welfare, Public Health Service, 1979) had originally categorized injuries, seeing them as resulting from "accidents" and placing them in the "health protection" category, along with other environmental problems considered to be beyond individual control. Inevitably, as injury prevention and health promotion become more closely aligned, the potential benefits of health promotion approaches to injury prevention strategies will become clearer and more widely accepted.

The immediate goals of health promotion for injury control include the following:

- Modifying individual risk behaviors
- Reducing exposure to hazardous environments
- Removing or modifying harmful products

Individual and community actions are required to succeed in these efforts, which are fostered by education stimulated by social and organizational change, and encouraged through public policy, legislation, and enforcement (Sleet & Gielen, 2004; Sleet, Wagenaar, & Waller, 1989).

Injury Prevention Strategies

Historically, planning for injury prevention and control has had to deal with a tension between *active* (behavioral) and *passive* (structural) strategies. The notion of passive protection arose from the unparalleled success of public health measures such as immunization and water fluoridation, which required a one-time intervention with few behavioral components. Passive approaches can also rely on changing products or environments to make them safer for all. Active approaches, in contrast, encourage or require people to take an active role in protecting themselves from encounters with the hazards around them. Adding to the controversy was the opinion expressed by some that a focus on changing individual behavior constitutes *blaming the victim* (Ryan, 1976). Yet one modern response to the victim-blaming assertion is that empowering individuals through behavioral change efforts can lead to the political or social action necessary to achieve structural changes (Bennet & Murphy, 1997; Gielen & Girasek, 2001).

Strategies in injury prevention, which are general plans of action used to reduce injuries, are distinct from *methods,* which are tactics used to implement the strategies. Whereas education is one strategy for preventing burns, clinical counseling is one method of implementing that strategy; another method is a mass media campaign to make the public aware of a burn hazard. There are three generally accepted strategies in injury prevention and many distinct methods for implementing each. The three strategies are

1. Education and behavioral change
2. Legislation and enforcement
3. Engineering and technology

A combination of strategies should be selected on the basis of an analysis of the situation, including a needs assessment, for the population being served. The strategy mix should also take into consideration local standards and the public acceptability of various behavioral, environmental, or engineering and infrastructural changes necessary to reduce injuries. In general the three types of strategies interact with the epidemiologic triad of host, agent (vector or vehicle), and environment in the manner described in Figure 11.3.

Figure 11.3 has two implications. First, strategy selection is influenced by the proposed target. Education and behavioral change may be used to target the host; legislation and law enforcement may target environmental change; and engineering

FIGURE 11.3. PREVENTION STRATEGIES APPLIED
TO THE EPIDEMIOLOGIC TRIAD OF INJURY CAUSATION.

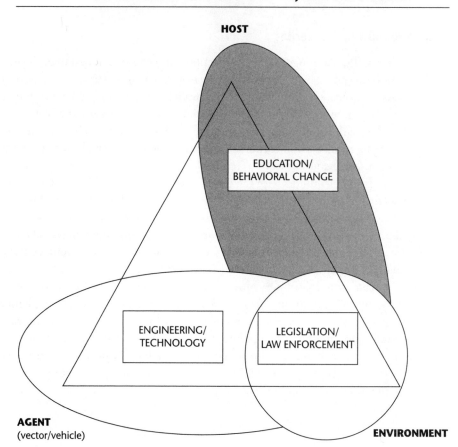

Source: Sleet, Egger, & Albany, 1991, by permission.

and technology may target changes in the agent to modify energy transfer. Second, strategies overlap (that is, one strategy may affect more than one target) (Sleet, Egger, & Albany, 1991).

Education and Behavioral Change. Education and behavioral change strategies are directed mostly toward decreasing the susceptibility of the host to injury by teaching or motivating individuals to behave differently. Some methods used to implement this strategy (for example, social marketing) may also affect social norms in the environment, as illustrated by the overlapping circles in Figure 11.3.

For example, the designated-driver campaigns aimed at modifying host drinking behaviors also affect attitudes in the community environment, resulting in drinking and driving being socially unacceptable.

Although the structural intervention paradigm might seem straightforward, there is rarely an environmental change that does not require human adaptation. For every technological advance, behavioral components need to be addressed. Children need to wear helmets while bicycling; parents need to correctly install child safety seats and booster seats; home owners need to check their smoke alarms and change the batteries; parents with four-sided fences around their backyard pools need to ensure that the gate to the pool is always closed; occupants alerted by a smoke alarm still need to find their way to safety. Even the fairly passive approach to poison prevention through using child-resistant closures—one of the great successes in injury control—requires active individual effort in replacing lids correctly (DiLillo, Peterson, & Farmer, 2002; Shields, 1997).

Although some controversy still remains about the benefits of educational approaches to injury control (O'Connor, 1982; Pless, 1978), there are numerous examples of successful applications of health promotion strategies for injury prevention (Dowswell, Towner, Simpson, & Jarvis, 1996; Sleet & Gielen, 2004). Discrepancies in the results of earlier studies can be attributed to a number of factors, including lack of control groups, use of varied methods of education, the absence of theory-based approaches to health education in the design of interventions, poorly designed methods for measuring change, and inadequate "doses" of education.

Behavioral modification techniques, however, have produced fairly consistent positive results (Roberts, Fanurik, & Layfield, 1987; Streff & Geller, 1986; Jones, van Hasselt, & Sisson, 1984), at least in short-term change. Such methods include incentives, social modeling, feedback, rewards, skills training, cognitive rehearsal, and competition to improve injury prevention behavior (Huesmann, Guerra, Miller, & Zelli, 1992; Farrell, Meyer, & Dahlberg, 1996; Geller, Elder, Hovell, & Sleet, 1991; Sleet, Hollenbach, & Hovell, 1986). Behavioral change methods such as these can be targeted to change the behavior of one person (for example, a juvenile's fire-starting behavior), of a particular group at risk (for example, the behavior of teenage drivers), or of an entire community (for example, the behavior of using the emergency 911 number). Behaviors for which behavioral change approaches have been successful include the following:

- Emergency fire safety skills for children in the home
- Child restraint and child safety belt use
- Adult safety belt use
- Worker behavior in hazardous occupations
- Impaired driving

Education and behavioral change approaches can also produce effects on those who make laws and design products, such as legislators and engineers, in ways that ultimately protect whole populations (Gielen, Sleet, & DiClemente, 2006).

Key factors necessary for education and behavioral change strategies to work are the following:

- The audience must be exposed to the information.
- The audience must understand and believe the information.
- The audience must have the resources and skills to make the proposed change.
- The audience must derive benefit (or perceive a benefit) from the change.
- The audience must be reinforced to maintain the change over time.

Legislation and Law Enforcement. Legislation and law enforcement strategies have their greatest effect when they make both the physical environment (for example, regulated highway signs and building codes) and the sociocultural environment (for example, social attitudes and policies supporting a safe community) safer. Laws and regulations can require changes in individual behavior or in product design or the alteration of environmental hazards. In each case there is an opportunity for the legislation and law enforcement strategies to work synergistically with the other two strategies. Laws that discourage individuals from drinking and driving (for example, laws that permit a maximum of 0.08 g/dL of alcohol in the blood of drivers) can also make individuals less tolerant of drinking and boating. Communities that raise the price of alcoholic beverages also stand a good chance of reducing overall alcohol consumption, thereby reducing many alcohol-related injuries.

Legislation can also be aimed at changing the environment, making it less hazardous for everyone. Regulations requiring residential pool fencing, safeguards against workplace hazards, or comprehensive trauma care systems are examples of how this strategy can benefit whole communities. Product safety regulations, such as those affecting toys, home appliances, sports equipment, and playgrounds, are other examples of the application of legislation and law enforcement to benefit multiple targets.

Key factors in assuring legislation enforcement strategies work are the following:

- The legislation must be widely known and understood.
- The public must accept the legislation and its enforcement provisions.
- The probability, or perceived probability, of being caught if one breaks the law must be high.
- The punishment must be perceived as swift and severe.

Engineering and Technology. Engineering and technology strategies are likely to have their greatest impact on the agent (vector or vehicle) of energy transfer, but they may also affect environmental factors contributing to injury. Hip pads designed to reduce hip fractures among the elderly by reducing the amount of energy transferred to the host during a fall led to the design of soft flooring materials to reduce environmental risks where risks for falls are high (for example, nursing homes). Technology and engineering contribute to injury reduction by the development of products that reduce the likelihood of sudden energy release. These strategies can affect the safety of environments as well and may even lead to safer behavior on the part of the host (for example, occupants may increase use of safety belts while riding in an air bag–equipped car).

Some of the many technological and engineering advances that reduce the host's risk for injuries and have also improved environmental safety are reflective clothing, bridged pedestrian paths, child-resistant cigarette lighters, household smoke alarms, institutional sprinkler systems, electrical insulation, swimming pool alarms, household fuses, machine guards, breakaway bases, tractor rollover protection, and soft playground surfaces.

Successfully implementing engineering and technology solutions that protect large populations, however, requires that the technology

- Be effective and reliable
- Be acceptable to the public and compatible with the environment
- Result in products that dominate in the marketplace
- Be easily understood and properly used by the public

Despite advances in technology, many protective devices (for example, swimming pool fences, stair gates, and antilock brakes) have had limited success because one or more of the factors just listed were ignored (for example, swimming pool fences were not environmentally aesthetic; the public did not know how to operate antilock brakes; stair gates were not closed after use).

Combining Strategies

The importance of using a mix of strategies to prevent and control injuries cannot be overemphasized. The examples already presented underscore the necessity of combining behavioral and environmental approaches to injury prevention (Sleet & Gielen, 1998; Gielen, 1992; Towner, 1995). This is the approach used in most other areas of disease prevention and health promotion (Green & Kreuter, 1999; McGinnis, Williams-Russo, & Knickman, 2002). Successes in both tobacco control and motor vehicle safety have taught us that an informed and supportive electorate facilitates the process by which legislative and other environmental strategies are adopted (CDC, 1999; Runyan, 1998).

A good example of combining education and behavioral change, engineering and technology, and legislative and law enforcement strategies to reduce injuries is the success in reducing injuries resulting from alcohol-impaired driving (Howat et al., 2004). Legislation controlling young drivers' access to alcohol was combined with legislation to lower blood alcohol concentration (BAC) limits and to impose stiff drunk-driving penalties. When the laws were enacted, a widespread public education campaign also began, through the news media and grassroots organizations, on the reasons for and benefits of the new laws and on the risks of drinking and driving. These strategies and methods were further enhanced through engineering, by the development of more sophisticated alcohol-sensing devices, Breathalyzer and roadside testing devices, and vehicle lockout devices for convicted drunken drivers (Trinca et al., 1988; Evans, 2004).

With these three strategies health promotion strategists can develop specific interventions that are targeted to specific populations and that use components of each strategy to design a comprehensive, community-based approach to injury prevention.

Clinical Health Promotion and Injury Prevention

Health care professionals have a special role in promoting injury prevention and control. First, they have direct and continuing access to persons whose safety is threatened. Second, standards of practice for most health care professions call for the provision of preventive services, including age-appropriate counseling about safety (American Academy of Pediatrics [AAP], 1996; U.S. Preventive Services Task Force, 1989, 1996; Murdock, 1994). Health promotion approaches need to consider developmental abilities of young audiences (Stevenson & Sleet, 1996–1997; Schieber & Thompson, 1996). Third, health care professionals are credible and important sources of information for clients and can influence client and parent health behaviors (Athey, 1995; Gielen et al., 2001). The remainder of this section provides examples and principles for promoting injury control in clinical settings, with an emphasis on counseling strategies.

Needs Assessment

Interventions, whether directed toward individuals or the community, should be developed based on needs assessments. Unless interventions are responsive to the specific needs of the target population, planners risk using limited program resources inefficiently or ineffectively (Green & Kreuter, 1999).

Needs assessment activities can range from simple to complex, depending on the situation. For example, before adding a new brochure on safety to a clinic's client education supply, the material should be tested with a subgroup of the intended audience to be sure that it is readable, understandable, attractive, culturally appropriate, and useful. Data on the magnitude of the injury problem in the population to be served are needed to determine which types of injuries and which subgroups most need to be addressed. The indicators used will depend on the specific setting but may include analyses of injury-related deaths, hospitalizations, emergency department visits, police reports, household or waiting room interviews, and surveys. Qualitative data on persons' perceptions of injury problems, as well as the benefits of and barriers to safer behavior, are critically important elements of a needs assessment that are commonly overlooked.

For example, for a clinic-based needs assessment study of injuries that occurred in the home to infants and toddlers, researchers interviewed mothers in a pediatric clinic waiting room (Gielen, Wilson, Faden, Wissow, & Harvilchuck, 1995). It was found that parents already had favorable beliefs about childproofing but lacked the resources and skills needed to undertake recommended safety measures. These findings and additional information collected through focus groups shaped the subsequent interventions (Gielen et al., 2001, 2002). The needs assessment indicated that safety supplies should be easily accessible to parents and that providing resource information and teaching specific safety skills would be more effective than delivering messages to increase general knowledge and to promote positive attitudes.

Persons responsible for safety education are often under pressure to "do something" to alleviate a perceived or real injury problem, which may make a needs assessment seem unnecessary. However, a needs assessment is important for at least three reasons. First, the data collected helps identify the injury that most needs to be addressed and the interventions most likely to be effective with the population being served, which facilitates efficient use of resources. Second, a needs assessment involves the target audience in program development. This *principle of participation* works well in health promotion (Green & Kreuter, 1999), because when the target population participates in defining its priority problems and in designing solutions, the programs are more likely to be effective. Third, a needs assessment provides baseline data for program evaluation.

Interventions in Clinical Settings

Clinical interventions for injury prevention typically include counseling, providing brochures or audiovisual materials, and arranging rental or low-cost distribution of safety supplies, such as smoke detectors. Which combination of interventions will be most effective in achieving safer behavior depends on the target population and the problem being addressed (Gielen, McDonald, Forrest, Harvilchuck, & Wissow,

1997). Programs determine which interventions are most appropriate, on the basis of the following factors:

- *Knowledge of what works.* Programs should base their intervention strategies on reviews of published reports on injury prevention, on descriptions of other successful programs, and on an understanding of the theories of behavioral change.
- *Availability of resources.* Obviously, the more resources (staff, funds, space) a program has, the more complex it can be.
- *Input from the target population.* For a program to be successful, participation by at least some members of the target population is essential. They can, for example, sit on planning committees or participate in focus groups, surveys, or personal interviews.
- *Access to the target population.* Programs must decide the most suitable method(s) for reaching the target population (for example, home visits, physicians' waiting rooms, or a mass media campaign).
- *Developmental staging.* If children are the target population or are affected by the intervention strategy, programs must ensure that the proposed intervention is developmentally appropriate and suitable for the age group targeted (Mercy, Sleet, & Doll, 2003).

Counseling. Counseling is an important component of any clinically based injury prevention program (Bass et al., 1993). In fact counseling about injury prevention is a recommended component of any preventive service, according to the U.S. Preventive Services Task Force Report (1996). Specifically, the task force recommends the following:

- Counsel all patients and the parents of young patients to use vehicle occupant restraints (lap and shoulder safety belts and child safety seats), to wear helmets when riding motorcycles, and to refrain from driving while under the influence of alcohol or other drugs.
- Periodically counsel the parents of children on measures to reduce the risk of unintentional household and recreational injuries.
- Counsel adolescents and adults on preventing household and recreational injuries.
- Identify, counsel, and monitor persons with alcohol or drug problems.
- Counsel elderly patients on specific measures to prevent falls.

The American Academy of Pediatrics recommends that pediatricians counsel parents on how to prevent childhood injuries resulting from motor vehicle crashes, falls from bicycles, other types of falls, fires and burns, electrical hazards, poisoning, aspiration, and firearm use and on how to prevent children from drowning or suffocating (AAP, 1996). Pediatricians should recommend specific preventive methods (for example, use child safety seats and bicycle helmets or install a smoke alarm in the home). Well-child visits provide a good opportunity to offer such counseling. Miller and Galbraith (1995) found that injury counseling by pediatricians produced a favorable cost-benefit result.

One major concern about counseling for injury prevention is the limited time available during a medical visit. However, through role-playing, McDonald and Gielen (1995) showed that counseling on a single topic takes less than five minutes. Research is currently under way to evaluate the effect of injury prevention counseling on parents' practices. Another concern is the need for health care professionals to have adequate information about the many facets of injury prevention. Health care professionals need specific training in the injury prevention practices being recommended. Experiential training (for example, actually installing a smoke alarm and changing its batteries) is a useful technique for providing the necessary knowledge and skills. Health care professionals also should have information on local resources that their clients need to carry out the recommended prevention practice (for example, how to obtain a bicycle helmet discount coupon). Finally, incorporating a counseling program into routine clinical practice is a behavioral change on the part of the health care professional. Thus, in addition to adequate preparation, knowledge, and skills, health care professionals need incentives and reinforcement for their own behavioral change. Adequate administrative support, supplementary client education materials, and ongoing feedback on the effectiveness of their counseling efforts will improve compliance with an injury prevention counseling program.

Compliance improves when health care professionals give adequate information, talk positively, and ask questions about behavioral compliance (Hall, Roter, & Katz, 1988; Roter & Hall, 1996). Because the desired outcomes of injury prevention counseling are behavioral (for example, compliance with recommendations to install smoke detectors), these communication skills should be used in injury prevention counseling.

Other principles of behavioral change also improve compliance when they are used during counseling. The U.S. Preventive Services Task Force (1989) recommends that health care professionals follow these principles:

- Develop a therapeutic alliance. Health care professionals should see themselves as expert consultants available to help clients.
- Ensure that clients understand the relationship between behavior and health. Inquire about what clients already know or believe.
- Work with clients to assess barriers to behavioral change.

- Gain a commitment from clients to begin the process of change.
- Involve clients in selecting risk factors to change.
- Design a behavior modification plan oriented toward changing clients' behaviors, not merely changing knowledge or attitudes.
- Monitor progress through follow-up contact. Reinforce successes through positive verbal feedback.

Brief Interventions. There is recent evidence that brief interventions and motivational interviewing are promising intervention methods for injury prevention. Although the distinction between types of clinic-based interventions may at times blur, brief interventions typically include having patients complete a short assessment of a health-related behavior, receive a written or spoken educational message, or participate in a motivational interview. Brief interventions have been applied to a variety of health-related behaviors, including domestic violence and alcohol use (Watson, 1999; Forsberg, Ekman, Halldin, & Ronnberg, 2000; Hungerford, Pollock, & Todd, 2000). The advent of computer tailoring technology allows assessment and feedback to be handled at a computer kiosk, with or without the involvement of the clinician. Two studies have offered promising results for the use of this technology in child injury prevention (Nansel et al., 2002; McDonald et al., 2005).

Community Health Promotion and Injury Prevention

Health promotion approaches work to reduce injury and chronic health conditions by changing not only the behavior of individuals but also the behavior and social norms of communities (Boutilier, Cleverly, & Labonte, 2000).

Community organization and mobilization and community-based participatory research focus on the active participation and development of communities to enable them to better evaluate and solve health and social problems (Minkler & Wallerstein, 1997). Early commentaries on the importance of community interventions in injury control described the difference between *community-wide* interventions and community-based programs (Gielen & Collins, 1993), and it was suggested that the effectiveness of community-wide programs could be enhanced by treating the community as the source and not simply the site of prevention programs (McLoughlin, Vince, Lee, & Crawford, 1982). Green and Kreuter (1999) have described the necessary components of community-level interventions: "Given reasonable resources, the chances are that a community intervention will succeed if the practitioner (1) builds from a base of community ownership of the problems and the solution, (2) plans carefully, (3) uses sound theory, meaningful data and local experience as a basis for problem decisions, (4) knows what types of interventions work best for specific populations and circumstances, and (5) has an organizational and advocacy plan to orchestrate multiple intervention strategies into a complementary cohesive program" (p. 261).

Recent systematic reviews of community-wide programs have focused on motor vehicle occupants (Zaza, Sleet, Shults, Elder, & Thompson, 2005), child pedestrians (Turner, McClure, Nixon, & Spinks, 2004), all injuries to children (Spinks, Turner, McClure, & Nixon, 2004), and poisoning (Nixon, Spinks, Turner, & McClure, 2004), and many of these reviews have reported positive impacts. One unique community intervention focused on alcohol-related unintentional and intentional injury prevention (Treno & Holder, 1997). This Community Trials Project is a community-research partnership formed to change the social and structural contexts of alcohol use. Participants worked to implement prevention policies and activities that were evidence based, and they asked communities to customize and prioritize their initiatives according to local concerns and interests. Specific components of the mobilization effort were directed toward responsible beverage service, drinking and driving, underage drinking, and alcohol access. Coalitions, task forces, and media advocacy were used to raise awareness and support for effective policies among the public and decision makers. An evaluation of the impact of the mobilization efforts demonstrated significant reductions in the following indicators: 6 percent in the reported quantity of alcohol consumed, 51 percent in driving over the legal blood alcohol limit, 10 percent in nighttime injury crashes, 6 percent in alcohol-related crashes, and 43 percent in alcohol-related assault injuries seen in emergency departments (Holder et al., 2000).

Many successful community-level approaches borrow heavily from the Swedish and WHO Safe Communities model, which includes organizing cross-sector planning groups or coalitions; reliance on existing local community networks; coverage of all ages, environments, and injury types; empowerment of the socially weak; and continuous tracking of high-risk environments and groups (Svanstrom, 2000). Often the community-led process is so compelling that it sustains itself, despite limited bureaucratic, political, or financial support.

Community-Based Approach to Injury Prevention

The following case study shows how using a comprehensive health promotion approach—including documenting the problem, educating others about its importance, seeking regulatory intervention, using consumer advocacy, and modifying technology—led to important changes affecting childhood burn injuries in the community.

Case Example: Burn Prevention and Child-Resistant Cigarette Lighters

After seeing many children suffering from burns, Diane Denton, a nurse in the Louisville, Kentucky, community, began asking these children's parents how their tragic injuries occurred. She learned that a large number of cases were the result of children playing with disposable cigarette lighters. The lighters are small enough to fit in the palm of the child's hand, are brightly colored, and become *sparking toys* when moved rapidly along a carpet or mattress. Denton documented these findings and petitioned the U.S. Consumer Product Safety Commission (CPSC) to investigate the risks posed by disposable cigarette lighters. Others in the burn prevention community joined her plea for action.

Impressed with the data Denton and others in her community had gathered, the CPSC funded research to examine cases in which children had been badly burned while playing with disposable cigarette lighters. Investigators found that children playing with lighters started residential fires that caused an annual average of 150 fatalities and 1,100 injuries. As many as 190 burn-related deaths among children younger than three years of age could be prevented by a simple and inexpensive childproof device, the CPSC estimated. Ten years after Denton's initial efforts, with CPSC prompting, the major cigarette lighter manufacturers complied with a request to make childproof disposable lighters, and they marketed them to the public as safer for the protection of children. CPSC finally set a standard (effective in 1994) requiring disposable and novelty lighters to be child resistant. Since this standard took effect, there has been a 58 percent reduction in fires caused by children under age five, representing the prevention of hundreds of deaths and injuries and thousands of fires. However, in a recent year there were still 2,400 fires resulting in 70 deaths and 480 injuries because of children under age five playing with lighters. As late as 2004, CPSC was still recalling novelty lighters, such as a digital wristwatch with a cigarette lighter incorporated into it, that are sold in the United States but do not meet the child-resistant standard. Manufacturers and marketers who disable the child-resistant feature in lighters or import nonstandard lighters have been jailed and fined (FindLaw for the Public, 2005).

In this example, the actions of one nurse and a small community of injury prevention advocates changed an entire industry, saving hundreds of lives and preventing thousands of children from being seriously burned (Sleet, 1989, 1995).

Summary

Although injury has plagued societies since humans first walked the earth, it has only recently been recognized as an important public health problem. Health promotion can help prevent injuries. Using an epidemiologic approach helps planners target interventions that modify the host, agent, or environment to prevent injury. A focus on behavioral, environmental, and technological solutions can help public health professionals prevent injuries by reducing or eliminating hazardous energy exchange. Injuries are not random events: they are predictable and preventable. Clinical approaches to injury control are an important health promotion intervention that can be delivered through existing public health and medical settings. Health promotion professionals can be instrumental in implementing interventions for injury prevention at the individual, family, and population levels.

Reductions in injuries and their associated medical costs can be made by using health promotion and community health approaches. These approaches involve strategies that target host, environmental, and agent factors. The three strategies are education and behavioral change, engineering and technology, and legislation and law enforcement. Using multiple strategies is most effective. Unintentional injuries and violence are major public health problems. Health promotion offers a comprehensive approach that can have life-saving benefits for all. (See Exhibit 11.1 on page 390 for a selection of helpful resources.)

References

American Academy of Pediatrics. (1996). *The Injury Prevention Program (TIPP)*. Chicago: Author.

Athey, A. M. (1995). Pediatric injury control: Strategies for the nurse practitioner. *Nurse Practitioner Forum, 6*(3), 99, 167–172.

Bass, J., Christoffel, K. K., Windome, M., Boyle, W., Scheidt, P., Stranwick, R., et al. (1993). Childhood injury prevention counseling in primary care settings: A critical review of the literature. *Pediatrics, 92*, 544–550.

Bennet, P., & Murphy, S. (1997). *Psychology and health promotion*. Philadelphia: Open University Press.

Boutilier, M., Cleverly, S., & Labonte, R. (2000). Community as a setting for health promotion. In B. D. Poland, L. W. Green, & I. Rootman (Eds.), *Settings for health promotion: Linking theory and practice* (pp. 250–301). Thousand Oaks, CA: Sage.

Centers for Disease Control and Prevention. (1999). Motor-vehicle safety: A 20th century public health achievement. *Morbidity and Mortality Weekly Report, 48*(18), 369–373.

Centers for Disease Control and Prevention. (2002). *Ten leading causes of death by age group, 2001* [Table]. Retrieved October 14, 2005, from http://www.cdc.gov/ncipc/wisqars

Centers for Disease Control and Prevention. (2004). Medical expenditures attributable to injuries—United States, 2000. *Morbidity and Mortality Weekly Report, 53*(1), 1–4.

Centers for Disease Control and Prevention. (2005a). *Number of deaths caused by injury and rates per 100,000 United States population—All ages and races, by sex, 2002* [Table]. Retrieved March 15, 2005, from http://www.cdc.gov/ncipc/wisqars

Centers for Disease Control and Prevention. (2005b). *Number of nonfatal injuries and rates per 100,000 United States population—all ages and races, by sex, 2003* [Table]. Retrieved March 15, 2005, from http://www.cdc.gov/ncipc/wisqars

Centers for Disease Control and Prevention. (2005c). *Ten leading causes of death* [Table]. Retrieved October 5, 2005, from http://www.cdc.gov/ncipc/wisqars

De Haven, H. (1942). Mechanical analysis of survival in falls from heights of fifty to one hundred and fifty feet. *War Medicine, 2,* 586–596.

DiLillo, D., Peterson, L., & Farmer, J. (2002). Injury and poisoning. In T. J. Boll, S. B. Johnson, N. W. Perry, & R. H. Rozensky (Eds.), *Handbook of clinical health psychology: Vol. 1. Medical disorders and behavioral applications.* Washington, DC: American Psychological Association.

Dowswell, T., Towner, E.M.L., Simpson, G., & Jarvis, S. N. (1996). Preventing childhood unintentional injuries: What works? A literature review. *Injury Prevention, 2,* 140–149.

Evans, L. (2004). *Traffic safety.* Bloomfield Hills, MI: Science Serving Society.

Farrell, A. D., Meyer, A. L., & Dahlberg, L. L. (1996). Richmond youth against violence: A school-based program for urban adolescents. *American Journal of Preventive Medicine, 12*(5, Suppl.), 13–21.

FindLaw for the Public. (2005). *Yongxin International Inc. to pay $50,000 civil penalty.* Retrieved April 18, 2005, from http://cobrands.public.findlaw.com

Forsberg, L., Ekman, S., Halldin, J., & Ronnberg, S. (2000). Brief interventions for risk consumption of alcohol at an emergency surgical ward. *Addiction and Behavior, 25*(3), 471–475.

Geller, E. S., Elder, J., Hovell, M., & Sleet, D. (1991). Behavioral approaches to drinking-driving interventions. In W. Ward & F. M. Lewis (Eds.), *Advances in health education and promotion* (Vol. 3, pp. 45–68). London: Jessica Kingsley Press.

Gielen, A. C. (1992). Health education and injury control: Integrating approaches. *Health Education Quarterly, 19*(2), 203–218.

Gielen, A. C., & Collins, B. (1993). Community-based interventions for injury prevention. *Family and Community Health, 15,* 1–11.

Gielen, A. C., & Girasek, D. C. (2001). Integrating perspectives on the prevention of unintentional injuries. In N. Schneiderman, M. A. Speers, J. M. Silva, H. Tomes, & J. H. Gentry (Eds.), *Integrating behavioral and social sciences with public health* (pp. 203–230). Washington, DC: American Psychological Association.

Gielen, A. C., McDonald, E. M., Forrest, C. B., Harvilchuck, J., & Wissow, L. (1997). Injury prevention counseling in an urban pediatric clinic: Analysis of audiotaped visits. *Archives of Pediatrics and Adolescent Medicine, 151*(2), 146–151.

Gielen, A. C., McDonald, E. M., Wilson, M.E.H., Hwang, W. T., Serwint, J. R., Andrews, J. S., et al. (2002). The effects of improved access to safety counseling, products and home visits on parents' safety practices. *Archives of Pediatrics and Adolescent Medicine, 156,* 33–40.

Gielen, A. C., & Sleet, D. A. (2003). Application of behavior-change theories and methods to injury prevention. *Epidemiologic Reviews, 25,* 65–76.

Gielen, A., Sleet, D. A., & DiClemente, R. (Eds.). (2006). *Injury and violence prevention: Behavioral science theories, methods, and applications.* San Francisco: Jossey-Bass.

Gielen, A. C., Wilson, M.E.H., Faden, R. R., Wissow, L., & Harvilchuck, J. D. (1995). In-home injury prevention practices for infants and toddlers: The role of parental beliefs, barriers, and housing quality. *Health Education Quarterly, 22*(1), 85–95.

Gielen, A. C., Wilson, M.E.H., McDonald, E. M., Serwint, J. R., Andrews, J. S., Hwang, W. T., et al. (2001). A randomized trial of enhanced anticipatory guidance for injury prevention. *Archives of Pediatrics and Adolescent Medicine, 155,* 42–49.

Girasek, D. C. (1999). How members of the public interpret the word accident. *Injury Prevention, 5,* 19–25.

Gordon, J. E. (1949). The epidemiology of accidents. *American Journal of Public Health, 39,* 504–515.

Green, L. W., & Kreuter, M. K. (1999). *Health program planning: An educational and ecological approach.* Mountain View, CA: Mayfield.

Haddon, W., Jr. (1970). On the escape of tigers: An ecologic note. *Technology Review (MIT), 72,* 44–53.

Haddon, W., Jr. (1980). Advances in the epidemiology of injuries as a basis for public policy. *Public Health Reports, 95,* 411–421.

Hall, J. A., Roter, D. L., & Katz, N. R. (1988). Meta-analysis of correlates of provider behavior in medical encounters. *Medical Care, 26,* 657–675.

Holder, H. D., Gruenewal, P. J., Ponicki, W. R., Treno, A. J., Grube, J. W., Saltz, R. F., et al. (2000). Effect of community-based interventions on high-risk drinking and alcohol-related injuries. *JAMA, 284,* 2341.

Howat, P., Maycock, B., Cross, D., Collins, J., Jackson, L., Burns, S., et al. (2003). Toward a more unified definition of health promotion. *Health Promotion Journal of Australia, 14*(2), 82–84.

Howat, P., Sleet, D. A., Elder, R., & Maycock, B. (2004). Preventing alcohol-related traffic injury: A health promotion approach. *Traffic Injury Prevention, 5*(3), 208–219

Huesmann, L., Guerra, N., Miller, L., & Zelli, A. (1992). The role of social norms in the development of aggression. In H. Zumkley & A. Fraczek (Eds.), *Socialization and aggression.* New York: Springer.

Hungerford, D. W., Pollock, D. A., & Todd, K. H. (2000). Acceptability of emergency department-based screening and brief intervention for alcohol problems. *Academic Emergency Medicine, 7*(12), 1382–1392.

Jones, R. T., van Hasselt, V. P., & Sisson, L. A. (1984). Emergency fire safety skills. *Behavior Modification, 8,* 59–78.

Mason, J. O., & Tolsma, D. (1984). Personal health promotion. *Western Journal of Medicine, 141,* 772–776.

McDonald, E. M., & Gielen, A. C. (1995, July). *Experiential training to improve pediatric counseling about injury prevention.* Paper presented at the Society for Public Health Education Midyear Scientific Conference, Little Rock, AR.

McDonald, E. M., Solomon, B., Shields, W., Serwint, J. R., Jacobsen, H., Weaver, N. L., et al. (2005). Evaluation of kiosk-based tailoring to promote household safety practices in an urban pediatric primary care practice. *Patient Education and Counseling, 59*(2), 168–181.

McGinnis, J. M., Williams-Russo, P., & Knickman, J. (2002). The case for more active policy attention to health promotion. *Health Affairs, 21*(2), 78–86.

McLoughlin, E., Vince, C., Lee, A., & Crawford, J. (1982). Project Burn Prevention: Outcome and implications. *American Journal of Public Health, 72,* 241–247.

Mercy, J., Sleet, D. A., & Doll, L. S. (2003). Applying a developmental approach to injury prevention. *American Journal of Health Education, 34*(5), S6–S12.

Miller, T. R., & Galbraith, M. (1995). Injury prevention counseling by pediatricians: A benefit-cost comparison. *Pediatrics, 96,* 1–4.

Minkler, M., & Wallerstein, N. (1997). Improving health through community organization and community building. In K. Glanz, F. M. Lewis, & B. K. Rimer (Eds.), *Health behavior and health education: Theory, research, and practice* (2nd ed., pp. 241–269). San Francisco: Jossey-Bass.

Murdock, M. A. (1994). Injury prevention: A nursing responsibility. *Orthopaedic Nursing, 13*(4), 7–11.

Nansel, T., Weaver, N., Donlin, M., Jacobsen, H., Kreuter, M., & Simons-Morton, B. (2002). Baby, be safe: The effect of pediatric injury prevention tailored communication provided in a primary care setting. *Patient Education and Counseling, 46*(3), 175–190.

National Academy of Sciences, National Research Council. (1988). *Injury control: A review of the status and progress of the injury control program at the Centers for Disease Control.* Washington, DC: Author.

National Center for Injury Prevention and Control. (2001). *1996 fact book.* Atlanta, GA: Centers for Disease Control and Prevention.

National Committee for Injury Prevention and Control. (1989). *Injury prevention: Meeting the challenge.* New York: Oxford University Press. Supplement to *American Journal of Preventive Medicine, 5*(3), 1–303.

Nixon, J., Spinks, A., Turner, C., & McClure, R. (2004). Community-based programs to prevent poisoning in children 0–15 years. *Injury Prevention, 10,* 43–46.

O'Connor, P. J. (1982). Poisoning prevention: Results of a public media campaign. *Australian Paediatrics Journal, 18,* 250–252.

Pan American Health Organization. (1996). *Health promotion: An anthology* (Publication No. 557). Washington, DC: Author.

Peden, M., Scurfield, R., Sleet, D. A., Mohan, D., Hyder, A. A., Jarawan, E., et al. (2004). *World report on road traffic injury prevention.* Geneva: World Health Organization.

Pless, I. B. (1978). Accident prevention and health education: Back to the drawing board? *Pediatrics, 62,* 431–435.

Roberts, M. C., Fanurik, D., & Layfield, D. A. (1987). Behavioral approaches to preventing childhood injuries. *Journal of Social Issues, 43*(2), 105–118.

Ross, H. (1984). *Deterring the drinking driver: Legal policy and social control.* Lexington, MA: Heath.

Roter, D. L., & Hall, J. A. (1996). Patient provider communication. In K. Glanz, F. M. Lewis, & B. K. Rimer (Eds.), *Health behavior and health education: Theory, research, and practice* (2nd ed., pp. 206–226). San Francisco: Jossey-Bass.

Runyan, C. W. (1998). Using the Haddon matrix: Introducing the third dimension. *Injury Prevention, 4,* 302–307.

Ryan, W. (1976). *Blaming the victim.* New York: Vintage.

Schieber, R. A., & Thompson, N. J. (1996). Developmental risk factors for childhood pedestrian injuries. *Injury Prevention, 2*(3), 228–236.

Sheinfeld Gorin, S., & Arnold, J. (Eds.). (1998). *Health promotion handbook.* St. Louis, MO: Mosby.

Shields, J. (1997). Have we become so accustomed to being passive that we've forgotten to be active? *Injury Prevention, 3,* 243–246.

Sleet, D. A. (Ed.). (1984). Occupant protection and health promotion [Special issue]. *Health Education Quarterly, 11.*

Sleet, D. (1989, May 3). Testimony before California Legislature, Assembly Bill #408, Child-proof Cigarette Lighters, Sacramento, CA.

Sleet, D. (1995). *Injury control 594.* [Course text material, teaching learning group (distance education)]. Perth, Australia: Curtin University of Technology.

Sleet, D. A., Egger, G., & Albany, P. (1991). Injury as a public health problem [Special issue on injury prevention]. *Health Promotion Journal of Australia, 1*(2), 4–9.

Sleet, D. A., & Gielen, A. C. (1998). Injury prevention. In S. Sheinfeld Gorin & J. Arnold (Eds.), *Health promotion handbook* (pp. 247–275). St. Louis, MO: Mosby.

Sleet, D. A., & Gielen, A. C. (2004). Developing injury interventions: The role of behavioral science. In R. McClure, M. Stevenson, & S. McEvoy (Eds.), *The scientific basis of injury prevention and control* (pp. 214–232). Victoria, Australia: IP Communications.

Sleet, D. A., Hollenbach, K., & Hovell, M. (1986). Applying behavioral principles to motor vehicle occupant protection. *Education and Treatment of Children, 9*(4), 320–333.

Sleet, D. A., & Rosenberg, M. L. (1997). Injury control. In D. F. Scutchfield & C. W. Keck (Eds.), *Principles of public health practice.* New York: Delmar.

Sleet, D. A., Wagenaar, A., & Waller, P. (Eds.). (1989). Drinking, driving, and health promotion. *Health Education Quarterly, 16,* 329–333.

Spinks, A., Turner, C., McClure, R., & Nixon, J. (2004). Community-based programs targeting all injuries for children. *Injury prevention, 10,* 180–185.

Stevenson, M. R., & Sleet, D. A. (1996–1997). Which prevention strategies for child pedestrian injuries? A review of the literature. *International Quarterly of Community Health Education, 16*(3), 207–217.

Streff, F. M., & Geller, E. S. (1986). Strategies for motivating safety belt use: The application of applied behavior analysis. *Health Education Research, 1,* 47–59.

Svanstrom, L. (2000). Building safe communities: A safety promotion movement entering 2000. In L. Norheim & M. Waller (Eds.), *Best practices: A selection of papers on quality and effectiveness of health promotion* (Presented at the 4th European IUHPE Conference, Helsinki, Finland, and Tallinn, Estonia). Helsinki: Finnish Centre for Health Promotion.

Towner, E.M.L. (1995). The role of health education in childhood injury prevention. *Injury Prevention, 1,* 53–58.

Treno, A. J., & Holder, H. D. (1997). Community mobilization: Evaluation of an environmental approach to local action, *Addiction, 92* (Suppl. 2), 173–187

Trinca, G. W., Johnston, I. R., Campbell, B. J., Haight, F. A., Knight, P. R., Mackay, G. M., et al. (1988). *Reducing traffic injury: A global challenge.* Melbourne: Royal Australasian College of Surgeons.

Turner, C., McClure, R., Nixon, J., & Spinks, A. (2004). Community-based programs to prevent pedestrian injuries in children 0–14 years: A systematic review. *Injury Control and Safety Promotion, 11*(4), 231–237.

U.S. Department of Health, Education and Welfare, Public Health Service. (1979). *Healthy people: The surgeon general's report on health promotion and disease prevention* (PHS Publication No. 79-55071). Washington, DC: Author.

U.S. Preventive Services Task Force. (1989). *Guide to clinical preventive services: An assessment of the effectiveness of 169 interventions.* Baltimore: Williams & Wilkins.

U.S. Preventive Services Task Force. (1996). *Guide to clinical preventive services* (2nd ed.). Baltimore: Williams & Wilkins.

Watson, H. E. (1999). A study of minimal interventions for problem drinkers in acute care settings. *International Journal of Nursing Standards, 36*(5), 425–434.

World Health Organization. (1984). *Health promotion: A discussion document on the concepts and principles.* Copenhagen: WHO Regional Office for Europe.

World Health Organization. (1986). *Ottawa Charter for Health Promotion.* Geneva: Author.

Zaza, S., Sleet, D. A., Shults, R. A., Elder, R. W., & Thompson, T. S. (2005). Motor vehicle occupant injury. In S. Zaza, P. A. Briss, & K. W. Harris; Task Force on Community Preventive Services (Eds.), *The guide to community preventive services: What works to promote health?* (pp. 329–384). New York: Oxford University Press.

EXHIBIT 11.1. HELPFUL RESOURCES.

Online Resources

Center for Rural Emergency Medicine, http://www.hsc.wvu/crem/crem.htm

This Web site of the CDC's Injury Control Training and Demonstration Center, at the University of West Virginia in Morgantown, includes lists of injury mechanisms (similar to E-codes), information on causes of injuries for which persons have sought treatment at the University of West Virginia Emergency Department, a hypertext map of West Virginia with extensive injury data by county, and links to other injury research centers.

Consumer Product Safety Commission (CPSC), http://www.cpsc.gov

CPSC is an independent federal regulatory agency that helps keep American families safe in their homes by reducing the risk of injury or death from consumer products. Its Web site can be used to report unsafe products and find out what consumer products are unsafe or have been recalled.

Injury Control Resource Information Network (ICRIN), http://www.injurycontrol.com/icrin

The ICRIN site provides a comprehensive list of injury control resources throughout the Internet. This Web site was developed by the CDC's Center for Injury Research and Control at the University of Pittsburgh.

National Center for Injury Prevention and Control (NCIPC), http://www.cdc.gov/ncipc

Resources available from the Web site of this Centers for Disease Control and Prevention (CDC) center include general information on the activities of NCIPC and its divisions, publications, research grants, WISQARS injury data, injury maps, funding opportunities, a "what's new" section, and links to other CDC centers.

National Program for Playground Safety, http://www.uni.edu/playground

This Web site presents information on playground injury, playground safety inspection, training, and materials distribution.

National SAFE KIDS, http://www.safekids.org

National SAFE KIDS is a nationwide movement to prevent unintentional childhood injury. The Web site has information in the Spanish and English languages. Subjects include a family safety checklist and a variety of injury topics affecting children.

Partnerships Against Violence Network Online, gopher//cyfer.esusda.gov:70/11/violence

This Web site offers information about federal resources related to violence prevention; it was developed by a coalition of federal agencies to improve speedy access to ideas and resources related to violence prevention.

State and Territorial Injury Prevention Directors Association (STIPDA), http://www.stipda.org

Resources on this Web site include state injury projects in member states, news and views on state and local injury initiatives, links to relevant individuals in each state, and state injury Web sites.

EXHIBIT 11.1. HELPFUL RESOURCES, Cont'd.

U.S. Department of Transportation, National Highway Traffic Safety Administration (NHTSA), http://www.nhtsa.dot.gov

NHTSA is a regulatory agency responsible for reducing deaths, injuries, and economic losses resulting from motor vehicle crashes through setting and enforcing safety performance standards for motor vehicles.

WHO Collaborating Centre on Community Safety Promotion, http://www.ki.se/phs/wcccsp/history.htm

This center is the headquarters for the *safe community* concept of community injury prevention and safety promotion.

World Health Organization, Department of Injuries and Violence Prevention, http://www.who.int/violence_injury_prevention/en

This Web site offers current information about violence and injury prevention efforts around the world, WHO publications on this topic, and a weekly review of the scientific literature on injury prevention.

Listserv

Sign up for the CDC's Injury Center listserv to receive current announcements and grant solicitations, http://www.cdc.gov/ncipc/email_list.htm; or visit the CDC injury Web site, CDC.gov/Injury.

Injury Control Research Centers

The CDC administers an extramural grant program for injury researchers and practitioners. The CDC also supports state and community injury prevention programs and injury control research centers throughout the United States. In addition to conducting research, surveillance, intervention, and evaluation studies, these centers serve as training centers and resources to the public, the media, and allied health professionals. The following are current as of 2005:

   Colorado State University, Fort Collins, Colorado Injury Control Research Center, (303) 491-3916.

   Harborview Injury Prevention and Research Center, Seattle, (206) 521-1530.

   Harvard Injury Prevention Research Center, Boston, (617) 432-4343.

   Johns Hopkins Center for Research and Policy, Baltimore, (410) 614-4026.

   Medical College of Wisconsin, Milwaukee, Wisconsin Injury Research Center, (414) 805-6453.

   University of Alabama-Birmingham Injury Control Research Center, (205) 934-7845.

   University of California, Los Angeles, Injury Prevention Research Center, (310) 825-7066.

   University of California, San Francisco, Injury Control Center, (415) 821-8209.

   University of Iowa, Iowa City, Injury Prevention Research Center, (319) 335-4189.

   University of North Carolina, Chapel Hill, Injury Prevention Research Center, (919) 966-3916.

   University of Pittsburgh, Center for Injury Research and Control, (412) 692-2800.

   West Virginia University, Morgantown, Injury Prevention Center, (304) 293-6682.

CHAPTER TWELVE

VIOLENCE PREVENTION

Lloyd B. Potter

Throughout human history, violence has been present. It takes many forms and varies as a function of many factors. The causes of violence and the prevention of violence are complex. In the World Health Organization's *World Report on Violence and Health* (Krug, Dahlberg, Mercy, Zwi, & Lozano, 2004), *violence* is defined as, "The intentional use of physical force or power, threatened or actual, against oneself, another person, or against a group or community, which either results in or has a high likelihood of resulting in injury, death, psychological harm, maldevelopment or deprivation." Therefore *violence* refers to interpersonal violence such as youth violence, rape and sexual assault, and violence against intimates, children, and elders, and it refers to self-harm that includes suicide and injuries sustained during suicidal behavior. Although violence is a worldwide problem, in this chapter the focus is on preventing violence in the United States.

Through the past few decades we have seen significant progress in our understanding of the causes and prevention of violence. The most prevalent strategy for addressing problems of violence has been and continues to be reactive. The focus has been mostly on a treatment approach after violent behavior and violence-related injury have been presented. Our justice and mental health treatment systems bear a significant burden in managing and treating persons who have acted-out violently toward others and themselves. Our society has done proportionately little to reduce this burden by scientifically identifying and implementing strategies to prevent violent behavior and injury before it occurs. Yet this proportion has been changing. We have seen a dramatic increase in research focused on understanding the causes of violent behavior and a corresponding increase in the research efforts to identify effective strategies to prevent this behavior.

Public health has led efforts to bring emphasis and commitment to identifying policies and programs that work to prevent violence. Public health draws on its tradition of collaboration among a broad spectrum of scientific disciplines, organizations, and communities to solve the problem of violence. The health sector, including primary care providers, emergency departments, and community health and mental health agencies, plays a prominent role in understanding the causes of and preventing violence. The public health approach also highlights the potential utility of applying a variety of scientific tools (for example, the tools of epidemiology, the behavioral and social sciences, and engineering) as we work to identify effective prevention strategies.

Significant advances have been made in understanding violence as a public health issue. In the late 1970s, federal public health officials announced their mission to reduce the rate of interpersonal violence among the most affected population subgroup—young African American males. The Centers for Disease Control and Prevention (CDC) began to document U.S. subgroup differences in the risk of becoming a homicide victim, disseminating the results to a large audience and attracting increased media coverage.

In 1985, the findings of the Task Force on Black and Minority Health of the secretary of the U.S. Department of Health and Human Services (USDHHS) marked the beginning of a sustained effort to address intentional injury among youths as a public health problem (USDHHS, 1986). By the late 1980s and early 1990s, violence surveillance, research, and the development of preventive interventions began to be integrated into the mandates of local and regional health departments.

Several comprehensive scholarly reviews on the occurrence and patterns of violence, the causes and consequences of violence, and violence intervention strategies have been published in the last decade. (For a synthesis of this research see USDHHS, 2001b; Thornton, Craft, Dahlberg, Lynch, & Baer, 2000; Krug et al., 2004). Informed by a broad range of disciplines, this research has contributed to a new level of assurance that violence can be both understood and prevented. These cumulative efforts have debunked myths and misperceptions about violence, generating new knowledge to shape informed policy and intervention development.

We have also seen advances in defining suicide as a public health issue. In 1996, the World Health Organization (WHO) issued *The Prevention of Suicide: Guidelines for the Formulation and Implementation of National Strategies* (United Nations, 1996). Recognizing the growing problem of suicide worldwide, WHO urged member nations to address this issue. In the United States, an innovative public-private partnership to seek a national strategy for this nation was established that brought agencies in the USDHHS (the CDC, Health Resources and Services Administration [HRSA], Indian Health Service [IHS], National Institute of Mental Health [NIMH], Office of the Surgeon General, and Substance Abuse and Mental Health Services Administration [SAMHSA]) together with the Suicide Prevention Advocacy Network (SPAN), a public grassroots advocacy organization made up of suicide survivors (persons close to someone who completed suicide), attempters of suicide, community activists, and health and mental health clinicians. In 1999, the U.S. Surgeon General's Office issued a brief report, *The Surgeon General's Call to Action to Prevent Suicide* (USDHHS, 1999), and in 2002, the Institute of Medicine published a report on the causes of suicide and recommended prevention strategies (Goldsmith, Pellmar, & Kleinman, 2002). The 2001 release of *The National Strategy for Suicide Prevention,* developed with public and private sector partners with leadership and support from the surgeon general, established a framework with specific goals and objectives that has guided the development of many state plans (USDHHS, 2001a).

A scientific approach to understanding and preventing violence is central to moving efficiently and effectively toward relief of this public health burden. *Science* refers to systematized knowledge derived from observation, study, and experimentation carried on in order to determine the nature and principles of what is being studied. The public health approach provides a multidisciplinary, scientific approach that is explicitly directed toward identifying effective approaches to prevention (Mercy, Rosenberg, Powell, Broome, & Roper, 1993). This perspective entails four interrelated steps: definition of the problem, identification of causes, development and testing of interventions, and implementation of effective interventions in affected populations. In this chapter the topic of violence is addressed from a public health perspective focused on prevention of injuries resulting from violent behavior.

Defining the Problem

The first step in the public health approach, defining the problem, includes delineating incidents of violence and related mortality and morbidity. This step goes beyond counting cases to include obtaining, analyzing, and presenting information on characteristics of violent events resulting in injury and also describing prevalence and trends of risk factors. Information on the demographic characteristics of the persons involved, the temporal and geographic characteristics of the incident, the victim-perpetrator relationship, the circumstances of the injury, and the severity and cost of the injury are important considerations in defining the problem. Every community is unique, and it is important to collect information that will give an accurate picture of violence and related problems in specific communities.

Violence is a complex phenomenon, and we easily discern subtypes of violence-related injury. One way to begin to delineate subtypes is to distinguish between interpersonal violence and self-inflicted violence. Interpersonal violence is often further delineated by the relationship between the *perpetrator* and the *victim*. Thus youth violence, intimate partner violence (including *domestic* violence), rape and sexual assault (adult and child), child abuse, and elder abuse are common delineations of violence. The perpetrator and victim are the same person in self-inflicted violence, though descriptions of suicidal behavior often address level of intent; these levels include self-mutilation (such as cutting and burning skin), suicidal *gestures*, serious self-inflicted injury, and completed suicide. Each of these categories is frequently subdivided in terms of other characteristics of perpetrators and victims and of the intent of the behavior. Inconsistently used terminology and definitional issues pose a significant barrier to our ability to use sublevels of specificity consistently in describing the problem of violence. Yet we are able to describe deaths and nonfatal injuries (morbidity) using a number of different sources of data.

Rates of violence in the United States have declined in recent years; however, homicide and suicide continue to be leading causes of death. In 2002, violence (homicide and suicide combined) was the ninth leading cause of death in the United States. There were 18,022 homicides (including legal intervention) and 31,655 suicides in 2002 (see Table 11.2, Chapter Eleven). Overall, the deaths from homicide and suicide in 2002 resulted in more than 1.2 million years of potential life lost in the United States. This accounts for almost 10 percent of the total years of potential life lost in that year.

Youth Violence

Much of the variation in violence is driven by changes in youth violence. Youth homicide rates have been particularly dynamic, despite recent declines. Although the homicide rate among adults aged twenty-five and older has been declining gradually since the early 1980s, the homicide rate among those aged ten to twenty-four increased 96 percent between 1985 and 1993. However, since 1993, the youth homicide rate has declined 45 percent. These temporal trends in homicide are generally apparent across data gathered on victims from death certificates (that is, National Vital Statistics data) and data gathered on perpetrators from police reports (Supplemental Homicide Reports). The National Violent Death Reporting System (NVDRS) is a new surveillance effort developed to merge these and other data sources in order to create a more comprehensive source of information about violent deaths in the United States. Preliminary data from 2003 for the first six states participating in the NVDRS suggest that the decline in youth homicide rates may be ending. Between 2002 and 2003, these six states experienced a 4.4 percent increase in homicide rates. This overall increase was attributable to an 18 percent increase in homicide rates among males younger than twenty-five.

Many survivors of violent injury are severely and often permanently injured. The National Spinal Cord Injury (SCI) Database has been in existence since 1973 and captures data from an estimated 13 percent of new SCI cases in the United States. Today, gunshot wounds are second only to motor vehicle accidents as the leading cause of traumatic quadriplegia and paraplegia (Smith, Simmonds, Alam, & Grant, 2003), disabilities that once resulted primarily from wartime injuries. Like many victims of violence in general, most of those sustaining spinal cord injuries due to violence are young and belong to minority groups. Of all the violence-related spinal cord injury victims during the 1973 to 1992 period, 69.8 percent were nonwhite (Garland, 1993). A current study of patients with spinal cord injury caused by gunshot wounds between 1993 and 1999 notes the continued predominance of young, minority patients (Smith et al., 2003).

Data from a nationally representative sample of U.S. emergency departments, collected by the National Electronic Injury Surveillance System (NEISS), provide an estimate of the number of nonfatal injuries due to self-directed violence or assaults that are treated in U.S. emergency departments. In 2002, there were an estimated 1,718,894 assault-related injuries (CDC, 2005). This means that for every homicide victim in 2002, there were approximately 97 persons treated in emergency departments for assault-related injury.

The Uniform Crime Reports produced by the Federal Bureau of Investigation (FBI) aggregate information on the characteristics of individuals arrested for violent crimes. These data indicate that persons under the age of twenty-five represent a significant proportion of those arrested for violent crimes. Although only 21.5 percent of the U.S. population is between the ages of ten and twenty-four, 48.9 percent of those arrested for murder and nonnegligent manslaughter, 39.9 percent of those arrested for aggravated assaults, 45.9 percent of those arrested for forcible rape, and 59.1 percent of those arrested for weapons carrying and possession offenses were younger than twenty-five (U.S. Department of Justice, 2003).

To fully understand the prevalence of youth violence it is necessary to look beyond deaths and hospitalizations and examine behavior. Self-report data allow us to better understand populations that engage in a variety of behaviors that put them or others at risk for violence-related injury. For example, data for the CDC's Youth Risk Behavior Surveillance System (YRBSS) are collected every other year from a large nationally representative sample of high school students through the Youth Risk Behavior Survey (YRBS). In the category of fighting behavior and fight-related injury, 40.5 percent of males and 25.1 percent of females reported being in at least one physical fight, and 5.7 percent of males and 2.6 percent of females reported needing medical care from a doctor or nurse for their fight-related injuries (Grunbaum et al., 2004). Longitudinal data from the YRBSS from 1991 to 2003 suggest significant decreases occurred in the percentage of students who had been in a physical fight (from 42.5 percent to 33.0 percent).

Public health efforts to assess the magnitude of weapon carrying and fighting among youths are fairly recent and the results are important as indicators of the potential for injury. The CDC's 2003 Youth Risk Behavior Survey asked high-school students, "During the past 30 days, how many times have you carried a weapon, such as a gun, knife, or club, for self-protection or because you thought you might need it in a fight?" Approximately 26.9 percent of males, 6.7 percent of females, and 17.1 percent of all surveyed students reported carrying a weapon (knife, razor, club, or firearm) at least once during the thirty days preceding the survey (Grunbaum et al., 2004). Approximately 6.1 percent of high school students reported carrying a firearm in the past thirty days. Although this may appear to be a small percentage, combined with other weapon-carrying behavior it suggests the potential for injury is of great concern. The percentage of students who carried a weapon decreased significantly from 1991 to 1997 (26.1 percent to 18.3 percent) and then remained constant from 1997 to 2003 (18.3 percent to 17.1 percent).

Intimate Partner Violence

It has been estimated that there are nearly 5.3 million incidents of intimate partner violence (IPV) each year that affect U.S. women aged eighteen and older and 3.2 million incidents that affect men. Most assaults are relatively minor and consist of pushing, grabbing, shoving, slapping, and hitting (Tjaden & Thoennes, 2000). However, IPV results in nearly 2 million injuries and 1,300 deaths nationwide every year (CDC, 2003a), and it accounted for 20 percent of nonfatal violence against women in 2001 and 3 percent of nonfatal violence against men (Rennison, 2003). From 1976 to 2002, about 11 percent of homicide victims were killed by an intimate partner. In 2002, 76 percent of IPV homicide victims were female; 24 percent were male (Fox & Zawitz, 2004). The number of intimate partner homicides has decreased 14 percent overall for men and women in the span of about twenty years, with a 67 percent decrease for men (from 1,357 to 388) and a 25 percent decrease for women (from 1,600 to 1,202) (Fox & Zawitz, 2004).

Child Maltreatment

Another form of interpersonal violence is violence against children. Data on the confirmed number of U.S. child maltreatment cases are available from child protective service agencies, but these data are generally considered underestimates (USDHHS, Administration on Children, Youth, and Families, 2003). Approximately 906,000 children were confirmed to have been maltreated in 2002. Among these children confirmed by child protective service agencies as being maltreated, 61 percent experienced neglect, 19 percent were physically abused, 10 percent were sexually abused, and 5 percent were emotionally or psychologically abused. An estimated 1,500 children were confirmed to have died from maltreatment; 36 percent of these deaths were from neglect, 28 percent from physical abuse, and 29 percent from multiple types of maltreatment.

Elder Maltreatment

The incidence and consequences of violent victimization are often assumed to be problems of young populations and not an area of concern among older populations. Limited data are available to monitor the incidence and consequences of violence-related injuries among older adults. To characterize serious injuries from physical assaults among older adults, CDC analyzed data from the NEISS-All Injury Program. Estimates from this study found that approximately 33,000 persons aged sixty or more were treated in U.S. hospital emergency departments for nonfatal assault–related injuries in 2001, with injuries occurring disproportionately among persons aged sixty to sixty-nine years (CDC, 2003b). Although this estimate indicates that violent injury among older adults is a significant issue, we know little about the contexts that led to these injuries.

Sexual Violence

Sexual violence is a serious problem that affects millions of people every year. Statistics about sexual violence vary due to differences in how sexual violence is defined and how data are collected. Sexual violence data usually come from police reports, clinical settings, nongovernmental organizations, and survey research. Available data greatly underestimate the true magnitude of the problem. Rape is one of the most underreported crimes. In 2002, only 39 percent of rapes and sexual assaults were reported to law enforcement officials (U.S. Department of Justice, 2003). An estimated 79,855 of the assaults treated in emergency departments (4.6 percent) were considered sexual assaults. Males represented 12.9 percent of the sexual assaults treated in emergency departments, but 60 percent of the victims of other assaults.

About 2 out of every 1,000 children in the United States were confirmed by child protective services agencies as having experienced sexual assault in 2003 (USDHHS, Administration on Children, Youth, and Families, 2003). Among high school youths nationwide, about 9 percent have reported that they had been forced to have sexual intercourse (Grunbaum et al., 2004). Female students are more likely than male students to report sexual assault (11.9 percent versus 6.1 percent). Overall, 12.3 percent of black students, 10.4 percent of Hispanic students, and 7.3 percent of white students reported that they had been forced to have sexual intercourse. Among college students nationwide, between 20 and 25 percent of women have reported experiencing completed or attempted rape (Fisher, Cullen, & Turner, 2000). Among adults nationwide, more than 300,000 women (0.3 percent) and over 90,000 men (0.1 percent) have reported being raped in the previous twelve months. One in six women (17 percent) and one in thirty-three men (3 percent) have reported experiencing an attempted or completed rape at some time in their lives. Among adults who report being raped, women experienced 2.9 rapes and men experienced 1.2 rapes in the previous year (Tjaden & Thoennes, 2000).

Suicide

From 1990 to 2002, the suicide rate in the United States has declined 12 percent, from 12.5 to 10.9 per 100,000. Suicide rates are generally higher than the national average in the Western states and lower in the Eastern and Midwestern states (CDC, 1997). In 2002, 132,353 individuals were hospitalized following suicide attempts; 116,639 were treated in emergency departments and released (CDC, 2005). In 2001, 55 percent of suicides were completed with a firearm (Anderson & Smith, 2003). Suicide rates are highest among whites and second highest among American Indian and Alaska Native men (CDC, 2005). Of the 24,672 suicide deaths reported among men in 2001, 60 percent involved the use of a firearm (Anderson & Smith, 2003). The injuries treated in emergency departments and considered self-directed have been fewer in number than those treated and considered to result from assault. An estimated 425,650 injuries were attributed to self-directed violence in 2002. Females (245,796) were more likely to be treated for injuries due to self-directed violence than males (179,735). Given that males are far more likely to die from suicide than females, the ratio of nonfatal injuries to suicides is far lower in males (13.6 to 1) than in females (117.2 to 1). YRBS data for 2003 indicate that approximately one in ten female high school students (11.5 percent) attempted suicide at least once in the past twelve months. About half as many males (5.4 percent) reported attempting suicide as females. Suicidal ideation was far more common, with 21.3 percent of females and 12.8 percent of males reporting having seriously considered suicide in the past twelve months. The percentage of students who made a plan to attempt suicide decreased significantly from 1991 to 2003 (from 18.6 percent to 16.5 percent) (Grunbaum et al., 2004).

Witnessing Violence

An important aspect of violence that has far-reaching consequences is witnessing violence. However, it is difficult both to measure the magnitude of its occurrence and to calculate its impact on witnesses. Numerous studies attempting to assess the prevalence of exposure to violence have been conducted, finding generally that inner-city youths both witness and are victims of violence at relatively higher rates than other groups (Richters & Martinez, 1993; Fitzpatrick & Boldizar, 1993; Bell & Jenkins, 1993; Gladstein, Rusonis, & Heald, 1992; Schubiner, Scott, & Tzelepis, 1993; Cooley, Turner, & Beidel, 1995). Also, the effects of witnessing or being victims of community violence have been examined by several researchers, with findings suggesting psychological and psychiatric effects that may severely hinder the life chances of these youths (Pynoos & Nader, 1989; Terr, 1990; Frederick, 1985; Fitzpatrick & Boldizar, 1993; Hinton-Nelson, Roberts, & Snyder, 1996; Berman, Kurtines, Silverman, & Serafini, 1996).

Identifying Causes

The second step in the public health approach involves identifying causes. This step may also be used to define populations at high risk and to suggest specific interventions. Some risk factors, such as alcohol and drug use and misuse, media violence, and social and economic influences, have been explored. However, many questions remain regarding the role that these and numerous other possible causes play in producing violent behavior and, more important, the ways in which these and other risk factors may be modified to prevent violent behavior.

The lack of definitive answers about the causes of violent behavior is probably due to both the infancy of scientific inquiry into the problem and the complexity of violence. As described earlier, many forms of violence appear to have multiple etiologies. This implies there is no simple answer to defining the cause or causes of violent behavior.

A fundamental question about violence is whether specific subtypes of violent behavior require multiple theories to explain a variety of etiologies. The alternative is that violence is a homogenous construct requiring one comprehensive theory to explain its etiology. Some of the difficulties in developing a precise taxonomy for violence and its causes result from our undeveloped understanding and agreement around this issue. Many use the term *violence* to refer to a fairly broad range of behaviors (or potential behaviors, or thoughts, or images) without providing much specification of these violent behaviors and how they differ from each other. This issue of taxonomy and specificity of language is a barrier to developing a better understanding of violence. It seems logical that there are subtypes of violence, with differing etiologies and that a first step is to begin to describe these various forms (Reiss & Roth, 1993). However, as data sources tend to collect inadequate information on the circumstances surrounding each violent event, it is difficult to describe the violence problem in terms of subtypes of violence. Inadequate data collection occurs partly because subtypes of violence are poorly articulated and partly because collection of information about circumstances is difficult.

It is impossible to understand the causes of violence without considering the interplay between the behavior of individuals, the immediate environments in which they act and are socialized, and the social and economic institutions that define norms for behavior and influence processes that define environments, that is, their ecology. The ecological perspective has been developed theoretically and employed empirically in a number of forms in a variety of scientific disciplines (see, for example, Hawley, 1950, 1986; Bronfenbrenner, 1977). Ecological analysis allows for assessment of relations within systems. In the case of humans and violent behavior, the focus is on the relationship between the individual and his or her immediate settings, as well as his or her larger social contexts, both formal and informal. The concept of the ecological environment is topological and involves a nested arrangement of systems, each contained within the next.

An ecological systems model of human development provides a useful framework for understanding the etiology of different forms of violence as well as identifying potential opportunities for intervention (Bronfenbrenner, 1977, 1988; Belsky, 1980; Cicchetti & Lynch, 1993). According to this model, intrapersonal, social, cultural, economic, and physical environments influence the development of violent behavior. In Bronfenbrenner's model (1977), the *microsystem* contains an individual's interpersonal relationships and includes relations with family and peers. Next is the *mesosystem*, which contains the interactions between the social systems found in the microsystem—for example, the relationships between the family and the individual's peer group. The *exosystem* is the larger social system within which the micro- and mesosystems exist. Finally, the *macrosystem* is the overarching institutional patterns of the culture or subculture, such as the economic, social, educational, legal, or political systems, of which the micro-, meso-, and exosystems are the concrete manifestations. Macrosystems are conceived and examined not only in structural terms but as carriers of information and ideology that both explicitly and implicitly endow meaning and motivation upon particular agencies, social networks, roles, and activities and their interrelations.

There are several implications of this ecological model for understanding violence. First it allows for the direct influence of environmental factors—familial, societal, and physical—on behavior. The model also explicitly acknowledges the multilevel determinants of behavior. Fitting the model to violence, it is not just family or neighborhood environments but all of these factors that contribute to the development of violence. Moreover, these factors interact with each other to influence whether or not individuals engage in violent behavior.

There are several studies that have attempted to employ an ecological framework to assess influences on behavior within and across levels of analysis. Brooks-Gunn, Duncan, Klebanov, and Sealand (1993) examined the effects of neighborhood characteristics on individual child outcomes. Also using an ecological framework, Richters and Martinez (1993) explored the effects of violent communities and family characteristics on the adaptational failure (in school performance and behavioral, using the the Child Behavior Checklist; Achenbach & Ruffle, 2000) of individual children. Another study combining data at multiple levels of analysis found that a measure of collective efficacy of communities was negatively associated with violence (Sampson, Raudenbush, & Earls, 1997).

Most etiologic research into violent behavior occurs at one level of analysis. Studies that are limited to one level of analysis are easier to conduct, though at higher levels of aggregation suffer from potential interpretation problems when attempting cross-level interpretation (Glick & Roberts, 1984; Richards, Gottfredson, & Gottfredson, 1990; Iversen, 1991).

The development and expression of violent behavior among individuals is likely to be partially determined by biological and other predisposing conditions. Though all human behavior has an important environmental component, it is also influenced in some way by genes (Carey & Goldman, 1997). The question emerging in genetic research in relation to antisocial behavior is not, "Is there genetic influence?" but, "What are the mechanisms for a genetic effect?" Numerous studies of the role of genetics and heritability in violent and aggressive behavior have been conducted in animal populations (Carey, 1994). In humans, there is some evidence that some personality traits and cognitive styles have some genetic component that may be associated with tendencies toward aggressive and violent behavior (Carey, 1994). There is also evidence that neurobiology, hormones, neurochemistry, and diet are related to antisocial behavior (Mirsky & Siegel, 1994; Kanarek, 1994; Miczek et al., 1994; Brain, 1994; Brain & Susman, 1997; Berman, Kavoussi, & Coccaro, 1997). Additionally, prenatal and perinatal factors may have some influence on potential for violence later in life (Lewis, Pincus, Bard, & Richardson, 1979; Mungas, 1983; Mednick & Kandel, 1988).

There is significant evidence that mental disorders are associated with violent behavior (Beck, 1994; Monahan, 1997; Mulvey, 1994; Hodgins, 1995). Antisocial personality disorder in particular has been associated with violent behavior (Robins & Regier, 1991). Alcohol use and abuse in relation to violence perpetration and victimization is a complicated issue, though there are clearly associations (White, 1997).

A number of studies have implicated hereditary factors and biological factors influencing the propensity for suicidal behavior (Arana & Hyman, 1989; Mann, 1987; Rainer, 1984). Substantial evidence has suggested that deficiencies in the serotonergic system are associated with suicidal behavior (Baldwin, Bullock, Montgomery, & Montgomery, 1991; Lowther et al., 1997; Mann, Arango, & Underwood, 1990; Ohmori, Arora, & Meltzer, 1992; Van Praag, 1991). A feeling of hopelessness is one characteristic that has been generally associated with suicidal behavior (Beck, Steer, Beck, & Newman, 1993; Hill, Gallagher, Thompson, & Ishida, 1988; Rotheram-Borus & Trautman, 1988; Shaffer et al., 1996; Weishaar & Beck, 1992). Additionally, a number of psychiatric disorders have been associated with suicidal behavior, such as depression (Brent, Kolko, Allan, & Brown, 1990; Brent, Perper, Moritz, Baugher, et al., 1993; Roy, 1986; Wolk & Weissman, 1996), bipolar affective disorder (Tondo, Jamison, & Baldessarini, 1997; Tondo et al., 1998), conduct disorder (Shaffer et al., 1996), and alcoholism and substance abuse (Marzuk et al., 1992; Roy, Dejong, Lamparski, Adinoff, et al., 1991; Roy, Dejong, Lamparski, George, & Linnoila, 1991; Shaffer et al., 1996; Stack & Wasserman, 1995), among others.

Although biological factors may play some role in the development and expression of violent behavior, at present it is also unclear how much influence environmental factors may have on biological factors. Thus, as biological factors associated with violent behavior are elucidated, we must also develop an understanding of how we can modify those factors or risks of developing violent behavior through environmental modifications.

Most research into the causes of violent behavior among individuals has focused on risk factors; however, some effort has also been made to address the issue from a resiliency perspective. Characteristics and experiences related to education, vocation, marriage, children, and social support were found to be associated with resilience (Werner, 1989). It was found that resilient children were those who exhibited good coping strategies with adult responsibilities (Werner & Smith, 1992). However, the concept of resilience as represented in research and the utility of this concept for violence prevention have been questioned (Tolan, 1996).

Characteristics of the family environment profoundly influence the development of individuals. The primary socializing agent for most children is the family. Many violent offenders appear to have experienced poor parental child rearing methods, poor supervision, or separations from their parents when they were children (Farrington, 1997), or they have experienced physical or sexual abuse and neglect (Widom, 1989; Tebbutt, Swanston, Oates, & O'Toole, 1997). It is also becoming more apparent that youths that witness violence in their homes are affected significantly by the experience (David, Steele, Forehand, & Armistead, 1996). Additionally, children's adaptational failure has been found to be related to unstable or unsafe homes (Richters & Martinez, 1993).

A number of family environment characteristics have been associated with suicide and suicidal behavior, including family conflict or discord (Brent et al., 1994; Campbell, Milling, Laughlin, & Bush, 1993), parental attachment (Dejong, 1992), poor family functioning (Adams, Overholser, & Lehnert, 1994), childhood separation from parents (Bagley & Ramsay, 1985), child abuse and neglect (Deykin, Alpert, & McNamara, 1985; Straus & Kantor, 1994), being a victim of intimate partner abuse or conflict (Deykin et al., 1985), and loss of a peer (Brent, Perper, Moritz, Friend, et al., 1993; Brent, Moritz, Bridge, Perper, & Canobbio, 1996).

Another factor that may operate at the level of family and peers, although it is clearly linked to community characteristics, is access to means. A number of studies have indicated, with varying degrees of rigor, that access to firearms increases the risk of suicide and homicide (Beautrais, Joyce, & Mulder, 1996; Boor & Bair, 1990; Brent, Perper, Moritz, Baugher, et al., 1993; Cummings, Koepsell, Grossman, Savarino, & Thompson, 1997; Medoff & Magaddino, 1983; Sloan, Rivara, Reay, Ferris, & Kellerman, 1990).

It is unclear what role peer influence plays in the development of violent behavior. Research has suggested that aggressive youths are frequently rejected by peers (Coie, Dodge, Terry, & Wright, 1991; Huesmann & Eron, 1986; Evans, Oates, & Schwab, 1992; Levy, 1992).

School environments appear to be relatively safe places, where homicide perpetration and victimization are rare (Kachur et al. 1996; Anderson et al., 2001), despite some recent dramatic exceptions. However, many students report being in fights and having been hit while in school (Grunbaum et al., 2004). There is also evidence that weapon carrying in schools is fairly common and even more common among high school youths outside of schools (Grunbaum et al., 2004). Thus, even though serious injury and homicide on school property appears to be rare, the realities of violence in the form of fighting and potential violent victimization appear to be significant for many youths. It is unclear how witnessing the fighting behavior of peers, knowing that peers are carrying weapons, or being a victim of violence in the school setting influences the violence potential of youths or how this may influence or be influenced by violence in the community. Violence prevention programs in elementary and middle schools appear to be associated with reduced risk for violent behavior, however (Cotten et al., 1994).

At a higher level of aggregation the mesosystem is focused on understanding how the microsystems of an individual's existence interact with each other. There appears to be little research into these interrelationships as they affect violence in communities. One possible exception is a study of the relationship between community efficacy and violence in Chicago (Sampson, Raudenbush, & Earls, 1997).

The social and economic conditions in which individuals, microenvironments, and mesoenvironments exist appear to have significant influence on the development of violent behavior. A number of neighborhood- or community-based studies have found community characteristics that appear to be associated with violence. Poverty is probably the most commonly studied variable in ecological analyses of violence. In fact, across studies, a number of indicators of poverty and income inequality have been found to be significant predictors of interpersonal violence (Shaw & McKay, 1942; Smith & Jarjoura, 1988; Messner & Tardiff, 1986; Harries, 1995; Taylor & Covington, 1988). Community stability, frequently measured through mobility, is another community characteristic that has been found to be associated with measures of violence (Smith & Jarjoura, 1988; Sampson, 1985; Taylor & Covington, 1988; Harries, 1995). Additionally, family structure and stability, housing and population density, and social organization factors have been found to be associated with community violence (Roneck, 1981; Sampson, 1985; Smith & Jarjoura, 1988; Sampson & Groves, 1989).

There has been significant discussion around the culture of violence in the United States and the role that this plays in promoting the acting out of violent behavior in our everyday lives. One important aspect of a culture of violence is the role played by the media. Significant evidence suggests that exposure to dramatic violence on television is associated with aggressive behavior (Huesmann & Miller, 1994). There is also evidence that this relationship is mediated by factors such as cultural norms (Landau, 1984), group norms (Huesmann & Bacharach, 1988), and family characteristics (Tangney & Feshbach, 1988). Some evidence suggests that even though the media may play a significant role in violence, direct models of interpersonal violence (witnessing real-life acts of violence) are much more influential than indirect models (dramatic presentations of violence in the media) (Friedlander, 1993).

A number of key concepts at several levels of aggregation (individual, family and peer, community, and macrosystem) appear to be central for understanding the causes of violence. Unfortunately, no research findings have yet simultaneously linked all these levels together to provide an understanding of the causes of violence that would allow us to develop and implement highly effective multisystemic interventions for the prevention of violent behavior. This fact highlights once again the issue of taxonomy. Reviewing the literature on suicide and interpersonal violence reveals that studies frequently use different definitions for like predictors and concepts. When it comes to prevention, we must be clear on exactly what is to be prevented. If the goal is to broadly prevent aggressive behavior (assuming we can agree on what we mean), our prospects are much more daunting than if our goal is to prevent something like firearm-related homicides in convenience stores in a specific city. Constructs that we use as proxies for or as predictive of violence are broad, as are those variables that actually measure violence. Thus we are left with a rapidly developing field of research that is struggling for both a more refined taxonomy and a more developed framework for understanding the causes of violence.

Developing and Testing Interventions

The third step in the public health model is to develop interventions based, in large part, on information obtained in the course of the previous steps and then to test these interventions. This step includes evaluating the efficacy of programs, policies, and interventions. Methods for testing include prospective randomized controlled trials, comparisons of prevention and other populations for occurrence of health outcomes, time series analyses of trends in multiple areas, and observational studies, such as case-control studies.

Preventive interventions are usually efforts to break a causal chain between the potential for a negative outcome and the achievement of that outcome. Thus development of preventive interventions is dependent on the second step in the public health model, in this case, gaining an understanding of causes of violent behavior. In practice, however, interventions are often implemented and occasionally evaluated with little or no specification of the causal chain or how the intervention will affect this chain.

Prevention must be based on the soundest, best evidence available. We have started to make significant advances to identify prevention strategies that have been followed by research to determine if these strategies work. Whenever we believe we have an effective strategy, we should explore the impact and cost of that strategy in community settings, and then work to improve it and its delivery.

Policymakers and program funders use information about effectiveness to set policy and funding priorities for violence prevention. They want to implement prevention strategies that work, and they generally consider the following issues when making decisions: potential to reduce or avoid violent injury or death: social, legal, and ethical impacts; economic impacts; and best methods of implemention. Each of these considerations is crucial to a successful violence prevention effort. It is best to consider these elements before starting a program. However, it is never too late to consider these elements within existing programs. Many violence prevention programs lack evidence about their effectiveness and could use the valuable information gleaned by evaluation to make immediate improvements in the program.

In violence prevention, *targeting* refers to focusing on modifying something that is causally related to violence-related injury in a specific population. The goal is to break the causal chain and prevent injury. There are two complementary ways to think about prevention targeting. One is to focus on the *level* of the prevention target. The other is to focus on the *injury stage*.

The Institute of Medicine report on reducing risks for mental disorders (Mrazek & Haggerty, 1994) suggests a framework for describing intervention approaches in terms of the intervention target; interventions may be indicated, selective, or universal (Gordon, 1983). Indicated interventions target identification and treatment and skill building among individuals and families. Selective interventions target high-risk groups, with a focus on screening and group prevention activities. Universal interventions target communities or larger aggregations and may involve media or educational campaigns and other broad, population-based prevention strategies.

This model of levels is congruent with an ecological model of human development (described previously). As we find characteristics of individuals that put these individuals at high risk of violent behavior, we can attempt to develop and evaluate indicated interventions to reduce this risk. Similarly, as we identify characteristics of groups that are indicative of member's potential to perpetrate or be a victim of violence and as we understand the causal pathways that may lead this group to experience violence, we can develop, test, and deliver selective interventions that may lead to reductions of community violence. Finally, as we understand more of societal influences on the development and expression of forms of violence, we will be able to implement universal interventions (laws, education, media images, and so forth).

Indicated interventions are highly targeted and frequently involve identification, treatment, and skill building among individuals and families. At this level the focus is on early detection, and frequently, intensive individual treatment relying on one-on-one, provider-to-patient interaction. Early-treatment programs are examples of indicated strategies. Indicated interventions tend to occur within the traditional health and mental health care delivery system and tend to be resource intensive per person served. Screening strategies can be employed to identify persons at high risk for which an indicated effort would be suggested.

Selective interventions are targeted at high-risk groups with a focus on screening and group prevention activities. Peer support programs for students with a number of risk indicators would be an example. Selective interventions are less resource intensive than indicated programs.

Universal interventions are targeted at communities or larger aggregations and may include media or educational campaigns and other broad population-based prevention strategies. Universal interventions may also be environmental prevention strategies that focus on physical changes that reduce risk. Reducing access to lethal means, especially firearms, is an example of an environmental strategy.

We can also conceptualize violence prevention in terms of stages of prevention. These stages correspond to before violent behavior occurs (primary prevention), as behavior occurs (secondary prevention), and after behavior occurs (tertiary prevention). Intervention strategies will vary depending on the stage being targeted.

Primary prevention refers to an effort that targets the *causes* of violent behavior and injury *before injury or violent behavior occurs.* Conduct disorder, depression, impulsive behavior, alcohol and drug abuse might be targets of primary prevention, usually through health and mental health services. Implementing programs that prevent alienation or isolation of youth, such as bullying prevention programs and programs that improve access to health and mental health care for individuals, is another example of a primary prevention strategy. Finally, efforts to reduce access to lethal means or to address media coverage of violence are also primary prevention strategies.

Secondary prevention attempts to target intervention *as behavior is occurring,* with the goal of minimizing any self-injury that may occur. Early detection of suicidal ideation or aggressive behavior and an appropriate referral and treatment for suicide risk is an example.

Tertiary prevention targets intervention *following a violent injury or behavior* to minimize the impacts and to reduce the likelihood of subsequent injury. For example, effective intervention in a suicidal crisis or criminal justice approaches to managing violent offenders with the intent to prevent future injuries or to reduce the severity of an injury.

By combining the level of intervention and the stage of intervention we can describe and compare different strategies. The efficacy, the effectiveness, and the cost of each prevention strategy are important pieces of information in this process. For example, comparing the effects of screening and treatment for depression or conduct disorder (indicated, primary) with training gatekeepers or delivering a social-cognitive curriculum in schools (selective, secondary), or comparing a particular clinical treatment for depression (indicated, primary) with a strategy to reduce access to firearms among youths (universal, primary), can provide sound data to help us choose or combine various strategies. The key is to consider the effectiveness of various strategies for reducing violence within the context of level and stage of prevention. With this information we can make decisions about the best use of scarce resources.

Assessing prevention effectiveness is a scientific approach for making sure that what we are doing or want to do will work. Basic steps in assessing prevention effectiveness include identifying which strategies will be most likely to reduce injury and death from violent behavior; determining the potential effects of those strategies, including social, legal, ethical, and economic factors; determining optimal methods for implementing those strategies; and assessing the effectiveness of each strategy periodically as it develops and is implemented.

With an understanding of the etiology of violent behavior it is possible to identify a target toward which an intervention or prevention strategy can be directed with the intent of breaking the causal chain. Use of a logic model that clearly specifies expected outcomes, inputs, and activities associated with a programmatic effort to prevent violence enables a program developer to understand and communicate the rationale behind the prevention approach. Clearly defining the logic of a program will also enable development of a strategy to evaluate the implementation and outcomes of that program.

Implementing Interventions

Compared to other public health areas, preventing violent behavior is an area in which relatively few programs or interventions have demonstrated efficacy and effectiveness. Most of the information we have has been focused on preventing interpersonal violence among youths. Efforts are now emerging for identifying effective programs for preventing suicide and other forms of violence.

A number of reviews and synthesis efforts have been aimed at advising both practitioners and policymakers about effective strategies for preventing violence. These include the Cochrane Collaboration, the U.S. Department of Education's new What Works Clearinghouse, the University of Colorado's Blueprints for Violence Prevention, the CDC's publications *Best Practices in Youth Violence Prevention* and *Youth Suicide Prevention Programs;* and SAMHSA's National Registry of Evidence-based Programs and Practices, among others.

The Cochrane Collaboration is discussed in Chapter Three. The What Works Clearinghouse was established in 2002 by the U.S. Department of Education's

Institute of Education Sciences to provide educators, policymakers, researchers, and the public with a central and trusted source of scientific evidence on what works in education. Currently, the What Works Clearinghouse is developing a topic area titled Interventions to Reduce Delinquent, Disorderly, and Violent Behavior in Middle and High Schools, and is anticipating publishing initial findings in 2006.

In 1996, the Center for the Study and Prevention of Violence (CSPV), based at the University of Colorado at Boulder, designed and launched a national violence prevention initiative to identify violence prevention programs that are effective. The project, Blueprints for Violence Prevention, has identified eleven prevention and intervention programs that meet a strict scientific standard of program effectiveness. Program identification is based on an initial review by the CSPV and a final review and recommendation from a distinguished advisory board made up of seven experts in the field of violence prevention. The eleven model programs, called *blueprints,* have been effective in reducing adolescent violent crime, aggression, delinquency, and substance abuse. Another eighteen programs have been identified as promising programs.

The CDC has produced a document titled *Best Practices of Youth Violence Prevention: A Sourcebook for Community Action* (Thornton et al., 2000). *Best Practices* examines the effectiveness of specific violence prevention practices in four key areas: parents and families, home visiting, social and conflict resolution skills, and mentoring. These programs are drawn from real-world experiences of professionals and advocates who have successfully worked to prevent violence among children and adolescents. As a CDC publication the sourcebook also documents the science behind each best practice and offers a directory of resources for more information about programs that have used these practices.

In addition, the CDC has reviewed and summarized a range of strategies intended to prevent suicidal behavior (CDC, 1992). A review of the suicide prevention efforts listed in the guide suggests that most suicide prevention programs embrace the high-risk model of prevention, where the goal is case finding and referral (Rose, 1985). Screening and referral, crisis centers, and community organization are common examples of this high-risk approach. Suicide awareness or education activities, media guidelines, and means restriction are examples of population-based interventions. Currently, neither one of these two prevention approaches can be said to be more effective than the other in addressing the problem of suicide. However, it is reasonable to expect that a combination of these approaches may be more effective than either approach by itself in affecting suicide rates and suicide-related morbidity. We could implement efforts to reduce suicide risk with a focus on a population or a population segment and combine those efforts with intensive efforts to identify and provide services for those at greatest risk. Some of the strategies reviewed are gatekeeper training, prevention education, screening, peer support programs, crisis intervention, restricting access to means, providing aftercare for those who experience significant loss, and educating families.

The Substance Abuse and Mental Health Services Administration is developing a National Registry of Evidence-based Programs and Practices (NREPP). This is a registry of programs that have been tested in communities, schools, social service organizations, and workplaces across America and have provided solid proof that they have prevented or reduced substance abuse and related high-risk behaviors. The NREPP rating criteria and process are currently being revised, and although the NREPP system is presently focused on alcohol and substance abuse prevention and treatment programs, the system will eventually include programs for mental health prevention and treatment and suicide prevention.

A number of model and promising programs for preventing violence have been identified, and more evidence is emerging for other programs. One of the major challenges we face is to ensure that the outcomes are appropriate to the populations on which they are focused.

At the implementation stage in the public health model the focus is on taking programs that have met criteria for effectiveness to scale in order to deliver the program to populations at risk. Data collection to evaluate a program's implementation and effectiveness is essential, particularly because an intervention that has been found effective in a clinical trial may perform differently in diverse settings. Another important component of this fourth stage is determining the cost effectiveness of such programs. Balancing the costs of a program against the cases prevented by the intervention can be very helpful to policymakers in determining optimal public health practice.

During the implementation phase it is important to develop guidelines and procedures for putting effective programs in place. Implementation guidelines are especially important for ensuring that programs will work on a large scale. Guidelines and technical assistance are also needed for adapting interventions for particular community values, cultures, and standards while allowing for and benefiting from racial and culturally diverse participation.

Implementation refers to how well a plan has been followed when put into practice. Implementation has been alternatively referred to as treatment adherence, fidelity, or integrity, or sometimes as a form of process evaluation that involves gathering data to assess the delivery of programs (Durlak, 1998). A good assessment of implementation will not only identify discrepancies between the planned and delivered programs but will also provide a thick description of the key players and components needed to attain the goals of a program.

Durlak (1998) notes that implementation varies across change agents (that is, program personnel and agencies) and settings and is sometimes seriously compromised. In a review of the literature, Durlak found that 23 to 81 percent of program activities may be omitted, with only a minority of programs implemented to a high degree of integrity or fidelity. Durlak also notes that preventionists, in general, should not expect the quantity or quality of implementation to be 100 percent. The level of implementation needed for maximum program impact is largely unknown for most violence prevention programs.

In most program models, process and outcome are closely intertwined (Reid & Hanrahan, 1988, p. 94). Monitoring program implementation is central to determining whether the quantity and quality of program delivery is consistent with the program model. Without periodic measurement of key program elements one can only assume that the program was being delivered. Unless we know what was truly delivered, we are hard pressed to say that we know what aspects of program delivery were associated with outcomes.

In addition to being an essential part of an outcome evaluation, effective and periodic program monitoring is a valuable management tool. An effective system for monitoring program delivery can assist with management decisions and with ensuring accountability of program staff. With periodic feedback about the program environment and the amount and quality of the program being delivered, program managers and line staff can make timely adjustments to improve the program.

Integration of Violence Prevention Efforts

Looking over the epidemiology of violence in different forms and learning about risk and protective factors, one is struck by the similarities in risk factors across forms of violence. Yet our approach to violence prevention is fragmented as we focus on specific forms of violence and create specific programs to address each form of violence separately. Recent efforts to study and prevent the co-occurrence of varied forms of violence have been made (Daro, Edleson, & Pinderhughes, 2004). Gaps in our understanding of how different types of violent behaviors are interrelated and whether they share common risk factors have limited our ability to design more cost-effective violence prevention and intervention efforts that could address multiple types of violence, however.

Research has begun to describe youth involvement in multiple forms of violent behavior, such as peer violence and suicide. One of the few studies that have specifically examined the overlap between physical peer violence and suicidal behaviors was based on the 1997 New York State Youth Risk Behavior Survey. This study found that 11 percent of high school students reported both suicidal and violent behavior in the past year (Cleary, 2000). Research based on the 2001 national Youth Risk Behavior Survey found that adolescents who report suicidal behavior are more likely to report involvement in physical fighting (Swahn, Lubell, & Simon, 2004). More specifically, high school students who reported attempting suicide were more likely to have been in a physical fight than were students who reported not attempting suicide (61.5 percent versus 30.3 percent) (Swahn et al., 2004). Higher proportions of both boys and girls who had attempted suicide (77.8 percent and 54.0 percent, respectively) reported fighting compared to the proportions of those boys and girls who had not attempted suicide (41.2 percent and 19.8 percent, respectively). Moreover, among those students who reported attempting suicide, the proportion who reported fighting was highest among ninth graders (64.5 percent) and decreased with each subsequent grade. Research has also found that youths who have attacked others with a weapon (Evans, Marte, Betts, & Silliman, 2001; Flannery, Singer, & Wester, 2001), engaged in dating violence (particularly for males; Coker et al., 2000), or perpetrated sexual violence (Borowsky, Hogan, & Ireland, 1997) have been shown to be at higher risk for suicidal behavior.

Advancing a complementary ecological model to help us think more clearly about how to create communities with a rich network of nurturing supportive relationships has been advocated by some neuroscientists, research scholars, pediatricians, and youth service professionals (Eccles & Gootman, 2002). In reviews of new research on the brain, human behavior, and social trends, networks of enduring, nurturing relationships have been shown to significantly strengthen brain development and diminish the likelihood of aggression, depression, and substance abuse. The characteristics of social groups—whether families or other social groups—that will produce good outcomes for children have begun to be identified and can be incorporated into community programs (Eccles & Gootman, 2002). This approach does not replace the focus on preventing problems but provides a broader view of activities in such areas as community service, school-to-work transition, parenting, mentoring, and arts and recreation, among others. In high-quality, comprehensive experimental and quasi-experimental evaluations, a few of these activities have been identified as effective in preventing delinquency, drug and alcohol use, high-risk sexual behavior, aggressive behavior, violence, truancy, and smoking, as well as effective in increasing psychological and social assets among youths (Catalano, Gainey, Fleming, Haggerty, & Johnson, 1999; Hawkins, Catalano, Kosterman, Abbott, & Hill, 1999). Much more collaborative, comprehensive, and longitudinal research is needed to evaluate which features of community programs influence development, which processes within each activity are related to these outcomes, and which combination of features are best for which outcomes to supplement family-based and school setting prevention efforts.

Summary

Using the public health approach as a framework, this chapter has provided a description of the problem of violence and suggested a means for understanding the causes and prevention of violent behavior. Although the spectrum of possible efforts is limited, several actions can advance violence prevention. First, we can advocate for investment in injury surveillance systems that will provide us with meaningful and timely information on magnitudes, trends, and affected populations. Second, we must further develop the taxonomy of violence and appropriate theoretical models to begin to move toward a comprehensive and thorough understanding of the causes of violence and the means to prevent violence. Third, we must take what we learn from conducting surveillance and research and apply it to developing and testing prevention strategies. Finally, we must streamline the pathway between science and program implementation by developing systems for rapidly and effectively disseminating information on the practice of violence prevention. As people die from violent behavior, we strive to understand the causes and to develop effective means to reduce the toll. Clearly, we have much work to do. (See Exhibit 12.1 on page 422 for a list of helpful resources.)

References

Achenbach, T. M., & Ruffle, T. M. (2000). The Child Behavior Checklist and related forms for assessing behavioral/emotional problems and competencies. *Pediatrics in Review, 21,* 265–271.

Adams, D. M., Overholser, J. C., & Lehnert, K. L. (1994). Perceived family functioning and adolescent suicidal behavior. *Journal of the American Academy of Child & Adolescent Psychiatry, 33,* 498–507.

Anderson, M. A., Kaufman, J., Simon, T. R., Barrios, L., Paulozzi, L., Ryan, G., et al. (2001). School-associated violent deaths in the United States, 1994–1999. *JAMA, 286,* 2695–2702.

Anderson, R. N., & Smith, B. L. (2003). Deaths: Leading causes for 2001. *National Vital Statistics Reports, 52*(9), 1–86.

Arana, G. W., & Hyman, S. (1989). Biological contributions to suicide. In D. Jacobs & H. N. Brown (Eds.), *Suicide: Understanding and responding.* Madison, CT.: International Universities Press.

Bagley, C., & Ramsay, R. (1985). Psychosocial correlates of suicidal behaviors in an urban population. *Crisis, 6,* 63–77.

Baldwin, D., Bullock, T., Montgomery, D., & Montgomery, S. (1991). 5-HT reuptake inhibitors, tricyclic antidepressants and suicidal behaviour. *International Clinical Psychopharmacology, 6* (Suppl. 3), 49–56.

Beautrais, A. L., Joyce, P. R., & Mulder, R. T. (1996). Access to firearms and the risk of suicide: A case control study. *Australian and New Zealand Journal of Psychiatry, 30*(6), 741–748.

Beck, J. (1994). Epidemiology of mental disorders and violence, beliefs and research findings. *Harvard Review of Psychiatry, 2,* 1–6.

Beck, A. T., Steer, R. A., Beck, J. S., & Newman, C. F. (1993). Hopelessness, depression, suicidal ideation, and clinical diagnosis of depression. *Suicide & Life-Threatening Behavior, 23,* 139–145.

Bell, C. C., & Jenkins, E. (1993). Community violence and children on Chicago's south side. *Psychiatry, 56,* 46–54.

Belsky J. (1980). Child maltreatment: An ecological integration. *American Psychologist,* pp. 320–335.

Berman, M. E., Kavoussi, R. J., & Coccaro, E. F. (1997). Neurotransmitter correlates of human aggression. In D. M. Stoff, J. Breiling, & J. D. Maser (Eds.), *Handbook of antisocial behavior* (pp. 305–313). New York: Wiley.

Berman, S. L., Kurtines, W. M., Silverman, W. K., & Serafini, L. T. (1996). The impact of exposure to crime and violence on urban youth. *American Journal of Orthopsychiatry, 66*(3), 329–336.

Block, R., & Zimring, F. E. (1973). Homicide in Chicago 1965–1970. *Journal of Research in Crime and Delinquency, 10,* 1–7.

Boor, M., & Bair, J. H. (1990). Suicide rates, handgun control laws, and sociodemographic variables. *Psychological Reports, 66,* 923–930.

Borowsky, I. W., Hogan, M., & Ireland, M. (1997). Adolescent sexual aggression, risk and protective factors. *Pediatrics, 100*(6), E7.

Brain, P. F. (1994). Biological-physiological. In M. Hersen, R. T. Ammerman, & L. A. Sisson (Eds.), *Handbook of aggressive and destructive behavior in psychiatric patients* (pp. 3–16). New York, Plenum.

Brain, P. F., & Susman, E. J. (1997). Hormonal aspects of aggression and violence. In D. M. Stoff, J. Breiling, & J. D. Maser (Eds.), *Handbook of antisocial behavior* (pp. 314–323). New York: Wiley.

Brent, D. A., Kolko, D. J., Allan, M. J., & Brown, R. V. (1990). Suicidality in affectively disordered adolescent inpatients. *Journal of the American Academy of Child & Adolescent Psychiatry, 29,* 586–593.

Brent, D. A., Moritz, G., Bridge, J., Perper, J., & Canobbio, R. (1996). The impact of adolescent suicide on siblings and parents. *Suicide & Life-Threatening Behavior, 26,* 253–259.

Brent, D. A., Perper, J. A., Moritz, G., Baugher, M., Schweers, J., & Roth, C. (1993). Firearms and adolescent suicide. *American Journal of Diseases of Children, 147,* 1066–1071.

Brent, D. A., Perper, J. A., Moritz, G., Friend, A., Schweers, J., Allman, C., et al. (1993). Adolescent witnesses to a peer suicide. *Journal of the American Academy of Child & Adolescent Psychiatry, 32,* 1184–1188.

Brent, D. A., Perper, J. A., Moritz, G., Liotus, T., Schweers, J., Roth, C., et al. (1993). Psychiatric impact of the loss of an adolescent sibling to suicide. *Journal of Affective Disorders, 28,* 249–256.

Bronfenbrenner, U. (1977). Toward an experimental ecology of human development. *American Psychologist, 32,* 513–531.

Bronfenbrenner, U. (1988). Interacting systems in human development, Research paradigms, Present and future. In N. Bolger, A. Caspi, G. Downey, & M. Moorehouse (Eds.), *Persons in context, developmental processes, human development in cultural and historical contexts* (pp. 25–49). New York, Cambridge University Press.

Brooks-Gunn, J., Duncan, G. J., Klebanov, P. K., & Sealand, N. (1993). Do neighborhoods influence child and adolescent development? *American Journal of Sociology, 99*(2), 353–395.

Campbell, N. B., Milling, L., Laughlin, A., & Bush, E. (1993). The psychosocial climate of families with suicidal preadolescent children. *American Journal of Orthopsychiatry, 63,* 142–145.

Carey, G. (1994). Genetics and violence. In A. J. Reiss, K. A. Klaus, & J. A. Roth (Eds.), *Understanding and preventing violence, Vol. 2. Biobehavioral influences.* Washington, DC: National Academies Press.

Carey, G., & Goldman, D. (1997). The genetics of antisocial behavior. In D. M. Stoff, J. Breiling, & J. D. Maser (Eds.), *Handbook of antisocial behavior* (pp. 243–254). New York: Wiley.

Catalano, R. F., Gainey, R. R., Fleming, C. B., Haggerty, K. P., & Johnson, N. O. (1999). An experimental intervention with families of substance abusers: One-year follow-up of the focus on families project. *Addiction, 94*(2), 241–254.

Centers for Disease Control and Prevention. (1992). *Youth suicide prevention programs: A resource guide.* Atlanta, GA: Author.

Centers for Disease Control and Prevention. (1997). Regional variations in suicide rates—United States, 1990–1994. *Morbidity and Mortality Weekly Report, 46,* 789–792.

Centers for Disease Control and Prevention. (2003a). *Costs of intimate partner violence against women in the United States.* Retrieved September 15, 2005, from http://www.cdc.gov/ncipc/pub-res/ipv_cost/ipv.htm

Centers for Disease Control and Prevention. (2003b). Public health and aging: Nonfatal physical assault—related injuries among persons aged >60 years treated in hospital emergency departments—United States, 2001. *Morbidity and Mortality Weekly Report, 52,* 812–816.

Centers for Disease Control and Prevention, National Center for Injury Prevention and Control. (2005). Web-Based Injury Statistics Query and Reporting System (WISQARS). Retrieved November 8, 2005, from http://www.cdc.gov/ncipc/wisqars/default.htm

Cicchetti, D., & Lynch, M. (1993). Toward an ecological/transactional model of community violence and child maltreatment: Consequences for children's development. *Psychiatry, 56,* 96–118.

Cleary, S. D. (2000). Adolescent victimization and associated suicidal and violent behaviors. *Adolescence, 35*(140), 671–682.

Coie, J. D., Dodge, K. A., Terry, R., & Wright, V. (1991). The role of aggression in peer relations: An analysis of aggression episodes in boys' play groups. *Child Development, 62*(4), 812–826.

Coker, A. L., McKeown, R. E., Sanderson, M., Davis, K. E., Valois, R. F., & Huebner, E. S. (2000). Severe dating violence and quality of life among South Carolina high school students. *American Journal of Preventive Medicine, 19,* 220–227.

Cooley, M. R., Turner, S. M., & Beidel, D. C. (1995). Assessing community violence, The children's report of exposure to violence. *Journal of the American Academy of Child and Adolescent Psychiatry, 34,* 201–208.

Cotten, N. U., Resnick, J., Browne, D. C., Martin, S. L., McCarraher, D. R., & Woods, J. (1994). Aggression and fighting among African-American adolescents: Individual and family factors. *American Journal of Public Health, 84*(4), 618–622.

Cummings, P., Koepsell, T. D., Grossman, D. C., Savarino, J., & Thompson, R. S. (1997). Association between the purchase of a handgun and homicide or suicide. *American Journal of Public Health, 87*(6), 974–978.

Daro, D., Edleson, J. L., & Pinderhughes, H. (2004). Finding common ground in the study of child maltreatment, youth violence, and adult domestic violence. *Journal of Interpersonal Violence, 19*(3), 282–298.

David, C., Steele, R., Forehand, R., & Armistead, L. (1996). The role of family conflict and marital conflict in adolescent functioning. *Journal of Family Violence, 11*(1), 81–91.

DeJong, M. L. (1992). Attachment, individuation, and risk of suicide in late adolescence. *Journal of Youth and Adolescence, 21,* 357–373.

Deykin, E. Y., Alpert, J. J., & McNamara, J. J. (1985). A pilot study of the effect of exposure to child abuse or neglect on adolescent suicidal behavior. *American journal of Psychiatry, 142,* 1299–1303.

Durlak, J. A. (1998). Why program implementation is important. *Journal of Prevention and Intervention in the Community, 17*(2), 5–18.

Eccles, J., & Gootman, J. A.; National Research Council and Institute of Medicine. (Eds.). (2002). *Community programs to promote youth development.* Washington, DC: National Academies Press.

Evans, W. N., Oates, W. E., & Schwab, R. M. (1992). Measuring peer group effects: A study of teenage behavior. *Journal of Political Economy, 100,* 966–991.

Evans, W. P., Marte, R. M., Betts, S., & Silliman, B. (2001). Adolescent suicide risk and peer-related violent behaviors and victimization. *Journal of Interpersonal Violence, 16*(12), 1330–1348.

Farrington, D. (1997). A critical analysis of research on the development of antisocial behavior from birth to adulthood. In D. M. Stoff, J. Breiling, & J. D. Maser (Eds.), *Handbook of antisocial behavior* (pp. 234–240). New York: Wiley.

Fisher, B. S., Cullen, F. T., & Turner, M. G. (2000). The sexual victimization of college women (Publication No. NCJ 182369). Washington, DC: U.S. Department of Justice, National Institute of Justice.

Fitzpatrick, K. M., & Boldizar, J. P. (1993). The prevalence and consequences of exposure to violence among African-American youth. *Journal of the American Academy of Child and Adolescent Psychiatry, 32,* 424–430

Flannery, D. J., Singer, M. I., & Wester, K. (2001). Violence exposure, psychological trauma, and suicide risk in a community sample of dangerously violent adolescents. *Journal of the American Academy of Child & Adolescent Psychiatry, 40*(4), 435–442.

Fox, J. A., & Zawitz, M. W. (2004). *Homicide trends in the United States.* Retrieved September 15, 2005, from http://www.ojp.usdoj.gov/bjs/homicide/homtrnd.htm

Frederick, C. (1985). *Children traumatized by catastrophic situations.* In J. Laube & S. A. Murphy (Eds.), *Perspectives on disaster recovery* (pp. 10–30). New York, Appleton-Century-Crofts.

Friedlander, B. Z. (1993). Community violence, children's development and the mass media: In pursuit of new insights, new goals, and new strategies. *Psychiatry, 56,* 66–81.

Garland, D. E. (1993). *Violence, prevalence, costs and prevention with emphasis on spinal cord injury.* Paper presented at the annual meeting of the American Spinal Cord Injury Association, Philadelphia, PA.

Gladstein, J., Rusonis, E. S., & Heald, F. P. (1992). A comparison of inner-city and upper-middle class youths' exposure to violence. *Journal of Adolescent Health, 13*(4), 275–280.

Glick, W. H., & Roberts, K. H. (1984). Hypothesized interdependence, assumed independence. *Academy of Management Review, 9*(4), 722–735.

Goldsmith, S. K., Pellmar, T. C., & Kleinman, A. M. (2002). *Reducing suicide: A national imperative.* Washington, DC: National Academies Press, 2002.

Gordon, R. (1983). An operational classification of disease prevention. *Public Health Reports, 98,* 107–109.

Grunbaum, J. A., Kann, L., Kinchen, S., Ross, J., Hawkins, J., Lowry, R., et al. (2004). Youth risk behavior surveillance—United States, 2003. *Morbidity and Mortality Weekly Report Surveillance Summaries, 53,* 2.

Harries, K. (1995). The ecology of homicide and assault: Baltimore City and County, 1989–91. *Studies on Crime & Crime Prevention, 4*(1), 44–60.

Hawkins, J. D., Catalano, R. F., Kosterman, R., Abbott, R., & Hill, K. G. (1999). Preventing adolescent health-risk behaviors by strengthening protection during childhood. *Archives of Pediatrics and Adolescent Medicine, 153*(3), 226–234

Hawley, A. (1950). *Human ecology: A theory of community structure.* New York: Ronald Press.

Hawley, A. (1986). *Human ecology: A theoretical essay.* Chicago: University of Chicago Press.

Hill, R. D., Gallagher, D., Thompson, L. W., & Ishida, T. (1988). Hopelessness as a measure of suicidal intent in the depressed elderly. *Psychology and Aging, 3,* 230–232.

Hinton-Nelson, M. D., Roberts, M. C., & Snyder, C. R. (1996). Early adolescents exposed to violence: Hope and vulnerability to victimization. *American Journal of Orthopsychiatry, 66*(3), 346–353.

Hodgins, S. (1995). Major mental disorder and crime: An Overview. *Psychology, Crime, and the Law, 2,* 5–17.

Huesmann, L. R., & Bachrach, R. S. (1988). Differential effects of television violence in kibbutz and city children. In R. Patterson & P. Drummond (Eds.), *Television and its audience: International research perspectives* (pp. 154–176). London: BFI.

Huesmann, L. R., & Eron, L. (1986). *Television and the aggressive child.* Mahwah, NJ: Erlbaum.

Huesmann, L. R., & Miller, L. S. (1994). Long-term effects of repeated exposure to media violence in childhood. In L. R. Huesmann (Ed.), *Aggressive behavior: Current perspectives* (pp. 153–186). New York: Plenum.

Iversen, G. R. (1991). *Contextual analysis* (Quantitative Applications in the Social Sciences, No. 81). Thousand Oaks, CA: Sage.

Kachur, S. P., Stennies, G. M., Powell, K. E., Modzeleski, W., Stephens, R., Murphy, R., et al. (1996). School-associated violent deaths in the United States, 1992–1994. *JAMA, 275,* 1729–1733.

Kanarek, R. B. (1994). Nutrition and violent behavior. In A. J. Reiss Jr., K. A. Miczek, & J. A. Roth (Eds.), *Understanding and preventing violence, Vol. 2. Biobehavioral influences* (pp. 515–539). Washington, DC: National Academies Press.

Krug, E. G., Dahlberg, L. L., Mercy, J. A., Zwi, A. B., & Lozano, R. (Eds.). (2004, May). *World report on violence and health.* Retrieved November 2005 from http://www.who.int/violence_injury_prevention/violence/world_report/wrvh1/en

Landau, S. F. (1984). Trends in violence and aggression: A cross-cultural analysis. *International Journal of Comparative Sociology, 25,* 133–158.

Levy, D. (1992). The liberating effects of interpersonal influence: An empirical investigation of disinhibitory contagion. *Journal of Social Psychology, 132*(4), 469–473.

Lewis, D. O., Pincus, J. H., Bard, B., & Richardson, E. (1979). Neuropsychiatric, psycho-educational, and family characteristics of 14 juveniles condemned to death in the United States. *American Journal of Psychiatry, 145,* 584–589.

Lowther, S., De Paermentier, F., Cheetham, S. C., Crompton, M. R., Katona, C. L., & Horton, R. W. (1997). 5-HT1A receptor binding sites in post-mortem brain samples from depressed suicides and controls. *Journal of Affective Disorders, 42*, 199–207.

Mann, J. J. (1987). Psychobiologic predictors of suicide. *Journal of Clinical Psychiatry, 48* (Suppl.), 39–43.

Mann, J. J., Arango, V., & Underwood, M. D. (1990). Serotonin and suicidal behavior. *Annals of the New York Academy of Sciences, 600*, 476–485.

Marzuk, P. M., Tardiff, K., Leon, A. C., Stajic, M., Morgan, E. B., & Mann, J. J. (1992). Prevalence of cocaine use among residents of New York City who committed suicide during a one-year period. *American Journal of Psychiatry, 149*, 371–375.

Mednick, S. A., & Kandel, E. (1988). Genetic and perinatal factors in violence. In T. E. Moffitt & S. A. Mednick (Eds.), *Biological contributions to crime causation* (pp. 121–131) (NATO Advanced Science Institutes Series D, Behavioral and Social Sciences, No. 40). Dordrecht, Netherlands: Martinus Nijhoff.

Medoff, M. H., & Magaddino, J. P. (1983). Suicides and firearm control laws. *Evaluation Review, 7*(3), 357–372.

Mercy, J. A., Rosenberg, M. L., Powell, K. E., Broome, C. V., & Roper, W. L. (1993). Public health policy for preventing violence. *Health Affairs, 12*(4), 7–29.

Messner, S., & Tardiff, K. (1986). Economic inequality and levels of homicide: An analysis of urban neighborhoods. *Criminology, 24*, 297–318.

Miczek, K. A., DeBold, J. F., Haney, M., Tidey, J., Vivian, J., & Weerts, E. M. (1994). Alcohol, drugs of abuse, aggression, and violence. In A. J. Reiss Jr., K. A. Miczek, & J. A. Roth (Eds.), *Understanding and preventing violence, Vol. 3. Social influences* (pp. 377–570). Washington, DC, National Academies Press.

Mirsky, A. F., & Siegel, A. (1994). The neurobiology of violence and aggression. In A. J. Reiss Jr., K. A. Miczek, & J. A. Roth (Eds.), *Understanding and preventing violence, Vol. 2. Biobehavioral influences* (pp. 59–172). Washington, DC, National Academies Press.

Monahan, J. (1997). Major mental disorders and violence to others. In D. M. Stoff, J. Breiling, & J. D. Maser (Eds.), *Handbook of antisocial behavior* (pp. 92–100). New York: Wiley.

Mrazek, P. J., & Haggerty, R. J. (Eds.). (1994). *Reducing risks for mental disorders: Frontiers for prevention intervention research*. Washington, DC: National Academies Press.

Mulvey, E. (1994). Assessing the evidence of a link between mental illness and violence. *Hospital and Community Psychiatry, 31*, 23–31.

Mungas, D. (1983). An empirical analysis of specific syndromes of violent behavior. *Journal of Nervous and Mental Disease, 171*(6), 354–361.

Ohmori, T., Arora, R. C., & Meltzer, H. Y. (1992). Serotonergic measures in suicide brain. *Biological Psychiatry, 32*, 57–71.

Pynoos, R. S., & Nader, K. (1989). Case study: Children's memory and proximity to violence. *Journal of American Academy of Child and Adolescent Psychiatry, 28*, 236–241.

Rainer, J. D. (1984). Genetic factors in depression and suicide. *American Journal of Psychotherapy, 38*, 329–340.

Reid, J. R., & Hanrahan, P. (1988). Measuring implementation of social treatment. In K. J. Conrad & C. Roberts-Gray (Eds.), *Evaluating program environments* (pp. 93–111). San Francisco: Jossey-Bass.

Reiss, A. J., & Roth, J. A. (Eds.). (1993). *Understanding and preventing violence: Panel on understanding and control of violent behavior*. Washington, DC: National Academies Press.

Rennison, C. (2003). *Intimate partner violence, 1993–2001* (Publication No. NCJ 197838). Washington, DC: Department of Justice, Bureau of Justice Statistics.

Richards, J. M., Gottfredson, D. C., & Gottfredson, G. D. (1990). Units of analysis and item statistics for environmental assessment scales. *Current Psychology, Research and Reviews, 9*(4), 407–413.

Richters, J. E., & Martinez, P. E. (1993). Violent communities, family choices, and children's chances: An algorithm for improving the odds. *Development and Psychopathology, 5*(4), 609–627.

Robins, L. N., & Regier, D. A. (Eds.). (1991). *Psychiatric disorders in America: The Epidemiologic Catchment Area study.* New York: Free Press.

Roneck, D. (1981). Dangerous places: Crime and residential environment. *Social Forces, 60,* 74–96.

Rose, G. (1985). Sick individuals and sick populations. *International Journal of Epidemiology, 14*(1), 32–38.

Rotheram-Borus, M. J., & Trautman, P. D. (1988). Hopelessness, depression, and suicidal intent among adolescent suicide attempters. *Journal of the American Academy of Child & Adolescent Psychiatry, 27,* 700–704.

Roy, A. (1986). Depression, attempted suicide, and suicide in patients with chronic schizophrenia. *Psychiatric Clinics of North America, 9*(1), 193–206.

Roy, A., Dejong, J., Lamparski, D., Adinoff, B., George, T., Moore, V., et al. (1991). Mental disorders among alcoholics. *Archives of General Psychiatry, 48,* 423–427.

Roy, A., Dejong, J., Lamparski, D., George, T., & Linnoila, M. (1991). Depression among alcoholics. *Archives of General Psychiatry, 48,* 428–432.

Sampson, R. J. (1985). Neighborhood and crime: The structural determinants of personal victimization. *Journal of Research in Crime and Delinquency, 22*(1), 7–40.

Sampson, R. J., & Groves, W. B. (1989). Community structure and crime: Testing social disorganization theory. *American Journal of Sociology, 94*(4), 774–802.

Sampson, R. J., Raudenbush, S. W., & Earls, F. (1997). Neighborhoods and violent crime, A multilevel study of collective efficacy. *Science, 277,* 918–924.

Schubiner, H., Scott, R., & Tzelepis, A. (1993). Exposure to violence among inner-city youth. *Journal of Adolescent Health, 14*(3), 214–219.

Shaffer, D., Gould, M. S., Fisher, P., Trautman, P., Moreau, D., Kleinman, M., et al. (1996). Psychiatric diagnosis in child and adolescent suicide. *Archives of General Psychiatry, 53,* 339–348.

Shaw, C. R., & McKay, H. D. (1942). *Juvenile delinquency and urban areas.* Chicago: University of Chicago Press.

Sloan, J. H., Rivara, F. P., Reay, D. T., Ferris, J. A., & Kellermann, A. L. (1990). Firearm regulations and rates of suicide: A comparison of two metropolitan areas. *New England Journal of Medicine, 322,* 369–373.

Smith, D. R., & Jarjoura, G. R. (1988). Social structure and criminal victimization. *Journal of Research in Crime and Delinquency, 25,* 27–52.

Smith, W., Simmonds, J. O., Alam, Z. S., & Grant, R. E. (2003). Spinal cord injury caused by gunshot wounds: The cost of rehabilitation. *Clinical Orthopaedics and Related Research, 408,* 145–151.

Stack, S., & Wasserman, I. M. (1995). Marital status, alcohol abuse and attempted suicide. *Journal of Addictive Diseases, 14*(2), 43–51.

Straus, M. A., & Kantor, G. K. (1994). Corporal punishment of adolescents by parents. *Adolescence, 29,* 543–561.

Swahn, M. H., Lubell, K. M., & Simon, T. R. (2004). Suicide attempts and physical fighting among high school students—United States, 2001. *JAMA, 292,* 428–429.

Tangney, J. P., & Feshbach, S. (1988). Children's television-viewing frequency: Individual differences and demographic correlates. *Personality and Social Psychology Bulletin, 14*(1), 145–158.

Taylor, R. B., & Covington, J. (1988). Neighborhood changes in ecology and violence. *Criminology, 26*(4), 553–589.

Tebbutt, J., Swanston, H., Oates, R. K., & O'Toole, B. I. (1997). Five years after sexual abuse: Persisting dysfunction and problems of prediction. *Journal of the American Academy of Child & Adolescent Psychiatry, 36*(3), 330–339.

Terr, L. (1990). *Too scared to cry: Psychic trauma in childhood.* New York, HarperCollins.

Thornton, T. N., Craft, C. A., Dahlberg, L. L., Lynch, B. S., & Baer, K. (2000). *Best practices of youth violence prevention: A sourcebook for community action* (Rev. ed.). Atlanta, GA: Centers for Disease Control and Prevention, National Center for Injury Prevention and Control.

Tjaden, P., & Thoennes, N. (2000). *Full report of prevalence, incidence, and consequences of violence against women: Findings from the national violence against women survey* (Publication No. NCJ 183781). Washington, DC: U.S. Department of Justice, National Institute of Justice.

Tolan, P. H. (1996). How resilient is the concept of resilience? *Community Psychologist, 29*(4), 12–15.

Tondo, L., Baldessarini, R. J., Hennen, J., Floris, G., Silvetti, F., & Tohen, M. (1998). Lithium treatment and risk of suicidal behavior in bipolar disorder patients. *Journal of Clinical Psychiatry, 59,* 405–414.

Tondo, L., Jamison, K. R., & Baldessarini, R. J. (1997). Effect of lithium maintenance on suicidal behavior in major mood disorders. *Annals of the New York Academy of Sciences, 836,* 339–351.

United Nations. (1996). *The prevention of suicide: Guidelines for the formulation and implementation of national strategies.* New York: United Nations, Department for Policy Coordination and Sustainable Development.

U.S. Department of Health and Human Services. (1986). *Surgeon General's Workshop on Violence and Public Health, Leesburg, Virginia, October 27–29, 1985.* Rockville, MD: U.S. Department of Health and Human Services, Bureau of Maternal and Child Health and Resources Development, Office of Maternal and Child Health.

U.S. Department of Health and Human Services. (1999). *The surgeon general's call to action to prevent suicide.* Retrieved November 10, 2005, from http://www.surgeongeneral.gov/library/calltoaction/default.htm

U.S. Department of Health and Human Services. (2001a). *National strategy for suicide prevention: Goals and objectives for action.* Rockville, MD: U.S. Department of Health and Human Services, Public Health Service.

U.S. Department of Health and Human Services. (2001b). *Youth violence: A report of the surgeon general.* Retrieved November 10, 2005, from http://www.surgeongeneral.gov/library/youthviolence

U.S. Department of Health and Human Services, Administration on Children, Youth, and Families. (2003). *Child maltreatment.* Retrieved November 10, 2005, from http://www.acf.hhs.gov/programs/cb/publications/cm03

U.S. Department of Justice. (2003). *Criminal victimization 2002* (Publication No. NCJ 199994). Retrieved November 10, 2005, from http://www.ojp.usdoj.gov/bjs/pub/pdf/cv02.pdf

Van Praag, H. M. (1991). Serotonergic dysfunction and aggression control. *Psychological Medicine, 21,* 15–19.

Vilhjalmsson, R., Kristjansdottir, G., & Sveinbjarnardottir, E. (1998). Factors associated with suicide ideation in adults. *Social Psychiatry and Psychiatric Epidemiology, 33*, 97–103.

Weishaar, M. E., & Beck, A. T. (1992). Hopelessness and suicide. *International Review of Psychiatry, 4*, 177–184.

Werner, E. E. (1989). High-risk children in young adulthood: A longitudinal study from birth to 32 years. *American Journal of Orthopsychiatry, 59*, 72–81.

Werner, E. E., & Smith, R. S. (1992). *Overcoming the odds.* Ithaca, NY: Cornell University Press.

White, H. R. (1997). Alcohol, illicit drugs, and violence. In D. M. Stoff, J. Breiling, & J. D. Maser (Eds.), *Handbook of antisocial behavior* (pp. 511–523). New York: Wiley.

Widom, C. S. (1989). Child abuse, neglect, and adult behavior: Research design and findings on criminality, violence, and child abuse. *American Journal of Orthopsychiatry, 59*(3), 355–367

Windle, R. C., & Windle, M. (1997). An investigation of adolescents' substance use behaviors, depressed affect, and suicidal behaviors. *Journal of Child Psychology and Psychiatry, and Allied Disciplines, 38*, 921–929.

Wolk, S. I., & Weissman, M. M. (1996). Suicidal behavior in depressed children grown up. *Psychiatric Annals, 26*, 331–335.

EXHIBIT 12.1. HELPFUL RESOURCES.

American Association of Suicidology (AAS)
4201 Connecticut Ave. NW, Ste. 408
Washington, DC 20008
Phone: (202) 237-2280
Web site: http://www.suicidology.org

The goal of the AAS is to understand and prevent suicide. AAS promotes research, public awareness programs, public education, and training for professionals and volunteers.

American College of Obstetricians and Gynecologists
409 Twelfth Street SW
PO Box 96920
Washington, DC 20090-6920
Phone: (202) 638-5577
Web site: http://www.acog.org

This Web site provides professional publications about violence against women, intimate partner violence, sexual violence, adolescent dating violence, and patient education materials, in both English and Spanish.

American Foundation for Suicide Prevention
120 Wall St., 22nd Flr.
New York, NY 10005
Phone: (888) 333-2377 or (212) 363-3500
Web site: http://www.afsp.org

The American Foundation for Suicide Prevention is dedicated to advancing knowledge of suicide and its preventable nature.

EXHIBIT 12.1. HELPFUL RESOURCES, Cont'd.

Center for the Study and Prevention of Violence (CSPV)
University of Colorado at Boulder
Institute of Behavioral Science
900 28th St., Ste. 107
439 UCB
Boulder, CO 80309-0439
Phone:(303) 492-1032
Fax: (303) 443-3297
Web site: http://www.colorado.edu/cspv/blueprints

CSPV offers eleven model programs, called *blueprints,* that have been effective in reducing adolescent violent crime, aggression, delinquency, and substance abuse; these are summarized, with a video segment, on the Web site. CSPV also offers training and technical assistance to help sites choose and implement these programs.

Children's Safety Network (CSN)
55 Chapel St.
Newton, MA 02458-1060
Phone: (617) 969-7100 x2722
Web site: http://www.childrenssafetynetwork.org

The Network provides resources and technical assistance to maternal and child health agencies and organizations seeking to reduce unintentional injuries and violence toward children and adolescents. There are two Children's Safety Network Resource Centers, funded by the Health Resources and Services Administration's Maternal and Child Health Bureau.

Clearinghouse on Abuse and Neglect of the Elderly
University of Delaware
Department of Consumer Studies
Alison Hall West, Rm. 211
Newark, DE 19716
Phone: (302) 831-3525
Web site: http://www.elderabusecenter.org

The Clearinghouse on Abuse and Neglect of the Elderly (CANE) is the nation's largest archive of published research, training, government documents, and other sources on elder abuse. The CANE collection is fully computerized and contains nearly 5,000 holdings. You can also search its database to obtain references pertaining to the many facets of elder mistreatment.

Family Violence Prevention Fund
383 Rhode Island St., Ste. 304
San Francisco, CA 94103-5133
Phone: (415) 252-8900
Web site: http://www.endabuse.org

The Family Violence Prevention Fund (FVPF) works to end violence against women and children around the world.

EXHIBIT 12.1. HELPFUL RESOURCES, Cont'd.

National Center for Injury Prevention and Control
Centers for Disease Control and Prevention
Mailstop K65
4770 Buford Hwy. NE
Atlanta, GA 30341-3724
Phone: (770) 488-1506
Fax: (770) 488-1667
Web site: http://www.cdc.gov/ncipc

The National Center for Injury Prevention and Control (NCIPC) works to reduce morbidity, disability, mortality, and costs associated with intentional and unintentional injuries.

National MCH Center for Child Death Review: Keeping Kids Alive
2438 Woodlake Circle, Ste. 240
Okemos, MI 48864
Phone: (800) 656-2434
Web site: http://www.childdeathreview.org

The National MCH Center for Child Death Review promotes, supports, and enhances child death review methodology and activities at the state, community, and national levels. It builds public and private partnerships to incorporate child death review (CDR) findings into efforts that improve child health. Building on the extensive knowledge of current CDR programs, the center actively involves states in the development of center services.

National Sexual Violence Resource Center
123 North Enola Dr.
Enola, PA 17025
Phone: (717) 909-0710 or (877) 739-3895
Web site: http://www.nsvrc.org

The National Sexual Violence Resource Center (NSVRC) identifies and disseminates information, resources, and research on all aspects of sexual violence prevention and intervention. The NSVRC Web site features links to related resources and information about conferences, funding, job announcements, and special events.

National Youth Violence Prevention Resource Center
PO Box 6003
Rockville, MD 20849-6003
Phone: (866) 723-3968
Web site: http://www.safeyouth.org

Developed by CDC in partnership with ten other Federal agencies, the National Youth Violence Prevention Resource Center (NYVPRC) provides current information pertaining to youth violence. The center is a gateway for professionals, parents, teens, and others interested in obtaining comprehensive information about youth violence and suicide prevention.

Office of Juvenile Justice and Delinquency Prevention
810 Seventh Street NW
Washington, DC 20531
Phone: (202) 307-5911
Web site: http://ojjdp.ncjrs.org

EXHIBIT 12.1. HELPFUL RESOURCES, Cont'd.

The Office of Juvenile Justice and Delinquency Prevention (OJJDP) provides national leadership, coordination, and resources to prevent and respond to juvenile delinquency and victimization. OJJDP supports states and communities in their efforts to develop and implement effective and coordinated prevention and intervention programs. OJJDP also works to improve the juvenile justice system so that it protects public safety, holds offenders accountable, and provides treatment and rehabilitative services tailored to the needs of juveniles and their families.

Office of Safe and Drug-Free Schools
U.S. Department of Education
400 Maryland Ave. SW
Washington, DC 20202
Phone: (800) USA-LEARN
Web site: http://www.ed.gov/about/offices/list/osdfs/index.html

The Office of Safe and Drug-Free Schools program is the Federal government's primary vehicle for reducing violence and the use of drugs, alcohol, and tobacco through education and prevention activities in our nation's schools.

Prevent Child Abuse America
200 S. Michigan Ave., 17th Flr.
Chicago, IL 60604-2404
Phone: (312) 663-3520
Web site: http://www.preventchildabuse.org
E-mail: mailbox@preventchildabuse.org

Prevent Child Abuse America builds awareness in, provides education to, and inspires hope in everyone involved in the effort to prevent the abuse and neglect of our nation's children. Working with chapters in thirty-nine states and the District of Columbia, Prevent Child Abuse America provides leadership to promote and implement prevention efforts at the national and local levels.

STOP IT NOW!
PO Box 495
Haydenville, MA 01039
Phone: (413) 268-3096
Web site: http://www.stopitnow.org

STOP IT NOW! is a national, public health–based organization working to prevent and ultimately eradicate child sexual abuse. Through public education, policy advocacy, and research and evaluation, STOP IT NOW! urges abusers and potential abusers to stop their behavior and seek help.

Substance Abuse and Mental Health Services Administration
Rm. 12-105 Parklawn Bldg.
5600 Fishers Ln.
Rockville, MD 20857
Phone: (301) 443-8956
Web site: http://www.samhsa.gov

EXHIBIT 12.1. HELPFUL RESOURCES, Cont'd.

The Substance Abuse and Mental Health Services Administration (SAMHSA) is the federal agency charged with improving the quality and availability of prevention, treatment, and rehabilitative services in order to reduce illness, death, disability, and cost to society resulting from substance abuse and mental illnesses.

Suicide Prevention Action Network
1025 Vermont Ave., NW, Ste. 1200
Washington, DC 20005
Phone: (202) 449-3600
Web site: http://www.spanusa.org

The Suicide Prevention Action Network (SPAN USA) is the nation's only suicide prevention organization dedicated to leveraging grassroots support among suicide survivors (those who have lost a loved one to suicide) and others in order to advance public policies that prevent suicide. The organization was created to raise awareness, build political will, and call for action with regard to creating, advancing, implementing, and evaluating a national strategy to address suicide in our nation.

Suicide Prevention Resource Center
Education Development Center, Inc.
55 Chapel St.
Newton, MA 02458-1060
Phone: (877) 438-7772
Web site: http://www.sprc.org

The Suicide Prevention Resource Center (SPRC) provides prevention support, training, and resources to assist organizations and individuals to develop suicide prevention programs, interventions, and policies and to advance the National Strategy for Suicide Prevention.

Violence Against Women Electronic Network
6400 Flank Dr., Ste. 1300
Harrisburg, PA 17113
Phone: (800) 537-2238
Web site: http://www.vawnet.org

The goal of the National Electronic Network on Violence Against Women (VAWnet) is to harness and use electronic communication technology as a resource for those working to end violence against women. To accomplish this goal, VAWnet staff and consultants collect, analyze, prepare, and electronically disseminate information and materials on domestic violence, sexual assault, and related issues via the Web site and facilitated listserv discussions.

What Works Clearinghouse
U.S. Department of Education
Web site: http://www.whatworks.ed.gov

The What Works Clearinghouse (WWC) promotes informed decision making in education through a set of easily accessible databases and user-friendly online materials.

CHAPTER THIRTEEN

DISASTER PREPAREDNESS

The concept of actively preparing for disasters is relatively new. Recent natural disasters and disasters resulting from deliberate acts of violence have shown that nations and communities still have much to learn about the factors that influence the consequences of disasters and how to prepare for these events. Today, disaster preparedness is an issue in the forefront of public health care professionals' attention, and this chapter offers two explorations of it. In the prologue, Sandro Galea and Craig Hadley discuss the social and ecological factors that may influence the consequences of disasters, how these factors intersect, and why consideration of these factors must be part of a comprehensive public health approach to mitigate the consequences of these events. Then, within this social and ecological context, Stephen Morse provides implementation strategies for health care professionals to adopt in preparation for and in response to disasters.

Prologue

Sandro Galea
Craig Hadley

Although definitions of disasters and the approaches used to study them may be quite disparate (Mileti, 1999; Quarantelli, 1995; Tierney, Lindell, & Perry, 2001; Hoffman & Oliver-Smith, 2002), the scientific literature generally recognizes that disasters are a relatively common human experience. In one survey of U.S. residents, 13 percent of the sample reported a lifetime exposure to natural or human-generated disaster (Burkle, 1996). In a large survey representative of the general population of the United States, 18.9 percent of men and 15.2 percent of women participants reported a lifetime experience of a natural disaster (Kessler, Sonnega, Bromet, Hughes, & Nelson, 1995). Although comparable international data are limited, large proportions of populations in many countries worldwide have been exposed to terrorism, forced relocation, and violence, suggesting that worldwide the overall prevalence of exposure to disasters is probably considerably higher than it is in the United States (Kessler, 2000; Corradi, Fagen, & Garreton, 1992).

Several recent, high-profile natural disasters (for example, the Southeast Asian tsunami of 2004 and the Gulf Coast hurricanes in the United States in 2005) and terrorist events (for example, the September 11, 2001, terrorist attacks in the United States and the March 11, 2004, train bombings in Madrid, Spain) in various parts of the world have heightened our awareness of disasters as determinants of population health. However, academic and public health interest in disasters remains episodic at best, surging when highly visible disasters occur and abating to a lower-level priority as these events fade in the public consciousness. In addition, much of the public health attention that is devoted to disasters frequently centers on a medical model of disaster preparedness. Such efforts highlight threat detection and development of elaborate protocols for evacuation, triage, and treatment.

We consider disasters to be traumatic events that are experienced by many people and may result in a wide range of mental and physical health consequences (Norris et al., 2002). We consider both acute onset, time-delimited events (for example, floods, transportation accidents) and events that take place over a longer period of time (for example, famines, conflicts, complex humanitarian emergencies) as disasters. This broad perspective, rooted in socioecological perspectives on the determinants of health (Krieger, 1994; Kaplan, 1999), highlights the range of contextual factors that contribute to population health after disasters.

Underlying Socioecological Vulnerability to the Consequences of Disasters

Briefly, socioecological perspectives suggest that factors at multiple levels of influence contribute to individual and to population health. These factors may include contextual factors, such as political structures, and individual-level factors, such as race or ethnicity. Building on this line of thinking, we suggest that multiple social and economic factors determine population vulnerability and play a role in shaping the population health consequences of disasters.

The study of vulnerability and its relation to disasters is certainly not limited to the realm of public health. When examining postdisaster outcomes, diverse academic disciplines have considered vulnerability a characteristic both of individuals and of populations (Bankoff, 2003; Turner et al., 2003; Cohen & Hamrick, 2003). Although definitions of *vulnerability* vary in the scientific literature, it is generally considered to be the capacity for harm in an individual or system in response to a stimulus. It has been postulated that different types of vulnerability exist, including genetic and biologic vulnerability at the individual level (Cohen & Hamrick, 2003; Heath & Nelson, 2002) and social vulnerability at the group level (McKeehan, 2000). Individuals who possess specific characteristics are frequently termed *vulnerable;* for example, children, homeless persons, and minority inner-city populations have been termed vulnerable in recent scientific publications, suggesting they are more likely to be harmed by external stressors than are others in the overall population (Stergiopoulos & Herrmann, 2003; Shi, 2000). In the study of disaster preparedness it has long been recognized that certain populations are also more vulnerable to the effects of disasters than are others (Oliver-Smith, 1996), although we are not aware of any systematic reviews that have considered how key social and ecological contextual factors may contribute to population vulnerability in the disaster context.

In the following discussion we adopt a population health perspective. Our primary focus is on factors that influence *rates* of disease after a disaster, rather than on how these factors may influence individual risk. Therefore we do not discuss individual-level factors (for example, individual race or ethnicity or individual socioeconomic position) that undoubtedly also contribute to the impact of disasters. We refer the reader to other, principally epidemiologic reviews (for example, Norris et al., 2002; Galea, Nandi, & Vlahov, 2005) that consider the role of individual-level factors in influencing individual health after disasters.

Contextual Determinants of Population Health After Disasters

We discuss nine determinants of population health in the wake of a disaster: geography, political structure and governance, community socioeconomic status, relative distribution of income and wealth, culture, health and social services infrastructure, physical environment, social environment, and civic society.

Geography

We start our discussion with a brief mention of the role of geography as a contextual determinant of disasters. Although disasters are a global phenomenon, the impact of disasters remains grounded in local context. Geographic factors render specific areas at particularly high risk of disasters. Areas below sea level or particularly close to bodies of water that change levels frequently (for example, the Gulf Coast region in the United States and river deltas in Bangladesh) are particularly prone to flooding. Similarly, human settlements in arid areas (for example, Southern Australia) are vulnerable to fires (Gillen, 2005). The threat of disasters in many such areas is endemic, and floods, bushfires, and earthquakes are recurrent events, with varying degrees of intensity in different seasons. In these areas the risk of recurrent disasters is virtually unavoidable, and the exigencies of geography highlight the fact that there is likely no solution for total elimination of these disasters, except, for example, complete resettlement of the at-risk human populations into lower-risk areas. Geography also plays an important role in structuring the postdisaster response. News of a disaster in isolated communities may take far longer to reach aid agencies or the media (as in the case of the Darfur famine in 2004 and 2005) than will news of disasters in more readily accessible locations. Similarly, the ability of agencies to actually provide aid may well be limited in geographically distant or difficult locales. For example, it took more than a week for domestic and international aid efforts to reach some victims of the devastating 2005 earthquakes in the Kashmir region of Pakistan that killed an estimated 54,000 people (Agence France Presse, 2005).

Political Structure and Governance

Political structures and systems of governance establish the parameters (for example, taxation, federal-state relations) that shape many of the other contextual factors that then shape health. Democratic governance is typically associated with greater government openness and responsiveness to domestic criticism, and there is some evidence that such regimes are less prone to state failures. For example, analyses of state failures in Liberia and Somalia that preceded disasters or predisposed these nations' citizens to disasters show that such events are far more likely to occur in partial as compared to fully democratic regimes (Esty & Ivanova, 2002). There is also evidence that disasters occurring in alternate political systems are substantially mitigated by effective governance. Perhaps a more consistent feature of political structures that relates directly to the mitigation of disaster consequences is the *effectiveness* of political structures and governance. Effectiveness of government can span a broad spectrum. At the extreme are a few societies worldwide without an effective government of any sort. For example, Somalia has not had a central government since 1993. In its stead, informal organizations, typically organized along clan lines, have emerged to provide a loose form of governance that typically organizes response to mass disasters such as famines, in terms of both providing relief for persons in affected communities and dealing with international aid organizations and outside offers of help. Less dramatically, within well-established national political structures there have been several recent examples of both effective and ineffective government response to disasters. Focusing on the United States as an example, during the past three decades subsequent U.S. federal administrations have devolved more government functions to state and local governments; taxes have been cut at the federal, state, and local levels; some environmental and consumer regulations have been loosened; and many previously public services (for example sanitation, water, and health care) have been privatized (Katz, 1989; Gans, 1995). Limited regulation of municipal water supplies has been considered at least in part responsible for water-borne disease outbreaks in various North American cities (Krewski et al., 2002; Corso et al., 2003; Garrett, 2000). Most recently, ineffective and uncoordinated U.S. government response to Hurricane Katrina in August and September 2005 has been widely attributed to devolvement of central government authority and to poor coordination between federal, state, and municipal levels of government (Nates & Moyer, 2005).

Community Socioeconomic Status

Postdisaster evidence has demonstrated an association between individual poverty and lower perception of disaster risk, poorer disaster preparedness, more limited communication of disaster warnings, greater physical and psychological impacts from disasters, and more limited access to emergency response after disasters (Forthergill & Peek, 2004). However, the disaster literature has focused almost exclusively on *individual* poverty rather than low community socioecological status (frequently also referred to as community deprivation). There is an abundance of research in public health demonstrating that aggregate community socioeconomic status is associated with health independent of individual socioeconomic position. Low community socioeconomic status encompasses multiple domains, including high rates of poverty (Berkman & Kawachi, 2000) and unemployment (Berkman & Kawachi, 2000) and low education and income levels (Krieger, 1994; Berkman & Kawachi 2000). Empirically, low community socioecological status is a determinant of health outcomes, including health-related behaviors, mental health, infant mortality rates, adult physical health, coronary heart disease, and mortality, even after accounting for individual-level factors (Diez-Roux, 2001; Pickett & Pearl, 2001; Diez-Roux et al., 1997). Community deprivation may also be associated with differential access to medical care (Mandelblatt, Yabroff, & Kerner, 1999) and with the limited availability of other salutary resources, such as healthy food (Cheadle et al., 1991; Sooman, Macintyre, & Anderson, 1993).

Low community socioeconomic status can affect residents' health by means of two primary mechanisms: (1) through limiting the availability of salutary resources that may be beneficial to residents' well-being and (2) through psychosocial stress accompanying chronic shortage of essential resources (Williams, Lavizzo-Mourey, & Warren, 1994). Both these mechanisms also explain how community socioeconomic status may influence health in the disaster context. After disasters, when both formal and informal resources are limited, societies with fewer resources to begin with are less likely than better-supplied societies to have access to salutary resources such as health and social services or food reserves. Similarly, postdisaster circumstances are likely to heighten preexisting stressors and may lead to poor coping health behaviors (for example, substance abuse). Evidence about the consequences of disasters across communities with different levels of deprivation comes, for example, from research after 1992 earthquakes in Humboldt County, California. Rio Dell, a more marginalized town, that had worse disaster response, a more limited and slower recovery, than Ferndale, an equally affected but more affluent community (Rovai, 1994).

Relative Distribution of Income and Wealth

Recent evidence, although controversial, suggests that inequalities in income distribution, as distinguished from outright material deprivation, may contribute to health differentials (Wilkinson, 1992; Kaplan, Pamuk, Lynch, Cohen, & Balfour, 1996;

Pappas, Queen, Hadden, & Fisher, 1993). Relative deprivation (frequently operationalized as degree of income inequality) has been shown to be an important correlate of homicide (Land, McCall, & Cohen, 1990; Kaplan et al., 1996; Cubbin, Williams Pickle, & Fingerhut, 2000) and mortality (Kaplan et al., 1996; Galea et al., 2003).

Psychosocial stress associated with living in communities with high income disparities may be associated with greater interindividual tension and likelihood of interpersonal violence. Also, perceived and actual inequality caused by the discrepancies in income distribution erodes the social trust and diminishes the social capital that shapes societal well-being and health (Kawachi, Kennedy, Lochner, & Prothrow-Stith, 1997) and may lead to underinvestment in public goods. Income inequality also may be associated with disinvestment in material resources in communities (Kaplan et al., 1996). Congruent with our discussion about the role of community socioeconomic status, these mechanisms also may be particularly relevant in the postdisaster context. Community income inequality may be associated with greater risk of psychopathology after a disaster, independent of the contribution of individual income.

Culture

The role of culture in shaping health in general and health in the postdisaster period in particular is difficult to quantify but probably pervasive. *Culture* as a notion lends itself to diverse definitions and interpretations. For the purposes of this discussion we consider *culture* to be "shared, learned behaviors and meanings that are transmitted socially" (Marsella & Christopher, 2004, p. 529). Therefore social relationships associated with formal social and religious institutions are elements of the cultural context that may shape health. Similarly, religiously sanctioned or endorsed behaviors and practices have the potential to influence health in the predisaster context. For example, a religious prohibition on alcohol use is associated with much lower rates of alcohol dependence among Muslims compared to non-Muslims (Cochrane & Bal, 1990). Evidence suggests that other manifestations of a dominant culture, such as patterns of social congregation in public places, are associated with social transmission of health behaviors and norms (Henrich & McElreath, 2003). Complex social security networks, which serve to minimize the risk of resource shortfalls, have also been identified as important informal sources of assistance that are called on during disasters (Shipton, 1990). It is important to note that this *moral economy* of sharing is also linked to community socioeconomic status, which in turn influences the efficacy of informal support networks. Less affluent communities may be less able than more affluent ones to mobilize material resources to assist others (Hadley, Borgerhoff Mulder, & Fitzherbert, under review), although this may or may not be true for other domains of social support. Strong cultural norms about societal organization and altruism may influence social cohesion in the postdisaster period and contribute to communal efforts to restore public places and other physical structures to their predisaster state. However, conversely, destruction of culturally significant places may be associated with communal grief (Bode, 1989), which has been associated with elevated rates of depression in the aftermath of disasters (Goenjian et al., 2001).

Health and Social Services Infrastructure

Predisaster availability of health and social resources is inextricably linked to postdisaster recovery. Rich countries and communities are characterized by an array of health and social services, particularly in comparison to poorer countries or communities (Casey, Thiede Call, & Klingner, 2001; Felt-Lisk, McHugh, & Howell, 2002). In the United States even the poorest communities often have dozens of social agencies, each with a distinct mission and service package. Many of the public health successes in wealthy countries over the past few decades, including reductions in HIV transmission and tuberculosis control, have depended in part on the efforts of these groups (Freudenberg et al., 2000). However, social and health services in poorer communities and countries are often limited. In poor communities and in less wealthy countries, social and health services are frequently susceptible to changing national and donor fiscal realities, with any resultant decreases in service frequently coinciding with times of greater need in the population (Felt-Lisk et al., 2002; Friedman, 1989). For example, in the United States in the past few decades the decline in the national economy and in tax revenues has forced many cities and states to reduce services at the very time unemployment and homelessness were increasing (National League of Cities, 2003; Freudenberg, Fahs, Galea, & Greenberg, in press).

Different disasters have varying scopes and magnitudes and may be associated with decimation of all, some, or none of the predisaster health and social services. When preexisting health and social services continue to function postdisaster, the contribution of these resources to preserving or restoring health in a population is self-evident. However, these preexisting resources are relevant even in devastating disasters where most formal resources are destroyed. Local health and social service practitioners have local knowledge, are accepted by local community members, and are much more likely to be able to provide continuity of care than are services provided by outside aid agencies (Fissel & Haddix, 2004).

Physical Environment

Multiple features of the physical environment are associated with health, with a vast empirical literature demonstrating links between the physical environment and well-being. The human built environment can influence both physical and mental health; empirical evidence about the relation between the built environment and health conditions has been discussed for, among other issues, asthma and other respiratory conditions, injuries, psychological distress, depression, and child development (Frumkin, 2002; Krieger & Higgins, 2002; Northridge, Sclar, & Biswas, 2003; Weich et al., 2002; Cohen et al., 2000). Other authors have linked various aspects of the built environment to specific health outcomes. For example, features of the built environment such as quality of housing, density of development, mix of land uses, scale of streets, aesthetic qualities of place, and connectivity of street networks may affect physical activity (Handy, Boarnet, Ewing, & Killingsworth, 2002) and in turn, all cause mortality (Diez-Roux, 2003; Pate et al., 1995). Infrastructure is also a critical part of the physical environment and determines how a city provides water, disposes of garbage, and provides energy (Melosi, 2000). Water scarcity and water pollution are serious problems in less wealthy countries. It is estimated that nearly 1.5 billion people lack safe drinking water and that at least 5 million deaths per year can be attributed to waterborne diseases (Krants & Kifferstein, 1998). The World Health Organization (WHO) estimates that the majority of urban populations in developing countries do not have access to proper sanitation (WHO, 1997). Inadequate provision for solid waste collection frequently results in contamination of water bodies, presenting a substantial risk for rapidly spreading epidemics (Alexander & Ehrlich, 2000; Chanthikul, Qasim, Mukhopadhyay, & Chiang, 2004; Satterthwaite, 2000).

The physical environment is perhaps one of the most obviously central features of the context for postdisaster recovery. Structures like buildings, bridges, and skyscrapers may be vulnerable to natural or human-made disasters, as recent earthquakes in Japan and Iran and as the September 11, 2001, terrorist attacks on New York City and Washington, D.C., demonstrated. Features of the physical environment can be immediately linked to the fatality rate after disasters (Daley et al., 2005). Recent earthquakes of comparable magnitude in Kobe, Japan, in 1995, and Bam, Iran, in 2003 were associated with 5,200 and 26,000 deaths, respectively. Much of this difference was attributed to differences in the quality of buildings; Japanese buildings had been reinforced to cope with earthquake tremors and did so, whereas much of the Iranian city of Bam collapsed with the earthquake, killing thousands of residents ("Major Earthquakes," 2005). Somewhat less immediately in terms of effects, infrastructure damaged in an earthquake or hurricane can strain already taxed systems and contribute to the spread of disease postdisaster. In the longer term, lengthy periods required for reconstruction of the local physical environment may contribute to prolonged community suffering after a disaster, limited job opportunities, and a slower recovery of population physical and mental health.

Social Environment

The social environment has been broadly defined to include "occupational structure, labor markets, social and economic processes, wealth, social, human, and health services, power relations, government, race relations, social inequality, cultural practices, the arts, religious institutions and practices, and beliefs about place and community" (Barnett & Casper, 2000, p. 465). This definition, by its very complexity, suggests that there are multiple ways in which the social environment may affect health. Social order, stability, and integration are conducive to conformity, whereas disorder is conducive to crime and poor integration into social structures (Shaw & McKay, 1969). Limited social cohesion may predispose persons to poorer coping and adverse health (Kawachi & Berkman, 2001; McLeod & Kessler, 1990). Social capital effects are thought to offer general economic and social support on an ongoing basis and also make specific resources available at times of stress. Social capital has been shown to be associated with lower all-cause mortality (Kawachi et al., 1997; Skrabski, Kobb, & Kawachi, 2004), reduced violent crime (Kennedy, Kawachi, Prothrow-Stith, Lochner, & Gupta, 1998), and self-reported health (Subramanian, Kim, & Kawachi, 2002). Spatial segregation of racial or ethnic and socioecological groups may enforce homogeneity in resources and social network ties, suppressing diversity that may benefit persons of lower socioeconomic status. Persons who live in segregated communities may have disproportionate exposure, susceptibility, and response to economic and social deprivation, toxic substances, and hazardous conditions (Williams & Collins, 2002).

Predisaster community cohesion is a base on which postdisaster recovery can be built (Torry, 1986; Oliver-Smith, 1996). In addition, preexisting social stressors, influenced by racial or ethnic and socioecological strains, may influence postcrisis interactions during the recovery phase. For example, strained relations between Somali and Somali Bantu groups have carried over into resettlement communities and forced resettlement agencies to tread carefully along these ethnic lines (Van Lehman & Eno, 2003). Preexisting social stressors may also influence social interactions between disaster-affected communities and those attempting to provide postdisaster aid. This was evident in the aftermath of Hurricane Katrina in New Orleans in September 2005, as racial tensions in the racially segregated city played out repeatedly on U.S. national television as clashes with military and paramilitary aid workers. Also, in the context of limited postdisaster resources, predisaster social relationships that enforce or reward equitable distribution of resources may be essential to ensure that resources are available to those individuals who are most vulnerable to the consequences of disasters.

Civic Society

Although related to features of the social and cultural environment, civic society frequently plays a distinct role in shaping a context that is beneficial to population health. Civic society defines the space, not controlled by government or the market, where residents interact to achieve common goals. Several participants in civil society influence the health of populations. For example, community-based organizations such as neighborhood associations and tenant groups provide services, mobilize populations, and advocate for resources. Community-based organizations (CBOs), or nongovernmental organizations (NGOs), have a long history of working to improve living conditions both in their home countries and internationally (Halpern, 1995). For example, in the 1960s and 1970s in the United States, sometimes with government support, CBOs promoted economic development, established health centers, advocated for improved public education, and built new housing (Halpern, 1995). In the 1980s and 1990s, CBOs were at the forefront of the struggle against the AIDS epidemic in the United States (Freudenberg & Zimmerman, 1995). Many of these organizations developed into effective international NGOs advocating for global AIDS control in the 1990s. Places of worship and faith-based organizations offer social support, safe space, and political leadership (Lincoln & Mamiya, 1990; Thomas, Quinn, Billingley, & Caldwell, 1994). In many instances, civic society in the aftermath of a disaster may well be the only formal societal structure standing that has the population's respect and trust. Particularly in human-made disasters, when population suspicion of formal government authority may be high, civic society can serve as an honest broker, delivering aid relief and helping to rebuild the social and physical environments. For example, during the extended conflict between Israel and Lebanon in the 1980s and 1990s, local civic institutions, many predating the conflict, played a central role in providing health and social services to local populations in contested territory.

Covariation of Contextual Factors That Influence Postdisaster Health

Although we have discussed contextual factors in isolation, this is not meant to suggest that these factors act in isolation from one another nor that they are likely to change independently of one another. In fact it is much more likely that a specific disaster will influence multiple elements of the local context and that these factors will conjointly influence postdisaster health. For example, the decline of an aging infrastructure coupled with declining local municipal resources may challenge communities' ability to continue to provide safe water and sanitation for their residents when the system is strained by an unexpected crisis (Glaab & Brown, 1976). In rapidly urbanizing areas too, frequently in less wealthy countries, cities are often challenged to maintain an adequate fresh water supply to the growing numbers of urban residents, and to transport the accumulating sewage and other waste. The likelihood of a breakdown of the sanitary infrastructure after disasters is much higher in systems that are already taxed, have no built-in redundancies, and no tradition of rapid response to remedy breakdowns. Other contextual factors that might also contribute to postdisaster population health include, but are not limited to, population demographics, urbanization, and migration.

Summary

The recognition that predisaster context is inextricably linked to postdisaster outcomes naturally raises questions for those interested in public health promotion about the course of action available to public health professionals that might influence the factors identified here. It might reasonably be argued that affecting features of the social environment that influence postdisaster health is a challenge beyond the scope of most public health practitioners. However, we suggest that although structural and systematic change to influence underlying context may seem daunting, a focus on the fundamental determinants of population health is inevitable if we are interesting in mitigating the consequences of disasters. Leonard Syme (1997) has argued effectively that interventions that take account of and act on only the individual level will doom public health to small positive effects. In addition, interventions that are misdirected (either at the wrong modifiable variable or at the wrong level) may well have unintended consequences and result in unanticipated changes in behavior and its consequences. It is critical for health care professionals to understand the *context* of disaster and to consider efforts to ameliorate this context, to change structures and ecologies, before a disaster occurs (Wodak & Des Jarlais, 1993).

We suggest that there are two primary implications of the observations drawn here for the role of those concerned with public health promotion. First, health care professionals interested in mitigating the consequences of disasters need to consider both policies that might improve the underlying determinants and practicable population-based interventions that might be implemented rapidly in the postdisaster period. Although policy change that influences some key underlying factors, such as income distribution in communities, may well be considered outside the realm of public health practice, we suggest that it is the role of public health to influence the determinants of health at all levels. For example, it was public health efforts to improve sanitary conditions in cities that led to sentinel improvements in European cities' infrastructure and attendant reductions in morbidity and mortality throughout the nineteenth century (Coleman, 1982). Effecting structural changes requires sentinel shifts in policies that may influence underlying determinants. The current increased awareness of disasters and their potential consequences creates an opportunity for advocacy and action to improve underlying features of context that may influence the health of populations after disasters. This then represents a plausible, and desirable, goal for those interested in health promotion.

Second, the role of multiple contextual determinants in shaping population health postdisaster is likely to be complex. Therefore, public health efforts to improve context to mitigate the consequences of disasters have to center around locally responsive population-based interventions, as detailed in the second half of this chapter. Emerging research methods such as community-based participatory research and emerging technologies such as Web-based communications may represent opportunities to ameliorate local context and to prepare communities for disasters and their potential consequences.

References

Agence France Presse. (2005). *Musharraf defends handling of devastating Pakistan quake.* Retrieved October 27, 2005, from http://web.lexis-nexis.com/universe/document?_m=6509211 fbe72cf882063e380faffa66e&_docnum=1&wchp=dGLbVlz-zSkVb&_md5=715c332 a1eb5c90f4eeb04ec85375da7

Alexander, S. E., & Ehrlich, P. R. (2000). Population and the environment. In W. G. Ernst (Ed.), *Earth systems: Processes and issues.* New York: Cambridge University Press.

Bankoff, G. (2003). Constructing vulnerability: The historical, natural and social generation of flooding in metropolitan Manila. *Disasters, 27,* 224–238.

Barnett, E., & Casper, M. (2001). A definition of "social environment." *American Journal of Public Health, 91,* 465.

Berkman, L., & Kawachi, I. (Eds.). (2000). *Social epidemiology.* New York: Oxford University Press.

Bode, B. (1989). *No bells to toll: Destruction and creation in the Andes.* New York: Scribners.

Burkle, F. M., Jr. (1996). Acute-phase mental health consequences of disasters: Implications for triage and emergency medical services. *Annals of Emergency Medicine, 28,* 119–128.

Casey, M. M., Thiede Call, K., & Klingner, J. M. (2001). Are rural residents less likely to obtain recommended preventive healthcare services? *American Journal of Preventive Medicine, 21,* 182–188.

Chanthikul, S., Qasim, S. R., Mukhopadhyay, B., & Chiang, W. W. (2004). Computer simulation of leachate quality by recirculation in a sanitary landfill bioreactor. *Journal of Environmental Science and Health. Part A, Toxic/Hazardous Substances & Environmental Engineering, 39,* 493–505.

Cheadle, A., Psaty, B. M., Curry, S., Wagner, E., Diehr, P., Koepsell, T., et al. (1991). Community-level comparisons between the grocery store environment and individual dietary practices. *Preventive Medicine, 20,* 250–261.

Cochrane, R., & Bal, S. (1990). The drinking habits of Sikh, Hindu, Muslim and white men in the west Midlands: A community survey. *British Journal of Addiction, 85,* 759–769.

Cohen, D. A., Spear, S., Scribner, R., Kissinger, P., Mason, K., & Wildgen, J. (2000). Broken windows and the risk of gonorrhea. *American Journal of Public Health, 90,* 230–236.

Cohen, S., & Hamrick, N. (2003). Stable individual differences in physiological response to stressors: Implications for stress-elicited changes in immune related health. *Brain, Behavior, and Immunity, 17,* 407–414.

Coleman, C. (1982). *Death is a social disease: Public health and political economy in early industrial France.* Madison: University of Wisconsin Press.

Corradi, J., Fagen, P. W., & Garreton, M. (1992). *Fear at the edge: State terror and resistance in Latin America.* Berkeley: University of California Press.

Corso, P. S., Kramer, M. H., Blair, K. A., Addiss, D. G., Davis, J. P., & Haddix A. C. (2003). Cost of illness in the 1993 waterborne cryptosporidium outbreak, Milwaukee, Wisconsin. *Emerging Infectious Diseases, 9,* 426–431.

Cubbin, C., Williams Pickle, L., & Fingerhut, L. (2000). Social context and geographic patterns of homicide among US black and white males. *American Journal of Public Health, 90,* 579–587.

Daley, R. W., Brown, S., Archer, P., Kruger, E., Jordan, F., Batts, D., et al. (2005). Risk of tornado-related death and injury in Oklahoma. *American Journal of Epidemiology, 161,* 1144–1150.

Diez-Roux, A. V. (2001). Investigating neighborhood and area effects on health. *American Journal of Public Health, 91,* 1783–1789.

Diez-Roux, A. V. (2003). Residential environments and cardiovascular risk. *Journal of Urban Health, 80,* 569–589.

Diez-Roux, A. V., Nieto, F. J., Muntaner, C., Tyroler, H. A., Comstock, G. W., Shahar, E., et al. (1997). Neighborhood environments and coronary heart disease: A multilevel analysis. *American Journal of Epidemiology, 146,* 48–63.

Esty, D. C., & Ivanova, I. (Eds.). (2002). *Global environmental governance: Options and opportunities.* New Haven, CT: Yale School of Forestry and Environmental Studies.

Felt-Lisk, S., McHugh, M., & Howell, E. (2002). Monitoring local safety-net providers: Do they have adequate capacity. *Health Affairs, 21,* 277–283.

Fissel, A., & Haddix, K. (2004). Traditional healer organizations in Uganda should contribute to AIDS debate. *Anthropology News, 45,* 10–11.

Forthergill, A., & Peek, L. A. (2004). Poverty and disasters in the United States: A review of recent sociological findings. *Natural Hazards, 32,* 89–110.

Freudenberg, N., Fahs, M., Galea, S., & Greenberg, A. (in press). The impact of New York City's 1975 fiscal crisis on the tuberculosis, HIV, and homicide syndemic. *American Journal of Public Health.*

Freudenberg, N., Silver, D., Carmona, J. M., Kass, D., Lancaster, B., & Speers, M. (2000). Health promotion in the city: A structured review of the literature on interventions to prevent heart disease, substance abuse, violence and HIV infection in US metropolitan areas, 1980–1995. *Journal of Urban Health, 77,* 443–457.

Freudenberg, N., & Zimmerman, M. (Eds.). (1995). *AIDS prevention in the community: Lessons from the first decade.* Washington, DC: American Public Health Association.

Friedman, F. (1989). Donor policies and Third World health. *International Health Development, 1,* 16–17.

Frumkin, H. (2002). Urban sprawl and public health. *Public Health Reports, 117,* 201–217.

Galea, S., Nandi, A., & Vlahov, D. (2005). The epidemiology of post-traumatic stress disorder after disasters. *Epidemiologic Reviews, 27,* 78–91.

Gans, H. (1995). *The war against the poor: The underclass and antipoverty policy.* New York: Basic Books.

Garrett, L. (2000). Betrayal of trust: The collapse of global public health. New York: Oxford University Press.

Gillen, M. (2005). Urban governance and vulnerability: Exploring the tensions and contradictions in Sydney's response to bushfire threat. *Cities, 22,* 55–64.

Glaab, C. N., & Brown, A. T. (1976). *A history of Urban America.* New York: Macmillan.

Goenjian, A. K., Molina, L., Steinberg, A. M., Fairbanks, L. A., Alvarez, M. L., Goenjian, H. A., et al. (2001). Posttraumatic stress and depressive reactions among Nicaraguan adolescents after Hurricane Mitch. *American Journal of Psychiatry, 158,* 788–794.

Hadley, C., Borgerhoff Mulder, M., & Fitzherbert, E. (under review). Seasonal food insecurity and perceived social support in rural Tanzania.

Halpern, R. (1995). *Rebuilding the inner city. A history of neighborhood initiatives to address poverty in the United States.* New York: Columbia University Press.

Handy, S. L., Boarnet, M. G., Ewing, R., & Killingsworth, R. E. (2002). How the built environment affects physical activity: Views from urban planning. *American Journal of Preventive Medicine, 23,* 64–73.

Heath, A. C., & Nelson, E. C. (2002). Effects of the interaction between genotype and environment: Research into the genetic epidemiology of alcohol dependence. *Journal of the National Institute on Alcohol Abuse and Alcoholism, 26,* 193–201.

Henrich, J., & McElreath, R. (2003). The evolution of cultural evolution. *Evolutionary Anthropology, 12,* 123–135.

Hoffman, S., & Oliver-Smith, A. (Eds.). (2002). *Catastrophe and culture.* Santa Fe, NM: School of American Research.

Kaplan, G. A. (1999). What is the role of the social environment in understanding inequalities in health? *Annals of the New York Academy of Sciences, 896,* 116–119.

Kaplan, G. A., Pamuk, E. R., Lynch, J. W., Cohen, R. D., & Balfour, J. L. (1996). Inequality in income and mortality in the United States: Analysis of mortality and potential pathways. *British Medical Journal, 312,* 1003.

Katz, M. (1989). *The undeserving poor: From the War on Poverty to the war on welfare.* New York: Pantheon.

Kawachi, I., & Berkman, L. F. (2001). Social ties and mental health. *Journal of Urban Health, 78,* 458–467.

Kawachi, I., Kennedy, B. P., Lochner, K., & Prothrow-Stith, D. (1997). Social capital, income inequality, and mortality. *American Journal of Public Health, 87,* 1491–1498.

Kennedy, B. P., Kawachi, I., Prothrow-Stith, D., Lochner, K., & Gupta, V. (1998). Social capital, income inequality, and firearm violent crime. *Social Science & Medicine, 47,* 7–17.

Kessler, R. C. (2000). Posttraumatic stress disorder: The burden to the individual and to society. *Journal of Clinical Psychiatry, 61,* 4–12.

Kessler, R. C., Sonnega, A., Bromet, E., Hughes, M., & Nelson, C. B. (1995). Post-traumatic stress disorder in the National Comorbidity Survey. *Archives of General Psychiatry, 52,* 1048–1060.

Krants, D., & Kifferstein, B. (1998). *Water pollution and society.* Retrieved October 27, 2005, from http://www.umich.edu/~gs265/society/waterpollution.htm

Krewski, D., Balbus, J., Butler-Jones, D., Haas, C., Isaac-Renton, J., Roberts, K. J., et al. (2002). Managing health risks from drinking water: A report to the Walkerton inquiry. *Journal of Toxicology and Environmental Health. Part A, 65,* 1635–1823.

Krieger, J., & Higgins, D. L. (2002). Housing and health: Time again for public health action. *American Journal of Public Health, 92,* 758–768.

Krieger, N. (1994). Epidemiology and the web of causation: Has anyone seen the spider? *Social Science & Medicine, 39,* 887–903.

Land, K. C., McCall, P. L., & Cohen, L. E. (1990). Structural covariates of homicide rates: Are there any invariances across time and social space? *American Journal of Sociology, 95,* 922–963.

Lincoln, C. E., & Mamiya, L. H. (1990). *The black church in the African American experience.* Durham, NC: Duke University Press.

Major earthquakes around the world over the past 80 years. (2005). *USA Today.* Retrieved November 2005 from http://www.usatoday.com/news/world/2005-10-08-quake-history_x.htm

Mandelblatt, J. S., Yabroff, K. R., & Kerner, J. F. (1999). Equitable access to cancer services: A review of barriers to quality care. *Cancer, 86,* 2378–2390.

Marsella, A. J., & Christopher, M. A. (2004). Ethnocultural considerations in disasters: An overview of research, issues, and directions. *Psychiatric Clinics of North America, 27,* 521–539.

McKeehan, I. V. (2000). A multilevel city health profile of Moscow. *Social Science & Medicine, 51,* 1295–1312.

McLeod, L., & Kessler, R. (1990). Socioeconomic status differences in vulnerability to undesirable life events. *Journal of Health and Social Behavior, 31,* 162–172.

Melosi, M. (2000). *The sanitary city: Urban infrastructure in America from colonial times to the present.* Baltimore: Johns Hopkins Press.

Mileti, D. S. (1999). *Disasters by design.* Washington, DC: Joseph Henry Press.

Nates, J. L., & Moyer, V. A. (2005). Lessons from Hurricane Katrina, tsunamis, and other disasters. *Lancet, 366,* 1144–1146.

National League of Cities. (2003). *City fiscal conditions in 2003.* Retrieved October 27, 2005, from http://www.nlc.org/nlc_org/site/files/reports/fbrief03.pdf

Norris, F., Friedman, M., Watson, P., Byrne, C., Diaz, E., & Kaniasty, K. (2002). 60,000 disaster victims speak: Part 1. An empirical review of the empirical literature, 1981–2001. *Psychiatry, 65,* 207–239.

Northridge, M. E., Sclar, E., & Biswas, P. (2003). Sorting out the connections between the built environment and health: A conceptual framework for navigating pathways and planning healthy cities. *Journal of Urban Health, 80,* 556–568.

Oliver-Smith, A. (1996). Anthropological research on hazards and disasters. *Annual Review of Anthropology, 25,* 303–328.

Pappas, G., Queen, S., Hadden, W., & Fisher, G. (1993). The increasing disparity in mortality between socioecological groups in the United States, 1960 and 1986. *New England Journal of Medicine, 328,* 103–109.

Pate, R. R., Pratt, M., Blair, S. N., Haskell, W. L., Macera, C. A., Bouchard, C., et al. (1995). Physical activity and public health: A recommendation from the Centers for Disease Control and Prevention and the American College of Sports Medicine. *JAMA, 273,* 402–407.

Pickett, K. E., & Pearl, M. (2001). Multilevel analyses of neighborhood socioecological context and health outcomes: A critical review. *Journal of Epidemiology and Community Health, 55,* 111–122.

Quarantelli, E. J. (1995). What is a disaster? Six views of the problem. *International Journal of Mass Emergencies and Disasters, 13,* 221–229.

Rovai, E. (1994). *The social geography of disaster recovery: Differential community response to the north coast earthquakes* (Yearbook 56). Association of Pacific Coast Geographers.

Satterthwaite, D. (2000). Will most people live in cities? *British Medical Journal, 321,* 1143–1145.

Shaw, C. R., & McKay, H. D. (1969). *Juvenile delinquency and urban areas.* Chicago: University of Chicago Press.

Shi, L. (2000). Vulnerable populations and health insurance. *Medical Care Research and Review, 57,* 110–134.

Shipton, P. (1990). African famines and food insecurity: Anthropological perspectives. *Annual Review of Anthropology, 19,* 353–394.

Skrabski, A., Kobb, M., & Kawachi, I. (2004). Social capital and collective efficacy in Hungary: Cross-sectional associations with middle-aged female and male mortality rates. *Journal of Epidemiology and Community Health, 58,* 340–345.

Sooman, A., Macintyre, S., & Anderson, A. (1993). Scotland's health: A more difficult challenge for some? The price and allocation of healthy foods in social contrasting localities in the west of Scotland. *Health Bulletin, 51,* 276–284.

Stergiopoulos, V., & Herrmann, N. (2003). Old and homeless: A review and survey of older adults who use shelters in an urban setting. *Canadian Journal of Psychiatry, 48,* 374–380.

Subramanian, S. V., Kim, D. J., & Kawachi, I. (2002). Social trust and self-rated health in US communities: A multilevel analysis. *Journal of Urban Health, 79,* S21–S34.

Syme, S. L. (1997). *Community participation, empowerment, and health: Development of a wellness guide for California.* Berkeley: University of California, Berkeley, School of Public Health.

Thomas, S. B., Quinn, S. C., Billingley, A., & Caldwell, C. (1994). The characteristics of northern black churches with community health outreach programs. *American Journal of Public Health, 84,* 575–579.

Tierney, K., Lindell, M. K., & Perry, R. W. (2001). *Facing the unexpected: Disaster preparedness and response in the United States.* Washington, DC: Joseph Henry Press.

Torry, W. I. (1986). Economic development, drought, and famine: Some limitations of dependency explanations. *Geojournal, 12,* 5–18.

Turner, B. L., 2nd, Kasperson, R. E., Matson, P. A., McCarthy, J. J., Corell, R. W., Christensen, L., et al. (2003). A framework for vulnerability analysis in sustainability science. *Proceedings of the National Academy of Sciences of the United States of America, 100,* 8074–8079.

Van Lehman, D., & Eno, O. (2003). *The Somali Bantu: Their history and culture.* Washington, DC: Center for Applied Linguistics.

Weich, S., Blanchard, M., Prince, M., Burton, E., Erens, B., & Sproston, K. (2002). Mental health and the built environment: Cross-sectional survey of individual and contextual risk factors for depression. *British Journal of Psychiatry, 180,* 428–433.

Wilkinson, R. G. (1992). National mortality rates: The impact of inequality? *American Journal of Public Health, 82,* 1082–1084.

Williams, D. R., & Collins, C. (2002). Racial residential segregation: A fundamental cause of racial disparities in health. In T. A. LaVeist (Ed.), *Race, ethnicity and health: A public health reader* (pp. 369–390). San Francisco: Jossey-Bass.

Williams, D. R., Lavizzo-Mourey, R., & Warren, R. C. (1994). The concept of race and health status in America. *Public Health Reports, 109,* 26–41.

Wodak, A., & Des Jarlais, D. C. (1993). Strategies for the prevention of HIV infection among and from injecting drug users. *Bulletin on Narcotics, 1,* 47–60.

World Health Organization. (1997). *Health and the environment in sustainable development: Five years after the earth summit.* Geneva: Author.

Yen, I. H., & Kaplan, G. A. (1999). Poverty area residence and changes in depression and perceived health status: Evidence from the Alameda County Study. *International Journal of Epidemiology, 28,* 90–94

Disaster Preparedness
Stephen S. Morse

All of us face emergencies in our daily lives. So too do public health agencies and their employees. The purpose of this part of the chapter is to give an overview of the kinds of emergencies to which public health responds and the basic principles of disaster preparedness and response.

Public Health as an Emergency Responder

Many people, including many who work in health departments, do not think of public health agencies as emergency responders. We tend to think of emergency responders as firefighters, police, and ambulances (as *emergency medical services* [EMS])—the people who wear uniforms and badges. Even within the public health community the appropriate emergency response role of public health is a subject of debate. But in reality public health has always responded to emergencies. The commonest and most obvious examples are, of course, responding to infectious disease outbreaks, but there are many less obvious examples of emergency response that have been carried out more or less routinely by public health. For example, during power outages, health department restaurant inspectors protect the safety of the food supply. During heat waves, health departments may provide group shelters for those lacking air conditioning. In some jurisdictions health departments are also responsible for the safety of the water supply and work to ensure water quality during floods or weather emergencies. State health departments are also often responsible for regulating health care institutions and may provide emergency assistance to hospitals, long-term care facilities, and home health care clients.

Despite this, the recognition that public health agencies are emergency responders has been relatively recent. And the emergency responder role has been expanding in recent years. For example, before 1993, the New York City Department of Health did not really consider itself an emergency response agency, even though it responded regularly to the sorts of emergencies described earlier. However, the 1993 bombing of the World Trade Center in New York made the health department acutely aware of its emergency response roles and led to a rethinking of these functions. This coincided with many other changes citywide in emergency response, such as the formation of the New York City Office of Emergency Management (OEM) to coordinate emergency response by different agencies. Most cities and states now have emergency management offices to coordinate response to all types of emergencies at the local and state levels.

Since the terrorist attacks of September 11, 2001 (9/11), emergency response roles have undergone further evolution. Public health is now more generally recognized as an emergency response agency (albeit one of many). In addition, public health played a major role in dealing with the anthrax attacks that followed 9/11 in the autumn and winter of 2001. Given the experience gained from the anthrax attacks, it is clear that public health will have a lead role in responding to bioterrorist events (which can be seen as an extension of the traditional public health role in responding to natural disease outbreaks) and will probably play a major supporting role in responding to terrorist events or accidents involving chemical agents or radiation. The CDC (Centers for Disease Control and Prevention, under the U.S. Department of Health and Human Services) has traditionally been the agency for the federal response to disease outbreaks, and the federal government's National Response Plan officially assigns responsibility for medical and public health functions to the Department of Health and Human Services.

Disaster Response

Definitions of key concepts in the field of disaster preparedness and response vary slightly among practitioners, researchers, and others, and of course the preparedness field continues to develop. In general, however, most disaster researchers would define an *emergency* as any event that requires the unanticipated use of additional community or agency resources, whereas a *disaster* is an emergency that requires resources beyond those available locally. In this discussion the term *emergency* will be used to mean both emergencies and disasters of all types. Emergencies may be natural (effects of weather or infectious disease outbreaks, for example) or human-made (transportation accidents, terrorist events).

All disaster preparedness and response must begin locally. In the United States, if the scope of an emergency exceeds the ability of local resources to handle the consequences, the local jurisdiction (city, county, or local municipality) may request help from the state (Figure 13.1). Under federal legislation known as the Stafford Act, federal assistance may be given upon request from a state governor and a declaration of emergency by the U.S. president. The lead agency for fed-

FIGURE 13.1. GENERAL RELATIONSHIPS
OF ORGANIZATIONS IN AN EMERGENCY.

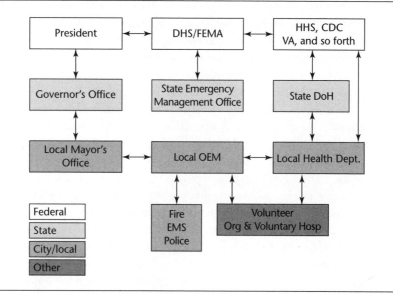

Note: The response to a natural emergency is shown. Response generally originates at the local level; local authorities may request assistance from the state, and the state may in turn request federal aid if needed. Terrorist events (for example, bioterrorism) differ somewhat in that additional agencies (including the FBI) would also take key roles.

Source: Adapted from a figure originally prepared by Linda Young Landesman and the author.

eral disaster response is usually FEMA (Federal Emergency Management Agency), now part of the U.S. Department of Homeland Security (DHS). Therefore DHS is the lead federal agency for emergency response and for federal coordination and standard setting. At this time the main document describing federal roles and responsibilities is the DHS National Response Plan. The U.S. Department of Health and Human Services is designated as the lead agency for public health and specific medical issues.

Traditionally, emergency management recognizes several key stages of a disaster (the definitions that follow are extracted from the U.S. Department of Homeland Security National Response Plan) (DHS, 2004b).

• *Preparedness* (pre-event phase). Preparedness describes the activities undertaken before a disaster. The DHS National Response Plan defines *preparedness* as "a continuous process involving efforts . . . to identify threats, determine vulnerabilities, and identify required resources." Preparedness, and how it is defined, is discussed in greater detail later in this chapter.

• *Response.* Response is "addressing the short-term, direct effects of an incident. These activities include immediate actions to preserve life, property, and the environment; meet basic human needs; and maintain the social, economic, and political structure of the affected community." The response phase typically lasts hours to a few days, depending on the nature of the emergency. (An influenza pandemic could last several months, for example.)

• *Recovery.* "Recovery involves actions needed to help individuals and communities return to normal, when feasible. Recovery actions include the development, coordination, and execution of service- and site-restoration plans and the reconstitution of government operations and services through individual, private-sector, nongovernmental, and public assistance programs." This phase is usually the longest. It begins after the initial response phase is over and can last for months (six months is usual for many major events) or even years (as in the case of the 9/11 attack in New York City and the 1995 Oklahoma City bombing).

• *Mitigation.* Emergency management officials and texts also refer to mitigation, efforts that may be taken either before, during, or after an emergency to lessen its effects. An example of mitigation is reinforcing buildings to withstand earthquakes or hurricanes.

The Incident Command System (ICS)

The *incident command system* (ICS) is widely used in the United States and a number of other countries for organizing responses to emergencies. ICS was originally developed for responding to wildfires in California but since then has been adopted by all types of response agencies as a national standard for emergency response. The term *incident management system* (IMS) may be used synonymously with ICS, or may be used to mean ICS plus additional systems that facilitate interagency or interjurisdictional coordination.

Although public health is always rising to the occasion in an emergency, this may occur at great personal or institutional expense. Therefore one important concept is that of emergency response functional roles. Applying this concept means breaking the emergency response into various functions, or duties, that people will perform. One purpose of ICS and of functional roles is to allow a more systematic (rather than ad hoc) response and to prevent any one individual from being totally indispensable to the effort. The emergency response functional role for a particular public health employee is the job he or she is expected to carry out in emergencies. Employees are generally asked to carry out only emergency response roles for which they are qualified by training or experience. It may be the same role that the employee normally fills, it may be different, or it may be the same except that the employee reports to a different supervisor. For example, an environmental health specialist who routinely does water testing may be doing exactly the same job during an emergency; during the same emergency, an immunization nurse may be providing immunizations at a mass immunization clinic but may now be reporting to the head of that clinic rather than to his or her usual supervisor.

The ICS has become the essential standard for all response. Advantages of the ICS include its flexibility and the clarity it provides in supervisory relationships. Despite the potential advantages of the ICS, health agencies are often uncomfortable with this system at first, because it uses a military-like organization and hierarchy, which is familiar to many uniformed agencies but culturally rather alien to public health. However, at its core the ICS is fairly simple and is designed to facilitate response to emergencies and interagency cooperation. In applying the ICS, each incident (a particular emergency) requires an incident commander, but other functions are activated, by the incident commander, only as needed. In health departments the incident commander may be the health commissioner or a designee. In the ICS each person ideally has no more than five to seven people reporting to him or her from below and has a designated person to report to above. Often operations are coordinated through an *emergency operations center* (EOC), where high-level representatives of the various organizations involved may be placed together to enhance communications and decision making. A large health department may have its own EOC to coordinate its own staff and (depending on the extent of the emergency) may simultaneously send representatives to other key agencies' emergency operations centers.

Figure 13.2 shows the basic top-level structure of an ICS. First comes the command function (the *incident commander* and several support officers, as needed; for a public health response these support officers might include a *liaison officer,* for communications with other sections or agencies; a *safety officer,* to ensure worker safety; and a *public information officer*). Next the ICS has four major sections (operations, planning, logistics, and finance/administration). For a relatively small incident only some of these sections may be activated. For a larger incident all of these sections may be activated, with additional functions (branches and units) as needed below each of these major sections. The ICS approach also offers the incident commander the flexibility to open or close portions of the ICS organization, or *tree,* in response to the way the emergency develops.

Many people think that the ICS is for "major" emergencies, but it can be used for all emergencies, including the "routine" emergencies to which local public health agencies are always responding. Using the ICS regularly makes it easier for the agency not only to manage the individual emergency but also to use the ICS effectively when it is needed for major emergencies.

FIGURE 13.2. GENERIC DIAGRAM OF
THE INCIDENT COMMAND SYSTEM (ICS).

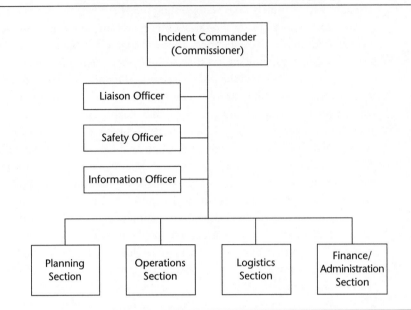

Hospital emergency departments are also required to apply the ICS, usually using a variant known as HEICS (hospital emergency incident command system). One feature of HEICS is the use of *job action sheets* (JASs) for each emergency response role. Models for public health ICSs generally include job action sheets customized to each health department's own staffing and emergency response roles, and we at the Mailman School of Public Health's Center for Public Health Preparedness at Columbia University have found them to be helpful. A detailed monograph on this public health ICS model, with sample JASs, has recently been completed (Qureshi, Gebbie & Gebbie, 2005). In our experience at the Center for Public Health Preparedness, a group exercise in which employees design job action sheets for their own or colleagues' anticipated functional roles makes a good interactive experience during emergency preparedness training.

Recently, the DHS promulgated the *National Incident Management System* (NIMS) for interagency and interjurisdictional coordination, as the national standard. It uses the ICS as the core for incident management and does not appear to be radically different from current ICS standards. DHS summarizes NIMS as follows: "NIMS establishes ICS as a standard incident management organization with five functional areas—command, operations, planning, logistics, and finance/administration—for management of all major incidents. To ensure further coordination, and during incidents involving multiple jurisdictions or agencies, the principle of unified command has been universally incorporated into NIMS. This unified command not only coordinates the efforts of many jurisdictions, but provides for and assures joint decisions on objectives, strategies, plans, priorities, and public communications." Public health and medical response remain as an *emergency support function* (ESF 8) in NIMS, with the Department of Health and Human Services as the lead agency at the federal level. In addition to the traditional public health agencies, there may be other governmental and nongovernmental organizations involved. Many locales have set up a *medical reserve corps,* to provide rapid volunteer assistance at the local level. At the national level, outside volunteer assistance may be provided through *disaster medical assistance teams* (DMATs) and the National Disaster Medical System (NDMS), which may also be used to track available hospital beds in the region and other resources.

What Is Preparedness?

After this introduction to emergency response, let us consider preparedness itself. Preparedness involves actions taken before emergencies, in order to be better able to respond to them. *Merriam-Webster's Collegiate Dictionary* defines *preparedness* as "the quality or state of being prepared." Preparedness is a constant and evolving process. Part of the DHS definition of preparedness was given in the previous section. In its NIMS document, the DHS (2004a) expands on this definition: "Preparedness incorporates a range of measures, actions, and processes accomplished before an incident happens . . . including planning, training, exercises, qualification and certification, equipment acquisition and certification, and publication management."

In public health terms preparedness comprises three main elements: having suitable emergency plans, training agency personnel for their specific roles within the plan, and practicing through drills and exercises (see Exhibit 13.1). In addition, of course, the appropriate materials and logistical support must be available, but people—good personnel and training—are the key and sine qua non of preparedness. The preparedness process is one of continuous quality improvement: what is learned from evaluations and exercises is used to refine the plans and training and then these plans and training are tried in new exercises.

One unique feature of public health preparedness is that some essential services of public health must be carried out even during emergencies. This is somewhat different from the situation facing regular emergency response agencies (such as police, fire, or EMS), for whom the normal and emergency functions generally

EXHIBIT 13.1. THE PREPAREDNESS CYCLE.

- Develop the emergency plan
- Develop and provide training, based on the plan
- Test the plan (series of drills and exercises)
  - Often, a graduated exercise sequence is used (tabletops/facilitated discussions, functional drills, full-scale drills)
- Use lessons learned to revise plans and training
- Repeat cycle

overlap. Therefore the challenge of maintaining essential services while responding appropriately to an emergency is an important issue that must be included in planning, so it can be carefully planned in advance.

Preparedness is an ongoing, indeed evolving, process. At present there is no "gold standard" for preparedness. Even if there were, the dynamic nature of the threats to the public's health would continue to make preparedness a moving target. Benchmarks are seriously needed. It can be expected that standards will continue to be developed and improved. In the United States the call for standardization was embodied in the Homeland Security Presidential Directive (HSPD-8) of December 2003. For public health and the health care response, some attempts have been made to produce a more specific definition and benchmarks. In public health the National Association of County and City Health Officials (NACCHO), which represents local health departments, recently began a program (in collaboration with the CDC, Kristine M. Gebbie [director, Center for Health Policy and Elizabeth Standish Gill Associate Professor, Columbia University School of Nursing], and other academic partners), called Project Public Health Ready, to help local health departments define minimum standards for emergency preparedness. Criteria are based on having an adequate plan, providing appropriate training on emergency preparedness to staff, and then testing agency preparedness through drills and exercises. Additional information and specific criteria can be obtained from NACCHO (2005).

For hospitals, federal bioterrorism funding, implemented through HRSA (the Health Resources and Services Administration), has set certain benchmarks for hospitals receiving these funds. The Joint Commission on Accreditation of Healthcare Organizations (JCAHO), a standard-setting organization for the United

States (see Chapter Three), has also set increasing standards for hospital emergency preparedness, beginning with having emergency plans and semiannual regular drills that also include the community.

In the public health community the federal Centers for Disease Control and Prevention (CDC), through a cooperative agreement with the Association of Schools of Public Health (ASPH), began establishing *Centers for Public Health Preparedness* (CPHPs) at schools of public health in 2000. The original impetus for the centers was to advance public health workforce development. The U.S. public health workforce consists of about half a million people, many of whom have limited formal training in public health. Ensuring that the entire public health workforce is well prepared to provide essential services and can respond effectively in any emergency is therefore critical. The general purpose of the academic centers for public health preparedness is to strengthen linkages between public health practice and academe in order to encourage the development and delivery of competency-based curricula in public health that address local needs and that could also serve as models for national replication. Since its original start as four academic centers (including the one at the Mailman School of Public Health), the network has grown to include about forty centers nationwide (twenty-two in schools of public health), all working together on developing the public health workforce in preparedness for emergencies, including bioterrorism and infectious diseases.

Let us now take a brief look at each of the elements of the *preparedness cycle* (planning, training, and drills and exercises) in turn.

Planning

Having a good emergency response plan is essential, because it serves as the basis for all subsequent activities. Unfortunately, there is no general standard for emergency plans. The general rule of thumb is that they should build on generic plans (sufficiently detailed to be useful but not overly detailed) and that they should have all major roles and responsibilities defined. As part of Project Public Health Ready, NACCHO has developed some guidelines for evaluating agency emergency plans, and some examples are available through NACCHO.

One subject of ongoing debate is whether plans, and training, should be highly specific or should build on an *all-hazards* approach. It should be noted that the FEMA model for emergency response uses an all-hazards approach. In training given by the Columbia Center for Public Health Preparedness we have generally favored the all-hazards approach as the foundation, using the Columbia University basic emergency preparedness competencies (discussed further later in this chapter). Specialized additional material (focused on bioterrorism, for example) can then be added to this foundation as needed. One advantage of the all-hazards approach is that it provides a general framework for emergency preparedness that can enhance the agency's response to the many emergencies that occur regularly. These "ordinary" emergencies provide good practice opportunities to test agency capacity and incorporate lessons learned in advance of catastrophic emergencies.

At the federal level, for all emergency response agencies, the DHS has developed the National Response Plan. The DHS (2004b) describes this plan as follows: "The National Response Plan establishes a comprehensive all-hazards approach to enhance the ability of the United States to manage domestic incidents. The plan incorporates best practices and procedures from incident management disciplines—homeland security, emergency management, law enforcement, firefighting, public works, public health, responder and recovery worker health and safety, emergency medical services, and the private sector—and integrates them into a unified structure. It forms the basis of how the federal government coordinates with state, local, and tribal governments and the private sector during incidents."

Training

Once appropriate emergency plans have been developed, a training plan is formulated, based on the functions articulated in the plan. A training needs assessment is usually done first. This may be a formal survey of the health department's workforce, covering the training status of the employees and identifying gaps, or may be done less formally through focus groups and interviews with key staff members and department leaders. The training needs assessment is keyed to the emergency plan and serves as the basis for training.

In order to train effectively, in addition to having a plan one needs to know what the employees are expected to be able to do. These expected abilities are usually referred to as *competencies*. Competency-based training is therefore one of the pillars of the CDC centers for public health preparedness and other recent programs. Relevant competency sets (available for downloading) include those for public health emergency preparedness and bioterrorism readiness developed at the Columbia University School of Nursing by Kristine Gebbie and colleagues (Columbia University School of Nursing, Center for Health Policy, 2002), and the basic competencies for public health developed by the Council on Linkages (n.d.). Additional information on the use of these competencies for developing training can be found in the Competency-to-Curriculum Toolkit, developed at the Columbia University School of Nursing (Columbia University School of Nursing, Center for Health Policy, & Association of Teachers of Preventive

Medicine, 2004). For those interested in competency sets for specific purposes (public health informatics, for example), an appendix in the toolkit contains an extensive listing of various other competency sets and where they can be obtained.

At the Mailman School of Public Health, the Columbia University emergency preparedness competencies for public health serve as the basic competency set for designing our training. These competencies are used for Basic Emergency Preparedness, an initial all-hazards introduction to emergency response roles of public health, which also introduces the ICS. More specialized training is then provided after this basic foundation has been established. Bioterrorism-related training uses the Columbia bioterrorism readiness competencies. After this initial training we usually provide some further introduction to ICS/ NIMS, at least for the senior agency leadership, and then develop customized training for groups of functional roles within the agency (such as epidemiology and surveillance, data entry, environmental testing, laboratory, logistics, and so on). Although many of the basics can be generic, specific courses and functional role training are customized for the specific procedures and staffing at each agency. Therefore, collaborating with the agency leaders, and obtaining their buy-in, is essential.

Each training should be evaluated. Many different models for evaluation are available. The simplest, which we use routinely, employs a paired pre- and posttest (with ten to twenty multiple-choice questions) together with a course evaluation (user satisfaction survey) filled out by each of the participants. We use paired numbered forms to keep input anonymous yet allow comparison of pre- and posttest results. Comments and other feedback are always invited, and often result in improvements to the training for future sessions.

Drills and Exercises

After training it is essential to test actively what has been learned. This is generally done through drills and exercises. Usually, using the FEMA model, a graduated sequence is followed, beginning with simple tabletop exercises or facilitated discussions, progressing through functional exercises, and ideally, ending in a full-scale drill. Before starting any exercise the facilitator or exercise developer should clearly define the exercise objectives, expectations, and duration, usually in consultation with the agency. A tabletop exercise brings together a group of people (such as the leaders of the health department or representatives of all the response agencies in a community) to discuss their response to an emergency scenario, provided by the exercise facilitator. Tabletop exercises typically last a couple of hours to half a day. The participants talk through what actions they might take and whom they might contact for additional information or help. Tabletop exercises are usually led by an outside facilitator and are good for helping the participants to clarify basic issues and to build teams.

The next step, limited functional exercises, is designed to test certain portions of the system under actual conditions (think of the fire drill for a familiar example). Notification drills, to test communications, are one very common exercise. These limited exercises may lead to larger functional exercises.

The last step in an exercise regime is the full-scale drill. The full-scale drill is the most stressful part of the testing, and it occurs basically in real time (or somewhat condensed real time). It involves all or most of the agency and often many response partners as well. Full-scale drills are the closest approximation to a real emergency response, but they also involve considerable expense. Such drills may last as long as three days and sometimes up to a week.

As it is for training, evaluation is an essential part of all drills and exercises. Usually the participants and facilitators will hold a discussion (an after-action session, often known colloquially as a *hot wash*) to identify lessons learned and areas for improvement. Larger exercises tend to have multiple evaluators, who look at different functional or geographic areas involved in the drill and note successes and areas for improvement. The end product is usually an after-action report, with lessons learned and recommendations, which can be used by the agency to improve response. The cycle then starts again with correcting identified weaknesses or gaps, improving the plan to take these into account, and adding or modifying training accordingly.

In response to HSPD-8, the Office of Domestic Preparedness in the Department of Homeland Security recently developed some fifteen standardized scenarios for drills and exercises for all responders, as well as exercise evaluation standards. The purpose is to facilitate agency response and interagency coordination. The scenarios and evaluation standards are for use by both first responders and other agencies. Some parts, although not necessarily all, will be obligatory for agencies receiving federal funding (for example, the standardized format for after-action reports will be obligatory).

One of the most frequent and important lessons learned in most exercises is the necessity of maintaining communication at all levels (internally within the agency and externally with response partners and other jurisdictions and with the media and the public). In a severe emergency, shortcomings in communications can have tragic consequences, as was demonstrated in 2005 during the emergency caused by Hurricane Katrina. Poor communications between the different levels of government, and conflicting expectations of the responsibilities of each, greatly added to the tragic events surrounding the response.

Good preparedness can save lives. Tragedies like Hurricane Katrina emphasize the importance of planning well in advance of a disaster and of ensuring that lines of communication are clearly delineated and that expectations for governments at the local, state, and federal levels are well defined and extensively practiced.

Personal Emergency Planning

In developing training for agencies, we have found that many employees are understandably concerned about the safety of their families and others who depend on them as caregivers, such as pets or elderly parents. Subsequent surveys conducted by the Mailman School of Public Health Center for Public Health Preparedness (Qureshi et al., 2004; Gershon et al., 2004; Qureshi, Merrill, Gershon, Calero-Breckheimer, 2002; Gebbie & Qureshi, 2002; Nandi et al., 2004) and others have found that these concerns can greatly inhibit the ability and willingness of employees to be available for emergency response, especially when the emergency duty is likely to involve extended hours. As a result, we have found it very helpful to distribute information on family emergency planning at our training sessions, and we recommend that all agencies should help their workforce members with their personal emergency planning. More information on personal and family emergency plans, with forms that individuals can fill out, can be obtained from the American Red Cross (2005) or the DHS.

Summary

Public health has long been responding to emergencies, but public health agencies have rarely considered themselves "real" emergency responders until recently. Public health is the front line in the nation's defense against bioterrorism, as it is for natural disease outbreaks, and it plays an essential role in many other emergencies. As such, public health agencies and traditional emergency responders must learn to speak each other's language and to work more closely together. It is clear that our increasingly complex world will continue to place increasing demands on public health as a responder. Good preparedness is therefore key to effective response, and people are key to preparedness. At the same time, public health performs many essential and life-saving services, including many health promotion activities, that should be supported and appropriately recognized. Disaster preparedness should therefore serve to reinforce, and not supplant, the capability of public health to carry out these core functions. (Exhibit 13.2 on page 459 offers some additional resources.)

References

American Red Cross. (2005). *Your family disaster plan.* Retrieved November 10, 2005, from http://www.redcross.org/services/disaster/beprepared/fdpall.pdf

Columbia University School of Nursing, Center for Health Policy. (2002). *Bioterrorism and emergency readiness: Competencies for all public health workers.* Retrieved October 20, 2005, from http://www.nursing.hs.columbia.edu/institutes-centers/chphsr/btcomps.html

Columbia University School of Nursing, Center for Health Policy, & Association of Teachers of Preventive Medicine. (2004). *Competency-to-curriculum toolkit.* Retrieved November 10, 2005, from http://www.cumc.columbia.edu/dept/nursing/institutes-centers/chphsr/toolkit.pdf

Council on Linkages. (n.d.). *Core competencies lists.* Retrieved November 10, 2005, from http://www.trainingfinder.org/competencies/list.htm

Gebbie, K. M., & Qureshi, K. (2002). Emergency and disaster preparedness: Core competencies for nurses. *American Journal of Nursing, 102,* 46–51.

Gershon, R. R., Qureshi, K. A., Sepkowitz, K. A., Gurtman, A. C., Galea, S., & Sherman, M. F. (2004). Clinicians' knowledge, attitudes, and concerns regarding bioterrorism after a brief educational program. *Journal of Occupational and Environmental Medicine, 46,* 77–83.

Nandi, A., Galea, S., Tracy, M., Ahern, J., Resnick, H., Gershon, R., et al. (2004). Job loss, unemployment, work stress, job satisfaction, and the persistence of posttraumatic stress disorder one year after the September 11 attacks. *Journal of Occupational and Environmental Medicine, 46,* 1057–1064.

National Association of County and City Health Officials. (2005). Retrieved November 10, 2005, from http://archive.naccho.org/Public-Health-Ready/Criteria.pdf

Qureshi, K. A., Gebbie, K. M., & Gebbie, E. N. (2005). *Public health Incident Command System: A guide for the management of emergencies or other unusual incidents within public health agencies.* Retrieved November 10, 2005, from http://www.ncdp.mailman.columbia.edu/video.htm

Qureshi, K. A., Gershon, R. R., Merrill, J. A., Calero-Breckheimer, A., Murrman, M., Gebbie, K. M., et al. (2004). Effectiveness of an emergency preparedness training program for public health nurses in New York City. *Family and Community Health, 27,* 242–249.

Qureshi, K. A., Merrill, J. A., Gershon, R. R., & Calero-Breckheimer, A. (2002). Emergency preparedness training for public health nurses: A pilot study. *Journal of Urban Health, 79,* 413–416.

U.S. Department of Homeland Security. (2004a, March). *National Incident Management System.* Retrieved November 10, 2005, from http://www.dhs.gov/interweb/assetlibrary/NIMS-90-web.pdf

U.S. Department of Homeland Security. (2004b, December). *National Response Plan.* Retrieved November 10, 2005, from http://www.dhs.gov/dhspublic/interapp/editorial/editorial_0566.xml

U.S. Department of Homeland Security. (2005). *Be ready.* Retrieved November 10, 2005, from www.ready.gov

EXHIBIT 13.2. HELPFUL RESOURCES.

Landesman, L. Y. (2005). *Public health management of disasters: The practice guide* (2nd ed.). Washington, DC: American Public Health Association.

Morse, S. S. (2003). Building academic-practice partnerships: The Center for Public Health Preparedness at the Columbia University Mailman School of Public Health, before and after 9/11. *Journal of Public Health Management and Practice, 9*(5), 427–432.

National Association of County and City Health Officials (NACCHO). *Project Public Health Ready* [and additional information and selected materials]. Available from http://www.naccho.org/topics/emergency/pphr.cfm

Noji, E. K. (Ed.). (1997). *The public health consequences of disasters.* New York: Oxford University Press.

U.S. Department of Homeland Security. *Homeland Security exercise evaluation program.* Available from http://www.ojp.usdoj.gov/odp/exercises.htm

U.S. Department of Homeland Security. In addition to the specific documents cited in the references, links to other publications are available at http://www.dhs.gov/dhspublic/theme_home1.jsp

CHAPTER FOURTEEN

ORGANIZATIONAL WELLNESS

Thomas Diamante
Samuel M. Natale
Manuel London

The workplace is under construction. Globalization, emerging technologies, newfound competition, customer demands, and legal and regulatory changes affect what companies do and how they do it. Strategically, the organization is moving toward an *organic* if not *digital* operational structure, relying on infrastructure and technologies to execute business. All of this happens (or not) because of people.

Organizations react to the endless, complex, global demands facing them. They prosper or decay. Are there human elements to business that accelerate business growth? What occurs *within* people when business demands and human capability do not align? Is health and well-being a by-product of work? The American Stress Institute estimates that $300 billion per year is lost on stress and stress-related illnesses. Are business health and human health on the same continuum? Can an organization foster individual and business wellness for mutual benefit?

Typically, the term *wellness*, when used in a business setting, calls to mind diet and exercise programs. Indeed, such initiatives are worthwhile. This chapter, however, does not limit its use of *wellness* to the typical definition. Instead, we define *wellness* in organizational settings as *the strategic integration of business, interpersonal, and individual needs to optimize overall human and organizational well-being* (see Figure 14.1).

FIGURE 14.1. PROPOSED MODEL OF FACTORS CONTRIBUTING TO INDIVIDUAL AND ORGANIZATIONAL WELLNESS.

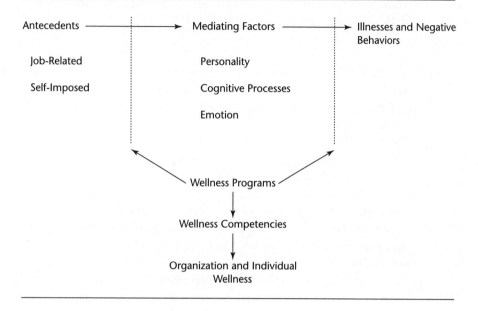

Understanding Wellness in the Business Environment

The National Institute for Occupational Safety and Health (NIOSH) defines the *healthy organization* as "one whose culture, climate and practices create an environment that promotes employee health and safety as well as organizational effectiveness" (see, for example, NIOSH, 2000). A wellness-focused organization contributes to its employees' physical, mental, spiritual, and social well-being. Such a system provides employees with tools to solve group conflicts maturely, a culture that prevents the release of harmful psychosocial elements, and a set of management practices that in general nurtures quality and management excellence in alignment with overall business strategy and customer demand.

A workplace promoting wellness brings job satisfaction, lower absenteeism and turnover, improved job performance, lower accident rates, and reduced health care and workers' compensation costs. The most important characteristics of a healthy organization are an organizational climate in which employees feel valued and are able to resolve group conflicts, management practices that reward workers for quality work, a sense of equity and support, and a learning-oriented and market-savvy leadership. Reduced demands for medical services, reduced absenteeism, reduced on-the-job injuries, reduced workers' compensation costs, and reduced disability-management costs are key metrics for health care cost reductions (U.S. Department of Health and Human Services [USDHHS], 2004).

If employers want to set new levels of excellence in the workplace, they need to strive for a holistic approach inclusive of wellness. This can be achieved by embedding healthy workplace goals into management practices. Not only will this nurture healthy relationships with contractors, suppliers, temporary workers, and customers but it will also contribute to building a healthy organizational community and will integrate business execution with employee well-being. It is also key that the workforce members attain *healthy competencies* that contribute to their own, their peers', and the organization's well-being. We propose a focus on *wellness competencies* as part of a leader's or manager's development plan. A wellness competency model brings benefits to the workplace as it places the burden of health development squarely on the individual and requires a supportive organizational context. Exhibit 14.1 defines seven competencies proposed to foster individual, interpersonal, and organizational wellness. These competencies are self-control, optimism, ability to form affiliations, ability to be nurturing, agreeableness, openness to new experiences, and ability to be self-directed. Individuals who have these characteristics, especially leaders, are likely to foster work environments that support wellness.

The Changing Workforce

The Families and Work Institute surveys a representative sample of the U.S. workforce every five years. Sponsored by the Alfred P. Sloan Foundation, IBM, Johnson & Johnson, and Motorola, the study includes an average 3,500 wage and salaried employees and self-employed workers. Findings from this national study, reported in 2002, illustrate the changing U.S. workforce (Bond, Thompson, Galinsky, & Prottas, 2002; see also Bond, Galinsky, & Hill, 2004):

- Dual earner couples increased from 66 percent in 1977 to 78 percent in the year 2002.
- Combined work hours for dual earner couples climbed by 10 hours a week (from 81 hours in 1977 to 91 hours in 2002).
- Fathers reduced time for themselves from 2.1 hours (twenty-five years ago) to 1.3 hours on workdays.
- Mothers reported even less time for themselves: 0.9 hours today versus 1.6 hours in 1977.
- Employees with families reported that work interferes with family life (45 percent today versus 34 percent twenty-five years ago).

EXHIBIT 14.1. WELLNESS COMPETENCIES DEFINED.

1. *Self-control.* The individual consciously monitors personal levels of stress or anxiety so that conscious decisions and actions can be taken to reduce anxiety levels and enhance work performance. She or he exhibits self-control under adversity or strain enabled by intrapsychic or environmental events.

2. *Positivism or optimism.* The individual interprets failures or the confrontation of obstacles in a manner that leads to rejuvenated effort and hope rather than stagnation, inaction, or depression. She identifies opportunities when in crisis and exhibits clarity and realism about the evaluation or meaning of events, without adding incorrect, unrealistic, or inappropriate elements to an event's meaning.

3. *Ability to form affiliations.* The individual has the desire to socialize, assist, or otherwise "be part of" a social unit, team, or organization where goals or objectives are shared and contributions of independent people bring added value to whole.

4. *Ability to be altruistic or nurturing.* The individual has the desire to help or to give for the sake of giving. He has a willingness to make a personal sacrifice for the good of someone else and is able to feel gratification from providing or doing for someone else without receiving any form of acknowledgment.

5. *Agreeableness.* The individual is able to negotiate or accommodate for the sake of progress. She is able to get along with others despite not seeing eye to eye. She is conversational, open, and easy to speak with, regardless of the subject matter or the potential to disagree.

6. *Openness to new experiences.* The individual is driven by curiosity and a willingness to experiment. He asks "why" and "why not" more often than wanting to follow rules. He is appreciative of new solutions, innovations, and possibilities.

7. *Ability to be self-directed.* The individual takes action to assess, plan, and act to make self-improvements or accomplish goals. She is goal-oriented and diligent. She takes deliberate action steps that lead to desired goals. She exhibits intrinsically motivated behavior.

Today the workforce is multicultural. The U.S. workforce is ethnically diverse, with 21 percent of workers being people of color versus 12 percent in 1977. There are almost equal numbers of men and women. The median age of all employees in 1988 was 35.9 rising to 38.7 in 1998 and projected to 40.5 as we approach 2008 (Fullerton, 1999). In 1995, the minority share of the workforce was 24 percent. Minority share of the workforce is projected to reach 32 percent by the year 2020. Hispanics are by far the fastest growing segment of the American workforce growing from 9 percent in 1995 to a projected 14 percent in the year 2020 (Judy & D'Amico, 1997).

Fullerton (1999) informs us that the U.S. population will look older in the years to come. The median age of workers was 35.9 in 1988, rising to 38.7 in

1998, and rising (it is expected) to 40.5 by the year 2008. Bond et al. (2002) states the fact that today only one in three fathers is the sole wage earner. Twenty-five years ago slightly more than one-half of all fathers were the sole wage earners in the family.

Expectations of job longevity have evaporated. Employees expect to be required to relocate and there are increased concerns for job insecurity. Bond et al. (2002) report that merely 36 percent of salaried workers feel secure in their jobs (meaning that they reported it was unlikely that they would lose their jobs within two years). Twenty-five years ago 45 percent of workers felt secure.

Working hours have expanded. Today men work 48.2 hours per week on average, and women 41.4 hours (including part-time employees). Twenty-five percent of workers report working one weekend day per week.

Technology has reinvented communications and personal, interpersonal, and organizational capabilities. Bond et al. (2002) inform us that almost half of all salaried workers are "connected" to work or are contacted on work matters outside the office or during "off" work hours regularly or occasionally.

Sadly, 67 percent of employed parents report a "time famine" (Bond et al., 2002, p. 2), referring to not having the time desired to spend with their children. In 1992, half of salaried workers reported not having enough time to spend with their spouses but today the number has escalated to 63 percent. Finally, 55 percent say they do not have enough time for themselves.

Organizations—and the health care professionals who work both in and with these organizations—need to face these challenges in order to design a workplace that is wellness oriented and effective.

Illnesses and Negative Behaviors at Work

Business requirements too often fail to consider human requirements. A focus on business execution and profitability to the neglect of psychosocial workplace elements is a poor business plan. The following section discusses ramifications (expected and not) of poor management practices on workers.

Behavioral Dysfunctions

Behavioral dysfunction in the workplace may take the form of aggression, hostility, sabotage, theft, violence (assault, stalking, battery, mobbing), and the withholding of output or knowledge (what could be called passive-aggressive behaviors). Passive aggressive-behaviors such as sabotage or theft may have an additional goal of *retaliating* against the employer for real or imagined injustices (Masterson, 2001).

Other dysfunctional behaviors in the workplace are underachievement, temporary production impediments, procrastination, fear of success, fear of failure, work addiction, and hostility or extreme or excessive behaviors. Behavioral dysfunction affects work, resulting in poor job performance and occupational stress and strain.

These aggressive acts are important because they point to employee *perception* as a legitimate territory for reducing health care costs. Further, these nonproductive situations are triggered, exacerbated, or mitigated by the relationship between the individual and the organization.

Behavior at Home Does Not Stay at Home

Abusive behavior that occurs at home may be carried into the workplace. Abusive behavior at home is often *domestic violence*, defined as any assault, battery, sexual assault, sexual battery, or stalking or any criminal offense resulting in physical injury to or the death of one family or household member by another who resides in the same single dwelling unit. Domestic violence can also include aggravated stalking, kidnapping, or false imprisonment. Almost 700,000 incidents of violence between partners were documented in the United States, and thousands more go unreported (The White House, 2002).

Domestic violence often becomes workplace violence in the form of assault, threat, harassment, bullying, emotional abuse, intimidation, battery, and other forms of conduct that create anxiety, fear, and a climate of distrust in the workplace. Assault, aggravated assault, battery, and aggravated battery include such acts as hitting, slapping, choking, burning, or threatening to do harm. Sexual assault and sexual battery include forcing unwanted sexual acts or intercourse and incest. The U.S. Department of Justice estimates that an average of 1.7 million violent victimizations were committed against persons aged twelve older while they were at work or on duty, according to the National Crime Victimization Survey (Duhart, 2001, p. 1).

Violence may be directed at employees by customers, clients, patients, students, inmates, or any others for whom an organization provides services. A present or former employee may foment violence against coworkers, supervisors, or managers. Criminals who are not employees may commit robbery or another crime. Violence may also be committed in the workplace by someone such as an abusive spouse or domestic partner who doesn't work there but who has a personal relationship with an employee (Di Martino & Musri, 2001). Zink and Sill (2004), examining a sample of thirty-two working mothers, found evidence demonstrating that intimate partner violence affects physical and mental health. In addition, intimate partner violence is related to poor job performance, increasing the likelihood of job loss.

Occupational Stress and Job Strain

Job stress can be defined as the harmful physical and emotional responses that occur when the requirements of the job do not match the capabilities, resources, or needs of the worker. According to the American Institute of Stress nearly half of all U.S. workers suffer from symptoms of burnout, a disabling reaction to stress on the job (*Stress,* 2001). Imagined threats affect individuals just as negatively as genuine threats do. Threats can be acute (that is, sudden—such as job loss or fearing job loss) or chronic (loneliness, isolation, relationship problems, financial worries, or incongruent person-work demands).

A number of organizational conditions may lead to occupational stress (NIOSH, 1999), including the design of tasks, heavy workloads, infrequent rest breaks, long work hours, and hectic and routine tasks that have little inherent meaning and provide little sense of control. A lack of participation by workers in decision making, poor communication in the organization, and a lack of family-friendly policies may increase organizational stress. Poor social environments and lack of support or help from coworkers and supervisors, as well as conflicting or uncertain job expectations, too much responsibility, and too many "hats to wear," may increase employees' feelings of stress.

Many employees experience career concerns owing to job insecurity and lack of opportunity for growth, advancement, or promotion. Often they experience rapid changes for which they are unprepared. These increase their feelings of stress. Environmental conditions, including unpleasant or dangerous physical conditions such as crowding, noise, air pollution, or ergonomic problems, can increase feelings of stress.

In general, stress is negatively related to psychological well-being (Schurman & Israel, 1995; Sauter, Murphy, & Hurrell, 1990) and positively related to psychosomatic symptoms and myriad other behavioral and psychological disorders affecting individuals and the organizations that employ them (Bocchino, Hartman, & Foley, 2003; Kenny & Cooper, 2003; Ivancevich, Matteson, Freedman, & Phillips, 1990). Mental disorders associated with occupational stress include anxiety, depression, and other mood disorders, maladaptive behavioral and lifestyle patterns, chemical dependencies, alcohol abuse, and sleep disorders (Israel, Baker, Goldenhar, & Heaney, 1996).

Differences between people, such as personality and copying style differences, are important predictors of stress; that is, what is stressful for one person may not be stressful for another (Benson, 1975; Williams & Williams, 1993). In both Europe and the United States coronary heart disease (CHD) has been linked to job strain when high job demands lead to small rewards or employees have little control over their work (Schat & Kelloway, 2000; Schnall & Landsbergis, 1994;

Theorell & Karasek, 1996). Among the other physical illnesses associated with occupational stress is immune system suppression (Haan, 1988, 1989; Marsland, Cohen, Rabin, & Manuck, 2001; Sauter et al., 1990).

Management practices or styles can reduce stress levels and their correlates by establishing support and by managing in humane ways that are considerate of self-esteem, social status, or the experience of shame (Gruenwald, Kemeny, Aziz, & Fahey, 2004) The only reason organizational stressors are not managed is simply that the concept of management wellness has not (yet) been introduced to the boardroom as a measure of health care cost management or a means of achieving employee health and well-being (Bond et al., 2002).

Antecedents of Workplace Illnesses and Negative Behavior

Factors that influence workplace illnesses and negative behaviors may be job related or self-imposed. Although these factors can be causes of negative reactions, they can also be adjusted or redesigned to be factors that contribute to wellness.

Job-Related Factors

Job-related factors reflect the work itself, organizational or supervisory practices, management control, culture and leadership, and the general human resource strategy.

Work Itself. Work and health are intimately connected, yet the complex association between the multiple features of employment arrangements and workers' health is not well understood. Given the dramatic labor supply and demand changes over the past decade, better identification of the employment characteristics that underlie the health of workers is of profound practical importance. The changing nature of jobs (for example, the shift from manufacturing to services), along with the aging and growing diversity of the workforce, makes workers' health requirements today different from what they were a generation ago. Therefore, in order to protect the health of workers and the health of the corporation, an examination of today's jobs and workers' health is an essential organizational requirement.

Research in occupational psychology has shown that psychological features (for example, decision latitude, demands) and psychosocial features (for example, relationships with coworkers, workplace culture) of workers' jobs promote or undermine health and well-being (see, for example, Israel et al., 1996). Psychosocial environmental stressors (for example, major life events, daily problems, chronic strains such as work overload, and deadlines) may be modified by variables that are social (for example, social support, control, socioeconomic status), psychological (for example, personality, coping strategies), biophysical (for example, age, sex, health status), behavioral (for example, relaxation skills, exercise, nutrition), or genetic (for example, family history of illnesses). Responses to workplace stress may be short term (for example, psychological reactions, behavioral reactions, physiological reactions) or longer term (for example, depression, coronary heart disease).

The workplace may alter workers' perceptions of their environment (for example, one might interpret solvable problems as catastrophes) and may yield enduring negative health outcomes (for example, poor cardiovascular disease, anxiety disorders, or alcoholism) (Israel et al., 1996; Israel, Schurman, & House, 1989). As one example, it is estimated that the cost of employees' suffering from depression is approximately $17 billion lost workdays per year (U.S. Preventive Services Task Force, 2002). Diamante and Primavera (2005) applied this research to practice by designing a feedback and coaching method that incorporates physiological, cognitive, emotional, and behavioral elements to effect changes in employees' perception of work and life events in order to improve employee self-control and positive health outcomes. These organizational change interventions involved an integration of business and human requirements (Diamante & Hyland, 2004).

Organizational and Supervisory Practices. Negative organizational and supervisory practices can adversely affect employees' wellness. Such actions include discrimination, harassment, and unfair treatment, to name a few. Positive practices can have the opposite effect, supporting and increasing wellness. Formal programs may encourage such practices. These programs can address diversity, networking and mentoring, stress management, employee assistance, and other performance enhancement issues, including continuous learning at all organizational levels. To support these programs, it is important that organizations begin to differentiate themselves not only in terms of their product offerings, separating what they offer to consumers from what competitors produce, but also in terms of their attention, care, and management of employees. Methods that supervisors can employ to increase employee wellness include providing job autonomy, creating learning opportunities, recognizing employees' successes, involving employees in decision making, and allowing flexibility in work hours.

Management Control. Today's dynamic world is witnessing an evolution to *organic* forms of organizations. These organic forms are self-organizing and rely on self-managed teams and intricately networked technological and social systems to be more responsive and adaptable to customer or client and employee demands than more rigid organizations are. In fact, these organic forms are so responsive and adaptable that many people react strongly against the term *management control* in this context because they think it sounds dominating, coercive, and heavy-handed; traditional control is thought to slow the speed of the networked and *learning* organization (Senge, 1994). Fast, cheap, and efficient are genuine descriptions of business execution, and managers who cannot get work done this way will not prosper. This organizational environment establishes new requirements for how employees think, work, and feel on the job.

Certainly, organizations, particularly businesses, are not going to stop the digital clock. Speed, functionality, and the call for "personalization" for customers and "tailoring" to clients are setting extreme demands on organizational capabilities. Today customers and clients want what they want, when they want it, and delivered on whatever device they prefer (or delivered in whatever manner they prefer). This sets new requirements on organizations and places new demands on the people who work in them.

Typical practices or tasks of a supervisor include carrying out basic management skills (decision making, problem solving, planning, delegating, and meeting management), organizing his or her department and teams, noticing the need for and designing new job roles in the group, hiring new employees, training new employees, conducting employee performance management (setting goals, observing, and giving feedback; addressing performance issues; firing employees; and so forth), and conforming to personnel policies and other internal and external regulations. These are challenging times for managers, who must deliver services and execute their functions in an increasingly complex, rapidly changing, and often-threatening global business environment. Managers are faced with shifting political, social, and economic conditions, as well as rapid technological developments and growing volumes of information.

Managers know that they need to address these changes head-on, adopting creative approaches and acquiring new skills. All levels of management are responsible for regularly communicating and interpreting business strategies and their implications for employees. In addition, managers must demonstrate support for continuous learning, respect individual needs and differences, and provide timely and supportive feedback.

Culture and Leadership. An organizational culture is the result of the values, beliefs, underlying assumptions, attitudes, and behaviors shared by the employees. Cultures arise from the employees' languages, symbols, stories, legends, and daily work practices (Schein, 2004). Leadership is determination, courage, confidence, and the ability to view a situation and respond to it. A globally competitive organization requires teamwork, collaboration, speed, learning environments, and the creation of an organizational culture that encourages expansiveness. Leadership today means continuous learning and growth of the organization and its capability.

The expansiveness of today's organizations requires new leadership behaviors. These behaviors should be directed at both pressing the organization to conquer markets in new ways while simultaneously working inside the organization to address the needs, values, and interpersonal relationships necessary for the organization to prosper (Diamante & London, 2002).

Autonomy and Job Design. Job design is the process by which managers plan and specify job tasks and the work arrangement through which these tasks are accomplished. Job design also involves the design of individual tasks in ways that make them more "fitting" to the company and to the employees, affecting employees' motivation and satisfaction in the workplace.

Among the various job design approaches are (1) job simplification; (2) job enlargement, which includes combining tasks to give a worker more of the same type of duties to perform; (3) job rotation, which involves moving workers through several jobs to increase experience and variety; and (4) job enrichment, which includes altering jobs by giving workers more autonomy and control over their own activities. These several techniques try to minimize the adverse consequences of task specialization, which include feelings of alienation, dissatisfaction, and lack of job involvement.

The best job design technique is the one that meets organizational requirements for high performance, offers a good fit with individual skills and needs, and provides opportunities for job satisfaction and employees' autonomy over their decision-making processes. For purposes of job satisfaction and wellness, the job enrichment technique is likely the most effective. Along with organizational support, proper design brings enormous motivational and performance benefits to individuals and work teams (Hackman, 2003). Autonomy and control are perceived as health enhancing.

Self-Imposed Factors

The fit between personal values and organizational mission, the ability to express oneself at work, and self-management will affect an individual's wellness. Making sense out of one's work environment is a complicated matter implicating perception, personality, thinking styles, and learning experiences.

Personal Values–Organizational Mission Fit. Mission is the purpose, value, or belief that is most meaningful to the company. It is also thought of as the purpose or reason for the organization's existence. Personal values are made up of the beliefs, missions, or philosophies that are meaningful to a person. Every individual has a number of personal values. The best way to create wellness is to have a match between key employees' personal values and the organization's mission or value. A mismatch will generate dysfunctional behaviors in the workplace, poor job performance, job dissatisfaction, stress, and other factors adverse to wellness.

Congruency between personal values and organizational mission will serve the best interests of shareholders, customers or clients, and employees. The organization's product offering or service reflects the values, practices, and culture of the company. There are many companies and they have varying missions (products or services), but in each of them congruency between the mission and management is key to organizational wellness (Bocchino et al., 2003). The organizational challenge, it appears, is to develop a goal commitment process that leads to high levels of acceptance (congruity) or an internalization of goals. The alignment of the product or service offering, customer or client expectations, management practices, and overall culture is the secret sauce for sustaining a competitive advantage.

Expressing the Self at Work. Every leader, manager, and supervisor has to learn the importance of communication and have a willingness to listen to what employees have to say. A culture that allows employees to "be themselves" is an enabling environment that reduces stress and strain. Organizational cultures that strategically enhance the opportunities to improve the fit between the employees and the organization benefit in terms of increased employee morale, lower strain, and potentially, increased overall effectiveness. Person-organization congruence can be improved through strategic planning, healthy dialogue, and conflict management (Bocchino et al., 2003). Self-expression, or emotional expression, is correlated with positive health effects (Sheese, Brown, & Graziano, 2003).

A workplace environment that honors diversity (particularly for populations such as newcomers who are at risk for slipping into the margins), seeks divergent ideas, allows room for respectful disagreement, and fosters continuous improvement nurtures human development and encourages altruism, autonomy, and thoughtful reflection. These elements breed healthy work cultures (Srivastva, Cooperrider, & Associates, 1990; Ivancevich & Lidwell, 2004).

Employee Physical Health. Science is discovering powerful connections between people's thoughts, feelings, and behaviors (Benson, 1975, 1984) in the placebo effect (expectations), personal beliefs, perceptions, sense of personal control, thinking styles, and proclivities toward being optimistic or pessimistic in attributing causes for failures or other events (Benson, 1984; Mailoo & Williams, 2004). When employees experience misalignment between their biopsychosocial and spiritual makeup and the external demands of the workplace and when this lack of fit leads to physical, mental, and behavioral problems, the costs to a business can be severe. Human organizations must wake up to the challenge of integrating the demands of business and people.

Programs or approaches to improve fit can include involving employees in community work, arranging sabbaticals in the workplace (where the manager spends time and effort with charitable organizations or university research on behalf of the employer), and personalizing the workplace to make everyone working there feel at home.

Mediating Factors

Job-related and self-imposed factors may affect the employees' and the organization's wellness. Mediators of the relationship between these antecedents and wellness include personality, cognitive, and emotional factors.

Personality Factors and Types

Personality variables such as having a tolerance for ambiguity, resilience, and hardiness, as well as whether a person is a type A or type B personality, will affect how a person reacts to difficult job situations.

Tolerance for Ambiguity. Tolerance for ambiguity is the ability to tolerate uncertainty. Intolerance for ambiguity has been associated with a number of anxiety-related problems, including worry, obsessions and compulsions, and panic sensations (Budner, 1962; Furnham & Ribchester, 1995; Kahn & Byosier, 1992). Organizational change demands the capacity to tolerate ambiguity. Many if not most businesses are experiencing the need to adapt their structures, their operations, and even their products and sevices to remain competitive. This affects what people do, and the ways they function are placed in a state of flux. Management "controls" this process, and so managing ambiguity becomes a new imperative for business managers.

Resilience. Collard, Epperheimer, and Saign (1996) inform us that the ability to adapt to changing circumstances, even when the circumstances are discouraging or disruptive, is the core of resilience. Resilience is a person's level of buoyancy, or how easily a person adapts; it is the ability to bounce back even after a "lifequake." It is the quality that enables a person to thrive during times of challenge, to recover quickly, and creatively turn adversity into advantage. Resilience calls for self-awareness about what one is facing and what one can do about it. A resilient individual is self-sufficient, determined, and harbors a sense that one's destiny is in one's own hands.

The characteristics of those who are career resilient—team-oriented, effective communicators, adaptable to change, holding positive and flexible attitudes, engaging in continuous learning, self-confident, willing to take risks, and committed to personal excellence—are also identified with employability. These characteristics are considered core competencies for jobs in highly networked, ever-changing business organizations (London, 1998a).

Hardiness. Hardiness connotes an ability to influence the situation; it is being committed to or fully engaged in one's activities and having a positive view of change (Rush, Schjoel, & Barnard, 1995). Hardy people are also resilient. Hardiness has also been associated with being open to new experiences, perseverance, innovation, and feelings of well-being (Kobasa, Maddi, Pucetti, & Zola, 1986; Maddi, 1998, 2002; Maddi & Hightower, 1999). Empirical research supports the importance of hardiness as a personality construct. For instance, recent research on military peacekeepers working in Bosnia used a structural equation modeling technique to demonstrate that hardiness improves capability to perform. Hardiness is advantageous to organizations and workers facing severe competition and constantly undergoing change.

Type A and Type B Personalities. The type A and type B labels describe two distinct personality types and behavioral patterns (Friedman & Rosenman, 1974). The characteristics of a type A personality include impatience, hostility, aggressiveness, irritability, impulsiveness, striving for achievement, and time urgency. The type B personality lacks these type A personality characteristics or shows lower levels of competitiveness and aggressiveness and is more easygoing. The type B individual is more relaxed, less competitive, and more patient than the type A individual.

Type A behavioral patterns have been linked to cardiovascular problems in some studies (Friedman & DiMatteo, 1989; Friedman & Rosenman, 1974). Recent evidence suggests that it is the *harboring of hostility*, a core component of the type A pattern, and *not* the type A behavioral pattern per se that leads to cardiovascular disease. Compared with low-hostility individuals, high-hostility individuals are less healthy, experience more anxiety and more interpersonal strain, and gain less social support (Williams & Williams, 1993; Dembroski, MacDougall, Costa, & Grandits, 1999; Hecker, Chesney, Black, & Frautschi, 1988; Smith, Pope, Rhodewalt, & Poulton, 1989; Smith, Haynes, Lazarus, & Pope, 1993).

Cognitive Processes

The cognitive processes that mediate job-related and self-imposed antecedents to wellness include perception of control, past learning, causal attribution, and learned helplessness and its converse, learned optimism.

Perception of Control. Perception refers to our interpretation of what we take in through our senses. The way we perceive our environment is what makes us different from other animals and different from each other. Viewing ourselves as autonomous or as having control over our work or life situation is a *prophylactic* against stress and subsequent physical disorders. Perceived control relates to somatic health, emotional well-being, and possibly the prevention of violence in the workplace (Schat & Kelloway, 2000). The belief that one has mastery over a situation or influence (real or imagined) is linked to more positive emotional states and somatic health (Schat & Kelloway, 2000). Even the *illusion* of benefit in a setting may be associated with the maintenance of psychological well-being (Taylor & Brown, 1988; Thompson, Sobolew-Shubin, Galbraith, Schwankovsky, & Cruzen, 1993).

This research suggests that it is advantageous to afford workers the perception of control—simply put, this might mean enabling workers to adjust their schedules, use technology to get things done, perform tasks on the basis of what works for them, make travel plans that take into account their overall lives. This can bring a sense of autonomy and a perception that one is controlling one's own work life.

Past Learning and Attribution. Past learning and attribution is concerned with how individuals interpret events that affect their current thinking and behavior. Attribution theory assumes that people try to determine why they do what they do, that is, they attribute causes to behavior (Heider, 1958; Weiner, 1974, 1986). Attributions are classified along three causal dimensions: locus of control, stability, and controllability (Weiner, 1974). The locus of control dimension has two poles: the locus may be internal or external. The stability dimension captures whether causes change over time or not. Controllability contrasts causes one can control, one's skill or efficacy, for example, with causes one cannot control, such as aptitude, mood, others' actions, and luck. What we learn, how we interpret or create our interpretation of our experiences, affects how we (or whether we) approach new challenges, contributes to our feeling awful or wonderful, and perhaps even plays a role in our physical and psychological well-being.

Continuous learning is a business requirement today. It is critical not only that workers learn but that they learn the right things. Past experiences can lead to learning but this does not ensure that the knowledge acquired is useful or beneficial to the person.

Learned Helplessness Versus Learned Optimism. Learned helplessness exists when individuals believe that their own behavior has no influence on consequent events (Seligman, 1991; Seligman & Csikszentmihalyi, 2000). The essential component of learned helplessness is exposure to conditions where response and outcome are independent. The opposite state of mind is self-efficacy, which occurs when people believe they control what happens to them. This is referred to as learned optimism (Seligman, 1991). Seligman (1991) suggests that learned helplessness produces three deficits: (1) an undermining of one's motivation to respond, (2) a retardation of one's ability to learn that responding works, and (3) an emotional disturbance, usually depression or anxiety.

When employees interpret work events (change) as inevitably leading to bad things, they will not continue to try. Management can help employees (and other managers) learn to interpret causes and the meaning of events in healthy, optimistic, resilient ways. Doing this may reduce unnecessary stress and anxiety in the organization and avoid productivity paralysis whenever a new executive or management team emerges (Seligman & Schulman, 1986).

Emotional Factors

Emotion is a powerful component of our being. It compels behavior as a response to external events and in itself *is* a response. Emotion is the connectivity between the world as we know it (or interpret it) and the world that we experience. To the extent that individuals can enhance well-being through self-awareness, emotion plays a key role. Business professionals can incorporate emotional characteristics into their strategies for attracting, selecting, retaining, and motivating human capital.

Hostility and Resentment. Cortina, Magley, Williams, and Langhout (2001) found that disrespect, condescension, and degradation (that is, incivility) were common among 1,180 surveyed public sector employees. Asked about incidences of such behaviors over the past five years, 71 percent reported an incident. By report, 33 percent of the uncivil acts were instigated by leadership (a high-power person). Both men and women were transgressed against although women were more often the target of an uncivil act. Uncivil acts were associated with greater psychological stress for both genders.

Insulting behavior can also be directed toward an individual by virtue of the individual's membership in a group that is subjected to stereotyping and rejection. Corporate efforts to promote inclusion through diversity programs are good examples of attempts to reduce these interpersonal sources of hostility. Diamante, Reid, and Giglio (1995) provide corporate training guidelines for the building of programs that identify deeply rooted, difference-based conflicts in the workplace.

Hostility brings social consequences by thwarting relationships that might serve to support, assist, or otherwise be useful to individuals as they cope with, solve, or resolve problems of work and life. Hostile individuals are not pleasant to be around, and a growing body of evidence suggests that negative emotions and behaviors may themselves be unhealthy (Belkic, Landsbergis, Schnall, & Baker, 2004; Dembroski, MacDougall, Williams, Haney, & Blumenthal, 1985). The linkage between hostility (typically understood as a personality trait) and coronary heart disease is receiving focused attention. Niaura et al. (2002) studied 774 older, unmedicated men free of cardiovascular disease as part of a collaborative research effort at Brown Medical School, Boston University School of Public Health, The Miriam Hospital, Brigham and Women's Hospital, and Harvard Medical School, among others. Tracking these patients for a three-year period the researchers were able to demonstrate the crucial, incremental risk hostility brings over and above the traditional risk factors, such as blood lipid profiles. Niaura et al. (2002) reviewed the literature and inform us that ". . . hostility is an independent psychosocial risk factor for coronary heart disease, hypertension and premature mortality" (p. 588). Although the research is clearly connecting hostility to medical problems, the intensity or "dosage" of the hostility remains ill-defined. It is likely that hostility-prone individuals exacerbate the intensity of the negative emotion—by making the emotion active more often, experiencing the emotion intensely, and failing to counteract its psychophysiologically mediated negative impact on health and well-being. Distinguishing the risks of *hostility* as a personality trait from *harboring* or *experiencing* the emotion for various amounts of time or under various levels of intensity awaits further investigation. Certainly, hostility as a trait is not advantageous to the individual or the business that employs the individual, and experiencing negative emotional states brings negative effects. Emotional support, through social relationships, may buffer any hypothesized effects of anger and hostility on stress (Hawkley, Burleson, Berntson, & Cacioppo, 2003) or coronary heart disease (Uchino, 2004).

The most common sources of resentment among workers in the workplace are inequitable benefit plans, failure to receive rewards to which they feel entitled, and heavy workloads without perceived resources or capabilities. The effort-reward imbalance, when workers perceive high demand and little control, leads to stress and anxiety (Tsutsumi & Kawakami, 2004).

Being resentful (having negative feelings but not expressing them) or harboring hostility (feeling hostile without expressing it) reflects underlying anger. Regardless of cause, anger is the underlying current (Williams & Williams, 1993; Smith et al., 1993). Employees who adopt a negative attitude or engage in hostile actions when they perceive the employment situation to be unfair lose support and make themselves unnecessarily vulnerable to continued performance declines and most certainly to less social support at work (Lepine & VanDyne, 2001; Pearson, Anderson, & Porath, 2000).

Anger. Anger is the internal emotion expressed by aggressive external behavior, which may be either verbal or physical. This emotion is caused by frustration, hostility, and disturbing actions such as insults, injuries, or threats not coming from a feared source (Williams & Williams, 1993; see also Job Stress Network, 2004). Cynicism, as a behavioral or verbal display of anger, has been found to undermine the positive effects of interpersonal support to reduce or mitigate the effects of anger on coronary heart disease (Lepore, 1995).

Effects of anger include increased blood pressure, muscle tension, scowling, teeth grinding, glaring, clenched fists, chills and shuddering, twitching, choking, flushing or paling, and numbness. Anger, anxiety, and other negative emotional states are accompanied by physiological and behavioral correlates that are counterproductive for performance, teamwork, and overall job involvement (Tavris, 1989; Williams & Williams, 1993). Destructive criticism from a manager can trigger anger and become an organization's recipe for interpersonal (as well as personal) disaster (Baron, 1998).

Workplace Interventions

A number of corporate programs and approaches support wellness and try to alleviate the negative effects of poor job conditions or difficulties that arise from employees themselves (their values, self-expression at work, and physical condition as well as their personality, cognitive processes, and emotions). These corporate efforts include employee assistance programs; diet and exercise programs; networking and mentoring programs; diversity programs; stress management, coaching, and feedback programs; and the use of a *wellness scorecard*. To implement some of these wellness approaches, management may partner with health care professionals who work within the organization or as consultants to it. In addition, these health care professionals may implement Occupational Safety & Health Administration (OSHA) standards for employee safety in the workplace, addressing ergonomics and enforcing accident and injury prevention and reduction interventions. (Readers interested in these topics should see the OSHA Web site [www.osha.gov].)

Employee Assistance Programs

An employee assistance program (EAP) is an *early intervention* strategy involving individual counseling for both work and personal problems (USDHHS, 2004).

Individual counseling assists not only employees but also their families with any personal or work-related difficulties they experience. EAPs were originally established in the late 1970s to deal with alcoholism but today provide an array of private and confidential services, in addition to substance abuse counseling, to deal with finances, stress, spousal relocation assistance, and legal needs and to offer marital and other counseling interventions and referrals (for more information see International Employees Assistance Professionals Association, 2005).

Employee assistance programs are designed to improve the physical and psychological health of a workforce. Financial savings and increased productivity are often claimed among the rewards, but there is little research on this topic in field settings and case studies flood the literature (Klarreich, DiGiuseppe, & DiMattia, 1987). Reviews of EAP research speak to how the stigma associated with such programs reduces their utilization (French, Dunlap, Roman, & Steel, 1997). Where individuals are referred by supervisors, rather than by themselves, the EAP becomes essentially a tool for management control.

Organizations provide EAP programs to reduce the human and financial costs derived from employee absenteeism and lateness for work, poor performance, high turnover, interpersonal frictions, and accidents in the workplace.

EAPs provide

- An independent, confidential, professional general counseling service that is accessible to all employees and their immediate families.
- Awareness briefings, training programs, and other services tailored to meet the needs of the client organization.
- Evaluation, in cooperation with the client organization, of the services provided in order to ensure high-quality services and to obtain data for reports to the client organization.

Employees can access the services of an EAP in three ways:

- Confidential self-referral. Employees call the EAP provider's telephone number confidentially.
- Recommended referral. A supervisor or other manager notices that a subordinate seems to be having problems and encourages the employee to seek assistance through the EAP.
- Mandatory referral. A supervisor or manager identifies work-related behavior that needs to be addressed and requires EAP counseling, to assist in the correction process.

Diet and Exercise Programs

More than thirty-four million Americans are overweight, and despite the population's increasing preoccupation with weight loss, the prevalence of overweight has increased 25 to 33 percent over the past ten years (Smith & McGhan, 1996). Furthermore, obesity leads to heart disease, this nation's number one killer, and to a total disease cost exceeding $39 billion, including $11 billion for diabetes, $22 billion for cardiovascular disease, $2.4 billion for gall bladder disease, and $1.9 billion for breast and colon cancer. These health effects are some of the reasons why organizations should vigorously promote diet and exercise programs.

Organizations implement diet programs by providing cafeterias that offer low-fat choices and that post nutritional information about food selections and by stocking snack machines with fruit and reduced-fat snacks. Companies establish fitness programs for employees by providing in-house gyms and other facilities and exercise equipment and by encouraging physical sports activities. A survey of Fortune 500 companies (with nearly 50 percent of companies responding) indicates that 66 percent have or soon plan to have fitness programs (Hollander & Lengermann, 1988). The most common corporate approach is to offer some form of on-site exercise facilities (rooms set aside for exercise bikes and treadmills) or stretching programs (which commonly take place just prior to the beginning of the workday or during breaks). Unfortunately, due to lack of standardization across programs and little measurement of program outcomes, it has been difficult to systematically capture the number of companies pursuing formal diet and exercise offerings or to estimate their level of success.

Networking and Mentoring Programs

Networking and mentoring are natural ways to deploy support in an organizational setting. Networks designed to increase social support in the workplace may involve employees, supervisors, and customers; participants may communicate through e-mails or one-to-one electronic correspondence, telephone conversations, archival journals and newsletters, professional meetings, paper mail, voice mail, chatting in the hallway, lectures and colloquia, job interviews, visits to other research sites, face-to-face meetings, conferences, seminars, and social events.

Organizations, colleges, and universities may provide mentors who counsel employees to help them grow personally and professionally. Mentoring programs may be one-on-one (one mentor working with one mentee), group based (one mentee working with two or more mentors), or team based (one mentor working with two or more mentees). Although employees have various potential sources of support in the workplace, including peers, coworkers, and subordinates, the level of trust, openness, and sincerity between mentor and mentee may optimize the prophylactic aspect of this particular supportive relationship. Mentoring programs can also be used to break down cultural barriers, foster diversity-friendly corporate environments, enhance employee commitment, promote teamwork, develop leadership qualities, and cultivate proactivity and creativity (Johnson, 2002). The efficacy of mentoring as a mechanism to promote wellness requires focused attention by researchers and practitioners.

Diversity Programs

Minorities, immigrants, and women constitute more than 50 percent of today's workforce. The United States is more ethnically diverse today than it was thirty years ago (Families and Work Institute, 2002).

Even in a relatively homogeneous society, not everyone is precisely the same. Employees will differ from each other in educational level, age, parental status, nationality, or physical attributes. Organizations look at diversity from both internal and external perspectives. It is particularly advantageous to view diversity from the customer's perspective, identifying and understanding the strategic competitive advantage that may be gained (Diamante et al., 1995). Developing diversity initiatives can therefore not only benefit human relations in the company but also create an advantage in market penetration.

Tactics on how to address diversity in a business context through effective training are available (Aronson, 2002; Diamante et al., 1995). Inclusion is core to diversity programs, coupled with business tactics that address competitive sales, marketing, or operations. Diversity has evolved into a new weapon in the war for the customer.

That said, there is little empirical evidence supporting the efficacy of diversity training. Applied research in this area is challenging due to variances in program characteristics and the elusiveness of outcome measures. Evaluation also requires that organizations allow an outsider to view a social and organizational issue that is volatile and sometimes potentially litigious. The National Study of the Changing Workforce (Families and Work Institute, 2002) conducts research every five years to get the pulse of workforce dynamics. It has found, for example, that men are more accepting of women in the workplace today than at any other time in the past. In 2002, 40 percent of men believed a woman's place is in the home. The job of family work, especially when dual-career couples are studied, falls on women.

The best diversity programs are developed through a partnership of internal employees (a diversity steering committee) and an external subject matter expert (a diversity consultant and trainer). The better programs have a senior-level advocate or champion in the organization president or CEO and are supported by sound research or experts in the field. In addition, weaving in psychological, social, and information-processing capabilities to evaluate the impact of managing diversity wisely on business outcomes is a distinct advantage to companies with these programs (Diamante et al., 1995).

Stress Management, Coaching, and Feedback Programs

Stress management programs teach workers about the nature and sources of stress, the effects of stress on health, and personal skills to reduce stress. Stress management training may rapidly reduce stress symptoms such as anxiety and sleep disturbances; they also have the advantage of being relatively inexpensive and easy to implement (Ivancevich et al., 1990).

Programs that integrate personal stress management strategies into cultural change initiatives, communications, action planning, and problem solving are likely to be most effective in the long term. Programs such as this are not easily found (or designed) but at times are used to assist with health and wellness and accelerate cultural shifts to support business objectives. Diamante and Hyland (2004), for example, offer one business case where a well-integrated "resilience" seminar was used both to convey the meaning of a shift in business strategy and to support executives in making the shift. The impact of existing stress on executives was measured using Osipow's Occupational Stress Index. The lead author of this chapter, as a consultant, conducted the nationwide series of seminars to senior management and measured the strain from job design or culture characteristics, the presence of psychological and physical ailments, and also the extent to which individuals practiced "healthful" strategies in terms of diet, exercise, cognitive control, and social support. Although not causal, the data from this study indicated that culture change hits management hard and that individual variation reflects differing levels of expertise in self-management under challenging conditions.

Spirituality and Positive Psychology in the Workplace

Spirituality is about meaningfulness in oneself and one's life works, about finding purpose in being. It is a basic feeling of "being connected" to oneself, others, and the entire universe (Mitroff & Denton, 1999; Moyers, 1993). In the workplace, spirituality is enhanced through bereavement programs, the distribution of wellness information, employee assistance programs, work and family balance policies and programs, and authentic corporate communications about business operations, missions, competitive threats, and the future of the company. A goal of enhancing spirituality also connects the company and its employees to socially responsible initiatives. For instance, companies may give employees paid time off to work on community projects or even to take sabbaticals.

Spirituality in the workplace may foster personal stability, a balance between work and personal life, higher performance expectations, clarification of work's meaning, workforce reduction, less interpersonal conflict, and connections between employees' personal values and those of the organization. When employees embrace or view their work as an expression of themselves and their values, it can unleash previously unrealized potential.

Helping behaviors (work and nonwork related) may confer benefits on both the individual (who may experience more positive affective states) and the organization (which may obtain increased commitment and organizational citizenship) (Organ & Ryan, 1995; Jex, Adams, Bachrach, & Sorenson, 2003). There is some evidence for these observations in the emerging field of *positive psychology*, which investigates the linkages between positive human thoughts, actions, beliefs, and personality and enduring health outcomes (Vaillant, 2000; see Chapter Two). The field of psychoneuroimmunology also connects the less tangible human elements of thoughts, actions, beliefs, and personality to immediate and long-term physical outcomes (Kiecolt-Glaser, McGuire, Robles, & Glaser, 2002). For example, influenza and cold viruses may flourish when the immune system is compromised, affecting business through absenteeism, lateness, and possibly decreased performance on the job.

The benefits of meditation, repetition, relaxation, and reflection are linked to positive emotional states, feelings of euphoria, and possibly immune system health and overall wellness (Benson, 1975, 1984; Maier & Laudenslager, 1985). These elements can be folded into seminars, expanding possibilities for the organization's operations and the people that make them happen. Clearly, programs bringing spirituality, a sense of personal and organizational meaningfulness that transcends mere job expectations, to the workplace are ripe for research.

Mediation and Litigation Consulting

It has been said that conflict is not negative. It is simply a natural part of living. Conflict exists between organizations, between organizations and employees, between employees, and between organizations or employees and customers. Mediation, along with arbitration, the shadow trial, the settlement conference, a private judge or ruling, and the mock jury trial, are forms of alternative dispute resolution (ADR) mechanisms to resolve conflicts that avoid costly litigation. Mediation is a voluntary, confidential, nonnegotiation process in which a neutral third party, chosen by both sides, helps both to reach a mutually satisfactory agreement. Unlike litigation, mediation is not adversarial. A mediator will try to find common grounds on which an agreement can be based. Therefore the process tends to reduce antagonism between the parties and allows them to resume their former relationships (Clarkson, Miller, Jentz, & Cross, 2003).

ADRs exist to save time and money, to protect the parties' image and morale, to avoid litigation expenses and time-consuming trials (the process of pretrial conferences, pretrial motions, motions, rulings on motions, discovery, a ruling, and sometimes appeals, can take years). ADRs allow the parties to discuss their stories in a less confrontational atmosphere than that of the courtroom.

In the courtroom, specifically, the foregoing research on human dynamics in organizations finds direct application in the professional service of litigation consulting. Wise counsel capitalizes on research in human capital assessment, interpersonal dynamics, and organizational culture in order to enable the jury to reach a desired decision.

Wellness Leadership and Support for Continuous Learning and Personal Growth

Overall, healthy organizations implement wellness programs by adopting comprehensive health approaches along with solid management practices (Ivancevich & Lidwell, 2004). Health promotion in organizations is an integrated, multidisciplinary challenge. In addition to sponsorship from senior management, it requires offering incentives and recognition for healthy behaviors, actively involving employees and middle management in decisions and change management, increasing individuals' sense of control, and building autonomy into jobs to bring competitive advantage to business operations (Srivastva et al., 1990).

Healthy organizations support continuous learners, individuals who recognize their own values and priorities and how they want to live and work. Continuous learners have personal vision and take an active role in the world and work; they continue to reflect on their experiences in the world (including work); seek ongoing feedback about the world (including work) and their activities in it; remain as open as possible to the feedback; and make ongoing adjustments, based on ongoing feedback, to the way they live their lives and conduct their work, in order to more closely meet their priorities and values (London, 1992, 1998a). Continuous learning is becoming increasingly critical for digitized organizations, that is, organizations run in a technology-drenched context employing technology-focused professionals (London & Diamante, 2002).

Continuous learning is achieved when managers support a climate where feedback is freely exchanged, employees have a clear and shared vision of the organizational goals and values, and employees are sent to seminars or training programs—most of the time with paid travel and expenses. There is genuine commitment to growth. A greater commitment to training may be reflected in the organization's adoption of 360-degree-feedback programs, leadership development activities, assessment centers, internal "universities," and other programs targeting self-awareness, interpersonal acumen, or related competencies that improve productivity by improving the person (London, 1992, 1998b).

The Wellness Scorecard

Continuous improvement at the individual and organization level enables a lifelong approach to business, management, and operations. Realizing that change is constant, there is no better way to ensure progress than to build a culture around human development and well-being. A sample wellness scorecard is presented in Exhibit 14.2 as guidance for building metrics useful for the implementation of and evaluation of wellness initiatives. Of course, there is nothing more important to an organization's bottom line than human capital, so the scorecard makes the issue of human health and well-being "digestable" to senior management.

The scorecard is easy to customize and can be used on departmental or organizational levels. Components of the organizational wellness scorecard can be linked to performance management or evaluation standards and objectives. Using the tactics on the scorecard collectively builds infrastructure that sustains a culture—and may drive the culture.

Summary

There are three basic steps to becoming a healthy organization:

1. *Examine the risk factors.* Organizational strategy must address both job and workplace factors. Job factors are the physical working conditions, the ergonomic aspects of a job, the temporal aspects of the workday and tasks, the actual work content, job autonomy, coworker relations, the quality of supervision, and the financial or economic aspects. Workplace factors are work climate and culture, communications, group dynamics that affect decisions, management practices, leadership, labor management relations, existing workplace health promotion, and occupational health and safety activities. Organizational health scans, we predict, will become commonplace as health care cost reduction becomes

EXHIBIT 14.2. SAMPLE ORGANIZATIONAL WELLNESS SCORECARD.

Rate each of the following elements in terms of the extent to which you see evidence that the company truly values them. Respond to each element with *Yes* or *No*.

Management Practices

1. Management instills a sense of inspiration.
2. Managers are focused on expanding themselves in entrepreneurial, creative ways to sustain competitive business advantage, while also journeying on an *internally expansive* path uncovering self and interpersonal insights.
3. Employees are provided multiple pathways to address professional and personal needs.
4. Management controls focus on business outcomes (rather than compliance behaviors).
5. Internal competition is avoided so that the focus can be on beating the competition, mastery learning, or the creation of mutually beneficial objectives.

Work Itself

1. Jobs promote a sense of meaningfulness.
2. Performance evaluation reflects genuine, valuable business outcomes.
3. Roles and responsibilities are clear.
4. Redundant or repetitive tasks are softened by the use of shifts, cognitive or physical breaks, and other ways of countering the ill effects of repetition.
5. Employee assessments reflect appreciation for the competencies needed by the business in relation to individuals' need to "express themselves" (knowledge, skills, abilities, personal characteristics, and interests).

Environment and Safety

1. Occupational health and safety standards are adhered to, trained against, and monitored.
2. Menu-driven benefit plans are implemented.
3. Employee assistance programs are integrated into the employee's day.
4. Employees are rewarded for identifying problems.
5. Active evaluations are conducted to improve the physical workplace.

Culture

1. The workforce participates in goal setting and gets a response from leadership.
2. Organizational deeds exemplify altruism.
3. The organization is designed to optimize user or consumer experiences at all points of the trade cycle.
4. Structure, rules, and policy are understood to be impermanent mechanisms, open to change or transformation when market demands dictate.
5. Conflict is managed to drive creativity and experimentation and to fuel curiosity aimed toward mutual, valuable business goals.

EXHIBIT 14.2. SAMPLE ORGANIZATIONAL WELLNESS SCORECARD, Cont'd.

Workforce Development

1. Stress management programs exist or are available.

2. Management workshops link personal and professional well-being.

3. Career paths, mentoring, supportive networks, customized educational programs, self-management workshops, and other *connective mechanisms* guard against isolation and loneliness and offer nurturance, social support, and other psychosocial elements that affect behavior.

4. Newcomer orientation establishes and aligns business goal expectations and cultural openness and adaptation.

5. Self-learning is separated from formal performance evaluation so that personnel decisions can reflect human potential and not merely performance in a given job.

Communication

1. The state of the business is communicated enterprise-wide, strategically.

2. Shifts in business strategy are accompanied by *town hall* meetings or localized communication.

3. Progress is measured and communicated within relevant teams and across teams that work together indirectly.

4. Bottom-up feedback mechanisms enable leaders to remain in the know.

5. The workforce feels free to express contrary viewpoints.

Leadership

1. Leadership monitors "bottom-line" (nonactuarial) indices of organizational performance—(a) voluntary turnover, (b) medical costs associated with stress-related disorders, and (c) costs of mismanaged conflict (litigation, stalled projects, slow implementation, failure to enhance product functionality, incongruent user or consumer experiences, lack of innovation)—gauging the human "cost" of profitability.

2. Executives lead by displaying balanced or holistic lifestyles, demonstrating the need to attend to human and social needs.

3. There are linkages between executives and *greater goods* in terms of their community involvement or roles in other, larger-than-oneself efforts.

4. The social construction of the organization optimizes technology that meets human and organizational needs.

5. The annual report speaks to intangible assets, to educating stakeholders, and to meeting investor expectations for wise growth through balanced management that mitigates risk to people and profit.

Scoring

This organizational wellness scorecard consists of a total of thirty-five (35) items, divided into seven (7) categories. The scorecard can be used to identify problem areas; compare perceptions of managers, departments, or levels; and accelerate the efficacy of strategic planning sessions. A *yes* scores 1 point, and a *no* scores 0 points:

EXHIBIT 14.2. SAMPLE ORGANIZATIONAL WELLNESS SCORECARD, Cont'd.

Score	Interpretation
25–35	Healthy Workplace

This workplace shows support for human and financial concerns. Wisely, the culture strengthens itself by valuing not only what the business does but how it does it. There is an understanding that enables *integration* between human and business requirements when establishing goals, methods, and results. The quality of management is top tier, and there is a constant focus on growth—for people and services or profit.

14–24	Diminished Health Workplace

An organizational environment that is torn in its desire to integrate organizational and human requirements. At times there is hope that integration of human and organizational needs is on the horizon, yet at other times this seems impossible. Strain, conflict, insecurity, and stress are unnecessarily pressing upon organizational execution—slowing things down, complicating operations, and placing strategy at risk. Policies and programs appear supportive of human concerns, but these initiatives are viewed as window treatments. Management talks a good game but likely does not walk the walk. Long-term organizational growth is at risk.

1–13	Unhealthy Workplace

An environment that is overly focused on generating organizational outcomes and is myopic about how such outcomes materialize. Human capital is viewed as a fungible asset. There is little or no thought given to optimizing human performance—other than establishing, expecting, and measuring organizational results. This is a short-term game—growth, if it occurs, is not sustainable.

essential. Practical checklists, organizational surveys, or other metrics with a list of "healthy ingredients" can be easily assembled, and managers can be held accountable for identifying deficiencies and acting on them. Indeed, this tactic of measurement, analysis, feedback, and action planning is routine in organization development practice. Over time, individual organizations can track their progress, compare departments, and indeed, embark on research of their own to identify the ingredients that appear most beneficial to morale and productivity. Perhaps in time, organizations can share their findings, creating a "Health Fortune" database useful to business executives, health practitioners, policy makers, and researchers committed to continuously improving the workplace.

2. *Zero in on desired outcomes.* Such outcomes can include improved individual health, return on investments, reduced litigation, reduced absenteeism, higher job work performance, and greater satisfaction among customers. Start with customer or client impact; keep everything aligned with customer or client expectations.

3. *Unleash health tactics.* Finally, identify the actions required to address underlying factors that threaten the achievement of desired outcomes. These actions are the aforementioned wellness programs, such as employee assistance programs; stress management programs; mentoring, conflict resolution, and diversity programs; diet and exercise programs; and customized programs to tackle special issues such as anger, hostility, and other emotions. Teach self-management so that personal accountability for individual wellness is high and incorporate spirituality (in terms of altruism, giving, community work, teaching and training, social responsibility, or faith-based, optional meditative opportunities) to compensate for leadership shortcomings. Encourage career development and continuous learning and build work and life balance plans that are customer-centric and valued by a culture equally driven to ensure that both people and profit grow. (Exhibit 14.3 on page 493 displays helpful resources supplemental to the references.)

References

Aronson, D. (2002). Managing the diversity revolution: Best practices for 21st century business. *Civil Rights Journal, 4,* 1–17.

Baron, R. A. (1998). Destructive criticism: Impact on conflict, self-efficacy and task performance. *Journal of Applied Psychology, 73,* 199–207.

Belkic, K. L., Landsbergis, P. A., Schnall, P. L., & Baker, D. (2004). Is job strain a major source of cardiovascular disease? *Scandinavian Journal of Work and Environmental Health, 30,* 85–128.

Benson, H. (1975). *The relaxation response.* New York: Avon.

Benson, H. (1984). *Beyond the relaxation response.* New York: Berkley.

Bocchino, C., Hartman, B. W., & Foley, P. F. (2003). The relationship between person-organization congruence, perceived violations of the psychological contract, and occupational stress symptoms. *Consulting Psychology Journal, 55,* 203–214.

Bond, J., Galinsky, E., & Hill, J. (2004). *When work works.* Retrieved, November 4, 2004, from www.familiesandwork.org

Bond, J., Thompson, C., Galinsky, E., & Prottas, D. (2002). *Highlights of the National Study of the Changing Workforce: Executive summary.* Retrieved October 26, 2005, from http://www.familiesandwork.org/summary/nscw2002.pdf

Budner, S. (1962). Intolerance of ambiguity as a personality variable. *Journal of Personality, 30,* 29–59.

Clarkson, K. W., Miller, R. L., Jentz, G. L., & Cross, F. B. (2003). *West's business law.* New York: Southwestern College/West.

Collard, B., Epperheimer, J. W., & Saign, D. (1996). *Career resilience in a changing workplace.* Columbus, OH: ERIC Clearinghouse on Adult, Career, and Vocational Education. (ED 396 191)

Cortina, L. M., Magley, V. J., Williams, J. H., & Langhout, R. D. (2001). Incivility in the workplace: Incidence and impact. *Journal of Occupational Health Psychology, 6,* 64–80.

Dembroski, T. M., MacDougall, J. M., Williams, R. B., Haney, T. L., & Blumenthal, J. A. (1985). Components of type A, hostility and anger: Relationship to angiographic findings. *Psychosomatic Medicine, 47*, 219–233.

Dembroski, T. M., MacDougall, J. M., Costa, P. T., & Grandits, G. A. (1999). Antagonistic hostility as a predictor of coronary heart disease in the multiple risk factor intervention trial. *Psychosomatic Medicine, 51*, 514–522.

Di Martino, V., & Musri, M. (2001). *Guidance for the prevention of stress and violence at the workplace.* Retrieved October 21, 2005, http://www.ilo.org/public/english/protection/safework/papers/malaysia/guide.pdf

Diamante, T., & Hyland, M. (2004, March). *Employees' response to a massive cultural change: Stress reactions in the workplace.* Presentation at the Eastern Academy of Management Annual Conference, Providence, Rhode Island.

Diamante, T., & London, M. (2002). Expansive leadership in an age of digital technology. *Journal of Management Development, 21*, 404–416.

Diamante, T., & Primavera, L. (2005). The professional practice of executive coaching: Principles, practices & key decisions. *International Journal of Decision Ethics, 1*, 85–115.

Diamante, T., Reid, C., & Giglio, L. (1995, March). Make the right training move: Designing diversity programs. *HR Magazine*, pp. 60–65.

Duhart, J. (2001). *Violence in the workplace, 1993–99* (Bureau of Justice Statistics special report). Washington, DC: Bureau of Justice Statistics.

Families and Work Institute. (2002). *National Study of the Changing Workforce: Executive summary.* Retrieved October 26, 2005, from http://www.familiesandwork.org/announce/2002NSCW.html

French, M. T., Dunlap, L., Roman, P. M., & Steel, P. D. (1997). Factors that influence the use and perception of employee assistance programs at six worksites. *Journal of Occupational Health Psychology, 2*, 312–324.

Friedman, M., & DiMatteo, M. R. (1989). *Health psychology.* Upper Saddle River, NJ: Prentice Hall.

Friedman, M., & Rosenman, R. H. (1974). *Type A behavior and your heart.* New York: Knopf.

Fullerton, H. N. (1999, November). Labor force projections to 2008: Steady growth and changing composition. *Monthly Labor Review*, pp. 19–32.

Furnham, A., & Ribchester, T. (1995). Tolerance of ambiguity: A review of the concept. *Current Psychology, 14*, 179–199.

Gruenwald, T. L., Kemeny, M. E., Aziz, N., & Fahey, J. L. (2004). Acute threat to the social self: Shame, social self-esteem and cortisol activity. *Psychosomatic Medicine, 66*, 915–924.

Haan, M. (1988). Job strain and ischaemic heart disease: An epidemiological study of metal workers. *Annals of Clinical Research, 20*, 143–145.

Haan, M. (1989). Job strain and cardiovascular disease: A ten year prospective study. *American Journal of Epidemiology, 122*, 532–540.

Hackman, J. R. (2003). *Leading teams.* Boston: Harvard Business School Press.

Hawkley, L. C., Burleson, M. H., Berntson, G. G., & Cacioppo, J. T. (2003). Loneliness in everyday life: Cardiovascular activity, psychosocial context and health behaviors. *Journal of Personality and Social Psychology, 85*, 105–112.

Hecker, M., Chesney, M., Black, G., & Frautschi, N. (1988). Coronary prone behaviors in the Western Collaborative Group Study. *Psychosomatic Medicine, 50*, 153–164.

Heider, F. (1958). *The psychology of interpersonal relations.* New York: Wiley.

Hollander, R. B., & Lengermann, J. J. (1988). Corporate characteristics and worksite health promotion programs: Survey findings from Fortune 500 companies. *Social Science & Medicine, 26,* 491–501.

International Employees Assistance Professionals Association. (2005). Home page. Retrieved October 20, 2005, from http://www.eapassn.org

Israel, B. A., Baker, E. A., Goldenhar, L. M., & Heaney, C. A. (1996). Occupational stress, safety, and health: Framework and principles for effective prevention interventions. *Journal of Occupational Health Psychology, 1,* 261–286.

Israel, B. A., Schurman, S. J., & House, J. S. (1989). Action research on occupational stress: Involving workers as researchers. *International Journal of Health Services, 19,* 135–155.

Ivancevich, J., & Lidwell, W. (2004). *Guidelines for excellence in management.* New York: Texere, Thomson.

Ivancevich, J., Matteson, M. T., Freedman, S., & Phillips, J. S. (1990). Worksite stress management interventions. *American Psychologist, 43,* 252–261.

Jex, S. M., Adams, G. A., Bachrach, D. G., & Sorenson, S. (2003). The impact of situational constraints, role stressors and commitment on employee altruism. *Journal of Occupational Health Psychology, 8,* 171–180.

Job Stress Network. (2004). *Hostility and coronary heart disease.* Retrieved November 4, 2004, from www.workhealth.org

Johnson, W. B. (2002). The intentional mentor: Strategies and guidelines for the practice of mentoring. *Professional Psychology: Research and Practice, 33,* 88–96.

Judy, R. W., & D'Amico, C. (1999). *Workforce 2020: Work and workers in the 21st century.* Indianapolis, IN: Hudson Institute.

Kahn, R. L., & Byosier, P. (1992). Stress in organizations. In M. D. Dunnette & L. Hough (Eds.), *Handbook of industrial & organizational psychology* (pp. 571–650). Palo Alto, CA: Consulting Psychologists Press.

Kenny, D. T., & Cooper, C. L. (2003). Occupational stress and its management. *International Journal of Stress Management, 10,* 275–279.

Kiecolt-Glaser, J. K., McGuire, L., Robles, T. F., & Glaser, R. (2002). Psychoneuroimmunology: Psychological influences on immune function and health. *Journal of Consulting and Clinical Psychology, 70,* 537–547.

Klarreich, S. H., DiGiuseppe, R., & DiMattia, D. (1987). Cost effectiveness of employee assistance programs with rational emotive therapy. *Professional Psychology, 18,* 140–144.

Kobasa, S. C., Maddi, S. R., Pucetti, M., & Zola, M. (1986). Relative effectiveness of hardiness, exercise and social support as resources against illness. *Journal of Psychosomatic Research, 29,* 525–533.

Lepine, J., & VanDyne, L. (2001). Peer responses to low performers: An attributional model of helping in the context of groups. *Academy of Management Review, 26,* 67–84.

Lepore, S. J. (1995). Cynicism, social support and cardiovascular reactivity. *Health Psychology, 14,* 210–216.

London, M. (1992). *Human resource development in changing organizations.* Westport, CT: Greenwood Press.

London, M. (1998a). *Career barriers.* Mahwah, NJ: Erlbaum.

London, M. (1998b). *Self and inter-personal insight.* New York: Oxford University Press.

London, M., & Diamante, T. (2002). Technology-focused expansive professionals: Continuous learning in the high-technology sector. *Human Resources Development Review, 1,* 500–524.

Maddi, S. R. (1998). Hardiness in health and effectiveness. In H. S. Friedman (Ed.), *Encyclopedia of mental health* (pp. 323–333). San Diego, CA: Academic Press.

Maddi, S. R. (2002). The story of hardiness: Twenty years of theorizing, research and practice. *Consulting Psychology Journal, 54,* 175–185.

Maddi, S. R., & Hightower, M. (1999). Hardiness and optimism as expressed in coping patterns. *Consulting Psychology Journal, 51,* 95–105.

Maier, S., & Laudenslager, M. (1985). Stress and health: Exploring links. *Psychology Today, 19,* 44.

Mailoo, V. J., & Williams, C. J. (2004). Psychoneuroimmunology: A theoretical basis for occupational therapy in oncology? *International Journal of Therapy and Rehabilitation, 11,* 7–12.

Marsland, A. L., Cohen, S., Rabin, B. S., & Manuck, S. B. (2001). Associations between stress, trait negative affect, acute immune reactivity and antibody response to hepatitis B injection in healthy young adults. *Health Psychology, 20,* 4–11.

Masterson, S. S. (2001). A trickle-down model of organizational justice: Relating employees' and customers' perception of and reactions to fairness. *Journal of Applied Psychology, 86,* 594–604.

Mitroff, I., & Denton, M. (1999). Spirituality in the workplace. *Sloan Management Review, 4,* 83–92.

Moyers, B. (1993). *Healing and the mind.* New York: Doubleday.

Niaura, R., Todaro, J. F., Stroud, L., Spiro, A., Ward, K. D., & Weiss, S. (2002). Hostility, the metabolic syndrome and incident coronary heart disease. *Health Psychology, 21,* 588–593.

National Institute for Occupational Safety and Health. (1999). *Stress at work* (DHHS [NIOSH] Publication No. 99-101). Retrieved November 4, 2004, from http://www.cdc.gov/niosh/pdfs/stress.pdf

National Institute for Occupational Safety and Health. (2000). Background. In *Creating healthy work organizations: Notice of availability of funds for fiscal year 1998.* Retrieved January 15, 2005, from http://www.cdc.gov/niosh/frn98024.html

Organ, D. W., & Ryan, K. (1995). A meta-analytic review of attitudinal and dispositional predictors of organization citizenship behavior. *Personnel Psychology, 48,* 775–802.

Pearson, C., Anderson, L., & Porath, C. (2000). Assessing and attacking workplace incivility. *Organizational Dynamics, 29,* 123–137.

Rush, M. C., Schjoel, W. A., & Barnard, S. M. (1995). Psychological resiliency in the public sector: Hardiness and pressure for change. *Journal of Vocational Behavior, 46,* 17–39.

Sauter, S. L., Murphy, L. R., & Hurrell, J. J. (1990). Prevention of work-related psychological disorders. *American Psychologist, 45,* 1146–1158.

Schat, A. C., & Kelloway, E. K. (2000). Effects of perceived control on the outcomes of workplace aggression and violence. *Journal of Occupational Health Psychology, 5,* 386–402.

Schein, E. H. (2004). *Organizational culture and leadership* (3rd ed.). San Francisco: Jossey-Bass.

Schnall, P. L., & Landsbergis, P. A. (1994). Job strain and cardiovascular disease. *Annual Review of Public Health, 15,* 381–411.

Schurman, S. J., & Israel, B. A. (1995). Redesigning work systems to reduce stress: A participatory action research approach to creating change. In L. R. Murphy, J. J. Hurrell Jr., S. L. Sauter, & G. P. Keita (Eds.), *Job stress interventions.* Washington, DC: American Psychological Association.

Seligman, M.E.P. (1991). *Learned optimism.* New York: Knopf.

Seligman, M.E.P., & Csikszentmihalyi, M. (2000). Positive psychology. *American Psychologist, 55,* 5–14

Seligman, M.E.P., & Schulman, P. (1986). Explanatory style as a predictor of quitting among sales agents. *Journal of Personality and Social Psychology, 50,* 832–838

Senge, P. (1994). *The fifth discipline: The art and practice of the learning organization.* New York: Doubleday.

Sheese, B. E., Brown, E. L., & Graziano, W. G. (2003). Emotional expression in cyberspace: Searching for moderators of the Pennebacker disclosure effect via e-mail. *Health Psychology, 23,* 457–464.

Smith, C. A., Haynes, K. N., Lazarus, R. S., & Pope, L. K. (1993). In search of the "hot" cognitions: Attributions, appraisals, and their relation to emotion. *Journal of Personality and Social Psychology, 65,* 916–929.

Smith, M., & McGhan, W. (1996). Flirting with the financials of fat in the workplace: Obesity. *Business and Health, 14*(7), 53–54.

Smith, T. W., Pope, M. K., Rhodewalt, F., & Poulton, J. L. (1989). Optimism, neuroticism, coping, and symptom reports: An alternative interpretation of the Life Orientation Test. *Journal of Personality and Social Psychology, 56,* 640–648.

Srivastva, S., Cooperrider, D. L., & Associates. (1990). *Appreciative management and leadership.* San Francisco: Jossey-Bass.

Stress. (2001, September). Retrieved November 22, 2004, from http://www.reutershealth.com/wellconnected/doc31.html

Tavris, C. (1989). *Anger: The misunderstood emotion.* New York: Simon & Schuster.

Taylor, S. E., & Brown, J. D. (1988). Illusion and well-being: A social psychological perspective on mental health. *Psychological Bulletin, 103,* 193–210.

Theorell, T., & Karasek, R. A. (1996). Current issues relating to psychosocial job strain and cardiovascular disease research. *Journal of Occupational Health Psychology, 1,* 9–26.

Thompson, S. C., Sobolew-Shubin, A., Galbraith, M. E., Schwankovsky, L., & Cruzen, D. (1993). Maintaining perceptions of control: Finding perceived control in low-control circumstances. *Journal of Personality and Social Psychology, 64,* 293–304.

Tsutsumi, A., & Kawakami, N. (2004). A review of empirical studies on the model of effort-reward imbalance at work: Reducing occupational stress by implementing a new theory. *Social Science & Medicine, 59,* 2335–2359.

Uchino, B. N. (2004). *Social support and physical health outcomes: Understanding the health consequences of our relationships.* New Haven, CT: Yale University Press.

U.S. Department of Health and Human Services. (2004). *Healthy people 2010: The cornerstone for prevention.* Rockville, MD: U.S. Department of Health and Human Services, Office of Disease Prevention and Health Promotion.

U.S. Preventive Services Task Force. (2002). *Screening for depression: What's new from the USPSTF* [fact sheet]. (AHRQ Publication No. APPIP02-0019). Rockville, MD: Agency for Healthcare Research and Quality.

Vaillant, G. E. (2000). Adaptive mental mechanisms and their role in positive psychology. *American Psychologist, 55,* 9–98.

Weiner, B. (1974). *Achievement motivation and attribution theory.* Morristown, NJ: General Learning Press.

Weiner, B. (1986). *An attributional theory of motivation and emotion.* New York: Springer-Verlag.

The White House. (2002). *National Domestic Violence Awareness Month.* Retrieved November 4, 2004, from http://www.whitehouse.gov/news/releases/2002/10/20021001-8.html

Williams, R., & Williams, V. (1993). *Anger kills.* New York: HarperCollins.

Zink, T., & Sill, M. (2004). Intimate partner violence and job instability. *Journal of the American Medical Women's Association, 59,* 32–35.

EXHIBIT 14.3. HELPFUL RESOURCES.

Adler, S. J. (1994). *The jury: Trial and error in the American courtroom.* New York: Times Books.

Argyris, C. (1999). *On organizational learning.* Malden, MA: Blackwell.

Das, S. (1997). *Awakening the Buddha within.* New York: Broadway Books.

Gates, B. (1999). *Business @ the speed of thought: Using a digital nervous system.* New York: Warner Books.

Harvard Business Review. (1979). *On human relations.* New York: HarperCollins

Lazurus, R. S. (1991). Cognition and motivation in emotion. *American Psychologist, 46,* 352–367.

Levinson, H. (1968). *The exceptional executive: A psychological approach.* Cambridge, MA: Harvard University Press.

McGrath, J. E., & Altman, I. (1966). *Small group research: A synthesis and critique of the field.* Austin, TX: Holt, Rinehart & Winston.

Pelletier, K. R. (1994). *Sound mind, sound body.* New York: Simon & Schuster.

Reece, B. L., & Brandt, R. (1993). *Effective human relations.* Boston: Houghton Mifflin.

Schneider, B. (1990). *Organizational climate and culture.* San Francisco: Jossey-Bass.

Westin, A. F., & Feliu, A. G. (1987). *Resolving employment disputes without litigation.* Washington, DC: Bureau of National Affairs.

CHAPTER FIFTEEN

ENHANCING DEVELOPMENT

Penelope Buschman Gemma
Joan Arnold

D evelopment is a dynamic lifelong process that by its nature is never complete. Transformative and evolving, it occurs within the context of every individual, family, group, and community as they interact with their environments and culture.

Development of the self is characterized by complexity and interaction, and often experienced with difficulty. In human development both healthy and unhealthy patterns are expressed. Families, groups, and communities also have their own developmental courses and dynamics, with the individual as the essential element of all these systems. Among the various systems with which the individual affiliates and in which the individual is nurtured, the family is surely the most significant. The support of families and the promotion of healthy family life are essential to self-development. Likewise, families and groups, with which individuals affiliate, are the essential building blocks of the community.

Families prepare their members to move into the outside world and to function beyond the familiar relationships within the family system. Yet families are often at risk and inadequately prepared or unable to endow their members with needed survival skills. Individuals who suffer from the absence of family unity and sustenance may find themselves isolated, alienated, and poorly prepared to enter and find successful ties to larger systems. These are overwhelming obstacles that thwart the development of healthy families and hence the developing self. Some individuals may also emerge from families where sustenance is unavailable with unexpected strengths and capacities.

Groups provide opportunities for people to affiliate through common goals, find support, accomplish various tasks, and realize values and beliefs. Groups may be, for example, schools, places of worship, social and political organizations, self-help entities, volunteer and service efforts, or professional and work-related organizations. Group work supports and extends personal development by providing a context in which group members gain new information, validation, insight, and assistance through their participation. The group becomes the context in which change and growth can occur. Groups also have identities of their own, which members reflect. Group mind, a phenomenon expressing shared ways of thinking, can be a powerful positive or negative force as individuals lose their personal identity and gain a shared identity.

Communities, the larger systems in which individuals, families, and groups interact, reflect and create a life force. Communities are composed of people and resources in interaction. A community depleted of resources cannot sustain its members and will not flourish. Communities have histories of their own, to which members contribute. Communities provide systems in which members can live, work, play, travel, learn, and feel safe. Never static, communities are always evolving and changing in demographics, systems of safety, education and health care, cultural influences, political factors, housing options, and recreational resources.

Development is context based, multidimensional, nonstatic, and process oriented (Leadbeater, Schellenbach, Maton, & Dodgen, 2004). Social, cultural, and historical contexts are influences that profoundly affect the development of individuals, families, groups, and communities.

Individual Development

Development of the individual is a gradually unfolding, dynamic process. No one theory has been constructed to encompass all aspects of growth. Theorists, as they strive to build frames of reference in which to order and interpret the facts and patterns of human development, differ in their views about the origin of behavior. Points of view based on the philosophies of John Locke (1964) and Jean-Jacques Rousseau (Boyd, 1962), such as nature versus nurture and heredity versus environment, continue to influence thinking and theory formation regarding individual development. The notion of self-generativity, the individual's ability to actively shape the self within the context of heredity and environment, has influenced developmental thinking (Schuster & Ashburn, 1992). More recently, development also has been considered within the context of culture (Coll & Magnuson, 2000). Resilience as a construct is shaping current research on human development (Glantz & Sloboda, 1999; Kaplan, 1999; Luthar & Zelazo, 2003; Masten, 2001; Rutter, 2000; Walsh, 2003). An awareness of disparity has also contributed greatly to an understanding of thwarted and limited development and unequal potential (Masten, 1999; U.S. Department of Health and Human Services, 2000; Gebbie, Rosenstock, & Hernandez, 2003). The field of genetics is revolutionizing thinking about the limitations and potentials of the human being and providing options for preventing and ameliorating conditions previously considered untreatable (Rutter, 1994).

Beginning with conception and ending with death, the development of the individual evolves over a lifetime. The first theorist to build upon the psychodynamic view of development postulated by Sigmund Freud (1935) was Erik Erikson (1963), who extended this theory to cover the life span of the individual. Erikson (1963) identified eight stages of development, each posing an essential task for growth. In each task are opposing dispositions that must be brought into balance for the individual to achieve the basic and necessary strength to move ahead. Erikson viewed each stage, or step, as a potential crisis (that is, a turning point or crucial period of vulnerability and potential) and as "the ontogenetic source of generational strength and maladjustment" (Erikson, 1968, p. 96).

Erikson proposed that development itself is an orderly process that is determined biologically and occurs within the context of family and community. He described the healthy individual as one who actively masters the environment, demonstrates a unified personality, and is able to perceive the self accurately in the world (Erikson, 1968). Personality, therefore, can be said to develop according to the steps predetermined in the human organism's readiness to be driven toward, to be aware of, and to interact with a widening radius of significant individuals and institutions (Erikson, 1968). The body of Erikson's work, which evolved over his lifetime, has significantly shaped the contemporary portrayal of human development as complex and psychobiological, an interactive process occurring across the life course. His framework set the stage for other theorists to postulate from his monumental contributions.

Robert Havighurst (1972), who was greatly influenced by Erikson's (1963) theory of psychosocial development, identified tasks crucial to the individual's growth. According to Havighurst, developmental tasks arise within certain time periods in an individual's life. Successful completion of these life phase tasks leads to satisfaction and future success, whereas failure leads to unhappiness, lack of future achievement, and ultimate social disapproval. Havighurst postulated that all human beings demonstrate a readiness to master life phase–related tasks, and that this readiness is based on a unique confluence of physical, psychological, and social factors. Havighurst proposed that development is a cognitive learning process. Tasks develop out of a combination of pressures arising from physical development, cultural expectations, and individual values and goals. He postulated the occurrence of *teachable moments,* when a special sensitivity or readiness to learn a task arises from a unique combination of physical, social, and psychic preparedness.

Many other theorists have contributed to an understanding of development in highly specific areas and during defined time periods. Piaget's seminal work in the study of cognition (Piaget, 1963; Piaget & Inhelder, 1969); Chess and Thomas's (1986) and Kagan's (1984, 1989) studies of temperamental patterns in young children; Gilligan's (1984) extensive research on gender-specific developmental issues; Piaget's (1965), Kohlberg's (1981), Gilligan's (1986), and Coles's (1997) contributions to an understanding of moral development; Maslow's (1968) description of self-actualization; and Rutter's (1994) exploration of turning points all address areas of development that significantly influence the health and well-being of the individual.

Identifying and analyzing the process of individual development is challenging. Many forces contribute to a healthy developmental process. Among these are genetic, physiological, physical, emotional, social, cultural, moral, and spiritual factors that, taken together, form the dimensions of the self. Genetic influences predetermine the potential for health, illness, disability, and death. Patterns of family risk for illness are found in the repeated incidence of health problems from one generation to the next. The profound impact of intergenerational transmission on human growth and development is being realized as genetic research advances (Rutter, 2000).

The idea that persons are whole beings and therefore must be perceived holistically runs counter to the notion that the individual can be reduced to component parts for analysis. When examining the parts, the health care professional must be mindful that this vantage point is necessarily myopic. This microscopic view must be mediated by the more expansive perspective of the whole system, but the holistic perspective is difficult to substantiate because of the lack of holistic indicators. It is possible to understand the smallest unit of human matter in all its intricacies, yet it is impossible to fully comprehend a particular human action. The whole being is also difficult to comprehend; therefore parameters are set as a reference range. Hence blood values for human biochemistry have been determined, just as patterns for behavior, termed *milestones,* have become markers for human development. Outliers, even though falling beyond the parameters set, are recognized for the uniqueness of their individual patterns. Each person is appreciated for the extent to which he or she manifests individuality while expressing shared characteristics with other human beings.

The trajectories of human development and of psychopathology have largely been understood as separate, antithetical processes; one is perceived as supporting growth and the other as thwarting growth. As a result, these patterns of behavior have been viewed from different perspectives, as though the origins of healthy growth and development were unrelated to the roots of pathology. However, development can no longer be viewed from this dichotomous perspective. Rather, development is a process profoundly influenced by the experience of loss. Myriad losses are enfolded and shape the individual in an unfolding of vulnerability, strength, and insight. Likewise, interaction is ongoing with forces found in the context of living, including family dynamics, community and environmental phenomena, cultural nuances, and societal demands. It is in moving through the continuum of life that emotions and behaviors emerge, which can be both health promoting and health depleting. In many cases they are both. Development results from the interplay of these forces. Resilience supports both healthy growth as well as the capacity to emerge from and with pathology. Surely, the ability to persevere in adversity and to survive despite horrific losses illustrates the resilient self. Resilience then may fuel development and therefore life itself.

How development evolves from conception to death has been well explicated in the human growth and development literature (Erikson, 1963; Havighurst, 1972; Maslow, 1968; Schuster & Ashburn, 1992). Underlying the concept of growth is the idea of a life span that traverses the life process and extends to death. No individual is guaranteed long life, but each person has a lifetime. For some the lifetime is quite limited. Prenatal, infant, and child death (Arnold & Gemma, 1994) are exquisitely painful losses that deepen our respect for the realization that lifetimes can be short. With this realization comes the awareness that each life, regardless of its length, is significant and affects the ever expanding circles of others connected to it.

It is anticipated that between the years 2000 and 2050, the shape of the population of the United States will become increasingly rectangular, reflecting the increasing numbers of elderly. It is also anticipated that by the year 2045, 95 percent of all deaths will occur between the ages of seventy-seven and ninety-three, with the average age of death being somewhere around eighty-five years (Schaie & Willis, 2002). The growth of an aging population calls not only for a new orientation to aged individuals and their development but also a new recognition of their contributions to family, group, and community life. When all ages are welcomed into the fabric of life, the weave becomes a healthier one (Pipher, 1999). Elders continue to contribute to the workforce as well as becoming sage advisers and mentors, teaching from the perspective of wisdom and experience. Further, retirement can be a dynamic time for fulfilling and exploring a multiplicity of interests. For those elders who are disabled or ill, this period of diminished health poses challenges in care and cost for an extended period of time. The accrued loss is felt by families, communities, and health institutions. Discussions of these population changes are under way at the federal level to reconfigure national guidelines for Social Security and insurance benefits and to accommodate an aging and graying workforce.

The individual develops and is nurtured in relationships throughout life; these relationships are critical to survival and growth. The infant is a competent and multitalented human being who is dependent on parents and other caregivers for existence. In the earliest phases of development the infant depends on the caregiver for nurture and safety, but as development proceeds the child grows in independent competencies and becomes more able to sustain the self. In addition, the child's connections to others are expanded beyond the immediate caregivers to significant others, from whom the child also derives nurturance. As growth continues, the individual enters into interdependent relationships and into a dynamic exchange, balancing need and want, as the recipient as well as the provider. With aging, individuals may be able to develop through disconnections and solitude as significant persons and support systems die, allowing new growth through memory and reminiscence. As throughout the life span, the enfolding of loss becomes a determining influence in development.

Family Development

A family, or cluster of persons living with and relating to one another, is the essential unit in which development occurs. Families grow and diminish as members are born or adopted, move away, and die. Families move through stages of development as the configurations and relationships among members change and grow and withstand and rebound from disruptive life challenges (Carter & McGoldrick, 1999; Walsh, 1998). A family is a system that challenges and nurtures the individual and provides the context that supports the healthy development of its members. A family is both a source of strength as well as a source of stress (Fogarty, 1985). Families may be described in many ways, as biological families, adoptive families, kinship networks, and families of choice (Weston, 1991).

Families influence development through the nature and consistency of support given to their members. When a family is depleted of its own resources, members' needs may be unmet unless alternate sources of support outside the family system can be located. A family milieu provides a source of *give and take*, and members quickly learn the capacities of a family to respond to their needs. The exchanges among members can be viewed as much like the steps of a dance, as members come together and then pull apart in an effort to connect with and to disengage from each other (Haley, 1980). Family life is a profound determinant of self-development; each member is affected individually by the myriad factors and forces found in a family.

Each family is held together by ties of history and experience that bind the members to each other and to the family as a whole (Carter & McGoldrick, 1999). Family ties are deep and long lasting, regardless of the stress and strife within the unit, and they influence the development of family members. Each family has a unique history, which traverses multigenerational family life cycles (Gerson, 1995; Leadbeater et al., 2004). Family history influences not only family values and beliefs but also the health potential of each member, as generational patterns are transmitted from one to the next.

Functional families tend to operate as open systems (Bowen, 1978). The boundaries that identify and define the family allow for mutual exchanges with the larger environment of the community and society. The boundaries also regulate input and output by filtering the amount and type of interchange with the environment. This kind of system regulation provides stability and enables the members of the family to experience constancy and predictable patterns, which facilitates a sense of security. Members derive satisfaction from the safety net provided by the family unit's ability to navigate its way through the daily challenges of family and community life. A family that adheres to its values and beliefs while also exhibiting flexibility provides a dependable structure for its members.

Families are the primary educators of their members. Families prepare their members to move outside the family system yet remain connected to it. They teach their members survival skills, including norms, values, roles, and communication and decision-making patterns. In addition, the transmission of family history and traditions, culture, religion, and spirituality provides members with a strong sense of family beliefs. It is the family belief system that provides the framework for the moral, ethical, and spiritual aspects of self-development.

The family tends to be goal directed, with its goals transmitted through the family's actions and efforts. Additionally, individual members learn to establish goals that may be self-enhancing, and they hope, attainable. Among these are goals related to health. The health patterns, behavioral choices, and coping strategies of the family are transmitted. Members may exhibit this learning in behaviors that are health enhancing and health depleting. The outcomes are often unpredictable.

Family roles and expectations contribute to the identities of individual members (Walsh, 1989) and are often carried on in contexts and relationships outside the family of origin. Roles are the expected behaviors that members assume to support the functions of the family. Roles permit orderly social interaction as well as balance and stability in the family. Roles that are flexible and reciprocal allow for growth, whereas roles that limit transactions and bind members to fixed behaviors limit growth and personal development.

Family communication patterns provide the foundation for the individual member to relate to others in the family and to the world. When communication is functional, the receiver gets the message that the sender intended. The family member is able to state his or her case; clarify and qualify the meaning of the message; ask for feedback; exhibit receptivity to the feedback; and accept responsibility for personal thoughts, feelings, and actions. Communication becomes a mutual process when clarity is the aim. Effective communication skills will support the member in all interactions and broaden the opportunities for gaining social support and a network of significant others (Watzlawick, 1978). Communication patterns that block, confuse, or manipulate limit authentic interactions with others and result in social distortion, alienation, and lack of support, thereby reducing the chances of maintaining a social network.

Family norms provide the developing self with rules that guide and regulate family behavior, whereas family values inculcate the inner convictions of what is right and wrong, good and bad, and desirable and undesirable. These family dynamics provide the developing self with guidelines to follow in deciphering the external world, evaluating the behavior of others, and reacting to observed behavior. A family also conveys values and beliefs concerning health and illness to its individual members. These shape the way the individual perceives and values health and its promotion. If the prospect for health is constrained by a lack of expectation for well-being, the individual will have an image of positive health as unattainable.

Family decision-making patterns provide skills in negotiating and methods for finding agreement on and demonstrating a commitment to a particular course of action (Minuchin, 1974). Families that allow issues to be processed and that arrive at decisions by consensus provide a rich foundation for their members in this area of skill development. Families that decide through compromise, a unilateral decision, or indecision confine the individual to giving in to others, rather than gaining from the perspective of others and the reformulation of personal thoughts. Effective decision making enables the individual to make choices about health and health care, thus fostering the development of the healthy self.

Self-care rests in the ability of individuals to meet their own needs, maximize their personal strengths, and become autonomous. The family supports the individual's development of personal boundaries and achievement of separation in order to become a distinct self (Minuchin & Nichols, 1993). Self-care enables members to identify and seek their own health agendas. Individuals possess personal health strengths that assist in dealing with health-depleting threats. The individual who learns dependency rather than self-care is more likely to turn control over to health care professionals rather than to negotiate and participate actively in decisions about health.

Evelyn Millis Duvall (1985) focused on family as a dynamic system whose individual members progress developmentally. Changes in one member necessitate changes in others and most certainly in the entire family system. Duvall maintains that as families develop, responsibilities remain constant but the focus shifts according to the specific stages. Duvall (1985) looks at the dynamics of development occurring in stages across the life span of a family. Each stage presents opportunities for individual members and families to make decisions, act on readiness, grow, and change.

A family provides an important context in which individuals learn and grow; a family is generally the primary context for individual development. A family nurtures and educates its members, providing a vital system of support that is identifiable by its own style and integrity. A family is also a stressful social and emotional system. Development is supported and thwarted as the family and its members interrelate. Family dynamics affect family members' development and prepare members for the larger world.

Group Development

Groups have their own organizational structures and dynamics. Individuals affiliate with myriad groups throughout their lives and grow and develop through and in these group relationships. Groups have identities of their own that significantly influence not only their members but also the larger circle of the community. Groups are a rich resource for individuals, families, and communities. Groups vary according to their intended purpose, style of leadership, phase of development, longevity, and interactional patterns. Each group is unique and balances the needs of its individual members with the group's own particular focus (Clark, 1994).

Groups may be informal or formal in their organization, depending on the type of the group and its leadership process. Friendships and a variety of other affiliations result as individuals bond together and form groups. These informal groupings may last throughout a lifetime or may be connected to developmental phases or purposefully short-lived goals. Groups serve to foster development beyond the family and to strengthen connections to schools, agencies, religious institutions, and other persons in the community. They protect against isolation and enable individuals to identify special interests and skills.

There are at least four types of formal groups: task, teaching, support, and psychotherapy. A task group focuses on the accomplishment of a given task and emphasizes decision making and problem solving. In most task groups there is pressure to complete the goal in an allocated time period, with the outcome being key. Examples of task groups include parent-teacher associations, committees to form a library, and volunteer community service groups. A teaching group is concerned with the processing of information and the teaching-learning exchange. Teaching groups abound and include scouting organizations, 4-H clubs, and health education groups. Support groups, which are commonplace in most communities, assist their members in dealing with emotional stress and focus on the expression of thoughts and feelings. These groups may be self-help or led by professionals. Support groups include Alcoholics Anonymous and Al-Anon, bereavement groups, and coalitions such as the National Alliance for the Mentally Ill (NAMI). Psychotherapy groups deal with intrapersonal and interpersonal aspects of personality (Ormont, 1992; Yalom, 1995). Psychotherapy groups may subscribe to a particular psychological theory or paradigm. These groups serve persons with diverse needs, such as families, partners, children, and those with common psychiatric problems.

Leadership is established within groups and may be shared among the members or may reside with a particular leader, either someone identified by the group or someone who emerges from the group. The style of leadership will differ with the type of group and will shift within each group as the process unfolds. When leadership is directed by an identified leader, it is considered authoritarian, or leader centered. When leadership is shared, the style is considered democratic, or group oriented. When less active, the leadership style is thought of as laissez-faire; in this case, consultation may be offered and information provided at timely interludes, with fewer actions expected from the leader.

Groups, being living systems, have a life span. Some groups may be intentionally short lived, whereas others may extend for months or years. Longevity influences the development of a group. Some groups may exist for a particular purpose and meet only once. Other groups may unfold and grow into different types for other purposes, taking on new form over time because of members' changing needs. Groups generally begin with an orientation phase in which common issues are discussed: namely, identity; control and power; the balancing of individual needs with group needs; and finally, acceptance and intimacy. Each of these issues is revisited again and again as the group develops. For the group to move into a working phase, many of these issues must be dealt with and assumptions stated so that members are clear about what the group stands for and what they believe. To arrive at the working phase, the group members must learn to work together cooperatively toward the intended purpose by accomplishing a given task, imparting knowledge, gaining support, or enabling intrapsychic analysis. As groups move toward termination, they evaluate and summarize the group experience.

A group is characterized by its purpose and dynamics, which include communication, conflict, decision making, bonding, and role identification; it is influenced by the individual members who compose the group as well as by forces outside the group that impinge on its development. Communication within a group occurs not only through what is said but also through behaviors, including body language and tone of voice (Watzlawick, 1978). Tension and anxiety exist in every group and reflect unexplained feelings of discomfort, especially when members' expectations are not being met. *Conflict* is a normal and necessary group dynamic that signifies opposing forces within a group. Conflict may be restricted to individual members, occur in subgroups, or take place for the entire group. Subgroups are subsystems of a group. These subgroups, referred to as coalitions, may occur when individual needs supersede the group's purpose so that small groups or pairs within the group compete and split off from the group as a whole (Yalom, 1995). Decision making is another important process in every group. Groups can make decisions through consensus (when all members agree), through accommodation (when members come to agreement through compromise), or through a de facto process (when members simply lack dissent). Groups make decisions and carry out their intended purpose with a strong orientation to shared norms, which are the rules that govern group behavior. Another dynamic, group bonding, creates a sense of belonging to something beyond the self and thus helps create the group's own identity. Cohesiveness, the attraction of group members for each other, is necessary for bonding to occur. Members of groups also experience role identification. Roles are expected behaviors of members. Members generally assume task roles, which help the group function through the accomplishment of group goals, or maintenance roles, which serve to keep members connected to each other and to keep the group functioning. In addition to these healthy roles, there are self-serving roles that impede group process. These anti-group roles (such as aggressor, blocker, recognition-seeker, self-confessor, help-seeker) serve the individual at the expense of the group. Finally, a pervasive destructive force found in some groups is apathy. Apathy is characterized by indifference and boredom in members and prevents the group from being able to mobilize energy to continue.

Community Development

The community consists of the wider circles of interaction that support the family, other groups, and individual members. The community supports the tangible resources that individuals use to grow and develop beyond the family and groups. These resources include schools, houses of worship, recreational facilities, health and social services, communication networks, safety and protective agencies, transportation systems, and political and economic structures (Anderson & McFarlane, 2004). Each community has its own particular identity and style of leadership (Warren, 1977; Loomis, 1957). Communities provide the broader context of living in which individuals, families, and groups may learn to become consumers and participants.

A community refers to "people in the context of their environment as they continuously interact with each other and the environment" (Arnold, 1998, p. 107). Communities can be viewed from a variety of perspectives in order to gain a fuller understanding of the nature of the community and the interactions that characterize it. A simple way to look at a community is through its structure and function. The structure of a community includes the persons who compose it and its physical characteristics. The function of a community includes the use of community resources by its members and the linkages between persons and resources. Other definitions of a community relate to the alignment or misalignment of resources and the nature of relationships within it (Loomis, 1957). Typologies (Warren, 1977) of community life have described the nature of community leadership, cohesiveness, self-sufficiency, and ties to the larger society. Communities can also be understood by their functional capacities, the things they provide, such as space utilization, livelihood, protection, education, participation, productivity, and linkages to other systems (Higgs & Gustafson, 1985).

Communities, like groups, are formed by affiliations as persons come together through something they have in common, which may be a geographic locale, an economic similarity, or a shared culture or value system. Some communities are created through membership or common experiences or causes. Communities are capable of self-care through effective partnerships (Anderson & McFarlane, 2004) or alliances (Klainberg, Holzemer, Leonard, & Arnold, 1998). Communities also possess capacities that enable them to be the providers of care and nurture for their members. Communities, to a great extent, define themselves. Each community forms its own image that is appreciative of its unique components, including the population of the community and its resources, culture, economics, and geography. A community is a system that develops and grows through the interaction of these component forces.

Within the community context, individuals and families develop and grow. The community provides multiple opportunities for socialization; the individual relates to neighbors, makes friendships, and forms acquaintances through routine tasks such as food shopping and obtaining necessary services. Through these tasks the individual becomes known and is afforded opportunities to participate in community life. Commitments, such as volunteering at the local hospital, fire department, library, or athletic events, enable the individual and the family to develop larger networks for socialization and to develop and use skills that may assist others and deepen involvement in the life of the community. Development is also fostered by the ability of individuals to locate work and earn a living within the community context. Working provides the individual with a means of livelihood and the ability to support an independent lifestyle. Development of self through work or professional identity expands the defining qualities of the person and fosters role assumption. The community, by providing the context for livelihood through employment, establishes an economic foundation to support services. "Both strengths and adversities must be examined from an ecological perspective, which places individuals, families, and communities in context. That context includes multiple systems, institutions, and environments that, interdependently, both affect people and are affected by them" (Perkins, Crim, Silberman, & Brown, 2004, p. 322).

The community is an educator, informing its members about resources and support systems that promote development (Werner, 2000). The community can protect its members through its resources, individuals, families, and social agencies. These protective factors nurture and support resilience, as illustrated in an excerpt from Jonathan Kozol's work. Kozol (1995), writing of children living in the crime- and drug-ridden community of Mott Haven in the South Bronx, describes Anthony, a bright, reflective twelve-year-old who presents himself as a "writer of novels." Befriended by the pastor of his community church, Anthony is introduced to Juan Castro, a poet and true intellectual who has lived in the South Bronx for more than fifty years, writing, teaching, and translating the works of Milton into Spanish. Under the protective wing of Castro, Anthony's image of himself as a writer is nurtured. He brings his work to Castro, who reads it carefully, responds to it, and introduces Anthony to the great writers and poets of the Western world. Castro said to Kozol: "The solitary figure of this child touches me tremendously. His mentality, as you have noticed, is not organized and that is part of his attraction. When he rings my bell, it pleases me. He reminds me by his earnestness of Don Quixote. He told me once, 'If I could not write, I would go crazy.' Children long for this—a voice, a way of being heard—but many sense that there is no one in the world to hear their words, so they are drawn to ways of malice" (p. 239).

Anthony is a rare child whose spirit and talent are nurtured by a significant adult in his community. Kozol describes this situation as a "little miracle" that happens infrequently as certain children create safe spaces for themselves that help them transcend the dreariness and danger of their lives (Kozol, 1995). These safe spaces can be filled with teachers, clergy, caregivers, and neighbors within a community who offer nurture and protection to the child with hopes and dreams, in the absence of family or family support. The nurture, protection, and support of a community can foster resilience and be life saving for both individuals and families.

Some communities are depleted of resources and have little to offer their members. Increased crime, limited services, insufficient leadership, and natural disasters contribute to the demise of communities. Withdrawal of government funding and private investment drains communities of the means to support services for members, thereby abandoning them. As publicly funded health and social services diminish and the public health infrastructure disappears, communities are at great risk. Communities may become so depleted and chaotic that members cannot access even limited services. Persons who live in poverty, homelessness, and chronic illness and disability, as well as recently arrived immigrant populations, are severely affected by the lack of community supports for individuals and families. Communities also become alienated from their members when they lose their unique flavors or identities, giving way to large, impersonal commercial areas.

The community's development is influenced by the availability of resources beyond it as well as by the needs and contributions of families and individuals within it (Earls & Buka, 2000). Harrison-Hale, McLoyd, and Smedley (2004) explore factors such as support from extended families, racial and ethnic socialization practices, and religion as protective factors—factors that facilitate positive outcomes among children, youths, families, and communities of color—and recommend policies to improve resilient outcomes among individuals in ethnic minority communities. "These include policies that enhance personal skills through existing institutions, strengthen family supports, and build the social capital of communities" (Harrison-Hale et al., 2004, p. 269).

Communities form, grow, die, or transform as their members and institutions change. There is potential in communities for transformation. For instance, surviving agencies and organized groups in communities depleted of most resources often open their doors to serve community needs. For example, a local house of worship may temporarily house a vulnerable member of the community and then become a shelter as the need grows and others seek assistance. In many communities, non–health care agencies and groups of individuals and families united by common bonds are extending their missions and boundaries and are becoming the community's social service agencies.

Vulnerabilities and Risks

The complex and dynamic process of development begins at conception and ends at death; a convergence of factors and events affects development along this trajectory. These factors and events include genetic, physiological, and intrapersonal factors; interpersonal connections; societal patterns; cultural traditions and variations; and the occurrence of significant life events and stressors. Separately and in combination, these factors and events may adversely affect development, contributing to vulnerability that thwarts potential (Garmezy, 1993; Luthar & Zelazo, 2003).

Recent advances in the complex and evolving field of genetics (Rutter, 2000) reveal linkages between specific genes or genetic patterns and the presence of health problems. Because of this, a new area for exploration and understanding is unfolding, contributing to a broader appreciation of the origins of some human conditions and behaviors. The affective, addictive, and psychotic disorders, which normally begin in adolescence and adulthood, are debilitating chronic mental disorders with genetic underpinnings that are not well understood. These conditions severely impair a person's self-perception and ability to make plans and choices for the present and future. Physical illnesses with strong genetic bases, such as cystic fibrosis, Huntington's chorea, and sickle-cell disease, can adversely affect development in childhood, adolescence, and throughout adulthood, depending on severity, age of onset, availability of treatment, family and community support.

Substance abuse, poor nutrition, and lack of prenatal care during pregnancy, separately and in combination, influence the growth of the fetus in utero and affect the health and well-being of the newborn, as well as having lasting effects on development as the infant evolves into a child, adolescent, and adult. Children born to substance-abusing mothers, including those born with fetal alcohol syndrome, are affected throughout their lives in areas of cognition and social and emotional development. Infants who are HIV infected as a result of being born to HIV-infected mothers, and other children who acquire or develop life-threatening illnesses during infancy or early childhood, run the risk that their disease, treatment, frequent hospitalizations, or separation from family will interfere with their normal development.

The death of a parent or sibling deeply affects the developing child. Interference in early relationships with parents and siblings because of mental or physical illness also adversely affects the child's development. Indeed, throughout the life span, human relationships that are broken or altered significantly can thwart or delay development at any age or at any stage and thus impede learning and growth.

There are also external factors that can impinge on the developing individual, family, and community. Societal patterns, including poverty, violence, racial discrimination, and oppression, contribute adversely to development. Violence within families, groups, and communities severs the trust between persons and erodes the foundations on which development is built. Violence within families and communities may result in the placement of children in foster care agencies or other homes, incarceration of adults, or death or injury to members young and old. Violence that can alter the ability of the family and community to protect and care for its members is a negative force, limiting options and opportunity.

A social and political climate that devalues and does not support education and health care for its population deprives individuals and families of opportunities to learn, grow, and maintain health. External events, including natural disasters, wars, and violent conflicts, contribute to the deprivation of all affected individuals, families, and communities by interfering with development and limiting opportunities for decision making and growth.

The individual, family, group, and community may be more vulnerable to certain stressors than others at specific times along the developmental trajectory. Consider the infant or young child, dependent on parents and adult caretakers for nurturance, sustenance, protection, and care, who is orphaned and set adrift with hundreds of refugee children. Without care, nurturance, and love, the young child will most certainly die. Consider the young adolescent sold into prostitution for a meager sum to support her family, moved from rural to urban surroundings away from known supports of family and community. Consider the elderly man or woman abandoned by family and placed without warning in a residential setting, deprived of loved ones and personal possessions. In these three situations the stressors are so profound and overwhelming and the individuals so deprived of external support, that development can be quite literally halted. Consider families left homeless by massive flooding and devastation. Consider groups and communities robbed of their resources and inhabitants in the wake of war, terrorism, or natural disaster. In these cases, mere survival becomes the goal of existence, and in the worst cases people may simply wish to die. Without intervention the effect of these stressors on the developing self at any stage is profound. The loss of potential in the individual, family, group, and community cannot be fully measured; development can be thwarted, altered, or halted, temporarily or forever.

Protecting, Replenishing, and Sustaining Development

There is within every human being, family, group, and community potential for fullness of development. This potential is realized as the person, family, group, and community participate in directing their development, choosing actions that reduce health risks and optimize health strengths, making informed decisions and choices, and assuming responsibility for self-care. This process occurs at both the microlevel, for individuals and families, and the macrolevel, for communities and larger systems. Development is not a steady, measured process. The healthy person, family, group, and community grow and develop through self-sustaining protective efforts (Werner, 2000). Effective strategies to promote self-development, family growth, and group and community strength focus on partnership and participation (Turnbull, Turbiville, & Turnbull, 2000). Social support is a recognized vehicle for promoting healthy development. Social support buffers and protects health from the effects of stress (Cohen & Willis, 1985; Sheinfeld Gorin, 1995).

The significant role of culture in development is just beginning to be recognized. Culture refers to a distinct system of meaning shared by a group of people. This system of meaning is learned and transmitted through generations. Culture is given form by values and beliefs that are evidenced in daily interactions (Coll & Magnuson, 2000). The family is most often recognized as the primary vehicle for cultural learning. Strengths are derived from cultural meanings and affiliations, which serve as foundations, grounding beliefs and behaviors (Harrison-Hale et al., 2004). It is essential that systems of health care become systems of cultural care, providing culturally competent and proficient care (Goode & Harrison, 2000).

Families develop through the accomplishment of tasks and functions that sustain and strengthen them. Some families grow through the need to separate or divorce. These actions are self-preserving and often serve to protect the members of the family. Divorce may lead to the possibility of blending or reconstituting a family with others (Carter & McGoldrick, 1999). The new family survives with the hope of creating its own identity and becoming a healthier support for its members. Some families survive and regenerate even with overwhelming stress, affirming their potential for self-repair and growth out of crisis and challenge (Walsh, 1998).

Groups change as their intended purposes are fulfilled and as phases of group development meld into each other and move toward termination with the establishment of new ties outside the group. Groups are replenished through the introduction of new members and the departure of existing members and through reshaping the group purpose. Groups expand and contract through the interactive processes of membership, desired affiliations, and inner dynamics.

Communities are replenished as they transform and develop, as populations and cultural groups enter and leave, as resources open and close, and as industrialization and housing expansion alter structure and function. Communities also change as their populations and resources shift; when resources are linked to human need, the community's development is enhanced. Communities are strengthened through crises, as members pull together to support each other and rebuild.

The interventions listed in Exhibit 15.1 protect, replenish and sustain development of the individual, family, and community.

Development is protected, replenished, and sustained through interaction among individuals, families, groups, and communities. "Individuals, families, and communities are viewed as interdependent systems that experience multidimensional changes over time in response to evolving risk and protective processes" (Leadbeater et al., 2004, pp. 15–16).

EXHIBIT 15.1. INTERVENTIONS FOR PROTECTING, REPLENISHING, AND SUSTAINING DEVELOPMENT.

- Maintaining relationships that provide nurture, protection, and support, and the opportunity for reciprocity
- Honoring cultural affiliations, traditions, and practices
- Participating in purposeful activity in the form of work, production of product and income, and provision of social support
- Securing and providing adequate resources for health, including primary care, nutrition, physical exercise, and rest
- Participating in and enhancing educational and recreational activities
- Enjoying aesthetic and cultural experiences; strengthening understanding of culture and cultural connection
- Discovering and fostering resilience
- Strengthening protective factors
- Enhancing spirituality
- Searching for meaning and finding hope
- Experiencing loss and expressing grief
- Engaging in introspection and appraisal

The process of growth encompasses times of triumph as well as struggle: challenges are met, adversity is translated into meaning, stressors are coped with, and pride is taken in valued choices. Inherent in growth is resilience. Spirituality provides hope in the time of adversity and affirms an inner core of support. Development also necessitates the integration of losses as well as gains, so that unmet challenges, adversity, and stress do not result in paralysis and apathy. Grieving assists in the healthy process of integrating loss and gain. The significance of social support, resilience, spirituality, and grieving to health and health promotion cannot be overestimated. Special attention must be directed to these powerful processes for replenishing and sustaining health.

Social Support

The social support system buffers and protects as development unfolds and as crises are experienced. From smaller circles of support to ever widening associations, social support is a changing dynamic providing nurture, resources, and protection. Embedded within a context of nested systems—families, groups, and larger communities—individuals create a network of unique relationships. In these relationships there is an exchange of support, which may be emotional (through esteem and trust, for example), may provide appraisal (through affirmation and social comparison, for example), or may be informational (offering advice and directives, for example) and instrumental (offering such things as money and time, for example) (Sheinfeld Gorin, 1997). These support sources shape norms and values and filter information influencing health behaviors.

Health is often viewed from an individual perspective in which lifestyle and personal choices shape health status. Yet individuals do not live in isolation. Every person has a multitude of relationships within a social and cultural environment in which there is constant and dynamic interaction. The social relationships that are strong and supportive influence the health of individuals in myriad ways. Berkman (1995) asserts that "for social support to be health promoting, it must provide not only a sense of belonging and intimacy, but it must also help people to be more competent and self-efficacious" (p. 251). Interventions to promote health cannot be planned for individuals without including this social context and, more specifically, without incorporating the social and cultural network (Finfgeld-Connett, 2005). An analysis of health-promoting environments emphasizes "the transactions between individual or collective behavior and the health resources and constraints that exist in specific environmental settings" (Stokols, 1992, p. 6). Without the inclusion of an individual's family and community, the potential for change is limited and the impact of change unsustainable.

Fostering Resilience

Understanding growth in the face of adversity leads to a consideration of resilience, strength forged through adversity (Walsh, 2003). "Resilience does not come from rare and special qualities, but from the everyday magic of ordinary, normative human resources in the minds, brains, and bodies of children, in their families and relationships, and in their communities" (Masten, 2001, p. 10). Resilience is rooted in protective factors within the individual, family, and environment. Individual protective factors include biological integrity, psychological predisposition, easy temperament, effective coping skills, and adequate cognition, sustained by social and emotional support systems (Werner & Smith, 2001). Resilience research has assumed that the factors promoting resilience are either embedded characteristics of the individual or derive from interaction between the person and the source of environmental risks. However, neither assumption is entirely supported. Rutter (2000) asserts that there is clear-cut evidence that growth or recovery, partial or complete, may derive from life experiences that take place well after the initial risk experience. Therefore resilience continues to be a force within the individual that can be activated at a later point in time, subsequent to stress or adversity. Resilience may now be best understood as an unfolding process rather than a trait.

Resilience at the family and community level is also not a static outcome. Families and communities may show multidimensional responses to ongoing challenges, risks, and protective factors over time (Leadbeater et al., 2004). "Resilient persons—and communities—often make the best of tragic situations by finding something to salvage and seeing new possibilities in the midst of wreckage" (Walsh, 1998, p. 73). Recognizing resilience as a dynamic process operating over time—and not as a fixed or embedded characteristic of human beings and human systems—opens possibilities for interventions. Research on resilience places an emphasis on nonnormative development or unexpected growth in the face of risk, which draws attention to populations most in need and provides lessons for promoting resilience (Reynolds & Ou, 2003). However, while recognizing that adversity may provide windows of opportunity for intervention, we need to continue to strive for a more complete understanding of the complexities and variables affecting the development, maintenance, and durability of the phenomenon of resilience (Fine, 1991; Luthar, Cicchetti, & Becker, 2000).

Enhancing Spirituality

Spirituality is a self-sustaining force within the individual, family, group, and community. As such, spirituality may nurture development. Erikson, Erikson, and Kivick (1986) identify the early development of the spiritual domain in the emergence of trust and hope in infancy. This essential strength matures over the life span and can sustain development of all subsequent strength. At the end of life, some form of this rudimentary hope may blossom into a mature faith in being that is closely related to essential wisdom (Erikson, Erikson, & Kivick, 1986, p. 218). All the basic virtues, including hope, will, purpose, competence, fidelity, love, care, and wisdom, that emerge from a successful resolution of the developmental tasks described by Erikson are components of the spiritual domain (Schuster & Ashburn, 1992). Schuster and Ashburn (1992) describe the spiritual domain as encompassing all the transcendental aspects of self. It is the center of awareness of existence. It is also hopefulness within the individual, the family, and community that sustains life in the face of adversity and loss. Spirituality can be experienced within or outside formal religious structures (Walsh, 1998).

Spirituality as a life force in the individual, family, group, and community is not well understood. Persons confronting dependencies and addictions often find strength through spiritual awakening during the struggles of detoxification and recovery. Spirituality is the life force that might help to sustain the resilience and courage of a grandmother as she realizes the task of raising her grandchildren bereft of their mother while she grieves for her daughter. Spirituality can help some find purpose in their suffering and in pain, and others will discover or rekindle spirituality in times of difficulty or painful loss. "Spirituality involves an active investment in internal values that bring a sense of meaning, inner wholeness, and connections with others" (Walsh, 1998, p. 70).

Many groups and communities hold to their spiritual beliefs and values in the face of poverty, oppression, and victimization, finding perseverance, emancipation, and repudiation possible. Survivors of disaster, when stripped of all, will exclaim, "All I have is my faith." In describing the horrific and dehumanizing experience of living in a concentration camp, Frankl (1984) writes of finding meaning in life even when a situation is hopeless, when facing a fate that cannot be changed: "For what then matters is to bear witness to the uniquely human potential at its best, which is to transform a personal tragedy into a triumph, to turn one's predicament into a human achievement" (p. 116). Spirituality is often discovered in living through painful experiences and can for some provide the purpose or meaning for suffering. Spirituality, as a life force (Coles, 1990), contributes to the self-esteem and strength of the individual; to the courage and resilience of the family; and to the energy, hope, and steadfastness of groups and the community. "Sustaining hope in the face of overwhelming odds enables us to carry on our best efforts. . . . Hope is a future-oriented belief; no matter how bleak the present, we can envision a better future" (Walsh, 1998, p. 62).

Expressing Grief

Grief is a vital function of human experience that facilitates healing and offers the potential for personal growth and development through the integration of loss into the self (Arnold, 1995). The facilitation of grief assists individuals, families, and even communities to live with losses inherent in the life process. Some losses are part of the natural experience of development and are expected. Other losses are unexpected. It is not uncommon for the grief associated with the myriad losses in life to be unacknowledged. Grieving can be a solitary experience and one that many persons try to put away and leave unattended because the pain of their loss may be unbearable. Loss may become a family secret and be denied. There are many reasons for grief being unacknowledged. For some people, time increasingly separates them from the loss and therefore from the opportunity to grieve. The health care professional will often encounter clients, whether individuals, families, or communities, who have experienced loss and have not had the opportunity to grieve or to recognize their need to grieve. Consider the impact of one person's death. This person may have been the partner of another who is now dealing with the pain of loss and emotional separation. This person may have had a family that now is not whole without this member. This person may have been part of a community that experiences the loss and seeks to protect its members from a similar death. Each individual touches others, and thus ever expanding circles of affected individuals are left to experience the emotions of loss through grief.

Life is filled with loss. Losses may be minor, almost imperceptible, or they may be significant and overwhelming. Individuals grieve as they leave childhood and move through adolescence into middle adulthood and old age. Individuals grieve as relationships change and end and when separation and divorce occur. Individuals grieve for jobs lost and positions changed. Individuals grieve at graduations, birthdays, celebrations of the new year, the changing seasons, and events marking a passage of time never regained. Individuals also grieve in their dying, and their survivors grieve for them (Arnold, 1996). The grieving process, although a universal response to loss, becomes individualized as each person reacts and copes using sources of strength and comfort. In this way, each person forms a unique mosaic of responses that become a pattern of grieving (Arnold, 1995). Some pieces of the mosaic are internal, whereas others reflect religion, culture, family belief systems, and traditions.

Memory fuels grief and helps to maintain the connection with the lost object, experience, or person. Grief is not a tragic episode or a pathological state, and it cannot be equated with illness. On the contrary, grief is a healthy process, in which one integrates loss and maintains a connection to the lost person or object and learns to live without (Arnold, 1995). This lasting connection through grief is recognized as a continuing bond (Klass, Silverman, & Nickman, 1996; Arnold & Gemma, 1994). Facilitating the grieving process assists individuals, families, and communities to learn to live with and integrate loss. It is never too late to acknowledge grief or to facilitate the expression of grief. Facilitation of grief is a therapeutic intervention that fosters development and growth throughout the continuum of life and at its end.

There are specific actions to support grief, a process that occurs throughout life as loss is experienced in its many forms. In therapeutic interactions there are responses that facilitate as well as those that hamper the ability of the health care professional to intervene. Exhibit 15.2 lists responses that enhance these interventions. Exhibit 15.3 lists responses that limit a health care professional's interventions in facilitating the grieving process.

Over the life span, efforts that facilitate therapeutic interaction will be sources of strength for the health care professional; they will encourage involvement with individuals, families, groups and communities living with loss and will guide therapeutic interventions that support development.

EXHIBIT 15.2. RESPONSES THAT
FACILITATE THERAPEUTIC INTERACTIONS FOR GRIEVING.

- *Shifting the paradigm of grief.* The health care professional who views grief as an integrative life process that continues throughout the life span and enables the client to gain insight as well as to grow can enhance the client's personal development. Closing the door on grief or containing it serves only to limit the potential for personal growth.

- *Case finding.* Health care professionals who are willing to recognize the importance of loss and grief as human experiences that facilitate growth and personal development are more likely to be open and available to clients for these discussions. The health care professional listens for experiences of loss and is particularly attuned to the possibility of unacknowledged grief. The health care professional also recognizes that losses are experienced not only by individuals but also by families and communities, so that family, group, and community meetings are just as feasible as a session with an individual client.

- *Expanding the comfort zone.* As the health care professional becomes astute in listening for experiences of loss and responding to them, she or he becomes more comfortable in dealing with loss. It is possible to become more comfortable in interacting with loss through clinical experience and with clinical supervision.

- *Supervision.* Health care professionals benefit from the opportunities for organized and consistent reflection and introspection that are available through supervision. Supervision can be contracted with colleagues or through case conferences. The intent is to allow the health care professional the opportunity to objectively analyze the case material and interpersonal interactions.

- *Professional development.* Health care professionals may desire to pursue continuing education about loss and grief through clinical literature and conferences and through seeking certification in the field of grief counseling and grief education.

- *Tool development.* Assessment tools for patterns of health and risk often neglect to address the incidence of loss and death in their individual and family health components. Use of the genogram (Pendagast & Sherman, 1973–1978) as a graphic representation of family connections can also reveal deaths and health problems, which should prompt the health care professional to explore with the client the meaning and significance of these losses in the client's history and family life. Further development of inventories of loss and the creation of clinical guidelines for attending to loss will enhance clinical practice.

- *Resource development.* It is necessary to accumulate resources that support the health care professional and the therapeutic process and that meet the specific and complex needs of clients. The health care professional providing grief support will require opportunities for personal reflection and replenishment as well as assistance from other professionals and agencies with special knowledge and services that can be mobilized to meet the needs of clients living with loss.

EXHIBIT 15.3. RESPONSES THAT
HAMPER THERAPEUTIC INTERACTIONS FOR GRIEVING.

- *Avoidance.* The health care professional may experience discomfort with discussing personal loss and may discourage or avoid, rather than encourage, authentic communication because the pain of the client provokes the health care professional's own sense of loss and pain.

- *Depletion.* The health care professional may experience emotional exhaustion and feel unable to be fully engaged. Therapeutic communication about grief rests in the health care professional's ability to engage in the therapeutic purpose. Health care professionals need to find ways to refuel themselves, particularly when their work immerses them in the experience of others' grief.

- *Anxiety.* Painful areas of discussion are often difficult to sustain. The health care professional may be anxious during these communications. Talking, rather than active listening, may be a sign that the health care professional is experiencing anxiety. Supervision and thoughtful analysis of the interaction is essential to give the health care professional a greater understanding of other means to meet personal needs and of ways to sustain a client-centered focus.

- *Forced resolution.* The health care professional may force resolution because he or she is uncomfortable with the emotions of the client and hopes the situation can end. Instead, the health care professional should be careful not to seek resolution, because grief is experienced as an ongoing process rather than as an event that must be resolved. Rather than offering reassurance the health care professional can offer acceptance and validation of the pain of the expression. This is experienced by the client as acceptance and validation of the self.

Development at the End of Life

At the end of life an individual will grieve for anticipated loss of life and for losses during life. Grieving facilitates transformative development. No system remains stable; all human systems experience loss, growth, and change. Loss and growth are interconnected, part of the same process of change. One cannot exist without the other; there is always a giving up in growth and growth in loss as they are inseparable in their transformative nature. Loss and growth are intrinsically linked at no time more so than at the end of life.

Consider the individual grieving for the end of life brought about by illness or old age. Consider the family grieving for its transformation through separation, divorce, reconstituted relationships, and the blending of families. Consider the group grieving as members leave and are replaced or as the group dissolves when goals are accomplished. Consider the community transformed by economic or political forces, such as a rural community unable to sustain the closing of a plant that has employed many members of the community, who now, unable to support their families, decide to move away. Consider a community devastated by natural disaster or an act of terrorism, where people disperse for safety or experience homelessness and wander in search of services to assist them in their plight. All human systems suffer losses and become transformed as they cope with the factors and forces that have disrupted their security or stability.

The human system, through the kindling of strengths and capacities, emerges transformed. Often this transformation results in added strengths and capacities for some, whereas for others development is thwarted and regression may occur. For some, at the end of life there is the hope that the human spirit will be transformed and continue in another form. For others, the transformation is a continuation of the human spirit in the lives of those who survive, transferring a legacy of history and values to the generation that follows.

Summary

Development is a dynamic, lifelong transformative process. Individuals, families, groups, and communities develop uniquely, with members intrinsically connected to each other. Each human system is characterized by diversity, risks, and protective factors. There is a synergy among these systems as they grow and develop, separately and together.

References

Anderson, E. T., & McFarlane, J. (2004). *Community as partner: Theory and practice in nursing* (4th ed.). Philadelphia: Lippincott Williams & Wilkins.

Arnold, J. (1995). *A reconceptualization of the concept of grief for nursing: A philosophical analysis.* Unpublished doctoral dissertation, New York University.

Arnold, J. (1996). Rethinking grief: Nursing implications for health promotion. *Home Healthcare Nurse, 14*(10), 777–783.

Arnold, J. (1998). The community as client. In M. Klainberg, S. Holzemer, M. Leonard, & J. Arnold, *Community health nursing: An alliance for health.* New York: McGraw-Hill.

Arnold, J. H., & Gemma, P. B. (1994). *A child dies: A portrait of family grief* (2nd ed.). Philadelphia: Charles Press.

Berkman, L. F. (1995). The role of social relations in health promotion. *Psychosomatic Medicine, 57,* 245–254.

Bowen, M. (1978). *Family therapy in clinical practice.* New York: Aronson.

Boyd, W. (Ed. & Trans.). (1962). *The Émile of Jean-Jacques Rousseau.* New York: Columbia University, Teachers College, Bureau of Publications.

Carter, B., & McGoldrick, M. (Eds.). (1999). *The expanded family life cycle: Individual, family and social perspectives* (3rd ed.). Needham Heights, MA: Allyn & Bacon.

Chess, S., & Thomas, A. (1986). *Temperament in clinical practice.* New York: Guilford Press.

Clark, C. C. (1994). *The nurse as group leader* (3rd ed.). New York: Springer.

Cohen, S., & Willis, T. A. (1985). Stress, social support, and the buffering hypothesis. *Psychological Bulletin, 98,* 310–357.

Coles, R. (1990). *The spiritual life of children.* Boston: Houghton Mifflin.

Coles, R. (1997). *The moral intelligence of children.* New York: Random House.

Coll, C. G., & Magnuson, K. (2000). Cultural differences as sources of developmental vulnerabilities and resources. In J. P. Shonkoff & S. J. Meisels (Eds.), *Handbook of early childhood intervention* (2nd ed., pp. 94–114). New York: Cambridge University Press.

Duvall, E.R.M. (1985). *Marriage and family development* (6th ed.). New York: HarperCollins.

Earls, F., & Buka, S. (2000). Measurement of community characteristics. In J. P. Shonkoff & S. J. Meisels (Eds.), *Handbook of early childhood intervention* (2nd ed., pp. 309–324). New York: Cambridge University Press.

Erikson, E. H. (1963). *Childhood and society* (2nd ed.). New York: Norton.

Erikson, E. H. (1968). *Identity, youth and crisis.* New York: Norton.

Erikson, E. H., Erikson, J. M., & Kivick, H. Q. (1986). *Vital involvement in old age.* New York: Norton.

Fine, S. (1991). Resilience and human adaptability: Who rises above adversity? *American Journal of Occupational Therapy, 45*(6), 493–503.

Finfgeld-Connett, D. (2005). Clarification of social support. *Journal of Nursing Scholarship, 37*(1), 4–9.

Fogarty, T. F. (1985). On stress. *The Family, 12*(2), 15–19.

Frankl, V. E. (1984). *Man's search for meaning: An introduction to logotherapy* (3rd ed.). New York: Simon & Schuster.

Freud, S. (1935). *A general introduction to psychoanalysis* (J. Riviere, Trans.). New York: Liveright.

Garmezy, N. (1993). Vulnerability and resilience. In D. C. Funder, R. D. Parke, C. Tomilson-Keasey, & K. Widaman (Eds.), *Studying lives through time: Personality and development* (pp. 377–398). Washington, DC: American Psychological Association.

Gebbie, K., Rosenstock, L., & Hernandez, L. M. (2003). *Who will keep the public healthy? Educating public health professionals in the 21st century.* Washington, DC: National Academies Press.

Gerson, R. (1995). The family life cycle: Phases, stages, and crises. In R. H. Mikesell, D. D. Lusterman, & S. H. McDaniel (Eds.), *Integrating family therapy: Handbook of family psychology and systems theory* (pp. 91–111). Washington, DC: American Psychological Association.

Gilligan, C. (1984). *In a different voice.* Cambridge, MA: Harvard University Press.

Gilligan, C. (1986). Remapping the moral domain: New images of the self in relationship. In T. C. Heller, M. Sosna, & D. E. Wellbery (Eds.), *Reconstructing individualism: Autonomy, individuality, and the self in western thought* (pp. 237–252). Stanford, CA: Stanford University Press.

Glantz, M. D., & Sloboda, Z. (1999). Analysis and reconceptualization of resilience. In M. D. Glantz & J. L. Johnson (Eds.), *Resilience and development: Positive life adaptations* (pp. 109–126). New York: Kluwer.

Goode, T. D., & Harrison, S. (2000, Summer). *Cultural competence in primary health care: Partnerships for a research agenda* (Policy Brief 3). Washington, DC: National Center for Cultural Competence.

Haley, J. (1980). *Leaving home.* New York: McGraw-Hill.

Harrison-Hale, A. O., McLoyd, V. C., & Smedley, B. (2004). Racial and ethnic status: Risk and protective processes among African American families. In K. I. Maton, C. J. Schellenbach, B. J. Leadbeater, & A. L. Solarz (Eds.), *Investing in children, youth, families, and communities: Strengths-based research and policy* (pp. 269–283). Washington, DC: American Psychological Association.

Havighurst, R. J. (1972). *Developmental tasks and education* (3rd ed.). New York: McKay.

Higgs, Z. R., & Gustafson, D. D. (1985). *Community as a client: Assessment and diagnosis.* Philadelphia: Davis.

Kagan, J. (1984). *The nature of the child.* New York: Basic Books.

Kagan, J. (1989). *Unstable ideas: Temperament, cognition, and self.* Cambridge, MA: Harvard University Press.

Kaplan, H. B. (1999). Toward an understanding of resilience: A critical review of definitions and models. In M. D. Glantz & J. L. Johnson (Eds.), *Resilience and development: Positive life adaptations* (pp. 17–83). New York: Kluwer.

Klainberg, M., Holzemer, S., Leonard, M., & Arnold, J. (1998). *Community health nursing: An alliance for health.* New York: McGraw-Hill.

Klass, D., Silverman, P. R., & Nickman, S. L. (Eds.). (1996). *Continuing bonds: New understandings of grief.* Bristol, PA: Taylor and Francis.

Kohlberg, L. (1981). *The philosophy of moral development.* San Francisco: HarperSanFrancisco.

Kozol, J. (1995). *Amazing grace.* New York: Crown.

Leadbeater, B. J., Schellenbach, C. J., Maton, K. I., & Dodgen, D. W. (2004). Research and policy for building strengths: Processes and contexts of individual, family, and community development. In K. I. Maton, C. J. Schellenbach, B. J. Leadbeater, & A. L. Solarz (Eds.), *Investing in children, youth, families, and communities: Strengths-based research and policy.* Washington, DC: American Psychological Association.

Locke, J. (1964). Some thoughts concerning education (abridged). In P. Gay (Ed.), *John Locke on education.* New York: Columbia University, Teachers College, Bureau of Publications.

Loomis, C. P. (Ed.). (1957). *Tönnies: Community and society (Gemeinschaft und Gesellschaft).* East Lansing: Michigan State University Press.

Luthar, S., Cicchetti, D., & Becker, B. (2000). The construct of resilience: A critical evaluation and guidelines for future work. *Child Development, 71*(3), 543–562.

Luthar, S. S., & Zelazo, L. B. (2003). Research on resilience: An integrative review. In S. S. Luthar (Ed.), *Resilience and vulnerability: Adaptation in the context of childhood adversities* (pp. 510–549). New York: Cambridge University Press.

Maslow, A. H. (1968). *Toward a psychology of being* (2nd ed.). New York: Van Nostrand Reinhold.

Masten, A. S. (1999). Resilience comes of age: Reflections on the past and outlook for the next generation of research. In M. D. Glantz & J. L. Johnson (Eds.), *Resilience and development: Positive life adaptations* (pp. 281–296). New York: Kluwer.

Masten, A. S. (2001). Ordinary magic: Resilience processes in development. *American Psychologist, 56*(3), 1–12.

Minuchin, S. (1974). *Families and family therapy.* Cambridge, MA: Harvard University Press.

Minuchin, S., & Nichols, M. (1993). *Family healing.* New York: Free Press.

Ormont, L. R. (1992). *The group therapy experience: From theory to practice.* New York: St. Martin's Press.

Pendagast, E. G., & Sherman, C. O. (1973–1978). A guide to the genogram. *The Family compendium: I. The best of The Family 1973–1978* (pp. 101–112). Washington, DC: Georgetown University Family Center.

Perkins, D. D., Crim, B., Silberman, P., & Brown, B. B. (2004). Community development as a response to community-level adversity: Ecological theory and research and strengths-based policy. In K. I. Maton, C. J. Schellenbach, B. J. Leadbeater, & A. L. Solarz (Eds.), *Investing in children, youth, families and communities: Strengths-based research and policy* (pp. 321–340). Washington, DC: American Psychological Association.

Piaget, J. (1963). *The origins of intelligence in children.* New York: Norton.

Piaget, J. (1965). *The moral judgment of the child.* New York: Free Press.

Piaget, J., & Inhelder, B. (1969). *The psychology of the child.* New York: Basic Books.

Pipher, M. (1999). *Another country.* New York: Riverhead Books.

Reynolds, A. J., & Ou, S.-R. (2003). Promoting resilience through early childhood intervention. In S. S. Luthar (Ed.), *Resilience and vulnerability: Adaptation in the context of childhood adversities* (pp. 436–459). New York: Cambridge University Press.

Rutter, M. (1994). Continuities, transitions and turning points in development. In M. Rutter & D. F. Hay (Eds.), *Development through life* (pp. 1–25). Oxford, England: Blackwell Science.

Rutter, M. (2000). Resilience reconsidered: Conceptual considerations, empirical findings, and policy implications. In J. P. Shonkoff & S. J. Meisels (Eds.), *Handbook of early childhood intervention* (2nd ed., pp. 651–682). New York: Cambridge University Press.

Schaie, K. W., & Willis, S. H. (2002). *Adult development and aging* (5th ed.). Upper Saddle River, NJ: Prentice Hall.

Schuster, C. S., & Ashburn, S. S. (1992). *The process of human development* (3rd ed.). Philadelphia: Lippincott.

Sheinfeld Gorin, S. (1995). Relationship enhancement intervention: Social support program for women survivors of breast cancer. *Program/Proceedings: American Society for Clinical Oncology, 14,* 236.

Sheinfeld Gorin, S. (1997). Outcomes of social support for women survivors of breast cancer. In E. Mullen & J. L. Magnobosco (Eds.), *Outcomes measurement in the human services: Cross-cutting issues and methods* (pp. 278–291). Washington, DC: NASW Press.

Stokols, D. (1992). Establishing and maintaining healthy environments: Toward a social ecology of health promotion. *American Psychologist, 47*(1), 6–22.

Turnbull, A. P., Turbiville, V., & Turnbull, H. R. (2000). Evolution of family-professional partnerships: Collective empowerment as the model for the early twenty-first century. In J. P. Shonkoff & S. J. Meisels (Eds.), *Handbook of early childhood intervention* (2nd ed., pp. 630–650). New York: Cambridge University Press.

U.S. Department of Health and Human Services. (2000). *Healthy people 2010: Understanding and improving health.* Washington, DC: Author.

Walsh, F. (1989). The family in later life. In B. Carter & M. McGoldrick (Eds.), *The changing family life cycle: A framework for family therapy* (2nd ed., pp. 312–327). Needham Heights, MA: Allyn & Bacon.

Walsh, F. (1998). *Strengthening family resilience.* New York: Guilford Press.

Walsh, F. (2003). Crisis, trauma, and challenge: A relational resilience approach for healing, transformation, and growth. *Smith College Studies in Social Work, 74*(1), 49–71.

Warren, D. I. (1977). Neighborhoods in urban areas. In R. L. Warren (Ed.), *New perspectives on the American community: A book of readings.* Skokie, IL: Rand McNally.

Watzlawick, P. (1978). *The language of change: Elements of therapeutic communication.* New York: Basic Books.

Werner, E. E. (2000). Protective factors and individual resilience. In J. P. Shonkoff & S. J. Meisels (Eds.), *Handbook of early childhood intervention* (2nd ed., pp. 115–132). New York: Cambridge University Press.

Werner, E. E., & Smith, R. S. (2001). *Journeys from childhood to midlife: Risk, resilience, and recovery.* Ithaca, NY: Cornell University Press.

Weston, K. (1991). *Families we choose: Lesbians, gays, kinship.* New York: Columbia University Press.

Yalom, I. D. (1995). *The theory and practice of group psychotherapy* (4th ed.). New York: Basic Books.

PART THREE

ECONOMIC APPLICATIONS AND FORECASTING THE FUTURE OF HEALTH PROMOTION

CHAPTER SIXTEEN

ECONOMIC CONSIDERATIONS IN HEALTH PROMOTION

Wendy Dahar
Duncan Neuhauser

Health promotion activities use resources. The client has a cost for the time taken up by the program and sometimes out-of-pocket payments. The professional provider expects to be paid and to have space to work in—paid from an organization's budget, revenue from patients, or grants. The organization's management wants to know that the organization is getting value for money. For a program to be viable everyone involved needs to believe that the effort and expense required is worth it and that the benefits exceed the costs or revenues exceed expenses. To provide the reader with an understanding of the role of economic considerations in health promotion, this chapter describes how to develop a health promotion plan. Such plans can be used to justify an organizational budget, apply for a grant, or draft a business plan to start a private practice. One solid approach to developing a convincing health promotion plan is to follow these seven steps:

1. Know your organization and who really makes the decisions there.
2. Understand the economic environment that affects your organization. This includes knowing the health insurance reimbursement for your services.
3. Define the content of your health promotion plan or program. This is the process of care as it relates to the type of prevention proposed.
4. Determine what your program will cost. Define the resources that you will need.

5. Identify the benefits of your program and determine who will benefit. This step relates in part to how good the evidence is that your program will improve health. You will also need to calculate when in the future these health benefits will occur. Smoking may satisfy an addiction but can result in lung cancer in the future. For most of us, future benefits are valued less than those same benefits today. Taking this time preference into account is called *discounting*. Understanding this trade-off between incurring costs in the present and gaining benefits in the future is important for understanding the acceptance of health promotion programs (Gold, Siegel, Russell, & Weinstein, 1996).

6. Measure the costs and outcomes compared to the next best use of the resources by the plan or program. Collecting this information will allow you to demonstrate the effectiveness of your program. Is it worth doing?

7. Combine this information and future projections into a business plan, budget, or grant proposal addressed to the relevant decision makers.

The rest of this chapter takes up these seven steps in more detail. By the end the reader should be able to see how to create a plan for a health promotion program.

1. Know Your Organization

Health promotion programs are found in many organizations: ambulatory clinics, public health departments, school health programs, health maintenance organizations (HMOs), government agencies, fitness centers, and corporate human resource programs, to name just a few. In order to convincingly advocate for a new prevention program within an organization, you have to understand the goals and values of that organization to make sure your program fits. The mission and agenda of the Sisters of Charity Homeless Shelter, for example, are different from the mission and agenda of an investor-owned, for-profit chain of fitness centers. You also need to know how organizational decisions are really made, and who the key decision makers are. Such knowledge is also needed for writing a successful grant application to a private foundation or government agency. Funders often have detailed policies about applications, their approval process, and the funding itself.

To understand your organization, know that it has its formal, official side and its informal, unwritten way of doing things. To understand the formal part, read the mission, vision, and value statements; corporate annual reports; financial statements; planning documents; organization charts; and Web site. To find out "how things really work" talk to people who know the organization about how decisions are really made, about personalities, social networks, office politics, and history (Kovner & Neuhauser, 2004).

2. Understand the Economic Context of Health Care

Who is going to pay for your health promotion program? With the large economic role played by Medicare, Medicaid, and private health insurance, the answer to this question can be a challenge. The growing number of uninsured Americans and the small but growing use of personal health savings accounts mean that compared to the recent past, relatively more care is being paid for today directly by patients rather than by third-party insurers.

It is important to know how the payments by third parties are made. Payment methods include fee-for-service, prospective payment, capitation, and for government agencies, fixed yearly budgets. As discussed more fully in Chapter Three, Medicare is a federal government program that pays for health care for people over the age of sixty-five and for people with some long-term chronic conditions, such as those needing renal dialysis. Medicaid is a federal and state program for the poor. Eligibility rules for who is covered and what services are covered vary by state. Private health insurance primarily pays for care for employees and their families. There are also government health care systems that are funded by fixed yearly budgets. These include the Indian Health Service and the systems run by the Veterans Administration and the active duty military services. Health maintenance organizations are paid a fixed amount per member enrolled per month, regardless of how much care is provided. Such HMOs have an economic reason for having healthy enrollees. Medicare and other insurers that make prospective payments to hospitals use a fixed payment for each diagnosis related group (DRG), whether the patient has more tests or less or a longer or shorter stay, giving hospitals an economic incentive to discharge patients sooner. If a government organization has a fixed budget allocation from year to year, then a new prevention program means that some other activity must be reduced. Out-of-pocket, or self-pay, payment takes several forms. Many people are willing to pay to use fitness centers and commercial products that are seen as promoting attractiveness, health, and well-being. People without health insurance may seek out lower-cost alternatives to medical care such as faith healing or traditional therapies. Health savings accounts coupled with a health insurance plan allow people to set money aside (tax-free) in a savings account to be used to pay for their own care, perhaps up to $5,000. When this amount is spent then the health insurance benefits start.

In summary, money is available for health promotion from many sources, but it is necessary to understand the revenue streams available for each proposed program.

3. Define the Health Promotion Program

Disease prevention can be divided into three types: environmental, behavioral, and clinical. Funding for important environmental prevention approaches typically comes from outside the health care field. Some examples of these approaches are efforts to construct safer highways, laws to control air and water pollution, programs for violence prevention, systems for air traffic control, use of car air bags and safety belts, and maintenance of a clean public drinking-water supply. Some programs, such as pasteurization of milk and restaurant sanitary inspections, are under the direction of health departments.

Behavioral prevention addresses both activities that are beneficial and activities that are harmful to individuals, such as, on the one hand, exercising, dieting, or using bicycle helmets and, on the other hand, smoking, drinking to excess, or taking part in high-risk sexual behavior.

Clinical health prevention includes activities such as disease screening and vaccinations, prenatal care, well-child visits, and periodic health checkups (U.S. Department of Health and Human Services, Public Health Service, 1991). Two of these vaccination efforts, for smallpox and polio, have been so successful that smallpox no longer exists in the open (outside the laboratory) and polio is no longer resident in all the Americas. At one time these diseases had a massive effect on health care costs, morbidity, and mortality (Daniel & Robbins, 1997; Hopkins, 1983).

A health promotion program proposal needs a clear definition of the content of the work to be done: who will do what for whom and where, when, and how. Answering these questions about the work to be done is the first step in calculating the costs of the program and developing a projected budget.

In developing a program two sources of information are especially valuable. One is assessing descriptions of successful programs in the published literature; program developers can learn from reviewing these accounts. The second is reviewing similar existing programs; program developers can gather valuable first-hand information from such programs.

4. Determine What the Program Will Cost

Here are some useful key concepts in managerial accounting:

Add-on incremental costs	How much more will have to be spent, beyond the current activities of the organization, to carry out the program?

Staffing costs	Salaries plus fringe benefits.
Supplies	This cost often depends on the number of clients served. This is a *variable* cost.
Equipment	This category of expenses is for expensive items that are used over several years. Their value depreciates over time.
Overhead	The program will need space, and there is a cost for this. There will also be costs for heat, light, electricity, and telephone services. Many organizations use standardized rates to calculate what each program costs in overhead.
Other costs	Depending on the program, travel costs or malpractice insurance may be included in the budget.

Look for examples of proposed budgets for other successful programs in your organization and learn from them.

5. Identify Program Benefits

Those who wish to advocate for more preventive services within the U.S. medical care system face a new imperative. It is no longer adequate to just say that prevention is good and therefore support is justified; ideals and virtue alone will not be persuasive. It is necessary to demonstrate that the preventive program being advocated really works. It must *give value for money.* Consider Louise B. Russell's summary of her 1986 review of screening efficacy: "A growing body of research indicates that the chronic, degenerative diseases of middle and old age can often be prevented or at least delayed many years. While prevention has great potential, it is neither riskless nor costless. The evidence also shows that, even after allowing for savings in treatment, prevention usually adds to medical expenditures, contrary to the popular view that it reduces them. Prevention cannot be assumed to be a better choice than cure in every case. Individual measures must be evaluated on their merits" (pp. 109–110). In her 1994 follow-up review, she stated: "The issue of first importance for any screening test is whether it accomplishes anything. A test may detect the condition accurately, but does anything need to be done about the condition, and if something needs to be done, are any of the available therapies effective? Are they more effective when applied early? Unless early treatment makes a difference, screening is pointless. . . . The high costs of screening are often ignored, indeed unrecognized, by those who develop recommendations" (pp. 77, 81).

There is a growing interest in evidence-based medicine, nursing, and health management. This means knowing what works and doing it. Increasingly the clinical literature for the health care professions includes careful evaluations of outcomes. This literature is the place to start. Can you show good evidence from previous studies that programs like yours make a difference? This requires knowing what good evidence is.

To show that a prevention effort works, a researcher should do the following: take two similar groups of persons who may benefit, and invite their participation. Involve one group in the prevention effort, and leave the other group alone. Then look at the results for both groups, and see whether the expected difference occurred (Riegelman & Hirsch, 1989; Meinyk & Fineout-Overholt, 2004; Bowers, House, & Owens, 2001; Downie, Fyfe, & Tannahill, 1990; see Chapter Two).

The necessary similarity of the study groups is best achieved by random assignment of persons to the groups. The study subjects should be similar to actual clients (for *generalizability* of the results) and numerous enough so that change can be observed (known as *power*). Participants are asked for informed consent, even though they may not know which group they are in (a *blind* study). For example, the intervention to be studied could be a screening test with follow-up treatment. The expected outcome should be clearly defined in advance (for example, cancers found, years of life saved), measurable, and posited to result from the preventive effort. The difference, if any, between the outcomes for the groups should be large enough so that they are unlikely to have occurred by chance (statistical tests of significance should be applied).

The U.S. Preventive Services Task Force (1996) used this approach to evaluate 169 clinical preventive services. The task force considered the best evidence to come from randomized controlled trials. Intermediate evidence came from other types of studies, and the lowest quality of evidence involved expert opinion alone (Battista & Lawrence, 1988; Canadian Task Force on the Periodic Health Examination, 1979).

If you have an understanding of the previous experiences of other similar programs, you may be able to use their results to estimate the benefits of your program. For example, an existing school-based program has been shown to reduce the number of teenage smokers by 10 percent. You plan to provide a similar program in five high schools in your city with 4,000 students. Therefore you predict that there will be 400 fewer smokers. Can you measure the number of smokers before and after your program starts to see if your program meets your expectations? Note that such a program makes sense for a public health agency that has the mission of improving the health of all the people in the area. Would an HMO in a competitive market do this? Why should it use member payments to help a group that includes people who are nonmembers, who may be members of a competing health plan? Nevertheless there are examples of such health plans joining together to share the costs and the health benefits of such community-wide health promotion programs.

6. Compare Costs and Value

Even if something is known to work, is it worth doing? To answer this broad question, a new set of tools is needed. These tools include technology assessment (Reiser & Anbar, 1984), clinical decision analysis (Petitti, 1994), and economic reasoning, including cost-benefit and cost-effectiveness analysis (Elixhauser, Luce, Taylor, & Reblando, 1993; Pelletier, 2001) (defined in Exhibit 16.1). The U.S. Preventive Services Task Force (whose function is described in Chapter Three) recognized the difference between showing that an effort worked versus showing that it is worth doing. Adding other information to its knowledge of efficacy (does it work), the task force developed an alphabetical summary score (based on earlier work of the Canadian Task Force on the Periodic Health Examination [now known as the Canadian Task Force on Preventive Health Care]): A is good evidence for use, B is fair evidence for use, C is poor evidence for use, D is fair evidence to reject, and E is good evidence

EXHIBIT 16.1. DEFINITIONS OF DECISION-MAKING TOOLS.

Medical technology assessment is the broadest of these concepts. It is the total evaluation of the social impact of a medical technology, such as a surgical procedure, laboratory test, or early cancer detection method.

Clinical decision analysis considers the choices; the consequences of those choices; the probability that those consequences will occur; how those consequences are valued; and given this information, how the right choice is made.

Cost-effectiveness analysis compares the costs of doing something and measures the outcomes in nonmonetary terms, such as years of life saved or cancers found. Cost per year of life saved is a typical outcome of such analysis.

Cost-benefit analysis compares the inputs, measured in costs, with the outputs (results or benefits), also measured in costs (or savings), to see whether the benefits are greater than the costs.

for exclusion from periodic health examinations. Preventive services with A ratings are generally the only ones that are promoted and paid for.

Clinical Decision Analysis

The U.S. Preventive Services Task Force and its Canadian counterpart paid particular attention to screening for disease. The following is a set of questions to ask to determine whether such screening tests are worth doing. These questions are associated with clinical decision analysis.

- What are the alternative choices? The major clinical choices are *test* or *not test* and *treat* or *not treat*.
- Who makes the decision: the client, health care professional, health plan, or society? All have slightly different interests at stake. One reason for these differences is the economic consequences of the decision. For example, an individual with health insurance may pay only a small part of the cost for an examination, whereas the insurer will pay for most of the cost. Deductibles and coinsurance payments are ways that health insurance plans share the costs of care with plan members. Such copayments have been shown to reduce the use of medical services. Today there are legislative proposals to allow family health savings accounts that are coupled with insurance and a $1,000 or even a $5,000 deductible. With such plans the family pays the first $1,000 or $5,000 of health care costs from its health savings account before health plan payments start. If this approach becomes widespread, it is expected to have a major effect on the use of medical services.
- What is the prevalence, or frequency, of the disease among the population being tested or screened? The rarer the condition, the greater the costs per case. There is considerable agreement that mammography is appropriate for women older than fifty years and generally not appropriate for use as a screening tool among those younger than forty years. There is a lively debate, however, about the appropriateness for all women aged forty to forty-nine years (Eddy, 1980). This debate focuses on the prevalence of the condition, the predictive value of screenings, and where to draw the line for a policy recommendation and reimbursement.
- How accurate is the test? There are two types of test errors—a test can be positive when the client is healthy, or a test can be negative when the client has the disease. There are four basic measures of how good a test is for a population being evaluated: sensitivity, specificity, predictive value positive, and predictive value negative. The relationships among these measures are best shown by a two-by-two matrix (Riegelman & Hirsch, 1989) (Figure 16.1).

FIGURE 16.1. FOUR MEASURES OF TEST USEFULNESS.

	Without Disease	With Disease
	b (false positives)	a (true positives)
	d (true negatives)	c (false negatives)
	b + d	a + c

Test is positive = a + b.
Test is negative = c + d.

Note: Sensitivity is $a/(a + c)$: the number of diseased patients with a positive test divided by all diseased patients.

Specificity is $d/(b + d)$: the number of healthy patients with negative test results divided by all healthy patients.

Predictive value positive is $a/(a + b)$: the number of true positives divided by the total number of patients testing positive.

Predictive value negative is $d/(c + d)$: the total number of true negatives divided by the total number of patients testing negative.

- What is the probability of obtaining a positive result?
- What is the next step if the test is positive?
- If action to treat is taken, what are the assurances that the treatment will be beneficial? What are the expected outcomes of treatment?

After answering this set of questions, the next steps in clinical decision making involve measuring the outcomes in a common metric (such as years of life saved, dollars spent or saved, or cancers found) and comparing the choices according to their average expected outcomes. The test (or treatment) with the better average outcome is selected. This is the basic structure of clinical reasoning.

Cost-Effectiveness Analysis

Cost-effectiveness analysis (CEA) relates the costs of the proposed program (efforts or inputs) to the outcomes (results or outputs) in the form of a ratio. Typical examples in health care are cost per cancer found, cost per auto accident avoided, cost per vaccination given, cost per life saved, cost per year of life saved, and cost per quality-adjusted life-year saved (QALYS).

Consider a study in which a large public awareness program aimed at reducing smoking is carried out in eleven communities (experimental communities) and is not conducted in eleven other similar communities (control communities). The results show that 10 percent of moderate smokers quit because of the program. The cost of the three-year program, including advertising and brochure costs, was $300,000 for each community. There were 5,000 moderate smokers in the study, and 500 of those quit as a result of the program (the program results show that 1,000 quit in the control communities and 1,500 quit in the communities with the program; thus the 500-person difference is presumed to be a result of the experimental program).

Were the costs (inputs) appropriately measured? Was everything included? On the output side the measure is the number of smokers who quit as a result of the program. The benefits derived because these individuals no longer smoke could be measured by total years of life saved, rather than just by the raw number of quitters. The years of life saved could be estimated from epidemiologic studies showing the life expectancy of smokers compared with the life expectancy of nonsmokers.

In this study the cost in each community per quitter is $600 ($300,000 total community program cost divided by 500 quitters equals $600). Should this preventive program be recommended? This question can only be answered by asking: How else could this money be spent? If the next best smoking cessation program has a cost-effectiveness ratio of $1,000 per quitter, then the $600 program is preferred. However, if another choice is to give influenza immunizations to the elderly at a cost of $50 per immunization, and only one program can be selected, it is difficult to decide which one it should be. It is necessary to transform the two different outcomes (quitters and immunizations) into a common metric, such as years of life saved, to make a comparison and a decision. One way to decide which program to select is to calculate years of life saved for both programs and assume that one year of life is valued the same for all, and then choose the program with the lowest cost per year of life saved. One should note that after doing so, one group will benefit and the other will not. This is called the *distribution effect*.

It is not necessary for health care professionals to engage in debates regarding the broader social, political, or economic outcomes of prevention choices (for example, young smokers are productively employed; the elderly are revered for their age and wisdom); however, it is important to be aware of this issue of distributive justice.

The last fifteen years have seen an explosion in the number of studies of the cost effectiveness of preventive and medical treatments. These studies calculate program costs per year of life saved. Tammy Tengs and associates (1995) have summarized the results of 500 life-saving interventions (a current list can be found at www.hsph.harvard.edu/cearegistry). In some instances the analyses show that the intervention saves both money and lives. An example is the use of fire detectors in homes. The cost of the detectors was more than made up by reduced fire damage, and the detectors saved lives. Some interventions showed a cost per year of life saved, but the cost was low, such as the chlorination of drinking water ($3,100 per year of life saved). Some interventions are beyond our society's resources to fund. A sampling of health promotion and disease prevention program results based on estimated cost per year of life saved are listed in Table 16.1. Studies such as the ones summarized in this table are conducted in specific settings and circumstances; change those settings and circumstances and the results could be different; also costs will change over time. The results in Table 16.1 evaluate only

TABLE 16.1. EXAMPLES OF HEALTH-RELATED COST-EFFECTIVENESS STUDY RESULTS.

Program Studied	Estimated Cost per Year of Life Saved
Fire detectors in homes	Saved lives and money
Mandatory motorcycle helmet laws	Saved lives and money
Reduced lead content in gasoline	Saved lives and money
Sickle-cell screening for African American newborns	$240
Influenza vaccination for high-risk persons	$570
Mammography for women aged 50 years	$180
Random motor vehicle inspection	$1,500
Smoking cessation advice for women aged 45–49 years	$1,900
Chlorination of drinking water	$3,100
National speed limit of 55 miles per hour	$6,600
Annual mammography versus current screening practices for women aged 40–49 years	$190,000
Preoperative chest X-rays to detect abnormalities in children	$360,000
Warning letters sent to problem drivers	$720,000
Asbestos ban in automatic transmission components	$66 million
Sickle-cell screening for nonblack, low-risk newborns	$34 billion

Source: Data from Tengs et al., 1995.

years of life saved and not the quality of those years. One method of combining these measures is to use quality-adjusted years of life saved. Another approach considers how much individuals themselves would be willing to pay to prolong their lives. This *willingness to pay* approach does not consider distributive justice (see Chapter Seventeen). When only one program can be funded, then one group benefits and the other groups needing other services do not benefit.

Cost-Benefit Analysis

Cost-benefit analysis (CBA) measures both inputs and outputs in dollar amounts. CBA allows decisions to be made in a way that is not possible using cost-effectiveness analysis. Cost-effectiveness analysis can rank order programs, but it does not define a cutoff point above which programs should be funded and below which programs should not be funded. In contrast, CBA defines approved programs as those where the benefits of a program exceed the costs. In the preceding example of a smoking cessation program, suppose the societal benefit of quitting smoking is $1,000 per person in terms of treatment costs avoided and productive life prolonged. Five hundred smokers stopped as a result of this program, which cost $300,000 per community. In this example, the costs total $300,000 but the benefits total $500,000 (500 quitters multiplied by $1,000 savings per quitter). Therefore this program should be implemented.

Cost-benefit analysis often requires translating years of human life into a dollar value. This is unnerving for many, and the translation is so imperfect that most analysts shy away from it. Table 16.2 gives examples of CBA in use.

Note that in the smoking cessation example, the costs and benefits accrue to different persons or organizations. Taxpayers may have paid for the program; smokers benefited with longer, better lives; and the smokers' employers saved on the cost of health care benefits. Note that the costs occur today and the benefits occur in the future. The concept of discounting is used to calculate the present value of future benefits.

7. Develop the Plan

The program plan is developed from the information gathered in the previous six steps. Program directors need to be able to explain their plan to others verbally and often in writing. The features of the description will depend on the decision makers being addressed. They could be funding agencies (grant proposal), organizational managers (budget justification), or bankers (business plan to start a private practice). With this information about the program and its costs and expected

TABLE 16.2. HEALTH PLAN
COST-BENEFIT ANALYSIS (HYPOTHETICAL COSTS).

Program	Description	Program Cost	Cost Savings	Net Savings	Area of Savings
Pediatric fever acute care	Use of fever education video and pamphlet for acute care	$150,000	$400,000	$250,000	Office
Influenza immunization	Mailed and telephone reminders	$3,000	$42,000	$39,000	Hospital
Asthma emergency department initiative	Identification of at-risk population; client and physician/staff education	$30,000	$200,000	$170,000	Emergency room
Diabetic amputation prevention	Identification of at-risk population; client education about foot care	$30,000	$165,000	$135,000	Hospital

outcomes (improved health, client satisfaction, revenue, and so forth), you can write up a plan of work. Your estimates can also become budget projections, which can be used to compare expected outcomes with actual performance.

Here are some other things to think about when developing a program:

- External performance evaluation of health care organizations is becoming widespread. Increasingly, health care organizations are having their outcomes evaluated and comparative performance information is being made available. One example of this information is HEDIS (Health Plan Employer Data and Information Set.) Another example is that hospitals are being asked to report referrals to smoking education programs by the Joint Commission on Accreditation of Healthcare Organizations (JCAHO).

- Some prevention saves money, but the reimbursement system may not capture these returns. Educating asthmatics in self-management can reduce expensive emergency visits and hospital admissions. In an HMO these savings are seen. For a hospital reimbursed for each admission, this same program could mean lost revenues.

- Some prevention benefits occur in the long run. When HMOs and employer health plans have a 20 to 30 percent yearly turnover of enrollees, then long-term health promotion will benefit other insurers. However, if all employers in an area can agree to provide support for health promotion, all will gain from benefits experienced by workers as long as these workers stay in the community, even if they change jobs.

- Some people prefer to work where there are active health promotion activities. Some people choose their health plans because they provide such programs. If evidence can be found that this is happening, it can be used to justify such programs for corporate employers.

Consider the following two plan development case studies.

Plan Development: Case Study One

A midsized managed care organization (an HMO) has 200,000 enrollees. It is committed to designing programs and services to improve the quality and decrease the costs of health care for its members. For example, these programs address smoking cessation to reduce heart disease mortality, eye screening for diabetics to reduce blindness, and education for asthmatics to reduce their need for emergency care. Outcomes of the health promotion programs are examined at three levels: enrolled members, employers, and society (see Exhibit 16.2).

EXHIBIT 16.2. POTENTIAL LEVELS AND TYPES OF BENEFITS FROM AN HMO'S HEALTH PROMOTION PROGRAMS.

Members
- Improved quality of life (for example, stress reduction)
- Less morbidity and disability (for example, back pain management)
- Lower mortality (for example, influenza immunizations for the elderly)
- Lower health care costs (for example, reduced emergency care for asthma)

Employers
- Reduced time lost from work (for example, from absenteeism)
- Improved productivity
- Lower health insurance premiums
- Increased employee satisfaction; better recruitment and retention of workers
- Ability to meet labor union contract requirements

Society
- Improved economic productivity
- Lower health costs
- Community benefits (for example, less risk of infectious disease)

Many disease care programs are aimed at improving quality and reducing costs. A process has been developed to assist the organization in the selection and prioritization of projects, or interventions. The projects are first considered by a quality project evaluation committee, which considers the value of the project and whether its outcomes can be tracked by an evaluator. An analysis is then conducted to determine the potential impact and applicability of each project to the managed care organization's population. The analysis has four stages: a review of the relevant literature, a review of available demographic databases, a determination of estimated cost savings, and a determination of each project's costs (Table 16.3 displays the hypothetical outcome of such an analysis).

The initial stage in determining the feasibility of a project is a review of the relevant literature, including peer-reviewed published literature. The literature is studied to determine the intervention's potential impact. For example, according to the literature, a program to encourage the use of aspirin in individuals with coronary artery disease (CAD) has shown fewer fatal and nonfatal events, improved quality of life, and lower costs. It has been reported that aspirin use can lead to a 34 percent reduction in nonfatal heart attacks, a 31 percent reduction in nonfatal stroke, and a 17 percent reduction in vascular deaths (Antiplatelet Trialists' Collaboration, 1994).

The second stage includes a review of demographic databases to determine the potential impact of an intervention for the population of interest. Membership systems can be used to determine the number of members in a particular age or gender group. A computerized client record system can be used to determine the number of hospital admissions or ambulatory visits in the population of interest with a particular diagnosis. For example, the number of members with a myocardial infarction or the number of office visits for depression can be obtained from the plan's computerized patient and member information system. Information about the demographics of the membership can be used to target and tailor the project to the group or subgroups of interest: for example, influenza immunizations for nursing home residents.

The next step includes a determination of potential savings and the incremental cost to the health care organization of treating a member with the disease in question. The literature can be used to help determine the cost per year of medical care for a member with the disease. For example, one $10,000 hospital admission avoided per 1,000 plan members reduces each member's average cost by $10.

The final step is a determination of the costs of the program. In Table 16.3 these costs are for the health plan. Costs could also be calculated for the patient, such as travel and waiting time costs. Costs could also be calculated for the employer, such as days lost from work.

These steps are summarized in Table 16.3 for coronary artery disease (CAD), diabetes, and depression. The literature review generated the findings on these potential interventions and their impact on health. The plan's demographic database was used to determine the prevalence (percentage of members with the condition and the 5,600 members of this HMO who are affected). The incremental program costs are calculated as a cost per year per member with the disease. In the case of CAD, a four-part intervention (lipid control, smoking cessation, beta blockers, and aspirin) was projected to

TABLE 16.3. HYPOTHETICAL DISEASE CARE PROGRAM TABLE: HMO WITH 200,000 ENROLLEES.

Disease Care Program	Prevalence	No. of Members Affected	Incremental Cost to the Health Care Organization of Treating Members with This Disease	Potential Interventions	Impact on Health Outcomes
Coronary artery disease (CAD)	2.8%	5,600	$5,169, based on plan information	Lipid-lowering medications	35% reduction in major CAD events; reduction in revascularization
				Smoking cessation	Reduced morbidity and mortality
				Use of beta blockers after a heart attack	Improved health in members
				Aspirin use	Fewer fatal and nonfatal events in members with CAD
Diabetes	7.1%	16,000	$4,150	Control of blood sugar	Fewer complications; improved control; delays onset and progression of long-term complications
				Lipid screening and lipid-lowering medications	Less CAD among diabetic members; delays onset and progression of MI and stroke
				Eye screening	Less blindness among diabetics
				Renal screening	Fewer renal failures; improved quality of life
Depression	5%	10,000	$1,900	Evidence-based treatment program with a clearly defined treatment coordinator	Improved depression diagnosis and follow-up; potentially improved patient compliance with medications
				Use of validated instruments for initial diagnosis and follow-up assessments	More accurate initial diagnosis; more appropriate treatment selection and medication levels

cost $5,169 per member with the disease (5,600 members times $5,169 would give the total program cost per year). The three outcomes of this CAD program are the combined results of all four interventions.

The potential savings from the programs for CAD, diabetes, and depression in reduced hospital use are not quantified in this table. The information in Table 16.3 is at the heart of the business plans developed by the staff of the HMO, however. These plans were presented to the clinical management committee that selects the programs that can be funded within the money available. In this case, all three programs were approved.

Plan Development: Case Study Two

Another similar health plan has taken this kind of analysis further. It has developed a list of programs estimating the total cost of each program (see Table 16.2, displayed earlier in this chapter). These programs are for pediatric fevers, influenza immunizations, asthma, and diabetes care. The health plan estimates the total program costs; the savings from fewer office visits, hospital admissions, and emergency service use; and the net savings from the perspective of the plan. These costs and savings become the target objectives for the program managers. A year later, the health plan managers will look to see if these goals have been met. Where families have a choice of health plans, competition can have its effects. If one plan offers a popular health promotion program, then its competitors may have to do so too or lose members and their premium revenue. This change in revenue can be compared to the costs of the program. For government programs the logic of politics may result in different decisions. More money may be spent in a "swing state" in hopes of winning the next election rather than on better programs.

Summary

In an era of evidence-based medicine, nursing, and management and an era of cost control, health promotion program managers will need to be able to justify their programs within the context of their organizations. This requires answering these questions: What is the evidence that a program works? What is the content of the program? What does it do and will it cost? How many people will benefit, in what ways, and by how much? The program manager should be able to combine this information into a plan, budget projection, and performance measurement system to show whether the program has met or will meet expectations.

Good intentions alone will not justify the continuing existence of a health promotion program.

References

Antiplatelet Trialists' Collaboration. (1994). Collaborative overview of randomized trials of antiplatelet therapy: I. Prevention of death, myocardial infarction, and stroke by prolonged antiplatelet therapy in various categories of patients. *British Medical Journal, 308,* 81–97.

Battista, R. N., & Lawrence, R. S. (Eds.). (1988). Implementing preventive services. *American Journal of Preventive Medicine, 4*(4, Suppl.), 1–194.

Bowers, D., House, A., & Owens, D. (2001). *Understanding clinical papers.* New York: Wiley.

Canadian Task Force on the Periodic Health Examination. (1979). The periodic health examination. *Canadian Medical Association Journal, 121,* 1193–1254.

Daniel, T. M., & Robbins, F. C. (Eds.). (1997). *Polio.* Rochester, NY: University of Rochester Press.

Downie, R. S., Fyfe, C., & Tannahill, A. (1990). *Health promotion models and values.* New York: Oxford University Press.

Eddy, D. (1980). *Screening for cancer: Theory, analysis and design.* Upper Saddle River, NJ: Prentice Hall.

Elixhauser, A., Luce, B. R., Taylor, W. R., & Reblando, J. (1993). Health care cost-benefit and cost-effectiveness analysis from 1979 to 1990: A bibliography. *Medical Care, 31*(7, Suppl.), JS1–JS149.

Gold, M. L., Siegel, J. E., Russell, L. B., & Weinstein, M. C. (1996). *Cost effectiveness in health and medicine.* New York: Oxford University Press.

Hopkins, D. R. (1983). *Princes and peasants: Smallpox in history.* Chicago: University of Chicago Press.

Kovner, A., & Neuhauser, D. (Eds.). (2004). *Health services management: Readings, cases and commentary* (8th ed.). Chicago: Health Administration Press.

Meinyk, B., & Fineout-Overholt, E. (2004). *Evidence-based practice in nursing and health care.* Hagerstown, MD: Lippincott, Williams and Wilkins.

Pelletier, K. R. (2001). A review and analysis of the critical and cost-effectiveness studies of comprehensive health promotion and disease management programs at the worksite: 1998–2000 update. *American Journal of Health Promotion, 16*(2), 107–116.

Petitti, D. (1994). *Meta-analysis, decision analysis, and cost-effectiveness analysis.* New York: Oxford University Press.

Reiser, S., & Anbar, M. (1984). *The machine at the bedside.* New York: Cambridge University Press.

Riegelman, R. K., & Hirsch, R. P. (1989). *Studying a study and testing a test: How to read the medical literature* (2nd ed.). Boston: Little Brown.

Russell, L. B. (1986). *Is prevention better than cure?* Washington, DC: Brookings Institution.

Russell, L. B. (1994). *Educated guesses: Making policy about medical screening tests.* Berkeley: University of California Press.

Tengs, T. O., Adams, M. E., Pliskin, J. S., Safran, D. G., Siegel, J. E., Weinstein, M. C., et al. (1995). Five-hundred life saving interventions and their cost effectiveness. *Risk Analysis, 15*(3), 369–390.

U.S. Department of Health and Human Services, Public Health Service. (1991). *Healthy people: National health promotion and disease prevention objectives* (DHHS Pub. No. [PHS] 91-50212). Washington, DC: U.S. Government Printing Office.

U.S. Preventive Services Task Force. (1996). *Guide to clinical preventive services* (2nd ed.). Baltimore: Williams & Wilkins.

CHAPTER SEVENTEEN

FUTURE DIRECTIONS FOR HEALTH PROMOTION

Sherri Sheinfeld Gorin

The landscape for health promotion will continue to change over the next ten years. More sociodemographic and economic changes will occur, including further growth in the aging population, increased diversity and urbanization in the U.S. population, community-based assessement and delivery of health care. In the future, as discussed in Chapter Three, communities will further increase their participation in the design, building, and evaluation of health promotion policies and programs worldwide.

Predicting the future generally rests in the realm of the soothsayer (or the strategic planner) rather than that of the health care professional. Nonetheless, a general guide to the most pronounced features of health promotion in the near future follows.

Demographic Shift Toward the Aging

The population of the developed world is aging, thus straining health care systems throughout this region. Further, populations are becoming increasingly diverse.

Worldwide, the projected rate of increase in the world's elderly population will be faster than that of the world's child population. Among the elderly worldwide, the segment of those aged eighty and older is the fastest growing. Most of these octogenarians live in developed countries now; however, it is projected that by 2020 the majority will live in developing countries (Organizacion Pan Americana de la Salud, 1992).

In America, persons aged sixty-five years and older constitute the fastest growing segment of the population. By 2020, more than sixty-four million Americans will be aged sixty-five years or older, constituting nearly 22 percent of the U.S. population. Women will predominate; minorities, however, will be underrepresented in this age group (Koplan & Livengood, 1994).

By the year 2020, the dependency ratio (that is, the proportion of persons not participating in the workforce to those who do participate) will increase because of the larger numbers of aged persons present (U.S. Senate Special Committee on Aging, 1991). This projection has obvious implications for changing health services and social support. As a result, in the United States the issue of reform in the Medicare and Social Security programs will continue to join the political agenda.

Policies and worldwide initiatives designed to encourage health promotion among older persons are being proposed at present (for example, the World Health Organization's Aging and Life Course initiative), and will no doubt continue to emerge as lawmakers themselves also age. Health promotion across the life span—from prenatal to elderly—will become important. To underpin these efforts the concept of *normality*, in the sense of a common or prevalent finding (for example, arthritis, root caries and periodontal disease, or an age-related increase in blood pressure), will require redefinition. Health care professionals will need to begin to view such normalities as risk factors for disease, rather than as immutable facts of aging.

Health promotion among older men and women will include efforts to maintain functional independence and add years of healthy life, rather than simply to elongate life. Increasingly, older Americans will be living alone and may need special assistance to retain their independent functioning. This assistance will involve help with performing activities of daily living (for example, bathing, dressing, and eating) so that individuals may remain residents in the community rather than being placed in long-term nursing care. Social support thus is a critical factor in the older person's ability to avoid institutionalization.

Chronic diseases are more common among the elderly than the young. A considerable number of the major causes of death among persons aged sixty-five and older—heart disease, cancer, stroke, chronic obstructive pulmonary disease, pneumonia, and influenza—are preventable or can be controlled. Changing certain health behaviors (for example, stopping smoking, eating a balanced diet, reducing sodium, losing weight if overweight, and increasing physical activity) can reduce the risk of disease among older adults (Institute of Medicine [IOM], 1990).

People age sixty-five and older consume about one-third of all prescriptions that are dispensed (Cassel et al., 2003). With the recent passage of "Medicare D" (The Medicare Prescription Drug, Improvement, and Modernization Act), the cost of these medications, particularly to low-income elderly, may be more fully covered by Medicare. The appropriate use of medications, both prescribed and over-the-counter, is critical to health promotion among older persons. Adverse reactions may be exacerbated by decreased kidney and liver functions as individuals age; these physiological alterations can change the way the body processes medications. Different drugs or lower doses may be used to offset these alterations.

The impact of medications and also general medical treatment on oral health, through increasing, for example, dry mouth (xerostomia) and orofacial pain, is increasingly important as individuals age (Narhi, Vehkalahti, Siukosaan, & Ainamo, 1998; Vargas, Kramarow, & Yellowitz, 2001; USDHHS, 2000). As detailed in Chapter Eight, oral health has considerable impact on medical health in assisting with nutritional adequacy and in moderating the advent or progression of type 2 diabetes, cardiovascular disease, stroke, and aspiration pneumonia (USDHHS, 2000; Budtz-Jørgensen, Chung, & Rapin, 2001).

Particularly among older individuals, health care professionals can monitor health status to detect early signs of health problems that would threaten independence, and can ensure accurate distinctions in diagnosis. For example, increased use of screening tools in primary care for the assessment of depression and early cognitive deficits, such as the deterioration of memory, orientation, general intellect, specific cognitive capacities, and social functioning—the clinical precursors to dementia and Alzheimer's disease—will become more important. As patients with Alzheimer's disease, particularly those with advanced disease, may be expected to deteriorate in function over time, regular discussions between family and health care professionals about appropriate medical care regimens as well as health promotive approaches to enrich quality of life are critical (Sheinfeld Gorin, Heck, Albert, & Hershman, 2005).

Clearly, increased resources will need to be devoted to the elderly; given a declining workforce, however, from where will the resources come? By 2013, if current U. S. trends continue, one out of every four dollars of personal consumption will be spent on health care (Heffler et al., 2004). An ethic of personal and family responsibility for health and the importance of lifestyle changes could again become an ideology to justify resource distributions. In contrast, an ideology that supports a fair, equitable distribution of bargaining power and resources among children, the young, working adults, and the old could be encouraged. A uniform political will, as well as economic munificence, will be required to support the chosen policy aims.

Health Insurance and Worksites

Three out of every five nonelderly Americans receive employer-based health insurance, either from their own employer or another family member's, and many
of these insurance plans cover preventive health care. Economic downturns, combined with less workplace insurance coverage of workers' families, have reduced
and will reduce that coverage, with serious consequences for the health of employees and their families, particularly low-wage earners, who are disproportionately African American or Latino.

Even among the insured, however, economic changes have altered the social
contract between employer and worker (particularly those workers shifted from
permanent to contractual or part-time jobs) and in many cases have eroded the
quality and scope of health insurance coverage and other employee benefits such
as employer-funded pensions. To reduce labor costs, employers are increasing the
portion of health insurance premiums paid by employees, especially for dependents, and are introducing other cost-sharing devices. The costs of increased employer efficiency thus continue to be borne by individual workers, and the effects
are felt by them, their families, and their communities.

As discussed in Chapter Fourteen, increased employer production efficiencies
leading to an outsourced or reduced labor force have also placed increased psychosocial demands on those who remain employed, because they must do more
work at their old level of compensation. Unpleasant or dangerous physical conditions such as crowding, noise, air pollution, or ergonomic problems, may delimit
productivity (National Institute for Occupational Safety and Health, 1999). Owing
to labor uncertainties, workers often stay in positions they dislike or perceive to
be below their level of competence, and these circumstances can lead to deleteri-
ous health consequences (Pelletier, 1994). Furthermore, employers, seeking better
locations or economic conditions, may rearrange the physical workspace or change
the location of the worksite, often requiring increased commuting from workers,
or may threaten workers with job elimination through out-sourcing the work to
other locales or further automation. As a result of fewer union protections, workers' concerns about job security and midlife career changes have increased
(Stokols, Churchman, Scharf, & Wright, 1990), often leading to psychological
stress, elevated blood pressure, performance decrements, and increased illness
symptoms (Novaco, Stokols, & Milanesi, 1990; Schaeffer, Street, Singer, & Baum,
1988; Bocchino, Hartman, & Foley, 2003; Kenny & Cooper, 2003).

Yet worksites have the potential to serve as centers for community-based
health promotion initiatives in the future: One study found that every dollar spent

on Citibank's worksite health promotion program saved nearly $5 in medical expenditures (Ozminkowski et al., 1999). Several other studies have found similarly high returns on investment for worksite health programs (Ozminkowski et al., 2002; for a review, see Aldana, 1998).

As detailed in Chapter Fourteen, organizations can enhance wellness by implementing *organizational health scans,* such as checklists or organizational surveys of the elements that seem most beneficial to morale and productivity. Changes can be tracked over time and among departments. Eventually, organizations can share their findings, creating a "Health Fortune" database useful to business leaders, policymakers, health providers, and researchers committed to continuously improving an increasingly diverse, health-insurance dependent and production-oriented workplace.

Growth in Community- and Evidence-Based Health Care

Communities will become a larger focus for health promotion in the future.

Focus on Health of the Community

As described in Chapter Three, health plans, such as Blue Cross Blue Shield and Group Health Cooperative of Puget Sound, have become more involved with the health of local communities. They have applied the techniques of managed care to insuring health care for a defined population (Manley, Griffin, Foldes, Link, & Sechrist, 2003). Because of their large size, these plans are likely to be active participants in the decisions regarding the provision of preventive services.

Most of these plans have implemented disease management programs that are designed to improve the clinical and economic outcomes for such chronically ill individuals as those with asthma, diabetes mellitus, depression, and rheumatoid arthritis. These programs often involve client self-management education, health care professional education, and screening, with routine reporting and regular feedback loops to support communication among these structures. Risk reduction through smoking cessation, for example, has been incorporated into many of these programs. Although programs are increasingly being asked to demonstrate improvement in clinical quality across several diseases, using uniform and clinical meaningful metrics, they have already demonstrated improved quality of care for depression (Neumeyer-Gromen, Thomas Lampert, Stark, & Kallischnigg, 2004).

Using disease management programs as a model, these programs may integrate clients, health care professionals, and varied health care sectors to enhance prevention in communities. They may also partner with others, using their power to encourage education, legislation, and regulations to, for example, prevent the initiation of tobacco use or encourage seat belt use among children and their parents. Alternatively, based upon the relative cost advantage of mortality for the most vulnerable, these plans may choose to fund fewer preventive services and thereby provide less care over an individual's shorter life span.

Evidence-Based Health Care

Accountability to consumers, providers, and regulators is an important feature of equitable health care. Generally, *evidence* is used to denote something that makes another thing evident; in clinical medicine the strongest evidence rests on a positivist base derived from a randomized clinical trial or a rigorous observational study (as described further in Chapter Two).

The application of evidence to health care, through evidence-based guidelines, offers advantages of consistency, predictability, and objectivity, as well as cost containment, that general advisory statements do not. The health care professional must balance, in the use of guidelines, the goal of standardization against the need for clinical flexibility. To achieve this balance, the Institute of Medicine (2003) has recommended that private accrediting entities and state regulatory bodies require that health plans publish their clinical practice protocols, along with the supporting evidence, thereby opening these protocols to professional and consumer review (Bloche, 2001).

Of late, employers have begun to review *report cards* from the Health Plan Employer Data and Information Set (HEDIS) and accreditation ratings from the Joint Commission on Accreditation of Healthcare Organizations (JCAHO) when making decisions about the health care services that they purchase. Further, many of these report cards, even those for individual health care professionals, have become available to consumers, on the Web (see, for example, State of California, Office of the Patient Advocate, 2005; Mukamel, Weimer, Zwanziger, Gorthy, & Mushlin, 2004/2005). Although few of these report cards highlight prevention, they can aid in patients' selection processes, lead to more informed choices, and improve access to the best providers for racial and ethnic minorities. If systems such as HEDIS continue to emphasize prevention and if useful information comparing providers on prevention becomes increasingly available, managed care entities and health plans will continue both to push for further evaluative mechanisms and to view the provision of cost-effective preventive services as a competitive tool for increasingly informed consumers.

The recommendations of the U.S. Preventive Services Task Force (USPSTF) and of the Task Force on Community Preventive Services (in *The Guide to Com-*

munity Preventive Services: What Works to Promote Health? by Zaza, Briss, & Harris, 2005) will continue to increase in importance in the United States. Both sets of recommendations use cost effectiveness as a consideration; given the certain growth in health care costs in the future, this concern will surely increase in importance alongside evidence-based outcomes. Explicit policy ramifications of health promotion programs will also become more important in the future.

The USPSTF is discussed in detail in Chapter Three. As *The Guide to Community Preventive Services* (the *Guide*) focuses on the community rather than the individual health care professional, its recommendations will be of particular interest to the field of health promotion as its guidelines increase (Briss et al., 2000). Given the pace of evidence-based recommendations, however, health promotion practice may outpace scientific guidance.

Choosing the Measures. It has been suggested that the focus of health promotion in the twenty-first century is finding the answer to the question, What makes people healthy? Policies and programs designed to build healthy communities and workplaces, strengthen social networks for health, and increase people's abilities to lead healthy lives are considered key to health promotion. The effects of health on wealth creation are yet to be fully measured.

A central question at the heart of these efforts, however, concerns obtaining a clear and consistent measurement of health. As discussed in Chapter One, health is a multifaceted concept. Measures of mortality, morbidity, and the use of health services are insensitive to short-term and small effects. Measures of health at the population level, such as the population attributable fraction or quality-adjusted life-years (that is, measures of the benefit of a health intervention in terms of a person's time spent in a series of quality-weighted health states) are imperfect. Local government measures of the determinants of health may rest on unreliable data sources. As discussed further in Chapter Twelve, indicators that are important to many community members, such as rates of violence, are difficult to quantify. Measures of the impact of important lifestyle factors such as diet, physical activity, and obesity are still less widely accepted, and so less useful, than are those for tobacco (see, for example, Royce, Sheinfeld Gorin, Edelman, Rendino-Perrone, & Orlandi, 1990a, 1990b), although, with funding support, these measures will improve in the future. It is difficult to select control populations against which to evaluate changes in programs and policies.

The challenge of developing tools to collect and evaluate evidence in response to the question of measuring health is daunting. A shift from measuring deficits to examining resilience and new models of community participation will move the field forward. As discussed in Chapter Two, theoretical models that incorporate multilevel concepts of health promotion and that explain changes in health over time are needed. Findings from studies using more comprehensive models of health promotion and better operationalized measures will, in time, be used both to evaluate and to enhance community planning, clinical programs, and health care professional and client dialogues.

In addition to the challenges of defining, choosing, and evaluating evidence, using the *Guide* as an exemplar, numerous methodological and political difficulties arise in consulting with stakeholders so that the findings from their participation are balanced and reliable. And, it is vital that outcomes that are simpler to understand and more reliably measured, such as costs, must not displace quality (or quality of life) as desirable community aims (Campbell, 1974; Sheinfeld Gorin, 1985).

Yet considerable methodological movement forward has been made—for example, with measures of "comprehensive community initiatives" (Weiss, 1995) and, in the field of social epidemiology, with the development of rigorous frameworks for triangulating qualitative and quantitative sources of evidence and for cluster randomization, time series measurement, and Bayesian and decision analysis modeling. These methods will continue to expand the repertoire of the health promotion researcher and further found practice (Parry & Stevens, 2001).

Developing Evidence for Health Promotion. Despite its increasing importance to all areas of health care, evidence-based practice is still relatively foreign to the change-oriented field of health promotion. Further, the use of the randomized clinical trial for evaluating health promotion programs has become a focus of debate. Although it is the gold standard of scientific evidence, many of the outcomes of interest to health promotion programs, such as intersectoral collaborations to improve quality of life, are nearly impossible to design and test using this methodology. In the future, new models will emerge to evaluate health promotion programs, often with more distal outcomes. Some may rely on the logic framework used by the *Guide*, that is, a diagram that maps out a chain of hypothesized causal relationships among determinants, intermediates (including mediators, which specify how or why effects hold; moderators or effect modifiers, which define under what conditions effects hold; and particularly in observational studies, confounders or predictors of outcome, which are associated with the exposure[s]), and health outcomes (Baron & Kenny, 1986; Bauman, Sallis, Dzewaltowski, & Owen, 2002; Gordis, 2000).

In addition to the qualitative approaches described briefly in Chapter Two, other, more novel approaches to evaluating evidence on the effectiveness of health promotion practice have been suggested. For example, in legal practice, evidence is often a mixture of stories, witness accounts, police testimony, expert opinions, and forensic science. It frequently comes from multiple sources and from persons of widely ranging expertise. Evidence requires interpretation of accounts that vary in their ontological origins (McQueen, 2001). These forms of evidence may be introduced into logic frameworks for the evaluation of health promotion programs.

Health Impact Assessments. The health consequences are explicit (and intended) in the programs addressed by the *Guide* and other evidence-based guidelines. However, public investments in other services and resources, ones that may span several sectors, such as building new highways or sports stadiums, also have implicit consequences on both health and health inequalities, and these consequences require elucidation. Such concerns may be addressed by a formal, systematic analysis (*health impact assessment,* or HIA) to prospectively assess the potential health impacts of proposed projects, programs, and policies. Uncommon in the United States but well accepted in Europe and Canada, the HIA has been widely used to increase community participation in decision making on issues that affect health or alongside environmental impact statements (Parry & Stevens, 2001; Cole et al., 2004). In the near future an HIA could examine the impact of intersectoral efforts to reduce obesity, or the effects of tax policies on the health of the entire population or on health disparities among subgroups (Cole et al., 2004). As discussed previously, increasing adoption of the HIA would require concurrent methodological advances to measure and assess community changes, and newer models of community participation.

The Role of Primary Care in Health Promotion

The most recent report of the Medicare Payment Advisory Commission (Medpac) (2005) has proposed that Congress should establish a quality incentive payment policy for physicians in Medicare. A pay-for-performance system is intended to improve the quality of care for beneficiaries. It could result in higher or lower payments for individual health care providers, depending on the quality of their care. Although the measures of quality to be used will expand, change, and improve over time, initially some measures of appropriate monitoring, follow-up, and coordination of patient care will be collected. As described in Chapter Three, primary care physicians in particular have not yet met all the *Healthy People 2010* goals for health promotion, and meeting these aims will be a challenge for many.

Academic Detailing

One promising strategy to increase physician compliance with evidence-based guidelines and to overcome physician barriers to health promotion is *academic detailing.* Academic detailing applies to physician involvement in health promotion the approach used by pharmaceutical salespersons. Academic detailers employ a brief, focused intervention, repeated at periodic intervals with the physician, in which they share materials and approaches that are tailored to the physician's barriers to, for example, preventive screening. Traditionally employed by pharmaceutical companies to promote prescription drug uptake among physicians, this approach has been found effective in many studies in which it has been evaluated (Shein-feld Gorin et al., 2000; Sheinfeld Gorin et al., in press; Honda & Sheinfeld Gorin, 2006; Thomson O'Brien et al., 2000; Schaffner, Ray, Federspiel, & Miller, 1983; Keys et al., 1995; Daly et al., 1993; Wyatt et al., 1998; Benincasa et al., 1996; Horowitz et al., 1996; Leninger et al., 1996; Dietrich, Sox, Tosteson, & Woodruff, 1994; Davis, Thompson, Oxman, & Haynes, 1995; Hulscher, Wensing, van der Weijden, & Grol, 2002).

Fundamentally, academic detailing seeks to change physicians' attitudes and beliefs toward prevention and health promotion through persuasive communications and to alter their knowledge (or cognitions) though tailored feedback and reinforcement. Concomitantly, it assists with the creation or maintenance of a prevention-oriented office, through staff training and through the provision of cues in office procedures (for example, flagged medical charts) to enrich the physician's memory of new information and to reinforce behavioral patterns.

Role of Informatics

To provide optimal care under a pay-for-performance program, physicians offices will need office-based systems capable of tracking numerous patient interactions over multiple settings of care, pharmaceutical use, test results, and continually evolving clinical guidelines. In fact, even manual office-based systems have been found to increase the provision of preventive care (Zapka, Puleo, Vickers-Lahti, & Luckmann, 2002; Dickey, Gemson, & Carney, 1999). Those offices that have put systematic processes, particularly computerized information technologies (IT) in place to improve care management, however, will be rewarded, so as to increase the use of electronic health records (Medpac, 2005).

Interactive media hold particular promise for enhancing the physician and patient interchange. A recent study suggests that Internet access is available to nearly three-quarters of all physicians (Kassirer, 2000; Jadad, Sigouin, Cocking, Whelan, & Brownman, 2001; Friedewald, 2000; Winkler, & Silberg, 1998; Glode, 1996). The Web is being used effectively to study disease, to educate, to train (Hayes & Lehmann, 1996; Harris, Salasche, & Harris, 2001; Chan, Leclair, & Kaczorowski, 1999), and to certify health care providers, even about the Web itself (Chi-Lum & Durkin, 1999). Interactive, digital programs offer promise both for enhancing health care provider understanding of evidence-based guidelines to improve the quality of care and for increasing providers' health promotion communication with patients.

In addition, the relatively new field of public health informatics—that is, the systematic application of information and computer science and technology to public health practice, research, and learning (Friede, Blum, & McDonald, 1995; Yasnoff, O'Carroll, Koo, Linkins, & Kilbourne, 2000)—suggests that information technology (IT) could enhance the health of communities and their populations as well. In particular, as described in Chapter Thirteen, new and improved information systems for public health will be necessary because of the risk of acts of chemical and biological terrorism, for which current national IT systems are either inadequate or nonexistent. Privacy concerns, however, will remain a challenge as these IT systems increasingly integrate and coordinate our health records and other data describing our lives.

Integration with Complementary and Alternative Medical Approaches

Interest in the integration of complementary and alternative medicine (CAM) with more orthodox medicine will continue to grow and expand over time. The CAM field has been legitimized by the formation of the National Institutes of Health National Center for Complementary and Alternative Medicine and the involvement of many noted scientific groups and universities in its study (for example, Columbia University's Richard & Hinda Rosenthal Center for Complementary & Alternative Medicine), and its formal integration into clinical practice (for example, the Integrative Medicine Service at Memorial Sloan-Kettering Cancer Center offers therapeutic massage, music therapy, meditation, acupuncture, and mind-body therapies as well as research, education, and training in the area).

Yet the two approaches to health care—orthodox and complementary—continue to reflect two different cultures, especially of science. Orthodox medical practice tends to view complementary approaches as placebos, or factors that are without specific activity for the condition being treated or evaluated (Shapiro & Morris, 1978). Orthodox medicine also views complementary and alternative medicine as using a less rigorous and a more qualitative approach to research. Several methodological obstacles to evaluating CAM remain, including the difficulty of defining a control or comparison condition for study and the variability of care from client to client, thus making treatment comparisons difficult (Levin et al., 1997). Further, the two approaches speak different languages in describing their health promotive activities. Nonetheless, in the future, more contact between the two sets of approaches will yield more integration in effective health promotive interventions, more consonance in their conduct of scientific inquiry, an expansion into spirituality, and the continued expansion of integrative clinical services, based on consumer demand.

Mental Health Promotion

According to a recent estimate from the World Health Organization, mental illness constitutes about 10 percent of the global burden of disease, suggesting the critical importance of mental health promotion. Depression will be one of the largest health problems worldwide by the year 2020 (Herrman, 2001). Depressive symptoms are associated with the development of ischemic disease as well as with poorer outcomes among patients who have preexisting cardiovascular disease (Glassman & Shapiro, 1998). In addition to cardiovascular risks, depressive symptoms are linked to higher morbidity and mortality in a number of other diseases, such as risk for cancer in older persons (Penninx et al., 1998); all-cause mortality in medical inpatients (Herrmann et al., 1998); risk for osteoporosis (Michelson et al., 1996); lessened physical, social, and role function; worse perceived current health; and greater bodily pain (Wells et al., 1989; IOM, 2000). As explored further in Chapter Fifteen and under the heading "Positive Psychology Perspective" in Chapter Two, mental health promotion involves an orientation toward health and not just treatment of illness. In the future, mental health promotion will involve a better understanding of the nature of mental health and mental illness as well as the development of policies and programs across multiple sectors, including law, social services, housing, and health, to alter the conditions that are conducive to health in its entirety.

Concern for Social Justice: Equity in Health Promotion

America's citizens who are poor—particularly poor children, the unemployed, and the economically marginal or exploited among racial and ethnic minorities—face social situations that place them at high risk for disease and premature death. In fact, poverty—partly because it is often associated with comparatively low levels of education—leads to poorer health prospects overall (Marmot et al., 1991; Tyroler, 1989; Salonen, 1982; Dayal, Power, & Chiu, 1982; Haan, Kaplan, & Camacho, 1987; Baquet, Horm, Gibbs, & Greenwald, 1991; Winkleby, Jatulis, Frank, & Fortmann, 1992; Guralink, Land, Blszer, Fillenbaum, & Branch, 1993; Charlton & White, 1995; Pappas, Queen, Hadden, & Fisher, 1993).

African Americans, in particular, have shown less movement toward health and are less likely to continue to move forward. For example, although white women have the highest incidence of breast cancer, black women have higher death rates from this disease. This finding is of particular concern for those committed to equitable health care.

Increasingly, the poor and underserved receive care through managed care organizations, Medicare, and Medicaid. A recent Institute of Medicine report urged that the same patient protections that apply to the privately insured should apply to those in publicly funded plans (Hashimoto, 2001). More and better insurance coverage for screening and counseling would encourage wider use of these services. Governments may encourage coverage for preventive services by commercial insurers and managed care entities by developing a market for such products and ensuring that they are financially viable. At present, many Americans have not received the clinical preventive services they need, in part due to financial barriers, thus contributing to the high levels of preventable morbidity and mortality in the population.

In addition, the number of individuals who are uninsured remains a problem, and that number may be increasing, particularly among children. As discussed in Chapter Three, forty-four million persons, including 11.2 million children, are without any health insurance because they are employed by firms that do not offer coverage or because they live below the poverty line and cannot afford it (U.S. Bureau of the Census, 2004). Uninsured children are more likely than the insured to lack a usual source of health care, to go without needed care, and to experience worse health outcomes (Institute of Medicine, 2002). Nearly 30 percent of children without coverage are under six years old, and one in three uninsured children lives in a family with an income below the poverty line (Mills & Bhandari, 2003; Employee Benefit Research Institute, 2004).

Of course, access to preventive services depends on more than insurance coverage. Access also depends on the provision of enabling services, such as transportation and the means to increase health literacy and reduce language barriers. National health policies could encourage equity in access to health services. These policies could be implemented by local coordinating bodies, such as the public health department, and overseen by a federal agency, such as the Centers for Disease Control and Prevention (CDC) or the Centers for Medicare and Medicaid Services (CMS) (CDC, 1995, 1996). Continued advocacy from the health care field, coupled with federal legislation and strong federal public health leadership, will be necessary to promote health among society's most vulnerable members.

Implications for Diverse Subpopulations

The well-documented disparities in morbidity and mortality from major diseases for blacks and Hispanics relative to whites, using varied measures, highlight the pressing need for health promotion programs that are culturally competent and tailored to relevant predisposing, enabling, and need-related factors as well as to the environmental conditions experienced by these populations. Of course black and Hispanic subgroups display considerable internal diversity as well, necessitating tailored, culturally relevant interventions both between and within subgroups. Some of the internal variations may be greater and more relevant to health promotion than the variations between the larger population groups.

For example, Latinos, the fastest growing population in the United States, are a highly diverse racial and ethnic subgroup. The U.S.–resident Latino population comprises Mexican Americans (66.9 percent of U.S. Latinos), mainland Puerto Ricans (8.6 percent), Central and South Americans (14.3 percent), Cubans (3.7 percent), and "other" Latinos (6.5 percent), a group that includes Latinos from the Dominican Republic and Spain, those with multiple Latino backgrounds, and those who do not identify with any one Latino group (U.S. Bureau of the Census, 2000).

Consequently, Latino subgroups vary in their disease (particularly, cancer) risk factors, including their rates of smoking and drinking alcohol and their patterns of dietary intake and exercise (Winkleby, Fortmann, & Rockhill, 1993; Loria et al., 1995; Gans et al., 2002; Cervantes, Gilbert, Salgado de Snyder, & Padilla, 1990; Epstein, Botvin, & Diaz, 2001; Gordon-Larsen, Harris, Ward, & Popkin, 2003; Perez-Stable et al., 2001). Overall, Latinos are less likely than whites to obtain recommended cancer screening services, due to economic, educational, cultural, and other structural barriers (Phillips, Morrison, Andersen, & Aday, 1998; National Center for Health Statistics, 2000; Sheinfeld Gorin & Heck, 2005). Psychosocial barriers, such as fear of screening and a sense of fatalism are important predictors of screening compliance among Latino subgroups (Sheinfeld Gorin, 2005). Their rates of disease (particularly cancer) morbidity and mortality also differ by subgroup (Mallin & Anderson, 1988; Rosenwaike & Shai, 1986; Warshauer, Silverman, Schottenfeld, & Pollack, 1986).

These findings suggest the vital importance of tailoring health promotion programs to population subgroups that are highly internally diverse.

Values for the Practice of Health Promotion

Because of major changes in the sociodemographics of the American populace and in the delivery of health care, in accountability, in technology, and in health promotion, ethical issues will emerge as critical to future practice. Some of the ethical questions to be answered in the near future are being posed now: for example, Should decisions about the allocations of monies from federal and foundation sources be made on the basis of the health of a community? Should health promotion interventions be targeted to those most in need or those in largest number? Is it morally acceptable (good) to smoke, to remain overweight? Should women at high risk for breast cancer undergo genetic testing? Who should see the results? How should the results be protected? What kinds of decisions about insurance, work, and family life should be made on the basis of these results?

Core Values

Given the challenges that the health care provider faces now and will face in the future, those who are working with clients toward health promotion must articulate their personal and collective vision of the *good life, health,* and the *good society.* They should make clear the values, models, and ideals they wish for individuals and for societies. For example, do they hold an individualist or a collectivist vision of society? They need "to explore and define what, very specifically, would be right. Toward what, stated as clearly as may be possible, should we aim?" (Galbraith, 1996, p. 1).

In the United States, liberal philosophies of self-determination and rugged individualism generate fears of moralizing others' actions or intruding into someone else's moral space (Etzioni, 1993; Sandel, 1996). Yet without moral direction, health care professionals' assumptions and practices may lead to abuses of power through their presuming to know best what clients need, stigmatizing clients with labels that imply deficits, or neglecting to consider social injustices (Prilleltensky, 1997).

A Dialogue on Values

In addition, health care professionals working to promote health may benefit from strategies for translating core values into action. The aim would be to generate a dialogue about the different conceptions of the good and how to arrive at them (Sheinfeld & Lord, 1981; Prilleltensky, 1997). Consensus would not be sought, nor would a particular conception of the good life, health, or the good society. An example of a structure for this dialogue is found in Chapter Sixteen of the *Health Promotion Handbook* (Sheinfeld Gorin & Arnold, 1998).

It is particularly important for the health care professional to seek consistency in the application of values to ethical questions. This is a difficult undertaking.

Commitment to Change

The ethical decisions health care professionals must continue to make emerge within a particular political context. At present, U. S. public policy for prevention is fragmented and fails to make use of the variety of strategies available to influence health-promoting behaviors of individuals and institutions. The current array of community programs, funded largely through federal categorical or block grants to state and local public health agencies and community organizations, is also fragmented, uncoordinated, and insufficient to improve the health of communities.

The political environment, increasingly conservative, reflects a move away from "comprehensive" governmental solutions and toward incremental approaches in which a few problems are tackled at a time and a bipartisan consensus is built. Congress itself tends to enforce this practice. In addition, when popular bills are proposed, lawmakers and lobbyists add amendments, thus slowing passage of the legislation. Further, seemingly small changes in health care can bring unintended effects. For example, many businesses and states fear a rise in premiums from any movement toward comprehensive efforts or an incremental federal derailing of state plans for health care reform. Finally, at present, little consensus exists regarding the direction of incremental changes.

Further, movement toward increased health has been slower among the more vulnerable. Although some political attention, both nationally and in many states, has of late been turned to the problems of health disparities, entirely new policies and programs designed to meet the needs of the most vulnerable members of society are few. Dissemination of recent influential Institute of Medicine reports (IOM, 2002, 2003, 2004) makes modifications of existing programs, such as increased access to managed care and expansion of the trial insurance programs for the poor who are uninsured, more likely. Yet various political agendas challenge each proposal. The traditional policy debate over the most efficient way to provide health care to the poor emerges during each administration. On one hand there are those who want to provide the poor with health insurance and leave it to them to obtain the care they need. On the other hand are advocates for special programs aimed directly at providing care for the poor (Fuchs, 1993). Comprehensive health care legislation is only successful under a unique set of historical forces, such as the push of the popularly rooted and widespread liberal Democratic groups of the 1960s for many of the Great Society legislative initiatives, which led to the original passage, in 1965, of the Health Insurance for the Aged Act (Medicare Act) (1994) and the Medicaid Act (1994) (Stocpol, 1996). In general, legislation attends to specialized aspects of health promotion or to narrow interests, such as nutrition or the health of older Americans, rather than to population-wide health.

Thus the leadership for comprehensive health promotion must arise from among those most interested in it. The health care provider must assess the impact of service delivery system alterations born of particular policy choices on both the provision of care *and* its outcome for the most vulnerable members of society. The focus of health care professionals concerned with health promotion must continue to move society toward the broadest aims of social justice (Rawls, 1971), so that all may be healthy.

Leadership in defining requisite action and necessary resources is needed. In some other parts of the developed world as well as in many U.S. cities, community lifestyle changes and multisectoral *healthy public policies* are burgeoning. A national health policy and appropriately funded programs are needed to achieve equity in access to health promotive care. Even more critical is an equitable sharing of society's basic health determinants: nutritious food, basic education, safe water, decent housing, secure employment, adequate income—and peace (McBeath, 1991). Leadership from all sectors—government, communities, health plans, and health care professionals in partnership with clients—is vital to ensuring fair allocation of these resources.

The Role of Government

Government may play an instrumental role in promoting health as a *public good* from which all benefit, rather than as a *commodity* to be bought and sold by self-interested entities (U.S. Senator D. P. Moynihan, personal communication, December 10, 1997). Government may support the activities of other entities, such as worksites and managed care companies, as well as lead efforts of its own. In particular the CDC may play an important role in building partnerships between managed care organizations, insurance purchasers, and public health agencies at all levels.

The Role of the Health Care Professional in Health Promotion

Given these potent forces for change, the role of the health care professional too will alter. Emerging partnerships with clients will continue to demand a new approach to the provision of care and a strong sense of the moral values underpinning actions within these relationships. As health care organizations become larger and more diverse and complex, the professional will need to listen more closely to the often solitary and unique voice of the client.

In an effort to further strengthen professional preparation in health education, the discipline in which the field of health promotion fits well, the Society for Public Health Education (SOPHE) and the American Association for Health Education (AAHE) have established the National Task Force on Accreditation in Health Education. The aim of this task force is to detail a plan for a coordinated accreditation system for undergraduate and graduate programs in health education. Its efforts are designed to enhance the profession and practice of health education and health promotion (Allegrante et al., 2004). In addition, through the enlargement of the professional base on which to rest practice, SOPHE will itself become a more potent intersectoral force, one that is capable of shaping the national policy agenda as well as creating an international presence (Allegrante, 1999). In so doing, it will provide a stronger platform from which professionals may advocate for health promotion and to meet the goals of *Healthy People 2010*.

The greatest potential for improving the health status of populations rests in policy change, community-based action, and research to improve effectiveness. These strategies will, however, require increased sophistication in their use, with health care professionals trained in community organization and group facilitation and skilled in collaborating with those from other disciplines. As health care professionals become more skilled at implementing policy change, the adversaries of health promotion (for example, tobacco manufacturers or large agribusinesses) will become more resolute. Health care providers will need tenacity to pursue health promotive strategies in the face of this opposition, and assistance in targeting these strategies to appropriate behaviors and groups.

Summary

In this final chapter the profound sociodemographic changes resulting from the aging and diversification of the population have been outlined. In addition, accountability for performance in the provision of services and applying evidence-based interventions will remain strong themes for future practice, as health care costs continue to rise. These changes will require that health care professionals clarify the values on which their field rests. Social justice—ensuring accessible and equitable care for society's most vulnerable—remains a core value for health promotion providers. To advance the value of social justice, change in the roles of government, communities, health plans, managed care organizations, and health care professionals is essential.

Take the challenge to promote health for all.

References

Aldana, S. G. (1998). Financial impact of health promotion programs: A comprehensive review of the literature. *American Journal of Health Promotion, 15,* 296–320.

Allegrante, J. P. (1999). SOPHE: At the intersection of education, policy, and science and technology. *Health Education and Behavior, 26,* 457–464.

Allegrante, J. P., Airhihenbuwa, C. O., Auld, M. E., Birch, D. A., Roe, K. M., & Smith, B. J.; National Task Force on Accreditation in Health Education. (2004). Toward a unified system of accreditation for professional preparation in health education: Final report of the National Task Force on Accreditation in Health Education. *Health Education and Behavior, 31,* 668–683.

Baquet, C. R., Horm, J. W., Gibbs, T., & Greenwald, P. (1991). Socioeconomic factors and cancer incidence among blacks and whites. *Journal of the American Cancer Institute, 83,* 553–557.

Baron, R. M., & Kenny, D. A. (1986). The moderator-mediator variable distinction in social psychological research: Conceptual, strategic, and statistical considerations. *Journal of Consulting and Clinical Psychology, 51,* 1173–1182.

Bauman, A. E., Sallis, J. F., Dzewaltowski, D. A., & Owen, N. (2002). Toward a better understanding of the influences on physical activity: The role of determinants, correlates, causal variables, mediators, moderators, and confounders. *American Journal of Preventive Medicine, 23*(2, Suppl.), 5–14.

Benincasa, T. A., King, E. S., Rier, B. K., Bloom, H. S., Balshem, A., & James, J., et al. (1996). Results of an office-based training program in clinical breast examination for primary care physicians. *Journal of Cancer Education 11,* 25–31.

Bloche, M. G. (2001). Race and discretion in American medicine. *Yale Journal of Health Policy, Law, and Ethics, 1,* 95–131.

Bocchino, C., Hartman, B. W., & Foley, P. F. (2003). The relationship between person-organization congruence, perceived violations of the psychological contract, and occupational stress symptoms. *Consulting Psychology Journal, 55,* 203–214.

Briss, P. A., Zaza, S., Pappaionaou, M., Fielding, J., Wright-DeAguero, L., Truman, B., et al.; The Task Force on Community Preventive Services. (2000). Developing an evidence-based guide to community preventive services: Methods. *American Journal of Preventive Medicine, 18,* 35–43.

Budtz-Jørgensen, E., Chung, J. P., & Rapin, C. H. (2001). Nutrition and oral health. Best practice and research. *Clinical Gastroenterology, 15,* 885–896.

Campbell, D. T. (1974, September). *Qualitative knowing in action research.* Kurt Lewin address, Society for the Psychological Study of Social Issues, Meeting with the American Psychological Association, New Orleans.

Cassel, C. K., Leipzig, R. M., Cohen, H. J., Larson, E. B., Meier, D. E., & Capello, C. F. (Eds.). (2003). *Geriatric medicine* (4th ed.). New York: Springer–Verlag.

Centers for Disease Control and Prevention. (1995). Prevention and managed care: Opportunities for managed care organizations, purchasers of health care, and public health agencies. *Morbidity and Mortality Weekly Report, 44*(RR-14), 1–12.

Centers for Disease Control and Prevention. (1996). *Inventory of managed care projects for FY 1995–1996.* Atlanta, GA: Author.

Cervantes, R. C., Gilbert, M. J., Salgado de Snyder, N., & Padilla, A. M. (1990). Psychosocial and cognitive correlates of alcohol use in younger adult immigrant and U.S.-born Hispanics. *International Journal of the Addictions, 25,* 687–708.

Chan, D. H., Leclair, K., & Kaczorowski, J. (1999). Problem-based small-group learning via the Internet among community family physicians: A randomized controlled trial. *MD Computing, 16,* 54–58.

Charlton, B. G., & White, M. (1995). Living on the margin: A salutogenic model for socioeconomic differentials in health. *Public Health, 109,* 235–243.

Chi-Lum, B. I., & Durkin, R. M. (1999). Physicians accessing the Internet: The PAI project. *JAMA, 282,* 633–634.

Cole, B. L., Wilhelm, M., Long, P. V., Fielding, J. E., Kominski, G., & Morgenstern, H. (2004). Prospects for health impact assessment in the United States: New and improved environmental impact assessment or something different? *Journal of Health Politics, Policy and Law, 29,* 1153–1186.

Daly, M. B., Balshem, M., Sands, C., James, J., Workman, S., & Engstrom, P. F. (1993). Academic detailing: A model for in-office CME. *Journal of Cancer Education, 8,* 273–280.

Davis, D. A., Thompson, M. A., Oxman, A. D., & Haynes, R. B. (1995). Changing physician performance: A systematic review of continuing medical education strategies. *JAMA, 274,* 700–705.

Dayal, H. H., Power, R. N., & Chiu, C. (1982). Race and socioeconomic status in survival from breast cancer. *Journal of Chronic Diseases, 35,* 675–683.

Dickey, L. L., Gemson, D. H., & Carney, P. (1999). Office system interventions supporting primary care-based health behavior change counseling. *American Journal of Preventive Medicine, 17,* 299–308.

Dietrich, A. J., Sox, C. H., Tosteson, T. D., & Woodruff, C. B. (1994). Durability of improved physician early detection of cancer after conclusion of intervention support. *Cancer Epidemiology, Biomarkers, and Prevention, 3,* 335–340.

Employee Benefit Research Institute. (2004). *Estimates from the March Current Population Survey, 2004 Supplement.* Retrieved November 2005 from http://covertheuninsuredweek.org/factsheets/display.php?FactSheetID=103

Epstein, J. A., Botvin, G. J., & Diaz, T. (2001). Alcohol use among Dominican and Puerto Rican adolescents residing in New York City: Role of Hispanic group and gender. *Journal of Developmental and Behavioral Pediatrics, 22,* 113–118.

Etzioni, A. (1993). *The spirit of community.* New York: Touchstone.

Friede, A., Blum, H. L., & McDonald, M. (1995). Public health informatics: How information age technology can strengthen public health. *Annual Review of Public Health, 16,* 239–252.

Friedewald, V. E., Jr. (2000). Why are physicians still turning their backs on the Internet? *Postgraduate Medicine, 108*(4, Suppl. 26).

Fuchs, V. R. (1993). *The future of health policy.* Cambridge, MA: Harvard University Press.

Galbraith, J. K. (1996). *The good society.* Boston: Houghton Mifflin.

Gans, K. M., Burkholder, G. J., Upegui, D. I., Risica, P. M., Lasater, T. M., & Fortunet, R. (2002). Comparison of baseline fat-related eating behaviors of Puerto Rican, Dominican, Colombian, and Guatemalan participants who joined a cholesterol education project. *Journal of Nutrition and Education Behavior, 34,* 202–210.

Glassman, A. H., & Shapiro, P. A. (1998). Depression in the course of coronary artery disease. *American Journal of Psychiatry, 155,* 4–11.

Glode, L. M. (1996). Challenges and opportunities of the Internet for medical oncology. *Journal of Clinical Oncology, 14,* 2181–2186.

Gordis, L. (2000). *Epidemiology.* Philadelphia: Saunders.

Gordon-Larsen, P., Harris, K. M., Ward, D. S., & Popkin, B. M. (2003). Acculturation and overweight-related behaviors among Hispanic immigrants to the US: The National Longitudinal Study of Adolescent Health. *Social Science and Medicine, 57,* 2023–2034.

Guralink, J. M., Land, K. C., Blszer, D., Fillenbaum, G. G., & Branch, L. G. (1993). Educational status and active life expectancy among older blacks and whites. *New England Journal of Medicine, 329,* 110–116.

Haan, M., Kaplan, G. A., & Camacho, T. (1987). Poverty and health: Prospective evidence from the Alameda County study. *American Journal of Epidemiology, 125,* 989–999.

Harris, J. M., Salasche, S. J., & Harris, R. B. (2001). Can Internet-based continuing medical education improve physicians' skin cancer knowledge and skills? *Journal of General Internal Medicine, 16*, 50–56.

Hashimoto, D. M. (2001). The proposed Patients' Bill of Rights: The case of the missing equal protection clause. *Yale Journal of Health Policy, Law, and Ethics, 1*, 77–93.

Hayes, K. A., & Lehmann, C. U. (1996). The interactive patient: A multimedia interactive educational tool on the World Wide Web. *MD Computing, 13*, 330–334.

Health Insurance for the Aged Act (Medicare Act), 42 U.S.C. §§ 301 et seq. (1994).

Heffler, S., Smith, S., Keehan, S., Clemens, M. K., Zezza, M., & Truffer, C. (2004). Health spending projections through 2013. *Health Affairs.* Retrieved February 2006 from http://content.healthaffairs.org/cgi/content/full/hlthaff.w4.79v1/DC1

Herrmann, C., Brand-Driehorst, S., Kaminsky, B., Leibin, E., Staats, H., & Ruger, U. (1998). Diagnostic groups and depressed mood as predictors of 22-month mortality in medical inpatients. *Psychosomatic Medicine, 60*, 570–577.

Herrman, H. (2001). The need for mental health promotion. *Australian and New Zealand Journal of Psychiatry, 35*, 709–715.

Honda, K., & Sheinfeld Gorin, S. (2006). A model of stage of change to recommend colonoscopy among urban primary care physicians. *Health Psychology, 25*, 65–73.

Horowitz, C. R., Goldberg, H. I., Martin, D. P., Wagner, E. H., Fihn, S. D., Christensen, D. B., et al. (1996). Conducting a randomized controlled trial of CQI and academic detailing to implement clinical guidelines. *Joint Commission Journal on Quality Improvement, 22*, 734–750.

Hulscher, M.E.J.L., Wensing, M., van der Weijden, T., & Grol, R. (2002). Interventions to implement prevention in primary care (Cochrane Review). *Cochrane Library, 2.*

Institute of Medicine. (1990). *The second fifty years: Promoting health and preventing disability.* Washington, DC: National Academies Press.

Institute of Medicine. (2000). *Promoting health: Intervention strategies from social and behavioral research.* Washington, DC: National Academies Press.

Institute of Medicine. (2002). *Health insurance is a family matter.* Washington DC: National Academy Press.

Institute of Medicine. (2003). *Unequal treatment: Confronting racial and ethnic disparities in health care.* Washington, DC: National Academies Press.

Institute of Medicine. (2004). *Insuring America's health: Principles and recommendations.* Washington, DC: National Academies Press.

Jadad, A. R., Sigouin, C., Cocking, L., Whelan, T., & Brownman, G. (2001). Internet use among physicians, nurses, and their patients. *JAMA, 286*, 12.

Joyce, C.R.B. (1994). Placebo and complementary medicine. *Lancet, 344*, 1279–1281.

Kassirer, J. P. (2000). Patients, physicians, and the Internet. *Health Affairs, 19*, 115–123.

Kenny, D. T., & Cooper, C. L. (2003). Occupational stress and its management. *International Journal of Stress Management, 10*, 275–279.

Keys, P. W., Goetz, C. M., Keys, P. A., Sterchele, J. A., Snedden, T. M., & Livengood, B. H. (1995). Computer-guided academic detailing as part of a drug benefit program. *American Journal of Health-System Pharmacy, 52*, 2199–2203.

Koplan, J. P., & Livengood, J. R. (1994). The influence of changing demographic patterns on our health promotion priorities. *American Journal of Preventive Medicine, 10* (Suppl. 1), 42–44.

Leninger, L. S., Finn, L., Dickey, L., Dietrich, A. J., Foxhall, L., Garr, D., et al. (1996). An office system for organizing preventive services: A report by the American Cancer Society Advisory Group on Preventive Health Care Reminder Systems. *Archives of Family Medicine, 5*, 108–115.

Levin, J. S., Glass, T. A., Kushi, L. H., Schuck, J. R., Steele, L., & Jonas, W. B. (1997). Quantitative methods in research on complementary and alternative medicine: A methodological manifesto. *Medical Care, 35*(11), 1079–1094.

Loria, C. M., Bush, T. L., Carroll, M. D., Looker, A. C., McDowell, M. A., Johnson, C. L., et al. (1995). Macronutrient intakes among adult Hispanics: A comparison of Mexican Americans, Cuban Americans, and mainland Puerto Ricans. *American Journal of Public Health, 85,* 684–689.

Mallin, K., & Anderson, K. (1988). Cancer mortality in Illinois Mexican and Puerto Rican immigrants, 1979–1984. *International Journal of Cancer, 41,* 670–676.

Manley, M. W., Griffin, T., Foldes, S. S., Link, C. C., & Sechrist, R.A.J. (2003). The role of health plans in tobacco control. *Annual Review of Public Health, 24,* 247–266.

Marmot, M. G., Smith, G. D., Stansfeld, S., Patel, C., North, F., Head, J., et al. (1991). Health inequalities among British civil servants: The Whitehall II study. *Lancet, 337,* 1387–1393.

McBeath, W. H. (1991). Health for all: A public health vision. *American Journal of Public Health, 81*(12), 1560–1565.

McQueen, D. V. (2001). Strengthening the evidence base for health promotion. *Health Promotion International, 16*(3), 261–268.

Medicare Payment Advisory Commission. (2005, March). *Report to the Congress: Medicare payment policy.* Washington, DC: Author.

Michelson, D., Stratakis, C., Hill, L., Reynolds, J., Galliven, E., Chrousos, G., et al. (1996). Bone mineral density in women with depression. *New England Journal of Medicine, 335,* 1176–1181.

Mills, R. J., & Bhandari, S. (2003). *Health insurance coverage in the United States: 2002.* Retrieved November 2005 from http://www.census.gov/prod/2003pubs/p60-223.pdf

Mukamel, D. B., Weimer, D. L., Zwanziger, J., Gorthy, S.F.H., & Mushlin, A. I. (2004/2005). Quality report cards, selection of cardiac surgeons, and racial disparities: A study of the publication of the New York State cardiac surgery reports. *Inquiry, 41,* 435–446.

Narhi, T. O., Vehkalahti, M. M., Siukosaan, P., & Ainamo, A. (1998). Salivary findings, daily medication and root caries in the old elderly. *Caries Research, 32,* 5–9.

National Center for Health Statistics. (2000). *2000 National Health Interview Survey cancer screening-public use.* Hyattsville, MD: Author.

National Institute for Occupational Safety and Health. (1999). *Stress at work* (DHHS [NIOSH] Publication No. 99-101). Retrieved November 2005 from http://www.cdc.gov/niosh/pdfs/stress.pdf

Neumeyer-Gromen, A., Thomas Lampert, D. S., Stark, K., & Kallischnigg, D. M. (2004). Disease management programs for depression: A systematic review and meta-analysis of randomized controlled trials. *Medical Care, 42,* 1211–1221.

Novaco, R. W., Stokols, D., & Milanesi, L. (1990). Objective and subjective dimensions of travel impedance as determinants of commuting stress. *American Journal of Community Psychology, 18,* 231–257.

Organizacion Pan Americana de la Salud. (1992). *Pronunciamiento de consenso sobre politicas de atencion a los ancianos en America Latina* [Consensus statements about the policies regarding the elderly in Latin America]. Santiago: Centro Latinoamericano de Demografia, Centrol Internacional del Envejecimiento.

Ozminkowski, R. J., Dunn, R. L., Goetzel, R. Z., Cantor, R. I., Murane, J., & Harrison, M. (1999). A return on investment evaluation of the Citibank, N.A., health management program. *American Journal of Health Promotion, 14,* 31–43.

Ozminkowski, R. J., Ling, D., Goetzel, R. Z., Bruno, J. A., Rutter, K. R., Issac, F., et al. (2002). Long-term impact of Johnson & Johnson's health & wellness program on health care utilization and expenditures. *Journal of Occupational and Environmental Medicine, 44,* 21–29.

Pappas, G., Queen, S., Hadden, W., & Fisher, G. (1993). The increasing disparity in mortality between socioeconomic groups in the United States, 1960 to 1986. *New England Journal of Medicine, 329,* 103–109.

Parry, J., & Stevens, A. (2001). Prospective health impact assessment: Pitfalls, problems, and possible ways forward. *British Medical Journal, 323,* 1177–1182.

Pelletier, K. R. (1994). *Sound mind—sound body: A new model for lifelong health.* New York: Simon & Schuster.

Penninx, B.W.J.H., Guralnik, J. M., Pahor, M., Ferrucci, L., Cehan, J. R., Wallace, R. B., et al. (1998). Chronically depressed mood and cancer risk in older persons. *Journal of the National Cancer Institute, 90,* 1888–1893.

Perez-Stable, E. J., Ramirez, A., Villareal, R., Talavera, G. A., Trapido, E., Suarez, L., et al. (2001). Cigarette smoking behavior among US Latino men and women from different countries of origin. *American Journal of Public Health, 91,* 1424–1430.

Phillips, K. A., Morrison, K. R., Andersen, R., & Aday, L. A. (1998). Understanding the context of healthcare utilization: Assessing environmental and provider-related variables in the behavioral model of utilization. *Health Services Research, 33,* 571–596.

Prilleltensky, I. (1997). Values, assumptions, and practices: Assessing the moral implications of psychological discourse and action. *American Psychologist, 52*(5), 517–535.

Rawls, J. (1971). *A theory of justice.* Cambridge, MA: Belknap Press, Harvard University Press.

Rosenwaike, I., & Shai, D. (1986). Trends in cancer mortality among Puerto Rican-born migrants to New York City. *International Journal of Epidemiology, 15,* 30–35.

Royce, J., Sheinfeld Gorin, S., Edelman, B., Rendino-Perrone, R., & Orlandi, M. (1990a). Student nurses and smoking cessation. In P. F. Engstrom & B. Rimer (Eds.), *Advances in cancer control VII* (pp. 49–71). New York: Alan Liss.

Royce, J., Sheinfeld Gorin, S., Edelman, B., Rendino-Perrone, R., & Orlandi, M. (1990b). Student nurses and smoking cessation. *Progress in Clinical and Biological Research, 339,* 49–71.

Salonen, J. T. (1982). Socioeconomic status and risk of cancer, cerebral stroke, and death due to coronary heart disease and any disease: A longitudinal study in eastern Finland. *Journal of Epidemiology and Community Health, 26,* 294–297.

Sandel, M. J. (1996). *Democracy's discontent: America in search of a public philosophy.* Cambridge, MA: Harvard University Press.

Schaeffer, M. H., Street, S. W., Singer, J. E., & Baum, A. (1988). Effects of control on stress reactions of commuters. *Journal of Applied Social Psychology, 18,* 944–957.

Schaffner, W., Ray, W., Federspiel, C. F., & Miller, W. O. (1983). Improving antibiotic prescribing in office practice: A controlled trial of three educational methods. *JAMA, 250,* 1732–1737.

Shapiro, A. K., & Morris, L. A. (1978). The placebo effect in medical and psychological therapies. In A. Bergin & S. Garfield (Eds.), *Handbook of psychotherapy and behavior change* (pp. 477–536). New York: Wiley.

Sheinfeld Gorin, S. (1985). Expect the unexpected: Consequences of the use of productivity indices. *Health Care Strategic Management, 3*(4), 12–15.

Sheinfeld Gorin, S. (2005). Colorectal cancer screening compliance among urban Hispanics. *Journal of Behavioral Medicine, 28,* 125–137.

Sheinfeld Gorin, S., & Arnold, J. (1998). *Health promotion handbook.* St Louis: Mosby.

Sheinfeld Gorin, S., Ashford, A., Lantigua, R., Hossain, A., Desai, M., Troxel, A., et al. (in press). Effectiveness of academic detailing on breast cancer screening among primary care physicians in an underserved community. *Journal of the American Board of Family Medicine.*

Sheinfeld Gorin, S., Gemson, D., Ashford, A., Bloch, S., Lantigua, R., Ahsan, H., et al. (2000). Cancer education among primary care physicians in an underserved community. *American Journal of Preventive Medicine, 19,* 53–58

Sheinfeld Gorin, S., & Heck, J. (2005). Cancer screening among Latino subgroups in the United States. *Preventive Medicine, 40,* 515–526.

Sheinfeld Gorin, S., Heck, J., Albert, S., & Hershman, D. (2005). Treatment for breast cancer among patients with Alzheimer's disease. *Journal of the American Geriatrics Society, 53,* 1897–1904.

Sheinfeld, S., & Lord, G. (1981). The ethics of evaluation researchers: An exploration of value choices. *Evaluation Review, 5*(3), 377–391.

State of California, Office of the Patient Advocate. (2005). *2005 HMO report card.* Retrieved November 2005 from http://www.opa.ca.gov/report_card

Stocpol, T. (1996). *Boomerang.* New York: Norton.

Stokols, D., Churchman, A., Scharf, T., & Wright, S. (1990). Workers' experiences of environmental change and transition at the office. In S. Fisher & C. L. Cooper (Eds.), *On the move: The psychology of change and transition* (pp. 231–249). New York: Wiley.

Thomson O'Brien, M. A., Oxman, A. D., Davis, D. A., Haynes, R. B., Freemantle, N., & Harvey, E. L. (2000). *Educational outreach visits: Effects on professional practice and health care outcomes* (Cochrane Review). *Cochrane Library, 2.*

Tyroler, H. A. (1989). Socioeconomic status in the epidemiology and treatment of hypertension. *Hypertension, 13* (Suppl. 1), 194–197.

University Center on Aging. (1993). Demographic transition and aging. In T. M. Schuman et al. (Eds.), *Population aging: International perspectives: Proceedings and recommendations of the international conference on population aging, San Diego, CA: 17–19 September 1992* (pp. 69–84). San Diego, CA: San Diego State University, University Center on Aging.

U.S. Bureau of the Census. (2000). *The Hispanic population of the United States: Population characteristics.* Washington, DC: Author.

U.S. Bureau of the Census. (2004). *Health insurance statistics: Low income uninsured by state.* Retrieved November 2005 from http://www.census.gov/hhes/hlthins/liuc03.html

U.S. Department of Health and Human Services. (2000). *Oral health in America: A report of the surgeon general.* Retrieved November 2005 from http://silk.nih.gov/public/hck1ocv.@www.surgeon.fullrpt.pdf

U.S. Senate Special Committee on Aging. (1991). *Aging America: Trends and projections.* Washington, DC: U.S. Government Printing Office.

Vargas, C. M., Kramarow, E. A., & Yellowitz, J. A. (2001). The oral health of older Americans. *Aging Trends, 3,* 1–8.

Warshauer, M. E., Silverman, D. T., Schottenfeld, D., & Pollack, E. S. (1986). Stomach and colorectal cancers in Puerto Rican–born residents of New York City. *Journal of the National Cancer Institute, 76,* 591–595.

Weiss, C. H. (1995). Nothing as practical as good theory: Exploring theory-based evaluation for comprehensive community initiatives for children and families. In J. P. Connell, A. C. Kubisch, L. B. Schorr, & C. Weiss (Eds.), *New approaches to evaluating community initiatives: Vol. 1. Concepts, methods, and contexts* (pp. 65–94). Washington, DC: Aspen Institute.

Wells, K. B., Stewart, A., Hays, R. D., Burnam, A., Rogers, W., Daniels, M., et al. (1989). The functioning and well-being of depressed patients. *JAMA, 262,* 914–919.

Winkleby, M. A., Fortmann, S. P., & Rockhill, B. (1993). Health-related risk factors in a sample of Hispanics and whites matched on sociodemographic characteristics: The Stanford Five-City Project. *American Journal of Epidemiology, 137,* 1365–1375.

Winkleby, M. A., Jatulis, D. E., Frank, E., & Fortmann, S. P. (1992). Socioeconomic status and health: How education, income, and occupation contribute to risk factors for cardiovascular disease. *American Journal of Public Health, 82,* 816–820.

Winkler, M. A., & Silberg, W. M. (1998). Computers, the Internet, and the practice of medicine. *JAMA, 279,* 66.

Wyatt, J. C., Paterson-Brown, S., Johanson, R., Altman, D. G., Bradburn, M. J., & Fisk, N. M. (1998). Randomised trial of educational visits to enhance use of systematic reviews in 25 obstetric units. *British Medical Journal, 317,* 1041–1046.

Yasnoff, W. A., O'Carroll, P. W., Koo, D., Linkins, R. W., & Kilbourne, E. M. (2000). Public health informatics: Improving and transforming public health in the information age. *Journal of Public Health Management, 6,* 67–75.

Zapka, J. G., Puleo, E., Vickers-Lahti, M., & Luckmann, R. (2002). Healthcare system factors and colorectal cancer screening. *American Journal of Preventive Medicine, 23,* 28–35.

Zaza, S., Briss, P. A., & Harris, K. W.; Task Force on Community Preventive Services (Eds.). (2005). *The guide to community preventive services: What works to promote health?* New York: Oxford University Press.

NAME INDEX

SUBJECT INDEX

A

AAHE (American Association for Health Education), 559

AAP (American Academy of Pediatrics), 92, 201, 378, 380–381

Absolute risk, 27

Abstinence-plus programs, 239–240

Academic detailing, 551–552

Accreditation agencies: JCAHO, 33, 76, 86, 87–88, 452–453, 537, 548; National Task Force on Accreditation in Health Education, 559–560; role in establishing standards, 86–88

Acheson Report, 36

Achieving Health for All: (Epp report) [Canada], 85

Acknowledgment of uncertainty, 27

ACT (Activity Counseling Trial), 199–200

Active for Life program, 214

Acupuncture smoking cessation treatment, 309

Ad Hoc Committee on Health Literacy for the Council on Scientific Affairs, 10

Addiction: nicotine, 287–288, 300, 330; sexual (or compulsivity), 224; substance abuse and, 342, 347–351. *See also* Alcohol abuse

Administration on Children, Youth, and Families, 398

Adolescents: oral health promotion for, 272*t*, 274, 277; physical activity counseling for, 212–213; reported rapes/sexual assaults against, 229; sexual health needs of, 229–230; smoking cessation counseling with, 307–308; suicide by, 415; tobacco control and youth access laws for, 295; unwanted pregnancies of, 228, 239–240; Youth Risk Behavior Surveillance System (YRBSS) on, 289, 295, 396–397, 399–400. *See also* Children

ADR (alternative dispute resolution), 482–483

Adults: individual development throughout lifespan, 495–499; oral health promotion for, 272*t*, 274–275. *See also* Older adults

AFDC (Aid to Families with Dependent Children), 104

African Americans: alcohol use by, 340–341; dental decay and, 257; equity in health promotion and, 554–555; factors affecting health protective activities by female, 31; substance-related health promotion for, 345–346; tobacco use of, 290; violence among young and male, 393. *See also* Ethnic/racial differences

Age differences: alcohol use and, 339*t*; deaths causes by injury, 367*t*; nonfatal injuries by, 368*t*; smoking and, 289; smoking cessation interventions and, 311*t*–312*t*; substance-related health promotion and, 346

Aggregates (or subpopulations), at risk of disease, 6

Aging: demographic shift toward, 543–545; individual development process and, 498–499; lifespan framework on, 8. *See also* Older adults